PET and SPECT in Neurology

Rudi A. J. O. Dierckx • Andreas Otte
Erik F. J. de Vries • Aren van Waarde
Editors

Klaus L. Leenders
Guest Editor

PET and SPECT in Neurology

Second Edition

Volume II

Springer

Editors
Rudi A. J. O. Dierckx
Nuclear Medicine and Molecular Imaging
University Medical Center Groningen
Groningen
The Netherlands

Erik F. J. de Vries
Nuclear Medicine and Molecular Imaging
University Medical Center Groningen
Groningen
The Netherlands

Andreas Otte
Faculty of Electrical Engineering,
Medical Engineering and Computer Science
Offenburg University
Offenburg
Germany

Aren van Waarde
Nuclear Medicine and Molecular Imaging
University Medical Center Groningen
Groningen
The Netherlands

Guest Editor
Klaus L. Leenders
Neurology
University Medical Center Groningen
Groningen
The Netherlands

ISBN 978-3-030-53170-6 ISBN 978-3-030-53168-3 (eBook)
https://doi.org/10.1007/978-3-030-53168-3

This Springer imprint is published by the registered company Springer Nature Switzerland AG
The registered company address is: Gewerbestrasse 11, 6330 Cham, Switzerland

Foreword

When in 2014 the editors published the first edition of this 3-volume series, dedicated to the use of PET and SPECT in the CNS, a major undertaking saw the light in print. These were significant multi-authored books, providing the most comprehensive review of this challenging field at the time.

Now, in 2020, a second edition is launched, demonstrating the success of this initial endeavour. With a further major effort, over 50% of the numerous chapters are either entirely novel or rewritten anew, by an impressive list of international contributors. The team deserves warm congratulations for this achievement.

In 2014, PET-MR had just emerged as a novel imaging modality, and the medical applications of machine learning, or artificial intelligence, had hardly surfaced. PET imaging of Tau had just made it.

Now, in 2020, amazing progress in the understanding of the brain is being made, and even dedicated brain PET and PET-MR imaging instruments are in development (Catana 2019). Yet, with its hundred billion neurons, the brain keeps its mystery and continues to engage and stimulate our enquiry.

Little by little progress is being made, from decoding consciousness (Sohn 2019) to growing neurons from reprogrammed skin fibroblasts (Kofler 2019). We now understand that protein deposits in the brain may precede clinical manifestations by years, great advances have been made in extracting quantitative data from such studies (as shown with PET-CT and amyloid and tau numerical data) and that we can intervene effectively, inter alia, in receptor deficiencies and in deep brain stimulation. The brain connectome is unravelling, with it, a greater understanding of, amongst others, pain and drug-induced addictions, the dementias and movement disorders. All of this and much more is being critically reviewed by 119 chapters spread into these 3 major volumes.

It is hence perfect timing that the Second Edition shines a new light at the significant progress made in PET and SPECT, describing and analysing latest information from novel biological radionuclide probes, neuroreceptors and the clinical progress achieved.

University College London
London, UK

Peter Josef Ell,

References

1. Catana C (2019) Development of Dedicated Brain PET Imaging Devices: Recent Advances and Future Perspectives. J Nucl Med 60:1044–1052.
2. Kofler N (2019) Brain in a Dish, Babies by Design: What It Means to Be Human. Nature 569:333–334.
3. Sohn E (2019) Decoding the Neuroscience of Consciousness. Nature 571:S2–S5.

Preface

Neuroscientists of today dispose of a powerful armament for functional, physiological and molecular imaging that has never made more impressive advances than before, helping to better understand the mechanisms of diseases and to develop and design drug treatment options with a superior efficacy and safety profile. Among these instruments, positron emission tomography (PET) and single-photon emission computed tomography (SPECT) have become forerunners in the *in vivo* imaging arena, and for this reason, the present trilogy, now in its second, completely revised and supplemented edition, is dedicated to PET and SPECT. The volumes of this trilogy are *PET and SPECT in Psychiatry, PET and SPECT in Neurology* and *PET and SPECT in Neurobiological Systems*. In all volumes, we have again assembled the combined expertise of the renowned authors of the first edition and expanded this by some new authors for the second edition, whose dedication to the investigation of psychiatric and neurological disorders or of neurobiological systems through nuclear medicine technology has achieved international recognition.

The editors, who are nuclear medicine specialists, radiochemists and biologists with a strong exposure to neurosciences, have again invited experts from the psychiatry, neurology, and medical physics fields to enhance the editorial board as guest editors for each volume of the trilogy. For *PET and SPECT in Psychiatry* this was Iris Sommer, professor of cognitive aspects of neurological and psychiatric disorders; for *PET and SPECT in Neurology* it remained Klaus (Nico) L. Leenders, emeritus professor of neurology; and for *SPECT in Neurobiological Systems* it was Adriaan A. Lammertsma, professor of medical physics and PET.

We are very happy that our trilogy has become a state-of-the-art compendium with top downloads already for the first edition. This is certainly also due to the production and distribution by one of the premier publishers in the field, guaranteeing a high quality of reproduction and allowing for the inclusion of many colour figures, which is essential in the field of neuroimaging. We are intrigued by the enthusiastic response from contributors from all over the world who made this endeavour successful and are confident that the second edition continues to live up to this onus. Finally, we would like to thank Mrs. Gesa Frese from *Springer-Verlag* for her continuous help and support during the development of the second edition of this book series.

We sincerely hope that the new trilogy will still serve as a key tool not only for all physicians in nuclear medicine, psychiatry, neurology, or geriatrics but also for all professionals working to understand or treat brain disorders. With today's ageing population, PET and SPECT imaging can provide new insights into the processes that may lead to unhealthy ageing of the brain. May this book series serve as a guide towards the present use of PET and SPECT in brain disorders and as a catalyst for future research. The progress achieved by PET and SPECT in the diagnosis of the many facets of diseases disposed in the neurosciences has been astounding. Nevertheless, in line with the Socratic paradox "*I know that I know nothing*", it seems that we are still at the beginning of understanding the brain. This book hopes to provide a renewed platform to further contribute to this quest, at the benefit of patients suffering from neurologic and psychiatric disorders.

Groningen, The Netherlands — Rudi A. J. O. Dierckx
Offenburg, Germany — Andreas Otte
Groningen, The Netherlands — Erik F. J. de Vries
Groningen, The Netherlands — Aren van Waarde

Contents

Part II Dementia

Part IV

Movement Disorders

Parkinson's Disease

24

Michele Matarazzo, Andre C. Felicio, and A. Jon Stoessl

Contents

M. Matarazzo · A. J. Stoessl (✉)
Pacific Parkinson's Research Center, University of British Columbia, Vancouver, BC, Canada
e-mail: jon.stoessl@ubc.ca

A. C. Felicio
Hospital Israelita Albert Einstein, São Paulo, Brazil

R. A. J. O. Dierckx et al. (eds.), *PET and SPECT in Neurology*,
https://doi.org/10.1007/978-3-030-53168-3_24

Abstract

A growing body of evidence supports the importance of functional imaging studies using single-photon emission tomography (SPECT) or positron emission tomography (PET) in neurology. In particular, Parkinson's disease (PD) and other neurodegenerative disorders are useful disease models to understand the contribution of modern functional neuroimaging techniques. In this chapter, our aim is to address the principles of molecular imaging and also its pitfalls, with a focus on PD motor and nonmotor symptoms. From brain pathology to neurochemical pathology, from clinically unclear cases of parkinsonism to non-dopaminergic ligands and, finally, taking into account experimental tracers, we hope to cover key issues regarding the contribution of SPECT and PET in PD.

24.1 Introduction

24.1.1 Parkinson's Disease Burden

Parkinson's disease (PD) is the second most prevalent neurodegenerative disorder after Alzheimer's disease (AD) worldwide. Recent epidemiological studies have shown an increase of its prevalence that has more than doubled in less than 30 years, affecting more than six million people worldwide in 2016 (GBD 2016 Parkinson's Disease Collaborators 2018). With the growing ageing population, along with potential contributions from other factors, the prevalence and worldwide burden of PD is estimated to increase even more in future years, with an expected doubling between 2010 and 2030 (Marras et al. 2018). This will boost the already very high social and economic burden of the disease with huge impact on the quality of life of millions of people and of their caregivers.

24.1.2 Clinical Manifestations

Currently, the diagnosis of PD is based on the combination of clinical manifestations, including bradykinesia and at least one other cardinal motor sign (rest tremor, rigidity, postural instability) (Gibb and Lees 1988; Postuma et al. 2015). However, the manifestations of PD extend beyond this spectrum, encompassing a wide variety of nonmotor symptoms, including neuropsychiatric disorders, autonomic dysfunction, olfactory loss and sleep disturbance, some of which may be present even before the onset of motor manifestations (Chaudhuri et al. 2011; Goldman and Postuma 2014; Postuma et al. 2015).

Additionally, at the time an affected PD patient is diagnosed, it is estimated that 30–50% of the nigrostriatal neurons are lost, associated with striatal dopamine loss of 50–80% (Bernheimer et al. 1973; Fearnley and Lees 1991; Kordower et al. 2013).

Despite the recent adoption of newer diagnostic criteria, such as the Movement Disorder Society Clinical Diagnostic Criteria for PD, the accuracy of the diagnosis is still suboptimal, with an estimated accuracy around 90% after extended clinical follow-up (lower at earlier stages), even though definitive clinicopathological validation is still strikingly lacking (Hughes et al. 2001; Postuma et al. 2018). The misdiagnosis in clinical practice, more so in a non-movement disorder specialized setting, is estimated to be even higher (Hughes et al. 1992, 2001).

Further, the high degree of variability in the clinical manifestations of PD and its long-term prognosis represent a major issue in clinical practice, with pragmatic consequences related to the unpredictability of the disease progression, at least at an individual level. To overcome this challenge, different phenotyping methods have been developed over time based on motor symptoms or, more recently, on a combination of motor and nonmotor symptoms (Fereshtehnejad et al. 2017; Hoehn and Yahr 1967; Stebbins et al. 2013). Additionally, early- versus late-onset PD may be associated with different epidemiological, clinical and genetic characteristics (Schrag and Schott 2006), which can also be assessed in part by in vivo studies using SPECT (Shih et al. 2007) and PET (de la Fuente-Fernández et al. 2011) ligands.

24.1.3 Brain Pathology

It is now known that clinical parkinsonism is just the tip of the iceberg in the complex cascade of events that takes place before the onset of motor symptoms in PD (Langston 2006). Indeed, long before the involvement of the substantia nigra *pars compacta* (SNc) and the loss of striatal dopamine, there is an ongoing neurodegenerative process. While the origin of the disease is still unclear, the prevailing hypothesis suggests a caudal-to-rostral spread of misfolded alpha-synuclein pathology that may start in the peripheral nervous system. The olfactory bulb is involved early, and the disease may actually onset in peripheral autonomic ganglia (Braak et al. 2003). Other theories have been recently proposed, and there is no definite evidence on the actual pathophysiological mechanism, especially in the earlier stages (Foffani and Obeso 2018). Even the toxic role of alpha-synuclein is now questioned, as this may represent a compensatory or even protective physiological reaction to an underlying neurodegenerative process (Espay et al. 2019). However, the hallmark pathology of this disease still relies on the identification of Lewy bodies in the SNc, which corresponds to intra-cytoplasmatic alpha-synuclein-positive staining inclusions (Spillantini et al. 1997).

The understanding of PD pathology is very important, especially when one considers the anticipated reality of disease-modifying therapies to come. Therefore, identifying individuals at earlier disease stages and preferably preclinical subjects would provide better therapeutic windows. Currently, there are available biomarkers, though with some drawbacks, but liable to be useful in identifying those subjects most likely to benefit from neuroprotective therapies, as well as in monitoring the effects of these interventions (Agarwal and Stoessl 2013; Merchant et al. 2019).

24.1.4 Neurochemical Pathology

Not only dopamine but also non-dopaminergic neurotransmitters such as acetylcholine, serotonin, GABA and glutamate are involved in the pathophysiology of PD and can potentially be assessed with in vivo molecular imaging approaches (Politis et al. 2017; Stoessl 2012; Stoessl et al. 2014). Additionally, other molecular targets that may shed insight into disease pathogenesis, such as aggregation of proteins known to participate in neurodegenerative processes (e.g. tau) and markers of neuroinflammation, may be of interest in PD, as well as other neurological conditions (Ghadery et al. 2019; Hammes et al. 2018; Narayanaswami et al. 2018).

24.1.4.1 Dopaminergic Dysfunction

Striatal dopamine denervation is the major neurochemical outcome of the relentless neurodegenerative process in PD, as it underlies the major clinical findings and it is the theoretical base for most of the treatment currently used. The dopaminergic denervation happens in the context of dysfunction in direct and indirect loops of the cortico-striato-pallido-thalamo-cortical pathway with secondary neurochemical, neurophysiological and functional changes in the brain at several anatomical network levels (Wichmann 2019; Wichmann et al. 2011).

Changes in dopamine metabolism are also related to changes in dopamine receptors and transporters during the course of PD. For example, in early PD at the presynaptic level, while dopamine transporters are downregulated, there is an upregulation in dopa-decarboxylase activity associated with a decrease in vesicular monoamine transporter type 2. However, at the postsynaptic level, D2 dopamine receptors are initially increased/upregulated, with a subsequent normalization, as disease progresses and dopamine-substitutive therapy is introduced (Antonini et al. 1997; Au et al. 2005). However, the interpretation of this latter finding might be biased by the reduced receptor occupancy due to reduced dopamine released at presynaptic level.

The equilibrium between the cellular and neuronal terminal loss and the compensatory mechanisms, likely influenced also by the treatment administered, undergoes a continuous biological adaptation over the course of the disease, which is more pronounced in the early phase. As a consequence, the neurophysiological and neurobiological profiles change in different stages of the disease.

24.1.4.2 Cholinergic Dysfunction

The main sources of cholinergic projection fibres in the forebrain are the *nucleus basalis* of Meynert and the septal nuclei. In the brainstem, the pedunculopontine and laterodorsal tegmental nuclei provide important cholinergic projections to the thalamus, hypothalamus, midbrain dopaminergic nuclei and the basal forebrain (Holmstrand and Sesack 2011). Both regions may be affected in PD (Rogers et al. 1985), with resulting cognitive impairment (Yarnall et al. 2011) and possible contributions to sleep disturbances. It is estimated that almost 85% of 20-year PD survivors are demented, pointing to the importance of cholinergic dysfunction in late stages of PD (Hely et al. 2008). The pedunculopontine tegmental nucleus

(PPN) involvement in PD has been established in neuropathological studies and represents the theoretical basis for the use of cholinesterase inhibitors in PD-related gait disorders, as well as for the trials of PPN deep brain stimulation (DBS), again for improving the gait dysfunction in people with advanced PD (Henderson et al. 2016; Moro et al. 2010). Also, symptoms of rapid eye movement (REM) sleep behaviour disorder (RBD) are associated with cholinergic denervation in PD (Kotagal et al. 2012), therefore showing the importance of the cholinergic system in nonmotor symptoms.

24.1.4.3 Serotonergic Dysfunction

Serotonin neurons have widespread projections in the brain, particularly in the brainstem, striatum, thalamus, hypothalamus, amygdala and cingulate cortex. A relationship between mood and serotonin deficiency is widely assumed, based on the response to tricyclic, tetracyclic, selective serotonin reuptake inhibitor and monoamine oxidase inhibitor antidepressants (Hung et al. 2011). However, serotonin has many other functions besides its effects on mood, and these rely in part on the 14 distinct serotonin receptors evident in mammals (Saulin et al. 2012). For example, body mass index changes and fatigue, both of which may be therapeutically challenging problems in PD, may be affected by serotonergic function (Pavese et al. 2010; Politis et al. 2011).

In addition, there is animal and human evidence showing the role of serotonin dysfunction in PD-related dyskinesias (Rylander et al. 2010). The machinery of a serotonergic neuron resembles that of the dopaminergic one. They both share dopa-decarboxylase and the vesicular monoamine transporter type 2. Therefore, it is proposed that dopamine may be released as a false neurotransmitter by serotonin terminals in PD patients. It is suggested that the absence of dopamine autoreceptors or dopamine transporters results in excessive nonphysiological and nonregulated dopamine release within the synaptic cleft, which contributes to the pathogenesis and expression of dyskinesias (Carta et al. 2007).

24.2 Brain Dopaminergic Imaging in PD

24.2.1 Targeting Dopaminergic Function

Molecular imaging studies depend on quantifying the distribution of radiotracers that bind to specific receptor sites or that reflect the activity of a particular enzyme or biochemical pathway, with minimal non-specific binding. These tracers are labelled with positron emitting or single-photon emitting radioisotopes. Radioisotopes labelled for PET have a much shorter half-life compared to those used in SPECT. This may permit studies using multiple tracers or multiple doses of the same tracer before and after a variety of interventions but on the other hand will also require a more well-structured dedicated facility, usually including an on-site cyclotron. Table 24.1 shows general characteristics of PET and SPECT techniques and their application in PD.

Table 24.1 General characteristics of positron emission tomography (PET) and single-photon emission tomography (SPECT) techniques and their application to Parkinson's disease

Technique	Pros	Cons	Radioisotopes	Application in Parkinson's disease
PET	– Unlimited depth penetration – Whole-body imaging – Co-registering with MRI or CT	– Irradiation exposure – Expensive – Intermediate spatial resolution (2–8 mm) – Long acquisition time	^{11}C ^{18}F ^{15}O	– Research – Dopamine-specific tracers not commercially available, fluorodeoxyglucose and amyloid tracers are
SPECT	– Unlimited depth penetration – Whole-body imaging – Co-registering with MRI or CT – Can combine imaging and radiotherapy	– Irradiation exposure – Low spatial resolution (5–10 mm) – Long acquisition time	^{99m}Tc ^{123}I	– Research – Commercially available to help with clinically unclear cases of parkinsonism, e.g. differentiation from essential tremor

Adapted from Pysz et al. (2010)

Both PET and SPECT techniques are capable of measuring the in vivo biodistribution of minute (<10^{-10} M) concentrations of radiolabelled biomolecules with resolution of a few millimetres and, with the application of appropriate models, of quantifying the molecular kinetic processes in which they participate (Felicio et al. 2009).

SPECT is similar to PET in its use of radioactive tracer material and detection of gamma rays (Pysz et al. 2010). In contrast with PET, however, the tracers used in SPECT emit single gamma rays, whereas PET tracers emit positrons that annihilate with electrons up to a few millimetres away, resulting in the emission of two gamma photons in opposite directions, whose simultaneous detection is required in order to be identified as an event.

The additional correction for degrading factors such as attenuation, scatter, random detection events, detector efficiencies and dead time allows for a quantitative image of the radiolabelled ligand's concentration to be generated. Spatial resolution is limited (SPECT > PET), but either the SPECT or PET data can be co-registered with structural data from computed tomography (CT) or MRI images to provide additional anatomical context to the functional PET data (Aiello et al. 2018; Owen et al. 2011; Sossi 2018; Tondo et al. 2019).

PET or SPECT data can be acquired and analysed using a variety of different approaches, including a simple ratio of target to background activity obtained from a single (static) image, or more complex analyses applied to dynamically acquired data. The application of tracer kinetic models to these data allows for the determination of quantitative measures of specific binding, which is aided by the presence of a reference region devoid of specific binding. If present, such 'reference regions' also facilitate modelling and may allow the investigator to bypass the requirement for arterial blood sampling (Tatsch and Poepperl 2012). Figure 24.1 shows the dopamine-related tracers most widely available and their binding sites.

24.2.2 Tracers for the Assessment of Presynaptic Dopamine Function

There are different binding sites at the presynaptic level, which can be assessed either by PET or SPECT ligands. This set of targets is of major interest in PD and parkinsonian disorders, as dopaminergic presynaptic terminals in the striatum presumably reflect the loss of nigrostriatal neurons, the pathophysiological hallmark of PD. Overall, these tracers provide useful information about the function of dopamine neurons while addressing key steps in dopamine turnover: dopamine synthesis, storage, release and reuptake (Stoessl 2011).

24.2.2.1 L-Aromatic Acid Decarboxylase (L-AADC)

The assessment of L-AADC through PET tracers such as ^{18}F-fluorodopa allows the estimate of dopamine synthesis and storage. Information derived from activity measured over the first 90–120 min of radiotracer administration provides evaluation of the uptake and conversion of fluorodopa to fluorodopamine by L-AADC (Martin et al. 1989). However, by measuring activity over a prolonged time (4 h following tracer administration), one can estimate the distribution volume and its inverse, dopamine turnover (Sossi et al. 2002). Hence, these prolonged scans can also be used to assess dopamine turnover.

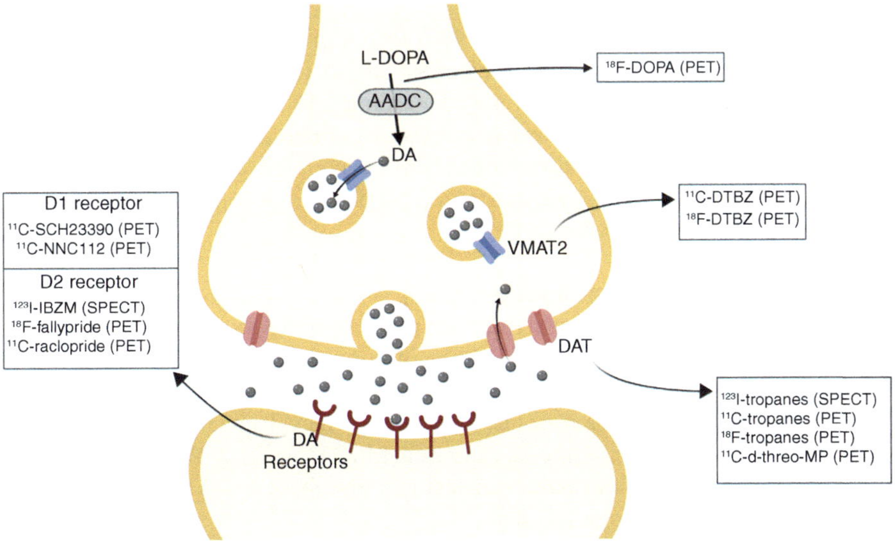

Fig. 24.1 Dopamine nerve terminal and dopaminergic radiotracer binding sites

AADC may be subject to compensatory upregulation, particularly in early PD, and F-dopa uptake is accordingly increased relative to dopamine nerve terminal density as assessed by vesicular monoamine transporter type 2 (VMAT2) binding (Lee et al. 2000; Nandhagopal et al. 2011). Hence, fluorodopa uptake may underestimate the degree of dopaminergic denervation, particularly in earlier stages of disease. Additionally, AADC is not specific to the dopaminergic neuron but is also expressed by serotonergic neurons, and F-dopa uptake is accordingly seen in non-dopaminergic regions (Moore et al. 2003, 2008; Pavese et al. 2012). In line with this, experimental evidence shows that dopamine may be released as a false neurotransmitter by serotonergic nerve terminals in parkinsonian rats (Carlsson et al. 2009; Carta et al. 2010; Muñoz et al. 2009, 2008; Rylander et al. 2010).

Another drawback of F-dopa scans is that some of its metabolites, which are formed by the action of the ubiquitous enzyme catechol-*O*-methyltransferase (COMT), can enter the brain and diminish image contrast. Therefore, an alternative agent is the related tracer 6-^{18}F-fluoro-meta-tyrosine (FMT). FMT is also a good substrate for L-AADC but is not metabolized by COMT and therefore has a higher sensitivity to represent L-AADC activity compared to F-dopa. However, FMT cannot be used to assess dopamine turnover (Asari et al. 2011; DeJesus et al. 1992, 2005; Doudet et al. 1999).

24.2.2.2 Vesicular Monoamine Transporter Type 2 (VMAT2)

VMAT2 promotes the transport of biogenic monoamines, such as serotonin and dopamine, from the cytoplasm to synaptic vesicles. It is assessed by PET with ^{11}C-dihydrotetrabenazine (^{11}C-DTBZ). While the VMAT2 is expressed by all monoaminergic neurons, striatal binding of DTBZ reflects mainly dopaminergic projections, and DTBZ PET is accordingly very useful to assess the density of dopamine nerve terminals. Although DTBZ binding is thought to be less subject to pharmacological effects (Vander Borght et al. 1995) or compensatory changes than either DAT ligands or fluorodopa, it is nonetheless subject to competition from endogenous intra-vesicular dopamine and may accordingly be increased in states of profound DA deficiency such as dopa-responsive dystonia (De La Fuente-Fernández et al. 2003) and early methamphetamine abstinence (Boileau et al. 2008a) and is reduced following levodopa administration in patients with advanced PD (de la Fuente-Fernández et al. 2009).

24.2.2.3 Dopamine Transporter (DAT)

The plasmalemmal DAT is located on the presynaptic terminals of dopaminergic neurons and is responsible for the reuptake of dopamine released into the synaptic cleft. In the healthy brain, this is the leading mechanism responsible for the termination of the actions of DA (Varrone and Halldin 2010). DAT imaging can be assessed using both PET and SPECT tracers as presented in Table 24.2. While the majority of DAT SPECT tracers are iodine- or technetium-labelled, DAT PET tracers are generally carbon- or fluorine-labelled.

Although DAT imaging is frequently used in PD as a surrogate imaging method to assess dopaminergic dysfunction, one should recognize the potential caveats of

Table 24.2 Commercially and research-available dopamine transporter ligands in Parkinson's disease studies

Binding site	SPECT	PET
DAT	^{99m}Tc-TRODAT-1[a]	^{11}C-dMP (d-threo-Methylphenidate)
	^{99m}Tc-Technepine	^{11}C-Cocaine
	^{123}I-FP-CIT[b]	^{11}C-Altropane
	^{123}I-PE2I	^{11}C/^{18}F-β-CFT
	^{123}I-β-CIT	^{11}C-RTI-32
	^{123}I-β-CIT-FE	^{11}C-β-CIT-FE
	^{123}I-Altropane	^{11}C-PE2I
		^{18}F-FE-PE2I

Adapted from Piccini (2003)
PET positron emission tomography, *SPECT* single-photon emission tomography
[a]Commercially available, non-FDA-approved
[b]Commercially available, FDA-approved

this methodology (Piccini 2003). Firstly, age-associated physiological DAT decline is estimated to range from 3% to 8% per decade and corresponds to nigrostriatal cell loss. This is substantially lower than the ~8% per year pathological DAT loss seen in PD (Volkow et al. 1994). Another major confounder is that DAT is subject to pharmacological regulation according to different medication intake, such as dopamine reuptake inhibitors (bupropion) or methylphenidate (Kägi et al. 2010). While this is an important theoretical concern, the significance of this in clinical trials with imaging outcome measures is less clear. Finally, DAT is also subject to compensatory changes, such as may occur in the early stages of PD. Downregulation of DAT should allow dopamine to interact for a longer time with pre- and postsynaptic receptors, by preventing its rapid reuptake (Lee et al. 2000). While several tracers are available for assessing DAT binding, it should be noted that their specificity for the DAT (as opposed to other plasmalemmal monoamine transporters) is variable, as are their pharmacokinetic properties.

24.2.3 Tracers for the Assessment of Postsynaptic Dopamine Function

Dopamine receptors are the primary targets in the treatment of many disorders such as PD, Huntington's chorea and schizophrenia. There are several radiotracers that can be used to access D1-like and D2-like dopamine receptors. ^{18}F-fallypride and ^{11}C-FLB-457, which are PET ligands, and ^{11}C-epidepride, a SPECT ligand, are ultrahigh affinity dopamine receptor antagonist radioligands, which allow quantification and visualization of low-density dopamine extrastriatal D2/D3 receptors as well as striatal receptors (de Paulis 2003). On the other hand, the radioligands ^{11}C-raclopride (or ^{11}C-RAC) for PET and ^{123}I-IBZM for SPECT are widely employed to assess striatal DA receptor availability. In contrast to the former, these ligands have lower D2/D3 receptor affinity; hence, quantification of extrastriatal receptors is not possible (Pinborg et al. 2007). However, RAC and IBZM are subject to competition from endogenous DA for in vivo binding to D2 receptors and can therefore be used to infer alterations in synaptic DA concentration, using multiple scans before and after a given intervention or, more recently, using models to dynamically quantify the synaptic dopamine in a single scan (Lippert et al. 2019).

Similar to DAT ligands, dopamine receptor binding is also influenced by age and, to a lesser extent, the stage of PD and therapy. While increased tracer binding is observed in the more affected putamen in early PD, probably reflecting a compensatory upregulation of dopamine receptors (Antonini et al. 1997), advanced PD and chronic treatment result in normalization of binding in the putamen and decreased binding in the caudate (Thobois et al. 2004). In contrast, D1 binding as assessed by ^{11}C-SCH23390 and PET is normal in PD (Rinne et al. 1990) but may be decreased in conditions characterized by loss of striatal neurons, such as multiple system atrophy (Shinotoh et al. 1993).

24.3 Brain Non-dopaminergic Sites

24.3.1 Other Neurotransmitters

24.3.1.1 Serotoninergic Tracers

5-Hydroxytryptamine (5-HT, serotonin) is a neurotransmitter widely distributed in the brain, and both pre- and postsynaptic tracers have been developed to study its involvement in vivo in different types of disorders, including PD.

Most studies of the serotonergic system in PD have focused on tracers that bind to the presynaptic serotonin reuptake transporter (SERT). The first SERT ligand developed in humans has been the ^{11}C-(+)-6β-(4-methylthiophenyl)-1,2,3,5,6α,10β-hexahydropyrrolo[2,1-a]isoquinoline (^{11}C-McN 5652) (Szabo et al. 1995). Over the next years, a second generation of ligands was developed to overcome some of the limitations of the ^{11}C-McN 5652, such as the relatively high non-specific binding and the protracted brain uptake (Frankle et al. 2004). The ^{11}C-3-amino-4-(2-dimethylaminomethylphenylthio)benzonitrile (^{11}C-DASB) has been vastly used in human studies in different neurological and psychiatric disorders. In PD, the analysis of ^{11}C-DASB binding has permitted the study of the role of serotonin in motor symptoms and complications as well as nonmotor symptoms, such as fatigue and mood disorders.

SERT binding has been found to be reduced in several areas (caudate, putamen, raphe nuclei, thalamus and cortical areas) of PD subjects with tremor-dominant phenotype as compared to the akinetic-rigid subtype, with a correlation with postural and action tremor, even though interestingly resting tremor was not correlated with DASB binding (Loane et al. 2013). The implication of serotonin in the tremor has been also suggested by a PET study using the $5HT_{1A}$ receptor ligand ^{11}C-WAY 100635 (^{3}H-(*N*-(2-(1-(4-(2-methoxyphenyl)-1-piperazinyl)ethyl)-*N*-(2-pyridyl) cyclohexane-carboxamide) that showed a reduction in PD subjects compared to healthy controls in the midbrain raphe, which correlated with the severity of resting tremor (Doder et al. 2003). As midbrain $5HT_{1A}$ receptors are somatodendritic autoreceptors, this is compatible with a loss of 5HT neurons. The role of serotonin in levodopa-induced dyskinesias finds its pathophysiological explanation in the possible aberrant levodopa uptake and unregulated dopamine release by serotonin terminals in the dopamine-denervated striatum (Carta et al. 2007). PET and SPECT studies have found an elevated SERT-to-DAT ratio in subjects with dyskinesias (Lee et al. 2015; Roussakis et al. 2016), as well as higher SERT preservation in the *globus pallidus* (Smith et al. 2015). The compensatory role of serotonin in the premotor stages of PD has also been hypothesized, as ^{11}C-DASB binding was found to be increased in premanifest *LRRK2* mutation carriers, compared to idiopathic PD subjects (hypothalamus and striatum) and to *LRRK2*-related PD (hypothalamus and brainstem) (Wile et al. 2017). In contrast, in premanifest *SNCA* A53T mutation carriers, ^{11}C-DASB binding was reduced even in the presence of normal SPECT dopaminergic imaging (Wilson et al. 2019). This difference between *LRRK2*-PD and *SNCA*-PD may be related to mutation-specific biological mechanisms, and therefore, particularly in the case of *LRRK2* mutations, the results might not be generalizable to idiopathic PD.

Serotonin innervation changes have been studied also in nonmotor symptoms related to PD. Correlation between ^{11}C-DASB binding and several nonmotor manifestations of the disease has been found, such as depression (increased SERT in limbic structures and raphe nuclei; Boileau et al. 2008b; Politis et al. 2010), body weight changes (Politis et al. 2011), fatigue, apathy and sleep problems (reduced SERT in basal ganglia and diencephalon; Maillet et al. 2016; Pavese et al. 2010; Wilson et al. 2018).

24.3.1.2 Cholinergic Tracers

The cholinergic system can be imaged with tracers for both SPECT and PET that bind to different targets related to acetylcholine storage and metabolism, including ligands for acetylcholinesterase (AChE), the presynaptic vesicular acetylcholine transporter (VAChT) and muscarinic or nicotinic acetylcholine receptors (Table 24.3).

The study of the cholinergic system is currently restricted to research, with limited clinical value on an individual basis. The interest for imaging this neurotransmitter originally derived from its implication in cognition, mainly to study in vivo the cholinergic neuronal loss in Alzheimer's disease. Along with the evidence of cognitive dysfunction and of implication of the cholinergic system in PD in neuropathological studies, starting from relatively early stages, several studies have focused on the role of the acetylcholine in PD. Acetylcholinesterase imaging shows widespread deficits in cortical and thalamic function in PD, more marked in those with cognitive impairment, but also associated with postural instability, REM sleep behaviour disorder and olfactory loss (Bohnen et al. 2003, 2009, 2012; Gilman et al. 2010; Hilker et al. 2005b; Hiraoka et al. 2012; Klein et al. 2010; Kotagal et al. 2012; Shimada et al. 2009; Shinotoh et al. 1999), even though the binding decline can vary significantly between subjects, and up to one third of the non-demented PD subjects

Table 24.3 Research-available acetylcholine transporter ligands in Parkinson's disease studies

Binding site	SPECT	PET
VAChT	(−)-5-^{123}I-Iodobenzovesamicol (^{123}I-IBVM)	^{18}F-Fluoroethoxybenzovesamicol (^{18}F-FEOBV)
AChE		^{11}C-Methyl-4-piperidyl acetate (^{11}C-MP4A)
		^{11}C-Methyl-4-piperidinyl propionate (^{11}C-PMP)
		^{11}C-Donepezil
Nicotinic receptors	5-^{123}I-Iodo-3-[2(*S*)-2-azetidinylmethoxy]pyridine (5-^{123}I-5-IA-85380)	2-^{18}F-FA-85380
		^{18}F-Flubatine
		^{11}C-Nicotine
		^{18}F-ASEM
Muscarinic receptors	^{123}I-Iodo-quinuclidinylbenzilate (^{123}I-QNB)	^{11}C-*N*-Methyl-4-piperidyl benzilate (^{11}C-NMPB)
		^{11}C-Benztropine

PET positron emission tomography, *SPECT* single-photon emission tomography, *VAChT* vesicular acetylcholine transporter, *AChE* acetylcholinesterase

may have values within the normal range (Bohnen et al. 2012). Interestingly, in subjects with *LRRK2* mutations (in whom cognitive impairment and RBD are less common), an increased AchE hydrolysis rate was shown compared to idiopathic PD, with higher values in non-manifesting carriers, suggesting a compensatory role at least in this subset of individuals (Liu et al. 2018).

Widespread cortical and subcortical reduction in nicotinic receptors has been observed in PD (Fujita et al. 2006; Kas et al. 2009; Meyer et al. 2009; Oishi et al. 2007), while the few muscarinic receptor-based studies have shown increased cortical binding, presumably reflecting upregulation in the face of cholinergic denervation (Asahina et al. 1995, 1998; Colloby et al. 2006). VAChT binding is decreased in PD dementia compared with PD subjects and in Lewy body dementia compared to healthy control (Kuhl et al. 1996; Mazère et al. 2017). A more recent study has shown a reduction of ^{18}F-FEOBV binding in PD with freezing of gait (striatum and limbic cortex) and falls (thalamus) compared to PD without gait impairment (Bohnen et al. 2019).

24.3.1.3 Noradrenergic Tracers

The lack until recently of a selective noradrenergic tracer that could cross the blood-brain barrier has limited the possibility of studying the role of the noradrenergic system in vivo. Only a few studies using non-selective monoaminergic synthesis or monoaminergic transporter-binding tracers have focused on this important neurotransmitter (Pavese et al. 2011; Remy et al. 2005).

More recently, selective reboxetine-based tracers that cross the blood-brain barrier and bind to the noradrenaline transporter (NET) have become available for the evaluation of the noradrenergic system in vivo. The (*S*,*S*)-^{11}C-2-(α-(2-methoxyphenoxy) benzyl)morpholine (^{11}C-MeNER) has been studied in PD showing BP reduction in several cortical (Sommerauer et al. 2018b) and subcortical regions, with higher reduction in PD subjects with RBD (Nahimi et al. 2018; Sommerauer et al. 2018a), confirming previous in vitro literature findings.

24.3.2 Brain Metabolism and Perfusion

The study of brain glucose metabolism and cerebral blood flow can provide valuable information in different diseases. Different SPECT tracers are used to measure brain perfusion, including ^{99m}Tc-ECD, ^{99m}Tc-HMPAO and ^{123}I-IMP. Usual findings show decreased perfusion in cortical regions in PD compared to controls, while subcortical perfusion is relatively increased in subcortical structures, including the basal ganglia (Imon et al. 1999). A relatively large number of studies have investigated the glucose metabolism in PD using the tracer ^{18}F-fluorodeoxyglucose (FDG). Similarly to the brain perfusion, a metabolism reduction has been observed in cortical regions, and it has been associated also with cognitive deficits. A diffuse involvement of lateral frontal, temporo-parietal and occipital cortex has been described in PD dementia (PDD), while no clear differences between PDD and dementia with Lewy bodies (DLB) are usually observed. Interestingly, the hypometabolism is correlated with neurocognitive measures and is significantly more pronounced in posterior regions in PDD compared with PD-related mild cognitive impairment (PD-MCI), and one study showed that lower values at diagnosis have prognostic value to predict lower cognition at 18 months (Firbank et al. 2017; Garcia-Garcia et al. 2012; Vander Borght et al. 1997; Wu et al. 2018). Relative hypermetabolism in cerebellum, pons, thalamus, paracentral gyrus and lentiform nucleus has also been described. Using FDG PET, Eidelberg et al. have developed an algorithm based on principal component analysis (PCA) to define a so-called PD-related pattern (PDRP) that has been proven to be accurate in the discrimination of PD from healthy controls, and, interestingly, it also has shown to be specific for PD, not being present in other types of parkinsonism (Fukuda et al. 2001; Tomše et al. 2017). Therefore, it has been suggested that it could be helpful in the differential diagnosis of parkinsonisms, especially at early stages. Also, the PDRP has been shown to correlate with disease progression (i.e. with clinical evaluations and with disease duration) and to be responsive to levodopa therapy and circuit-based treatment, such as STN DBS (Asanuma et al. 2006; Feigin et al. 2001). This algorithm-based approach has been used by the same group to define other neurometabolic network patterns, specifically associated with different aspects of the disease, such as tremor (PD tremor-related metabolic network, PDTP) and cognition (PD-related cognitive pattern, PDCP). The PDTP shows only a partial overlap with the PDRP, being mainly a different independent network, manifesting with a relative increased metabolic activity in the primary motor cortex, anterior cerebellum/dorsal pons and the caudate/putamen. In one study, it was significantly associated with tremor in PD subjects and responded to STN DBS, as well as DBS of the ventral intermediate nucleus (Vim) of the thalamus, while the PDRP responded only to STN DBS but not to stimulation of the Vim (which is a DBS target for tremor but not for other parkinsonian features) (Mure et al. 2011). The PDCP is characterized by hypometabolism in premotor and supplementary motor areas and posterior parietal regions and relative hypermetabolism of the cerebellar vermis and dentate nuclei. Its expression is increased in PDD and PD-MCI, and, contrary to the PDRP, it does not change significantly with dopaminergic or DBS treatment (Huang et al. 2007a, 2008).

24.3.3 Protein Aggregation

Parkinson's disease pathology is characterized by the accumulation of alpha-synuclein in the brain, but, as is the case in other neurodegenerative conditions, aggregation of other misfolded proteins, as well as mixed pathology, is well recognized (Constantinides et al. 2017; Irwin et al. 2013; Winer et al. 2017). To date, there is still no radiolabeled tracer available that binds selectively and consistently to alpha-synuclein that has been tested in humans, but other tracers that bind to other misfolded proteins, such as tau and amyloid beta, have been assessed. The possible role of this type of imaging in PD is to clarify the effect of mixed pathology in the phenotype of the disease, to be used as a predictor of specific characteristics or symptoms and to assess disease progression and the impact of disease-modifying therapies. Also, this may help in clinical practice for the differential diagnosis of doubtful cases, where there are overlapped or mixed symptoms.

24.3.3.1 Tau Imaging

Tau protein, in its different isoforms, is the pathological hallmark of different neurodegenerative diseases, including atypical parkinsonian syndromes. Tau imaging has been used especially to study the most common neurodegenerative disorder, Alzheimer's disease (AD), but it has also been investigated in tau-related forms of parkinsonism, such as PSP and corticobasal degeneration (CBD), in which the aggregated tau is in a different isoform compared to AD (Buée et al. 2000).

The tracer ^{18}F-AV1451, also known as flortaucipir, has been intensively studied in different conditions, including PD. Interestingly, it was shown that the binding in the substantia nigra is decreased in PD compared to controls and likely related to off-target binding of this ligand to neuromelanin that is reduced in PD subjects compared to controls. Also, flortaucipir, as well as other tau tracers, has off-target binding to monoamine oxidase enzymes, which may alter the interpretation of the results, especially when the tau load is not very high, as in AD (Murugan et al. 2019). A more recent ligand, called ^{11}C-PBB3 (2-((1*E*,3*E*)-4-(6-(^{11}C-methylamino) pyri-din-3-yl)buta-1,3-dienyl)benzo[d]thiazol-6-ol), has shown a higher affinity for pure 4R isoforms of tau, which may be beneficial in non-AD tauopathies. However, it appears to have off-target binding to alpha-synuclein both in vitro (Koga et al. 2017) and in vivo (Perez-Soriano et al. 2017). This tracer could therefore potentially be used to study alpha-synuclein aggregation and could be a potential biomarker for PD, even though this dual protein-binding may complicate the interpretation of the results.

24.3.3.2 Amyloid Beta Imaging

Amyloid beta (Aβ) PET imaging has been proposed as a biomarker for Alzheimer's disease (AD). Neuropathological studies have reported varying amounts of amyloid pathology in PDD and more so in DLB (Hughes et al. 1993; Hurtig et al. 2000; Jellinger 2003). Therefore, PET with amyloid ligands has been used to investigate its relationship with the clinical phenotype of Lewy body-related disorders in vivo.

The ^{11}C-Pittsburgh compound B (PiB) is the most investigated Aβ tracer. Other tracers include ^{18}F-florbetaben (FBB), ^{18}F-florbetapir, ^{18}F-flutemetamol and fluoroethyl-methylamino-2-naphthylethylidene malononitrile (^{18}F-FDDNP). Studies in subjects with PD, PD-related mild cognitive impairment (PD-MCI) and PDD have shown variable results, ranging from no differences compared to healthy controls in all PD groups (PD, PD-MCI and PDD) to increase binding in up to 37% of the PD sample, with cortical and striatal involvement (Akhtar et al. 2017; Jokinen et al. 2010; Mashima et al. 2017; Melzer et al. 2019; Petrou et al. 2015; Shah et al. 2016).

The negative results in most PD subjects, even with cognitive dysfunction, have suggested that the cognitive decline in PD is not mainly driven by Aβ deposition. Furthermore, the cases of positive PET studies may be related with a mixed pathology with overlap of Lewy bodies and AD-type pathology (Maetzler et al. 2008), showing the typical AD CSF characteristics and a higher prevalence of ApoE4 genotype, and therefore probably represent the manifestation of a different coincident pathological condition (Maetzler et al. 2009).

24.3.4 Neuroinflammation

Neuroinflammation has been implicated in the process of neurodegeneration in PD and in other neurodegenerative disorders. The interest in this area has grown in the last years, linked to the hope that this may result in new therapeutic targets that could potentially alter the progression of the disease. Having reliable in vivo data on neuroinflammation is vital to further explore the role of this process in the progression of the disease, possibly also in its premotor phase, and as a biomarker to study new drugs.

The main molecular target for the study of neuroinflammation with molecular imaging has been the mitochondrial translocator protein (TSPO), which is upregulated in activated microglia (but is also expressed in astrocytes). A large number of studies have assessed the expression of this protein in vivo, in several neurological conditions, but several problems have limited the interpretation of the findings achieved with tracers that target this protein. The first-generation tracer ^{11}C-(R) PK11195 shows a high level of non-specific binding, with a relatively poor signal-to-noise ratio, and reduced penetration of the brain-blood barrier. Also, the second-generation radioligands (e.g. ^{11}C-PBR28, ^{18}F-PBR-111) have shown high between-subject binding variability in healthy controls as well as people with PD, reflecting a variable binding affinity related to a polymorphism (rs6971) in the gene encoding *TSPO*. This complicates the interpretation of the findings, despite adjusting the results according to the genetic status (Owen et al. 2014). Thirdly, there is no consistently good reference region for TSPO binding, which further complicates scan analysis. Despite these limitations, some studies have shown an increase in TSPO binding (measured with ^{11}C-PK 11195) in PD compared to healthy controls in different brain regions, including midbrain, substantia nigra, striatum and cortical regions (Gerhard et al. 2006; Iannaccone et al. 2013; Terada et al. 2016), with midbrain binding inversely correlated with striatal dopaminergic denervation (measured by ^{11}C-CFT PET) (Ouchi et al. 2005), and cortical binding inversely correlated with hippocampal volume and metabolism and with cognitive scores (Edison et al. 2013; Fan et al. 2015; Femminella et al. 2016). Increased ^{11}C-PK 11195 binding has also been demonstrated in the substantia nigra of patients with idiopathic REM sleep behaviour disorder (Stokholm et al. 2017). However, studies performed with second-generation TSPO ligands such as ^{18}F-FEPPA (Koshimori et al. 2015) or ^{11}C-PBR28 (Varnäs et al. 2019) have failed to demonstrate a consistent increase in PD brain.

To overcome some of the limitations of the TSPO imaging, newer neuroinflammation tracers that target different molecules, such as the P2X7 receptor, reactive oxygen species or the colony-stimulating factor-1 receptor, are under investigation (Horti et al. 2019; Narayanaswami et al. 2018). In a pilot study, ^{11}C-JNJ54173717, a radioligand that binds to the P2X7 receptor, found no differences between PD subjects and healthy controls. Furthermore, the investigators observed a relationship between total volume of distribution (V_T) and a polymorphism of the *P2X7R* gene, raising the question of whether genotyping will also be needed with this target (Van Weehaeghe et al. 2019).

24.3.5 Phosphodiesterase 10A

Phosphodiesterase 10A (PDE10A) is an intracellular enzyme highly expressed in the medium spiny neurons of the striatum, involved in several neuronal functions through the hydrolysis of the cyclic nucleotides adenosine monophosphate (cAMP) and guanosine monophosphate (cGMP) (Bollen and Prickaerts 2012). It has a role in the signalling of dopamine receptors in the striatum (Nishi et al. 2008), and mutations in the *PDE10A* gene have been associated with genetically driven movement disorders, including childhood-onset chorea and one case of adult-onset parkinsonism (Mencacci et al. 2016). Furthermore, a downregulation of PDE10A has been demonstrated in the striatum of animal models of parkinsonism (Sancesario et al. 2014). For these reasons, there has been an increasing interest in the study of this pathway, which has also been postulated as a possible therapeutic target for diseases that affect the basal ganglia, including Huntington's disease and PD. Its evaluation in vivo is therefore considered of high relevance in this subset of diseases, and a relatively high number of ligands have been tested in human studies (Boscutti et al. 2019). In PD subjects, the ligand ^{11}C-IMA107 has reduced binding compared to controls in the striatum but also in the GP, correlating positively with disease duration and motor severity (Niccolini et al. 2015). Indeed, longer disease duration and increased motor deficit correlate with reduced PDE10A binding in both caudate and putamen, whereas in the case of dopamine transporter binding, this correlation is seen in putamen only (Pagano et al. 2019). Another study did not find significant differences in caudate or putamen binding between PD subjects and healthy controls, using a different tracer (^{18}F-JNJ42259152), but this could be due to the small sample size and to the relatively early stage of the disease of the subjects scanned. Interestingly, though, the same study found that PD but also PSP patients had a lower caudate-to-putamen binding ratio compared to healthy controls (Koole et al. 2017). Further investigation is needed to define the utility of this interesting target as a biomarker and to understand its potential role in the therapy of the disease, and the molecular imaging is certainly an ideal way to study it.

24.4 Peripheral Nuclear Imaging

Parkinson's disease is a multisystemic disorder that affects the CNS but also the peripheral and enteric nervous system. An increasing body of evidence has shown the peripheral involvement in the early stages of the disease, even before the first motor symptoms are detected that may be responsible of some of the nonmotor features, such as the gastrointestinal and genitourinary symptoms. It has been hypothesized that the disease may even start in the peripheral nervous system and then spread to the CNS, as alpha-synuclein deposits have been detected in the gastrointestinal tract and other peripheral tissues. Nuclear imaging in PD has mainly focused on the brain, but some recent studies have shown the usefulness of imaging the periphery both for clinical purposes and also in research for better understanding of the progression of the disease.

Cardiac sympathetic denervation has been detected using ^{123}I-meta-iodobenzylguanidine (^{123}I-MIBG) scintigraphy and SPECT. About 80–90% of PD and DLB subjects have reduced uptake compared to controls (Chung and Kim 2015; Orimo et al. 1999, 2012). Interestingly, this feature is specific of PD, while there is no uptake decline in PSP or MSA subjects (Tateno et al. 2011; Yoshita et al. 1998). As a consequence, this test can be used in clinical practice to help differentiate the PD from other non-Lewy body parkinsonisms. It is necessary to keep in mind that the cardiac sympathetic denervation is not specific for PD, but it can be observed also in diabetes and chronic heart failure, and therefore the interpretation of results must be cautious in this subset of subjects.

A cholinergic tracer, ^{11}C-donepezil, has been used to study AChE density in peripheral organs, as a surrogate to quantify in vivo vagal innervation by one group. A reduced cholinergic innervation has been observed in colon, small intestine and pancreas of early PD subjects, possibly reflecting the parasympathetic involvement of PD (Fedorova et al. 2017; Gjerløff et al. 2015).

24.5 Clinical Implications

24.5.1 Diagnosis and Differential Diagnosis

In clinical practice, the diagnosis of PD is still based on clinical criteria (Postuma et al. 2018), with no required investigations in the vast majority of cases. In some clinically doubtful cases, though, the differential diagnosis may benefit from objective tests. This is especially useful to differentiate secondary parkinsonisms (e.g. iatrogenic parkinsonism) or cases of tremor with mixed characteristics or overlapped mild parkinsonism. In these cases, several approaches have been suggested to help the differential diagnosis, including smell tests, SN ultrasound and molecular neuroimaging. PET and SPECT dopaminergic imaging are able to show dopaminergic denervation that follows the typical posterior-to-anterior pattern and is usually asymmetric (Fig. 24.2). SPECT DAT imaging is probably the most commonly used investigation in Europe and North America and has consistently shown its usefulness in this specific setting.

Unfortunately, DAT imaging performance in differentiating PD from other types of neurodegenerative parkinsonism, such as progressive supranuclear palsy (PSP), multiple system atrophy (MSA) or dementia with Lewy bodies (LBD), is low, and therefore it is not useful in clinical practice. For this problem, multiple-step approaches have been suggested, in which a DAT imaging for the initial diagnosis of a neurodegenerative parkinsonism is followed by a dopaminergic postsynaptic imaging or by FDG PET, which shows better results in differentiating PD from other non-Lewy body parkinsonisms (Hellwig et al. 2012). The cardiac MIBG imaging has also been proposed as a useful test to differentiate PD from other

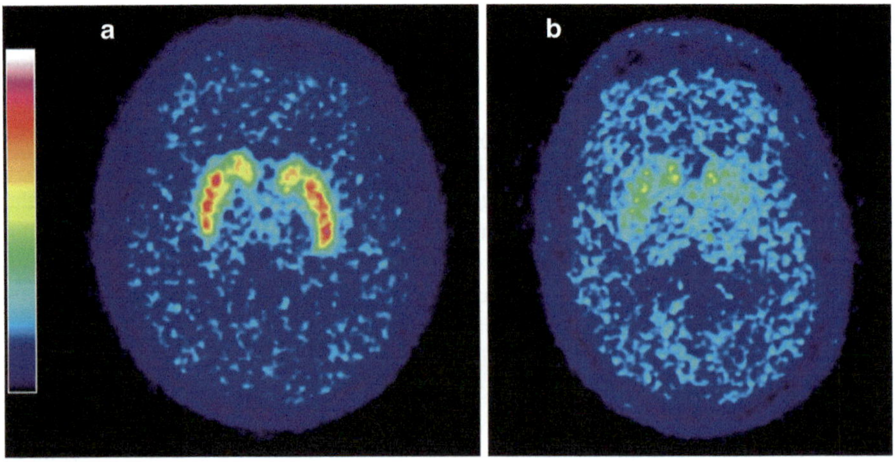

Fig. 24.2 ^{11}C-DTBZ imaging in PD. The figure shows normal striatal binding of the ^{11}C-DTBZ in a healthy subject (**a**) and the striatal binding reduction in a PD subject, which follows the typical posterior-to-anterior pattern of involvement in the putamen, in an asymmetric fashion (**b**)

clinically similar conditions, as the cardiac sympathetic denervation is seen in PD but is usually absent in other types of parkinsonism. In the future, we may envision the use of tau protein-based tracers to diagnose tauopathies, but they still need further validation, and therefore their role in the clinical practice is still to be defined.

At present, these investigations have several limitations. First of all, they are not widely available, and their cost is high when compared to possible clinical benefit. Also, their usefulness is mostly in the early stages of the disease, as the longitudinal progression and the response to medication are usually sufficient to define an operational diagnosis. And finally, in the absence of disease-modifying drugs for any of these diseases, the importance of a specific and early diagnosis is limited, as it does not imply a different management of the patients in clinical practice.

24.5.2 Tracking Disease Progression

Molecular neuroimaging would be an ideal biomarker to track disease progression, as it is a relatively noninvasive technique and it can provide an insight at multiple functional and molecular levels (Strafella et al. 2017). In the earliest stages of PD, presynaptic dopamine tracer uptake is most severely decreased in the dorsal part of the caudal putamen, but a significant reduction of uptake is also seen throughout the striatum. The rate of loss of FD uptake is much higher in PD than in age-matched normal controls (Nurmi et al. 2001; Vingerhoets et al. 1994). In patients with unilateral disease, the clinically unaffected putamen is still abnormal, as one would expect with a subclinical loss of dopaminergic function (Marek et al. 1996).

A posterior-to-anterior gradient of dopaminergic dysfunction has been demonstrated in the putamen, with side-to-side asymmetry in tracer uptake between the less and more severely affected striatal structures that normally correspond to the clinical findings (more severely affected side contralateral to clinically most affected limbs). This asymmetry is also a supporting feature in the diagnosis of PD, when compared to other forms of parkinsonism, or normal ageing. As disease progresses, the antero-posterior gradient is maintained, suggesting a similar relative rate of decline throughout the putamen, while the degree of asymmetry between less and more severely affected putamen diminishes (Brück et al. 2009; Nandhagopal et al. 2009). Thus, when ^{18}F-dopa PET was used to assess the annual rate of decline of tracer uptake in different striatal subregions over a 5-year period, the annual reduction in uptake was found to be 10.3% in posterior putamen, 8.3% in anterior putamen and 5.9% in caudate compared to baseline values. However, the absolute rate of decline was similar in all striatal subregions (Nurmi et al. 2001). Other studies have found similar results (Brück et al. 2006).

These findings are consistent with the view that while factors responsible for the initiation of PD affect striatal subregions in a differential fashion, once disease has started, progression may occur due to non-specific mechanisms such as oxidative stress/free radical elaboration, excitotoxicity, mitochondrial damage and inflammation (Muchowski 2002; Schapira et al. 1998) that would affect striatal subregions to a similar degree.

Analysis of longitudinal data with multitracer PET has revealed that at symptom onset, there is a substantially greater loss of putaminal DTBZ binding in younger, compared with older, PD patients. Further, the rate of reduction in tracer uptake is slower in younger compared to older patients, and the estimated presymptomatic disease phase spans more than 20 years in younger patients compared to one decade in older cases. This suggests that younger PD patients' symptoms progress more slowly and they are able to endure more damage to the dopaminergic system before the appearance of motor symptoms, both possibly due to more efficient compensatory mechanisms (de la Fuente-Fernández et al. 2011).

Autopsy studies in PD have shown a 45% decrease in nigral cell counts during the first 10 years of PD, ten times greater than the loss associated with normal ageing, with a tendency to approach the normal age-related linear decline in the later stages. A number of PET studies support this non-linear pattern of nigral cell loss (Brück et al. 2009; Nandhagopal et al. 2009). Dopaminergic hypofunction in the putamen, as demonstrated by decline in uptake of dopaminergic tracers, is more rapid in early disease than in later stages, supporting the hypothesis of negative exponential decline (Kuramoto et al. 2013; Nandhagopal et al. 2009) as also shown in neuropathological post-mortem analysis of loss of striatal TH staining (Kordower et al. 2013).

Estimation of preclinical duration in PD based on FD PET studies varies according to the model that is used as well as other technical factors but is approximately 6 years with estimated losses ranging from approximately 30% (Hilker et al. 2005a; Morrish et al. 1998) to 55% (Lee et al. 2000) of normal putaminal FD uptake at the time of symptom onset, in general agreement with post-mortem studies. Longitudinal analysis of DTBZ data also suggests that the preclinical interval varies depending on the age of onset, with longer duration in subjects with a younger age of onset. For DTBZ, this preclinical interval is approximately 17 years (for age of onset 53), but at this same age of onset, the interval is shorter when other tracers are used (13 years for DAT binding, 6 years for FD uptake; de la Fuente-Fernández et al. 2011).

PET with DA tracers is a sensitive means of detecting striatal DA dysfunction. This has been used in clinically unaffected mutation carriers from families with LRRK2 mutations (Adams et al. 2005), and progression in these families has been associated with further decline in dopaminergic tracer uptake, with clinical involvement appearing to correspond to progression of impaired FD uptake (Nandhagopal et al. 2008). Interestingly, abnormalities of DA turnover can be seen very early in LRRK2 mutation carriers, many years prior to the expected age of disease onset and earlier than changes in other markers of DA function (Sossi et al. 2010). Once PD becomes manifest in LRRK2 mutation carriers, the rate of decline in presynaptic dopaminergic tracer uptake is indistinguishable from that seen in sporadic disease (Wile et al. 2017).

Changes in metabolic network activity can also be used to track PD progression (Huang et al. 2007b). PDRP expression has been found to be elevated at baseline relative to healthy control subjects and to increase linearly with disease progression, with increasing metabolism in the STN, GPi, dorsal pons and primary motor cortex and declining metabolism in prefrontal and inferior parietal regions with advancement of disease. Changes in PDRP activity correlated with concurrent declines in striatal DAT binding and increases in motor ratings. However, PDRP is also expressed in the asymptomatic striatum in patients with unilateral disease and progresses symmetrically and in parallel with the symptomatic striatum, with no difference in values between the two sides. A relatively short preclinical period is indicated, in which dissociation of the normal relation between metabolic activity and age occurred about 5 years prior to the onset of PD symptoms (Tang et al. 2010).

24.5.3 Monitoring Therapeutic Effects

Imaging has been used as an in vivo biomarker to assess the effect of treatment on disease progression in various clinical trials. These studies include the comparison of the agonist pramipexole with levodopa on motor complications of Parkinson's disease (CALM-PD) study (Parkinson Study Group 2000) which used ^{123}I-β-CIT SPECT (a measure of DAT binding) to compare the effects of L-dopa versus pramipexole in early PD, REAL-PET (Whone et al. 2003) that compared ropinirole and L-dopa in de novo PD patients with FD PET as the primary outcome measure and the earlier versus later levodopa in Parkinson's disease (ELLDOPA) study (Fahn 1999) in which the effects of L-dopa on clinical progression of PD were studied, and ^{123}I-β-CIT SPECT was included, and studies on foetal nigral transplantation and intraputaminal glial cell line-derived neurotrophic factor (GDNF) on clinical and imaging end points have also been reported with FD PET as a secondary outcome measure (Gill et al. 2003; Lang et al. 2006; Nakamura et al. 2001; Olanow et al. 2003; Whone et al. 2019).

All the above studies found discordance in results between clinical outcome and estimated disease progression, as determined by SPECT or PET. Imaging findings suggested a slower rate of disease progression with pramipexole in the CALM-PD study and with ropinirole in REAL-PET. However, clinical improvement, as measured by the unified Parkinson's disease rating scale (UPDRS), was more in the levodopa treatment group. In ELLDOPA, the L-dopa treatment group had a slower rate of clinical progression compared with the placebo group when clinical assessments were performed after a washout period of two weeks. Although this probably reflects inadequate washout of symptomatic effects, a more rapid rate of decline in DAT binding was noted with imaging in the L-dopa treatment group. In the studies of foetal nigral transplantation and intraputaminal GDNF, although there was a significant increase in striatal FD uptake, there was no significant change in the clinical outcomes.

This discrepancy between clinical progression and imaging findings could reflect many factors, including potentially confounding effects of dopaminergic medication or other therapy on the imaging biomarkers rather than on the disease process. Levodopa may act to depress DAT binding and AADC activity relative to DA agonists. Also, if DA agonists are indeed neuroprotective or levodopa neurotoxic, this effect might be masked by the higher symptomatic efficacy of levodopa, especially when using short washout periods. It must also be noted that clinical progression was measured using the UPDRS that reflects a composite of dopaminergic and non-dopaminergic dysfunction in PD; the clinical sign that best reflects the severity of the nigrostriatal lesion is bradykinesia. Clinical rating scales also remain vulnerable to both patient and evaluator subjectivity. In the case of cell-based therapy such as transplantation, grafts may survive but fail to form synaptic connections with the host striatum, there may be other deficits in reintegration of a repaired nigrostriatal system into the cortico-striato-pallido-thalamo-cortical network and, finally, many of the deficits of advanced PD may be related to non-dopaminergic abnormalities. Thus, assessment of the nigrostriatal DA system alone may be inadequate to assess the overall disease progression in PD.

Further trials are hence needed to define the contribution of possible confounding factors and to better validate imaging outcomes as biomarkers of PD progression (Agarwal and Stoessl 2013). Attention to study design and analysis are imperative, and functional imaging outcomes must be interpreted with caution and in the context of the clinical result.

The above concerns notwithstanding, functional imaging still offers an objective method of assessing disease progression in PD. In trials of implantation of foetal DA cells (Brundin et al. 2000) into putamen, ^{18}F-dopa PET provided proof of mechanism by detecting increased DA storage capacity after treatment. Similarly, changes in glucose metabolism with PET, while not providing a direct evaluation of DA function, can also be used to infer re-establishment of physiological connections. This approach has been successfully used to study the effects of STN DBS, response to levodopa and glutamic acid decarboxylase (GAD) gene transfer in the STN (Kaplitt et al. 2007). The disadvantage of this approach is that while it may track the outcome of a therapy, it is related to its symptomatic effect, and it may therefore be difficult to determine the degree to which it reflects a disease-modifying component.

Acknowledgements Dr. M. Matarazzo was supported by a Clinical Research Fellowship Award from Parkinson Canada. Dr. A. J. Stoessl is supported by the Michael J. Fox Foundation, the Weston Brain Institute and the Canada Research Chairs Program. We gratefully acknowledge the assistance of Nasim Vafai for the image processing and generating the figures.

References

Adams JR, van Netten H, Schulzer M, Mak E, Mckenzie J, Strongosky A et al (2005) PET in LRRK2 mutations: comparison to sporadic Parkinson's disease and evidence for presymptomatic compensation. Brain 128(Pt 12):2777–2785. https://doi.org/10.1093/brain/awh607

Agarwal PA, Stoessl AJ (2013) Biomarkers for trials of neuroprotection in Parkinson's disease. Mov Disord 28(1):71–85. https://doi.org/10.1002/mds.25065

Aiello M, Cavaliere C, Marchitelli R, D'Albore A, De Vita E, Salvatore M (2018) Hybrid PET/MRI methodology. Int Rev Neurobiol 141:97–128. https://doi.org/10.1016/bs.irn.2018.07.026

Akhtar RS, Xie SX, Chen YJ, Rick J, Gross RG, Nasrallah IM et al (2017) Regional brain amyloid-β accumulation associates with domain-specific cognitive performance in Parkinson disease without dementia. PLoS One 12(5):e0177924. https://doi.org/10.1371/journal.pone.0177924

Antonini A, Schwarz J, Oertel WH, Pogarell O, Leenders KL (1997) Long-term changes of striatal dopamine D2 receptors in patients with Parkinson's disease: a study with positron emission tomography and [11C]raclopride. Mov Disord 12(1):33–38. https://doi.org/10.1002/mds.870120107

Asahina M, Shinotoh H, Hirayama K, Suhara T, Shishido F, Inoue O, Tateno Y (1995) Hypersensitivity of cortical muscarinic receptors in Parkinson's disease demonstrated by PET. Acta Neurol Scand 91(6):437–443

Asahina M, Suhara T, Shinotoh H, Inoue O, Suzuki K, Hattori T (1998) Brain muscarinic receptors in progressive supranuclear palsy and Parkinson's disease: a positron emission tomographic study. J Neurol Neurosurg Psychiatry 65(2):155–163. https://doi.org/10.1136/jnnp.65.2.155

Asanuma K, Tang C, Ma Y, Dhawan V, Mattis P, Edwards C et al (2006) Network modulation in the treatment of Parkinson's disease. Brain 129(Pt 10):2667–2678. https://doi.org/10.1093/brain/awl162

Asari S, Fujimoto K, Miyauchi A, Sato T, Nakano I, Muramatsu S (2011) Subregional 6-[18F]fluoro-L-m-tyrosine uptake in the striatum in Parkinson's disease. BMC Neurol 11:35. https://doi.org/10.1186/1471-2377-11-35

Au WL, Adams JR, Troiano AR, Stoessl AJ (2005) Parkinson's disease: in vivo assessment of disease progression using positron emission tomography. Brain Res Mol Brain Res 134(1):24–33. https://doi.org/10.1016/j.molbrainres.2004.09.028

Bernheimer H, Birkmayer W, Hornykiewicz O, Jellinger K, Seitelberger F (1973) Brain dopamine and the syndromes of Parkinson and Huntington. Clinical, morphological and neurochemical correlations. J Neurol Sci 20(4):415–455. https://doi.org/10.1016/0022-510X(73)90175-5

Bohnen NI, Kaufer DI, Ivanco LS, Lopresti B, Koeppe RA, Davis JG et al (2003) Cortical cholinergic function is more severely affected in parkinsonian dementia than in Alzheimer disease: an in vivo positron emission tomographic study. Arch Neurol 60(12):1745–1748. https://doi.org/10.1001/archneur.60.12.1745

Bohnen NI, Müller MLTM, Koeppe RA, Studenski SA, Kilbourn MA, Frey KA, Albin RL (2009) History of falls in Parkinson disease is associated with reduced cholinergic activity. Neurology 73(20):1670–1676. https://doi.org/10.1212/WNL.0b013e3181c1ded6

Bohnen NI, Müller MLTM, Kotagal V, Koeppe RA, Kilbourn MR, Gilman S et al (2012) Heterogeneity of cholinergic denervation in Parkinson's disease without dementia. J Cereb Blood Flow Metab 32(8):1609–1617. https://doi.org/10.1038/jcbfm.2012.60

Bohnen NI, Kanel P, Zhou Z, Koeppe RA, Frey KA, Dauer WT et al (2019) Cholinergic system changes of falls and freezing of gait in Parkinson's disease. Ann Neurol 85(4):538–549. https://doi.org/10.1002/ana.25430

Boileau I, Rusjan P, Houle S, Wilkins D, Tong J, Selby P et al (2008a) Increased vesicular monoamine transporter binding during early abstinence in human methamphetamine users: is VMAT2 a stable dopamine neuron biomarker? J Neurosci 28(39):9850–9856. https://doi.org/10.1523/JNEUROSCI.3008-08.2008

Boileau I, Warsh JJ, Guttman M, Saint-Cyr JA, McCluskey T, Rusjan P et al (2008b) Elevated serotonin transporter binding in depressed patients with Parkinson's disease: a preliminary PET study with [11C]DASB. Mov Disord 23(12):1776–1780. https://doi.org/10.1002/mds.22212

Bollen E, Prickaerts J (2012) Phosphodiesterases in neurodegenerative disorders. IUBMB Life 64(12):965–970. https://doi.org/10.1002/iub.1104

Boscutti GA, Rabiner E, Plisson C (2019) PET radioligands for imaging of the PDE10A in human: current status. Neurosci Lett 691:11–17. https://doi.org/10.1016/j.neulet.2018.08.006

Braak H, Del Tredici K, Rüb U, de Vos RAI, Jansen Steur ENH, Braak E (2003) Staging of brain pathology related to sporadic Parkinson's disease. Neurobiol Aging 24(2):197–211. https://doi.org/10.1016/S0197-4580(02)00065-9

Brück A, Aalto S, Nurmi E, Vahlberg T, Bergman J, Rinne JO (2006) Striatal subregional 6-[18F]fluoro-L-dopa uptake in early Parkinson's disease: a two-year follow-up study. Mov Disord 21(7):958–963. https://doi.org/10.1002/mds.20855

Brück A, Aalto S, Rauhala E, Bergman J, Marttila R, Rinne JO (2009) A follow-up study on 6-[18F]fluoro-L-dopa uptake in early Parkinson's disease shows nonlinear progression in the putamen. Mov Disord 24(7):1009–1015. https://doi.org/10.1002/mds.22484
Brundin P, Pogarell O, Hagell P, Piccini P, Widner H, Schrag A et al (2000) Bilateral caudate and putamen grafts of embryonic mesencephalic tissue treated with lazaroids in Parkinson's disease. Brain 123(Pt 7):1380–1390. https://doi.org/10.1093/brain/123.7.1380
Buée L, Bussière T, Buée-Scherrer V, Delacourte A, Hof PR (2000) Tau protein isoforms, phosphorylation and role in neurodegenerative disorders. Brain Res Brain Res Rev 33(1):95–130. https://doi.org/10.1016/S0165-0173(00)00019-9
Carlsson T, Carta M, Muñoz A, Mattsson B, Winkler C, Kirik D, Björklund A (2009) Impact of grafted serotonin and dopamine neurons on development of L-DOPA-induced dyskinesias in parkinsonian rats is determined by the extent of dopamine neuron degeneration. Brain 132(Pt 2):319–335. https://doi.org/10.1093/brain/awn305
Carta M, Carlsson T, Kirik D, Björklund A (2007) Dopamine released from 5-HT terminals is the cause of L-DOPA-induced dyskinesia in parkinsonian rats. Brain 130(Pt 7):1819–1833. https://doi.org/10.1093/brain/awm082
Carta M, Carlsson T, Muñoz A, Kirik D, Björklund A (2010) Role of serotonin neurons in the induction of levodopa- and graft-induced dyskinesias in Parkinson's disease. Mov Disord 25(Suppl 1):S174–S179. https://doi.org/10.1002/mds.22792
Chaudhuri KR, Odin P, Antonini A, Martinez-Martin P (2011) Parkinson's disease: the non-motor issues. Parkinsonism Relat Disord 17(10):717–723. https://doi.org/10.1016/j.parkreldis.2011.02.018
Chung EJ, Kim SJ (2015) (123)I-Metaiodobenzylguanidine myocardial scintigraphy in lewy body-related disorders: a literature review. J Mov Disord 8(2):55–66. https://doi.org/10.14802/jmd.15015
Colloby SJ, Pakrasi S, Firbank MJ, Perry EK, Piggott MA, Owens J et al (2006) In vivo SPECT imaging of muscarinic acetylcholine receptors using (R,R) 123I-QNB in dementia with Lewy bodies and Parkinson's disease dementia. NeuroImage 33(2):423–429. https://doi.org/10.1016/j.neuroimage.2006.07.026
Constantinides VC, Paraskevas GP, Emmanouilidou E, Petropoulou O, Bougea A, Vekrellis K et al (2017) CSF biomarkers β-amyloid, tau proteins and a-synuclein in the differential diagnosis of Parkinson-plus syndromes. J Neurol Sci 382(September):91–95. https://doi.org/10.1016/j.jns.2017.09.039
De La Fuente-Fernández R, Furtado S, Guttman M, Furukawa Y, Lee CS, Calne DB et al (2003) VMAT2 binding is elevated in dopa-responsive dystonia: visualizing empty vesicles by PET. Synapse (New York, NY) 49(1):20–28. https://doi.org/10.1002/syn.10199
de la Fuente-Fernández R, Sossi V, McCormick S, Schulzer M, Ruth TJ, Stoessl AJ (2009) Visualizing vesicular dopamine dynamics in Parkinson's disease. Synapse (New York, NY) 63(8):713–716. https://doi.org/10.1002/syn.20653
de la Fuente-Fernández R, Schulzer M, Kuramoto L, Cragg J, Ramachandiran N, Au WL et al (2011) Age-specific progression of nigrostriatal dysfunction in Parkinson's disease. Ann Neurol 69(5):803–810. https://doi.org/10.1002/ana.22284
de Paulis T (2003) The discovery of epidepride and its analogs as high-affinity radioligands for imaging extrastriatal dopamine D(2) receptors in human brain. Curr Pharm Des 9(8):673–696
DeJesus OT, Holden JE, Endres C, Murali D, Oakes TR, Shelton S et al (1992) Visualization of dopamine nerve terminals by positron tomography using [18F]fluoro-beta-fluoromethylene-m-tyrosine. Brain Res 597(1):151–154. https://doi.org/10.1016/0006-8993(92)91518-j
DeJesus OT, Flores LG, Murali D, Converse AK, Bartlett RM, Barnhart TE et al (2005) Aromatic L-amino acid decarboxylase turnover in vivo in rhesus macaque striatum: a microPET study. Brain Res 1054(1):55–60. https://doi.org/10.1016/j.brainres.2005.06.086
Doder M, Rabiner EA, Turjanski N, Lees AJ, Brooks DJ, 11C-WAY 100635 PET Study (2003) Tremor in Parkinson's disease and serotonergic dysfunction: an 11C-WAY 100635 PET study. Neurology 60(4):601–605

Doudet DJ, Chan GL, Jivan S, DeJesus OT, McGeer EG, English C et al (1999) Evaluation of dopaminergic presynaptic integrity: 6-[18F]fluoro-L-dopa versus 6-[18F]fluoro-L-m-tyrosine. J Cereb Blood Flow Metab 19(3):278–287. https://doi.org/10.1097/00004647-199903000-00006
Edison P, Ahmed I, Fan Z, Hinz R, Gelosa G, Ray Chaudhuri K et al (2013) Microglia, amyloid, and glucose metabolism in Parkinson's disease with and without dementia. Neuropsychopharmacology 38(6):938–949. https://doi.org/10.1038/npp.2012.255
Espay AJ, Vizcarra JA, Marsili L, Lang AE, Simon DK, Merola A et al (2019) Revisiting protein aggregation as pathogenic in sporadic Parkinson and Alzheimer diseases. Neurology 92(7):329–337. https://doi.org/10.1212/WNL.0000000000006926
Fahn S (1999) Parkinson disease, the effect of levodopa, and the ELLDOPA trial. Earlier vs later L-DOPA. Arch Neurol 56(5):529–535. https://doi.org/10.1001/archneur.56.5.529
Fan Z, Aman Y, Ahmed I, Chetelat G, Landeau B, Ray Chaudhuri K et al (2015) Influence of microglial activation on neuronal function in Alzheimer's and Parkinson's disease dementia. Alzheimers Dement 11(6):608–21.e7. https://doi.org/10.1016/j.jalz.2014.06.016
Fearnley JM, Lees AJ (1991) Ageing and Parkinson's disease: substantia nigra regional selectivity. Brain 114(Pt 5):2283–2301. https://doi.org/10.1136/jnnp.2007.131045
Fedorova TD, Seidelin LB, Knudsen K, Schacht AC, Geday J, Pavese N et al (2017) Decreased intestinal acetylcholinesterase in early Parkinson disease: an 11C-donepezil PET study. Neurology 88(8):775–781. https://doi.org/10.1212/WNL.0000000000003633
Feigin A, Fukuda M, Dhawan V, Przedborski S, Jackson-Lewis V, Mentis MJ et al (2001) Metabolic correlates of levodopa response in Parkinson's disease. Neurology 57(11):2083–2088. https://doi.org/10.1212/wnl.57.11.2083
Felicio AC, Shih MC, Godeiro-Junior C, Andrade LAF, Bressan RA, Ferraz HB (2009) Molecular imaging studies in Parkinson disease: reducing diagnostic uncertainty. Neurologist 15(1):6–16. https://doi.org/10.1097/NRL.0b013e318183fdd8
Femminella GD, Ninan S, Atkinson R, Fan Z, Brooks DJ, Edison P (2016) Does microglial activation influence hippocampal volume and neuronal function in Alzheimer's disease and Parkinson's disease dementia? J Alzheimers Dis 51(4):1275–1289. https://doi.org/10.3233/JAD-150827
Fereshtehnejad S, Zeighami Y, Dagher A, Postuma RB (2017) Clinical criteria for subtyping Parkinson's disease: biomarkers and longitudinal progression. Brain 140(7):1959–1976. https://doi.org/10.1093/brain/awx118
Firbank MJ, Yarnall AJ, Lawson RA, Duncan GW, Khoo TK, Petrides GS et al (2017) Cerebral glucose metabolism and cognition in newly diagnosed Parkinson's disease: ICICLE-PD study. J Neurol Neurosurg Psychiatry 88(4):310–316. https://doi.org/10.1136/jnnp-2016-313918
Foffani G, Obeso JA (2018) A cortical pathogenic theory of Parkinson's disease. Neuron 99(6):1116–1128. https://doi.org/10.1016/j.neuron.2018.07.028
Frankle WG, Huang Y, Hwang D, Talbot PS, Slifstein M, Van Heertum R et al (2004) Comparative evaluation of serotonin transporter radioligands 11C-DASB and 11C-McN 5652 in healthy humans. J Nucl Med 45(4):682–694
Fujita M, Ichise M, Zoghbi SS, Liow J-S, Ghose S, Vines DC et al (2006) Widespread decrease of nicotinic acetylcholine receptors in Parkinson's disease. Ann Neurol 59(1):174–177. https://doi.org/10.1002/ana.20688
Fukuda M, Mentis MJ, Ma Y, Dhawan V, Antonini A, Lang AE et al (2001) Networks mediating the clinical effects of pallidal brain stimulation for Parkinson's disease: a PET study of resting-state glucose metabolism. Brain 124(Pt 8):1601–1609. https://doi.org/10.1093/brain/124.8.1601
Garcia-Garcia D, Clavero P, Gasca Salas C, Lamet I, Arbizu J, Gonzalez-Redondo R et al (2012) Posterior parietooccipital hypometabolism may differentiate mild cognitive impairment from dementia in Parkinson's disease. Eur J Nucl Med Mol Imaging 39(11):1767–1777. https://doi.org/10.1007/s00259-012-2198-5
GBD 2016 Parkinson's Disease Collaborators (2018) Global, regional, and national burden of Parkinson's disease, 1990–2016: a systematic analysis for the Global Burden of Disease Study 2016. Lancet Neurol 17(11):939–953. https://doi.org/10.1016/S1474-4422(18)30295-3

Gerhard A, Pavese N, Hotton G, Turkheimer F, Es M, Hammers A et al (2006) In vivo imaging of microglial activation with [11C](R)-PK11195 PET in idiopathic Parkinson's disease. Neurobiol Dis 21(2):404–412. https://doi.org/10.1016/j.nbd.2005.08.002

Ghadery C, Best LA, Pavese N, Tai YF, Strafella AP (2019) PET evaluation of microglial activation in non-neurodegenerative brain diseases. Curr Neurol Neurosci Rep 19(7):38. https://doi.org/10.1007/s11910-019-0951-x

Gibb WR, Lees AJ (1988) The relevance of the Lewy body to the pathogenesis of idiopathic Parkinson's disease. J Neurol Neurosurg Psychiatry 51(6):745–752. https://doi.org/10.1136/jnnp.51.6.745

Gill SS, Patel NK, Hotton GR, O'Sullivan K, McCarter R, Bunnage M et al (2003) Direct brain infusion of glial cell line-derived neurotrophic factor in Parkinson disease. Nat Med 9(5):589–595. https://doi.org/10.1038/nm850

Gilman S, Koeppe RA, Nan B, Wang C-N, Wang X, Junck L et al (2010) Cerebral cortical and subcortical cholinergic deficits in parkinsonian syndromes. Neurology 74(18):1416–1423. https://doi.org/10.1212/WNL.0b013e3181dc1a55

Gjerløff T, Fedorova T, Knudsen K, Munk OL, Nahimi A, Jacobsen S et al (2015) Imaging acetylcholinesterase density in peripheral organs in Parkinson's disease with 11C-donepezil PET. Brain 138(Pt 3):653–663. https://doi.org/10.1093/brain/awu369

Goldman JG, Postuma R (2014) Premotor and nonmotor features of Parkinson's disease. Curr Opin Neurol 27(4):434–441. https://doi.org/10.1097/WCO.0000000000000112

Hammes J, Drzezga A, van Eimeren T (2018) The role of Tau imaging in parkinsonian disorders. Curr Neurol Neurosci Rep 18(12):86. https://doi.org/10.1007/s11910-018-0898-3

Hellwig S, Amtage F, Kreft A, Buchert R, Winz OH, Vach W et al (2012) [^{18}F]FDG-PET is superior to [^{123}I]IBZM-SPECT for the differential diagnosis of parkinsonism. Neurology 79(13):1314–1322. https://doi.org/10.1212/WNL.0b013e31826c1b0a

Hely MA, Reid WGJ, Adena MA, Halliday GM, Morris JGL (2008) The Sydney multicenter study of Parkinson's disease: the inevitability of dementia at 20 years. Mov Disord 23(6):837–844. https://doi.org/10.1002/mds.21956

Henderson EJ, Lord SR, Brodie MA, Gaunt DM, Lawrence AD, Close JCT et al (2016) Rivastigmine for gait stability in patients with Parkinson's disease (ReSPonD): a randomised, double-blind, placebo-controlled, phase 2 trial. Lancet Neurol 15(3):249–258. https://doi.org/10.1016/S1474-4422(15)00389-0

Hilker R, Schweitzer K, Coburger S, Ghaemi M, Weisenbach S, Jacobs AH et al (2005a) Nonlinear progression of Parkinson disease as determined by serial positron emission tomographic imaging of striatal fluorodopa F18 activity. Arch Neurol 62(3):378–382. https://doi.org/10.1001/archneur.62.3.378

Hilker R, Thomas AV, Klein JC, Weisenbach S, Kalbe E, Burghaus L et al (2005b) Dementia in Parkinson disease: functional imaging of cholinergic and dopaminergic pathways. Neurology 65(11):1716–1722. https://doi.org/10.1212/01.wnl.0000191154.78131.f6

Hiraoka K, Okamura N, Funaki Y, Hayashi A, Tashiro M, Hisanaga K et al (2012) Cholinergic deficit and response to donepezil therapy in Parkinson's disease with dementia. Eur Neurol 68(3):137–143. https://doi.org/10.1159/000338774

Hoehn MM, Yahr MD (1967) Parkinsonism: onset, progression and mortality. Neurology 17(5):427–442

Holmstrand EC, Sesack SR (2011) Projections from the rat pedunculopontine and laterodorsal tegmental nuclei to the anterior thalamus and ventral tegmental area arise from largely separate populations of neurons. Brain Struct Funct 216(4):331–345. https://doi.org/10.1007/s00429-011-0320-2

Horti AG, Naik R, Foss CA, Minn I, Misheneva V, Du Y et al (2019) PET imaging of microglia by targeting macrophage colony-stimulating factor 1 receptor (CSF1R). Proc Natl Acad Sci U S A 116(5):1686–1691. https://doi.org/10.1073/pnas.1812155116

Huang C, Mattis P, Tang C, Perrine K, Carbon M, Eidelberg D (2007a) Metabolic brain networks associated with cognitive function in Parkinson's disease. NeuroImage 34(2):714–723. https://doi.org/10.1016/j.neuroimage.2006.09.003

Huang C, Tang C, Feigin A, Lesser M, Ma Y, Pourfar M et al (2007b) Changes in network activity with the progression of Parkinson's disease. Brain 130(Pt 7):1834–1846. https://doi.org/10.1093/brain/awm086

Huang C, Mattis P, Perrine K, Brown N, Dhawan V, Eidelberg D (2008) Metabolic abnormalities associated with mild cognitive impairment in Parkinson disease. Neurology 70(16 Pt 2):1470–1477. https://doi.org/10.1212/01.wnl.0000304050.05332.9c

Hughes AJ, Daniel SE, Kilford L, Lees AJ (1992) Accuracy of clinical diagnosis of idiopathic Parkinson's disease: a clinico-pathological study of 100 cases. J Neurol Neurosurg Psychiatry 55(3):181–184. https://doi.org/10.1136/jnnp.55.3.181

Hughes AJ, Daniel SE, Blankson S, Lees AJ (1993) A clinicopathologic study of 100 cases of Parkinson's disease. Arch Neurol 50(2):140–148. https://doi.org/10.1001/archneur.1993.00540020018011

Hughes AJ, Daniel SE, Lees AJ (2001) Improved accuracy of clinical diagnosis of Lewy body Parkinson's disease. Neurology 57(8):1497–1499. https://doi.org/10.1212/WNL.57.8.1497

Hung ASM, Tsui TYM, Lam JCY, Wai MSM, Chan WM, Yew DT (2011) Serotonin and its receptors in the human CNS with new findings - a mini review. Curr Med Chem 18(34):5281–5288

Hurtig HI, Trojanowski JQ, Galvin J, Ewbank D, Schmidt ML, Lee VM et al (2000) Alpha-synuclein cortical Lewy bodies correlate with dementia in Parkinson's disease. Neurology 54(10):1916–1921. https://doi.org/10.1212/wnl.54.10.1916

Iannaccone S, Cerami C, Alessio M, Garibotto V, Panzacchi A, Olivieri S et al (2013) In vivo microglia activation in very early dementia with Lewy bodies, comparison with Parkinson's disease. Parkinsonism Relat Disord 19(1):47–52. https://doi.org/10.1016/j.parkreldis.2012.07.002

Imon Y, Matsuda H, Ogawa M, Kogure D, Sunohara N (1999) SPECT image analysis using statistical parametric mapping in patients with Parkinson's disease. J Nucl Med 40(10): 1583–1589

Irwin DJ, Lee VM-Y, Trojanowski JQ (2013) Parkinson's disease dementia: convergence of α-synuclein, tau and amyloid-β pathologies. Nat Rev Neurosci 14(9):626–636. https://doi.org/10.1038/nrn3549

Jellinger KA (2003) Neuropathological spectrum of synucleinopathies. Mov Disord 18(S6):S2–S12. https://doi.org/10.1002/mds.10557

Jokinen P, Scheinin N, Aalto S, Någren K, Savisto N, Parkkola R et al (2010) [(11)C]PIB-, [(18)F]FDG-PET and MRI imaging in patients with Parkinson's disease with and without dementia. Parkinsonism Relat Disord 16(10):666–670. https://doi.org/10.1016/j.parkreldis.2010.08.021

Kägi G, Bhatia KP, Tolosa E (2010) The role of DAT-SPECT in movement disorders. J Neurol Neurosurg Psychiatry 81(1):5–12. https://doi.org/10.1136/jnnp.2008.157370

Kaplitt MG, Feigin A, Tang C, Fitzsimons HL, Mattis P, Lawlor PA et al (2007) Safety and tolerability of gene therapy with an adeno-associated virus (AAV) borne GAD gene for Parkinson's disease: an open label, phase I trial. Lancet (London, England) 369(9579):2097–2105. https://doi.org/10.1016/S0140-6736(07)60982-9

Kas A, Bottlaender M, Gallezot JD, Vidailhet M, Villafane G, Grégoire MC et al (2009) Decrease of nicotinic receptors in the nigrostriatal system in Parkinson's disease. J Cereb Blood Flow Metab 29(9):1601–1608. https://doi.org/10.1038/jcbfm.2009.74

Klein JC, Eggers C, Kalbe E, Weisenbach S, Hohmann C, Vollmar S et al (2010) Neurotransmitter changes in dementia with Lewy bodies and Parkinson disease dementia in vivo. Neurology 74(11):885–892. https://doi.org/10.1212/WNL.0b013e3181d55f61

Koga S, Ono M, Sahara N, Higuchi M, Dickson DW (2017) Fluorescence and autoradiographic evaluation of tau PET ligand PBB3 to α-synuclein pathology. Mov Disord 32(6):884–892. https://doi.org/10.1002/mds.27013

Koole M, Van Laere K, Ahmad R, Ceccarini J, Bormans G, Vandenberghe W (2017) Brain PET imaging of phosphodiesterase 10A in progressive supranuclear palsy and Parkinson's disease. Mov Disord 32(6):943–945. https://doi.org/10.1002/mds.27005

Kordower JH, Olanow CW, Dodiya HB, Chu Y, Beach TG, Adler CH et al (2013) Disease duration and the integrity of the nigrostriatal system in Parkinson's disease. Brain 136(Pt 8):2419–2431. https://doi.org/10.1093/brain/awt192

Koshimori Y, Ko J-H, Mizrahi R, Rusjan P, Mabrouk R, Jacobs MF et al (2015) Imaging striatal microglial activation in patients with Parkinson's disease. PLoS One 10(9):e0138721. https://doi.org/10.1371/journal.pone.0138721

Kotagal V, Albin RL, Müller MLTM, Koeppe RA, Chervin RD, Frey KA, Bohnen NI (2012) Symptoms of rapid eye movement sleep behavior disorder are associated with cholinergic denervation in Parkinson disease. Ann Neurol 71(4):560–568. https://doi.org/10.1002/ana.22691

Kuhl DE, Minoshima S, Fessler JA, Frey KA, Foster NL, Ficaro EP et al (1996) In vivo mapping of cholinergic terminals in normal aging, Alzheimer's disease, and Parkinson's disease. Ann Neurol 40(3):399–410. https://doi.org/10.1002/ana.410400309

Kuramoto L, Cragg J, Nandhagopal R, Mak E, Sossi V, de la Fuente-Fernández R et al (2013) The nature of progression in Parkinson's disease: an application of non-linear, multivariate, longitudinal random effects modelling. PLoS One 8(10):e76595. https://doi.org/10.1371/journal.pone.0076595

Lang AE, Gill S, Patel NK, Lozano A, Nutt JG, Penn R et al (2006) Randomized controlled trial of intraputamenal glial cell line-derived neurotrophic factor infusion in Parkinson disease. Ann Neurol 59(3):459–466. https://doi.org/10.1002/ana.20737

Langston JW (2006) The Parkinson's complex: parkinsonism is just the tip of the iceberg. Ann Neurol 59(4):591–596. https://doi.org/10.1002/ana.20834

Lee CS, Samii A, Sossi V, Ruth TJ, Schulzer M, Holden JE et al (2000) In vivo positron emission tomographic evidence for compensatory changes in presynaptic dopaminergic nerve terminals in Parkinson's disease. Ann Neurol 47(4):493–503. https://doi.org/10.1002/1531-8249(200004)47:4<493::AID-ANA13>3.0.CO;2-4

Lee J-Y, Seo S, Lee JS, Kim H-J, Kim YK, Jeon BS (2015) Putaminal serotonergic innervation: monitoring dyskinesia risk in Parkinson disease. Neurology 85(10):853–860. https://doi.org/10.1212/WNL.0000000000001909

Lippert RN, Cremer AL, Edwin Thanarajah S, Korn C, Jahans-Price T, Burgeno LM et al (2019) Time-dependent assessment of stimulus-evoked regional dopamine release. Nat Commun 10(1):336. https://doi.org/10.1038/s41467-018-08143-4

Liu S-Y, Wile DJ, Fu JF, Valerio J, Shahinfard E, McCormick S et al (2018) The effect of LRRK2 mutations on the cholinergic system in manifest and premanifest stages of Parkinson's disease: a cross-sectional PET study. Lancet Neurol 17(4):309–316. https://doi.org/10.1016/S1474-4422(18)30032-2

Loane C, Wu K, Bain P, Brooks DJ, Piccini P, Politis M (2013) Serotonergic loss in motor circuitries correlates with severity of action-postural tremor in PD. Neurology 80(20):1850–1855. https://doi.org/10.1212/WNL.0b013e318292a31d

Maetzler W, Reimold M, Liepelt I, Solbach C, Leyhe T, Schweitzer K et al (2008) [11C]PIB binding in Parkinson's disease dementia. NeuroImage 39(3):1027–1033. https://doi.org/10.1016/j.neuroimage.2007.09.072

Maetzler W, Liepelt I, Reimold M, Reischl G, Solbach C, Becker C et al (2009) Cortical PIB binding in Lewy body disease is associated with Alzheimer-like characteristics. Neurobiol Dis 34(1):107–112. https://doi.org/10.1016/j.nbd.2008.12.008

Maillet A, Krack P, Lhommée E, Météreau E, Klinger H, Favre E et al (2016) The prominent role of serotonergic degeneration in apathy, anxiety and depression in de novo Parkinson's disease. Brain 139(Pt 9):2486–2502. https://doi.org/10.1093/brain/aww162

Marras C, Beck JC, Bower JH, Roberts E, Ritz B, Ross GW et al (2018) Prevalence of Parkinson's disease across North America. NPJ Parkinsons Dis 4(1):21. https://doi.org/10.1038/s41531-018-0058-0

Martin WR, Palmer MR, Patlak CS, Calne DB (1989) Nigrostriatal function in humans studied with positron emission tomography. Ann Neurol 26(4):535–542. https://doi.org/10.1002/ana.410260407

Mashima K, Ito D, Kameyama M, Osada T, Tabuchi H, Nihei Y et al (2017) Extremely low prevalence of amyloid positron emission tomography positivity in Parkinson's disease without dementia. Eur Neurol 77(5–6):231–237. https://doi.org/10.1159/000464322

Mazère J, Lamare F, Allard M, Fernandez P, Mayo W (2017) 123I-Iodobenzovesamicol SPECT imaging of cholinergic systems in dementia with lewy bodies. J Nucl Med 58(1):123–128. https://doi.org/10.2967/jnumed.116.176180

Melzer TR, Stark MR, Keenan RJ, Myall DJ, MacAskill MR, Pitcher TL et al (2019) Beta amyloid deposition is not associated with cognitive impairment in Parkinson's disease. Front Neurol 10(April):391. https://doi.org/10.3389/fneur.2019.00391

Mencacci NE, Kamsteeg E-J, Nakashima K, R'Bibo L, Lynch DS, Balint B et al (2016) De novo mutations in PDE10A cause childhood-onset chorea with bilateral striatal lesions. Am J Hum Genet 98(4):763–771. https://doi.org/10.1016/j.ajhg.2016.02.015

Merchant KM, Cedarbaum JM, Brundin P, Dave KD, Eberling J, Espay AJ et al (2019) A proposed roadmap for Parkinson's disease proof of concept clinical trials investigating compounds targeting alpha-synuclein. J Parkinsons Dis 9(1):31–61. https://doi.org/10.3233/JPD-181471

Marek KL, Seibyl JP, Zoghbi SS, Zea-Ponce Y, Baldwin RM, Fussell B, Charney DS, van Dyck C, Hoffer PB, Innis RP (1996) [123I] beta-CIT/SPECT imaging demonstrates bilateral loss of dopamine transporters in hemi-Parkinson's disease. Neurology 46:231–237

Meyer PM, Strecker K, Kendziorra K, Becker G, Hesse S, Woelpl D et al (2009) Reduced alpha4beta2*-nicotinic acetylcholine receptor binding and its relationship to mild cognitive and depressive symptoms in Parkinson disease. Arch Gen Psychiatry 66(8):866–877. https://doi.org/10.1001/archgenpsychiatry.2009.106

Moore RY, Whone AL, McGowan S, Brooks DJ (2003) Monoamine neuron innervation of the normal human brain: an 18F-DOPA PET study. Brain Res 982(2):137–145. https://doi.org/10.1016/s0006-8993(03)02721-5

Moore RY, Whone AL, Brooks DJ (2008) Extrastriatal monoamine neuron function in Parkinson's disease: an 18F-dopa PET study. Neurobiol Dis 29(3):381–390. https://doi.org/10.1016/j.nbd.2007.09.004

Moro E, Hamani C, Poon Y-Y, Al-Khairallah T, Dostrovsky JO, Hutchison WD, Lozano AM (2010) Unilateral pedunculopontine stimulation improves falls in Parkinson's disease. Brain 133(Pt 1):215–224. https://doi.org/10.1093/brain/awp261

Morrish PK, Rakshi JS, Bailey DL, Sawle GV, Brooks DJ (1998) Measuring the rate of progression and estimating the preclinical period of Parkinson's disease with [18F]dopa PET. J Neurol Neurosurg Psychiatry 64(3):314–319. https://doi.org/10.1136/jnnp.64.3.314

Muchowski PJ (2002) Protein misfolding, amyloid formation, and neurodegeneration: a critical role for molecular chaperones? Neuron 35(1):9–12

Muñoz A, Li Q, Gardoni F, Marcello E, Qin C, Carlsson T et al (2008) Combined 5-HT1A and 5-HT1B receptor agonists for the treatment of L-DOPA-induced dyskinesia. Brain 131(Pt 12):3380–3394. https://doi.org/10.1093/brain/awn235

Muñoz A, Carlsson T, Tronci E, Kirik D, Björklund A, Carta M (2009) Serotonin neuron-dependent and -independent reduction of dyskinesia by 5-HT1A and 5-HT1B receptor agonists in the rat Parkinson model. Exp Neurol 219(1):298–307. https://doi.org/10.1016/j.expneurol.2009.05.033

Mure H, Hirano S, Tang CC, Isaias IU, Antonini A, Ma Y et al (2011) Parkinson's disease tremor-related metabolic network: characterization, progression, and treatment effects. NeuroImage 54(2):1244–1253. https://doi.org/10.1016/j.neuroimage.2010.09.028

Murugan NA, Chiotis K, Rodriguez-Vieitez E, Lemoine L, Ågren H, Nordberg A (2019) Cross-interaction of tau PET tracers with monoamine oxidase B: evidence from in silico modelling and in vivo imaging. Eur J Nucl Med Mol Imaging 46(6):1369–1382. https://doi.org/10.1007/s00259-019-04305-8

Nahimi A, Sommerauer M, Kinnerup MB, Østergaard K, Winterdahl M, Jacobsen J et al (2018) Noradrenergic deficits in Parkinson disease imaged with 11C-MeNER. J Nucl Med 59(4):659–664. https://doi.org/10.2967/jnumed.117.190975

Nakamura T, Dhawan V, Chaly T, Fukuda M, Ma Y, Breeze R et al (2001) Blinded positron emission tomography study of dopamine cell implantation for Parkinson's disease. Ann Neurol 50(2):181–187

Nandhagopal R, Mak E, Schulzer M, McKenzie J, McCormick S, Sossi V et al (2008) Progression of dopaminergic dysfunction in a LRRK2 kindred: a multitracer PET study. Neurology 71(22):1790–1795. https://doi.org/10.1212/01.wnl.0000335973.66333.58

Nandhagopal R, Kuramoto L, Schulzer M, Mak E, Cragg J, Lee CS et al (2009) Longitudinal progression of sporadic Parkinson's disease: a multi-tracer positron emission tomography study. Brain 132(Pt 11):2970–2979. https://doi.org/10.1093/brain/awp209

Nandhagopal R, Kuramoto L, Schulzer M, Mak E, Cragg J, McKenzie J et al (2011) Longitudinal evolution of compensatory changes in striatal dopamine processing in Parkinson's disease. Brain 134(Pt 11):3290–3298. https://doi.org/10.1093/brain/awr233

Narayanaswami V, Dahl K, Bernard-Gauthier V, Josephson L, Cumming P, Vasdev N (2018) Emerging PET radiotracers and targets for imaging of neuroinflammation in neurodegenerative diseases: outlook beyond TSPO. Mol Imaging 17:1536012118792317. https://doi.org/10.1177/1536012118792317

Niccolini F, Foltynie T, Reis Marques T, Muhlert N, Tziortzi AC, Searle GE et al (2015) Loss of phosphodiesterase 10A expression is associated with progression and severity in Parkinson's disease. Brain 138(Pt 10):3003–3015. https://doi.org/10.1093/brain/awv219

Nishi A, Kuroiwa M, Miller DB, O'Callaghan JP, Bateup HS, Shuto T et al (2008) Distinct roles of PDE4 and PDE10A in the regulation of cAMP/PKA signaling in the striatum. J Neurosci 28(42):10460–10471. https://doi.org/10.1523/JNEUROSCI.2518-08.2008

Nurmi E, Ruottinen HM, Bergman J, Haaparanta M, Solin O, Sonninen P, Rinne JO (2001) Rate of progression in Parkinson's disease: a 6-[18F]fluoro-L-dopa PET study. Mov Disord 16(4):608–615. https://doi.org/10.1002/mds.1139

Oishi N, Hashikawa K, Yoshida H, Ishizu K, Ueda M, Kawashima H et al (2007) Quantification of nicotinic acetylcholine receptors in Parkinson's disease with (123)I-5IA SPECT. J Neurol Sci 256(1–2):52–60. https://doi.org/10.1016/j.jns.2007.02.014

Olanow CW, Goetz CG, Kordower JH, Stoessl AJ, Sossi V, Brin MF et al (2003) A double-blind controlled trial of bilateral fetal nigral transplantation in Parkinson's disease. Ann Neurol 54(3):403–414. https://doi.org/10.1002/ana.10720

Orimo S, Ozawa E, Nakade S, Sugimoto T, Mizusawa H (1999) (123)I-metaiodobenzylguanidine myocardial scintigraphy in Parkinson's disease. J Neurol Neurosurg Psychiatry 67(2):189–194. https://doi.org/10.1136/jnnp.67.2.189

Orimo S, Suzuki M, Inaba A, Mizusawa H (2012) 123I-MIBG myocardial scintigraphy for differentiating Parkinson's disease from other neurodegenerative parkinsonism: a systematic review and meta-analysis. Parkinsonism Relat Disord 18(5):494–500. https://doi.org/10.1016/j.parkreldis.2012.01.009

Ouchi Y, Yoshikawa E, Sekine Y, Futatsubashi M, Kanno T, Ogusu T, Torizuka T (2005) Microglial activation and dopamine terminal loss in early Parkinson's disease. Ann Neurol 57(2):168–175. https://doi.org/10.1002/ana.20338

Owen DRJ, Piccini P, Matthews PM (2011) Towards molecular imaging of multiple sclerosis. Mult Scler 17(3):262–272. https://doi.org/10.1177/1352458510390070

Owen DR, Guo Q, Kalk NJ, Colasanti A, Kalogiannopoulou D, Dimber R et al (2014) Determination of [(11)C]PBR28 binding potential in vivo: a first human TSPO blocking study. J Cereb Blood Flow Metab 34(6):989–994. https://doi.org/10.1038/jcbfm.2014.46

Pagano G, Niccolini F, Wilson H, Yousaf T, Khan NL, Martino D et al (2019) Comparison of phosphodiesterase 10A and dopamine transporter levels as markers of disease burden in early Parkinson's disease. Mov Disord 34(10):1505–1515. https://doi.org/10.1002/mds.27733

Parkinson Study Group (2000) Pramipexole vs levodopa as initial treatment for Parkinson disease: a randomized controlled trial. Parkinson Study Group. JAMA 284(15):1931–1938. https://doi.org/10.1001/jama.284.15.1931

Pavese N, Metta V, Bose SK, Chaudhuri KR, Brooks DJ (2010) Fatigue in Parkinson's disease is linked to striatal and limbic serotonergic dysfunction. Brain 133(11):3434–3443. https://doi.org/10.1093/brain/awq268

Pavese N, Rivero-Bosch M, Lewis SJ, Whone AL, Brooks DJ (2011) Progression of monoaminergic dysfunction in Parkinson's disease: a longitudinal 18F-dopa PET study. NeuroImage 56(3):1463–1468. https://doi.org/10.1016/j.neuroimage.2011.03.012

Pavese N, Simpson BS, Metta V, Ramlackhansingh A, Chaudhuri KR, Brooks DJ (2012) [^{18}F]FDOPA uptake in the raphe nuclei complex reflects serotonin transporter availability. A combined [^{18}F]FDOPA and [^{11}C]DASB PET study in Parkinson's disease. NeuroImage 59(2):1080–1084. https://doi.org/10.1016/j.neuroimage.2011.09.034

Perez-Soriano A, Arena JE, Dinelle K, Miao Q, McKenzie J, Neilson N et al (2017) PBB3 imaging in Parkinsonian disorders: evidence for binding to tau and other proteins. Mov Disord 32(7):1016–1024. https://doi.org/10.1002/mds.27029

Petrou M, Dwamena BA, Foerster BR, Maceachern MP, Bohnen NI, Müller ML et al (2015) Amyloid deposition in Parkinson's disease and cognitive impairment: a systematic review. Mov Disord 30(7):928–935. https://doi.org/10.1002/mds.26191

Piccini PP (2003) Dopamine transporter: basic aspects and neuroimaging. Mov Disord 18(Suppl. 7):S3–S8. https://doi.org/10.1002/mds.10571

Pinborg LH, Videbaek C, Ziebell M, Mackeprang T, Friberg L, Rasmussen H et al (2007) [123I]Epidepride binding to cerebellar dopamine D2/D3 receptors is displaceable: implications for the use of cerebellum as a reference region. NeuroImage 34(4):1450–1453. https://doi.org/10.1016/j.neuroimage.2006.11.003

Politis M, Wu K, Loane C, Turkheimer FE, Molloy S, Brooks DJ, Piccini P (2010) Depressive symptoms in PD correlate with higher 5-HTT binding in raphe and limbic structures. Neurology 75(21):1920–1927. https://doi.org/10.1212/WNL.0b013e3181feb2ab

Politis M, Loane C, Wu K, Brooks DJ, Piccini P (2011) Serotonergic mediated body mass index changes in Parkinson's disease. Neurobiol Dis 43(3):609–615. https://doi.org/10.1016/j.nbd.2011.05.009

Politis M, Pagano G, Niccolini F (2017) Imaging in Parkinson's disease. Int Rev Neurobiol 132(C):233–274. https://doi.org/10.1016/bs.irn.2017.02.015

Postuma RB, Berg D, Stern M, Poewe W, Olanow CW, Oertel WH et al (2015) MDS clinical diagnostic criteria for Parkinson's disease. Mov Disord 30(12):1591–1601. https://doi.org/10.1002/mds.26424

Postuma RB, Poewe W, Litvan I, Lewis S, Lang AE, Halliday G et al (2018) Validation of the MDS clinical diagnostic criteria for Parkinson's disease. Mov Disord 33(10):1601–1608. https://doi.org/10.1002/mds.27362

Pysz MA, Gambhir SS, Willmann JK (2010) Molecular imaging: current status and emerging strategies. Clin Radiol 65(7):500–516. https://doi.org/10.1016/j.crad.2010.03.011

Remy P, Doder M, Lees A, Turjanski N, Brooks D (2005) Depression in Parkinson's disease: loss of dopamine and noradrenaline innervation in the limbic system. Brain 128(Pt 6):1314–1322. https://doi.org/10.1093/brain/awh445

Rinne JO, Laihinen A, Någren K, Bergman J, Solin O, Haaparanta M et al (1990) PET demonstrates different behaviour of striatal dopamine D-1 and D-2 receptors in early Parkinson's disease. J Neurosci Res 27(4):494–499. https://doi.org/10.1002/jnr.490270409

Rogers JD, Brogan D, Mirra SS (1985) The nucleus basalis of Meynert in neurological disease: a quantitative morphological study. Ann Neurol 17(2):163–170. https://doi.org/10.1002/ana.410170210

Roussakis A-A, Politis M, Towey D, Piccini P (2016) Serotonin-to-dopamine transporter ratios in Parkinson disease: relevance for dyskinesias. Neurology 86(12):1152–1158. https://doi.org/10.1212/WNL.0000000000002494

Rylander D, Parent M, O'Sullivan SS, Dovero S, Lees AJ, Bezard E et al (2010) Maladaptive plasticity of serotonin axon terminals in levodopa-induced dyskinesia. Ann Neurol 68(5):619–628. https://doi.org/10.1002/ana.22097

Sancesario G, Morrone LA, D'Angelo V, Castelli V, Ferrazzoli D, Sica F et al (2014) Levodopa-induced dyskinesias are associated with transient down-regulation of cAMP and cGMP in the caudate-putamen of hemiparkinsonian rats: reduced synthesis or increased catabolism? Neurochem Int 79:44–56. https://doi.org/10.1016/j.neuint.2014.10.004

Saulin A, Savli M, Lanzenberger R (2012) Serotonin and molecular neuroimaging in humans using PET. Amino Acids 42(6):2039–2057. https://doi.org/10.1007/s00726-011-1078-9

Schapira AH, Gu M, Taanman JW, Tabrizi SJ, Seaton T, Cleeter M, Cooper JM (1998) Mitochondria in the etiology and pathogenesis of Parkinson's disease. Ann Neurol 44(3 Suppl 1):S89–S98

Schrag A, Schott JM (2006) Epidemiological, clinical, and genetic characteristics of early-onset parkinsonism. Lancet Neurol 5(4):355–363. https://doi.org/10.1016/S1474-4422(06)70411-2

Shah N, Frey KA, Müller MLTM, Petrou M, Kotagal V, Koeppe RA et al (2016) Striatal and cortical β-amyloidopathy and cognition in Parkinson's disease. Mov Disord 31(1):111–117. https://doi.org/10.1002/mds.26369

Shih MC, Felicio AC, de Oliveira Godeiro-Junior C, de Carvalho Aguiar P, de Andrade LAF, Ferraz HB, Bressan RA (2007) Molecular imaging in hereditary forms of parkinsonism. Eur J Neurol 14(4):359–368. https://doi.org/10.1111/j.1468-1331.2007.01691.x

Shimada H, Hirano S, Shinotoh H, Aotsuka A, Sato K, Tanaka N et al (2009) Mapping of brain acetylcholinesterase alterations in Lewy body disease by PET. Neurology 73(4):273–278. https://doi.org/10.1212/WNL.0b013e3181ab2b58

Shinotoh H, Inoue O, Hirayama K, Aotsuka A, Asahina M, Suhara T et al (1993) Dopamine D1 receptors in Parkinson's disease and striatonigral degeneration: a positron emission tomography study. J Neurol Neurosurg Psychiatry 56(5):467–472. https://doi.org/10.1136/jnnp.56.5.467

Shinotoh H, Namba H, Yamaguchi M, Fukushi K, Nagatsuka S, Iyo M et al (1999) Positron emission tomographic measurement of acetylcholinesterase activity reveals differential loss of ascending cholinergic systems in Parkinson's disease and progressive supranuclear palsy. Ann Neurol 46(1):62–69. https://doi.org/10.1002/1531-8249(199907)46:1<62::AID-ANA10>3.0.CO;2-P

Smith R, Wu K, Hart T, Loane C, Brooks DJ, Björklund A et al (2015) The role of pallidal serotonergic function in Parkinson's disease dyskinesias: a positron emission tomography study. Neurobiol Aging 36(4):1736–1742. https://doi.org/10.1016/j.neurobiolaging.2014.12.037

Sommerauer M, Fedorova TD, Hansen AK, Knudsen K, Otto M, Jeppesen J et al (2018a) Evaluation of the noradrenergic system in Parkinson's disease: an 11C-MeNER PET and neuromelanin MRI study. Brain 141(2):496–504. https://doi.org/10.1093/brain/awx348

Sommerauer M, Hansen AK, Parbo P, Fedorova TD, Knudsen K, Frederiksen Y et al (2018b) Decreased noradrenaline transporter density in the motor cortex of Parkinson's disease patients. Mov Disord 33(6):1006–1010. https://doi.org/10.1002/mds.27411

Sossi V (2018) Advances in PET methodology. In: International review of neurobiology, vol 141, 1st edn. Elsevier Inc., Amsterdam, pp 3–30. https://doi.org/10.1016/bs.irn.2018.07.034

Sossi V, de La Fuente-Fernández R, Holden JE, Doudet DJ, McKenzie J, Stoessl AJ, Ruth TJ (2002) Increase in dopamine turnover occurs early in Parkinson's disease: evidence from a new modeling approach to PET 18 F-fluorodopa data. J Cereb Blood Flow Metab 22(2):232–239. https://doi.org/10.1097/00004647-200202000-00011

Sossi V, de la Fuente-Fernández R, Nandhagopal R, Schulzer M, McKenzie J, Ruth TJ et al (2010) Dopamine turnover increases in asymptomatic LRRK2 mutations carriers. Mov Disord 25(16):2717–2723. https://doi.org/10.1002/mds.23356

Spillantini MG, Schmidt ML, Lee VM, Trojanowski JQ, Jakes R, Goedert M (1997) Alpha-synuclein in Lewy bodies. Nature 388(6645):839–840. https://doi.org/10.1038/42166

Stebbins GT, Goetz CG, Burn DJ, Jankovic J, Khoo TK, Tilley BC (2013) How to identify tremor dominant and postural instability/gait difficulty groups with the movement disorder society unified Parkinson's disease rating scale: comparison with the unified Parkinson's disease rating scale. Mov Disord 28(5):668–670. https://doi.org/10.1002/mds.25383

Stoessl AJ (2011) Neuroimaging in Parkinson's disease. Neurotherapeutics 8(1):72–81. https://doi.org/10.1007/s13311-010-0007-z

Stoessl AJ (2012) Neuroimaging in Parkinson's disease: from pathology to diagnosis. Parkinsonism Relat Disord 18(Suppl 1):S55–S59. https://doi.org/10.1016/S1353-8020(11)70019-0

Stoessl AJ, Lehericy S, Strafella AP (2014) Imaging insights into basal ganglia function, Parkinson's disease, and dystonia. Lancet (London, England) 384(9942):532–544. https://doi.org/10.1016/S0140-6736(14)60041-6

Stokholm MG, Iranzo A, Østergaard K, Serradell M, Otto M, Svendsen KB et al (2017) Assessment of neuroinflammation in patients with idiopathic rapid-eye-movement sleep behaviour disorder: a case-control study. Lancet Neurol 16(10):789–796. https://doi.org/10.1016/S1474-4422(17)30173-4

Strafella AP, Bohnen NI, Perlmutter JS, Eidelberg D, Pavese N, Van Eimeren T et al (2017) Molecular imaging to track Parkinson's disease and atypical parkinsonisms: new imaging frontiers. Mov Disord 32(2):181–192. https://doi.org/10.1002/mds.26907

Szabo Z, Kao PF, Scheffel U, Suehiro M, Mathews WB, Ravert HT et al (1995) Positron emission tomography imaging of serotonin transporters in the human brain using [11C](+)McN5652. Synapse (New York, NY) 20(1):37–43. https://doi.org/10.1002/syn.890200107

Tang CC, Poston KL, Dhawan V, Eidelberg D (2010) Abnormalities in metabolic network activity precede the onset of motor symptoms in Parkinson's disease. J Neurosci 30(3):1049–1056. https://doi.org/10.1523/JNEUROSCI.4188-09.2010

Tateno F, Sakakibara R, Kishi M, Ogawa E, Terada H, Ogata T, Haruta H (2011) Sensitivity and specificity of metaiodobenzylguanidine (MIBG) myocardial accumulation in the diagnosis of Lewy body diseases in a movement disorder clinic. Parkinsonism Relat Disord 17(5):395–397. https://doi.org/10.1016/j.parkreldis.2011.02.001

Tatsch K, Poepperl G (2012) Quantitative approaches to dopaminergic brain imaging. Q J Nucl Med Mol Imaging 56(1):27–38

Terada T, Yokokura M, Yoshikawa E, Futatsubashi M, Kono S, Konishi T et al (2016) Extrastriatal spreading of microglial activation in Parkinson's disease: a positron emission tomography study. Ann Nucl Med 30(8):579–587. https://doi.org/10.1007/s12149-016-1099-2

Thobois S, Vingerhoets F, Fraix V, Xie-Brustolin J, Mollion H, Costes N et al (2004) Role of dopaminergic treatment in dopamine receptor down-regulation in advanced Parkinson disease: a positron emission tomographic study. Arch Neurol 61(11):1705–1709. https://doi.org/10.1001/archneur.61.11.1705

Tomše P, Jensterle L, Grmek M, Zaletel K, Pirtošek Z, Dhawan V et al (2017) Abnormal metabolic brain network associated with Parkinson's disease: replication on a new European sample. Neuroradiology 59(5):507–515. https://doi.org/10.1007/s00234-017-1821-3

Tondo G, Esposito M, Dervenoulas G, Wilson H, Politis M, Pagano G (2019) Hybrid PET-MRI applications in movement disorders. Int Rev Neurobiol 144:211–257. https://doi.org/10.1016/bs.irn.2018.10.003

Van Weehaeghe D, Koole M, Schmidt ME, Deman S, Jacobs AH, Souche E et al (2019) [11C]JNJ54173717, a novel P2X7 receptor radioligand as marker for neuroinflammation: human biodistribution, dosimetry, brain kinetic modelling and quantification of brain P2X7 receptors in patients with Parkinson's disease and healthy volunteers. Eur J Nucl Med Mol Imaging 46(10):2051–2064. https://doi.org/10.1007/s00259-019-04369-6

Vander Borght TM, Kilbourn MR, Koeppe RA, DaSilva JN, Carey JE, Kuhl DE, Frey KA (1995) In vivo imaging of the brain vesicular monoamine transporter. J Nucl Med 36(12):2252–2260. https://doi.org/10.1096/fj.00-0204rev

Vander Borght T, Minoshima S, Giordani B, Foster NL, Frey KA, Berent S et al (1997) Cerebral metabolic differences in Parkinson's and Alzheimer's diseases matched for dementia severity. J Nucl Med 38(5):797–802

Varnäs K, Cselényi Z, Jucaite A, Halldin C, Svenningsson P, Farde L, Varrone A (2019) PET imaging of [11C]PBR28 in Parkinson's disease patients does not indicate increased binding to TSPO despite reduced dopamine transporter binding. Eur J Nucl Med Mol Imaging 46(2):367–375. https://doi.org/10.1007/s00259-018-4161-6

Varrone A, Halldin C (2010) Molecular imaging of the dopamine transporter. J Nucl Med 51(9):1331–1334. https://doi.org/10.2967/jnumed.109.065656

Vingerhoets FJG, Snow BJ, Lee CS, Schulzer M, Mak E, Calne DB (1994) Longitudinal fluorodopa positron emission tomographic studies of the evolution of idiopathic parkinsonism. Ann Neurol 36(5):759–764. https://doi.org/10.1002/ana.410360512

Volkow ND, Fowler JS, Wang GJ, Logan J, Schlyer D, MacGregor R et al (1994) Decreased dopamine transporters with age in health human subjects. Ann Neurol 36(2):237–239. https://doi.org/10.1002/ana.410360218

Whone AL, Watts RL, Stoessl AJ, Davis M, Reske S, Nahmias C et al (2003) Slower progression of Parkinson's disease with ropinirole versus levodopa: the REAL-PET study. Ann Neurol 54(1):93–101. https://doi.org/10.1002/ana.10609

Whone A, Luz M, Boca M, Woolley M, Mooney L, Dharia S et al (2019) Randomized trial of intermittent intraputamenal glial cell line-derived neurotrophic factor in Parkinson's disease. Brain 142(3):512–525. https://doi.org/10.1093/brain/awz023

Wichmann T (2019) Changing views of the pathophysiology of Parkinsonism. Mov Disord 34(8):1130–1143. https://doi.org/10.1002/mds.27741

Wichmann T, DeLong MR, Guridi J, Obeso JA (2011) Milestones in research on the pathophysiology of Parkinson's disease. Mov Disord 26(6):1032–1041. https://doi.org/10.1002/mds.23695

Wile DJ, Agarwal PA, Schulzer M, Mak E, Dinelle K, Shahinfard E et al (2017) Serotonin and dopamine transporter PET changes in the premotor phase of LRRK2 parkinsonism: cross-sectional studies. Lancet Neurol 16(5):351–359. https://doi.org/10.1016/S1474-4422(17)30056-X

Wilson H, Giordano B, Turkheimer FE, Chaudhuri KR, Politis M (2018) Serotonergic dysregulation is linked to sleep problems in Parkinson's disease. NeuroImage Clin 18:630–637. https://doi.org/10.1016/j.nicl.2018.03.001

Wilson H, Dervenoulas G, Pagano G, Koros C, Yousaf T, Picillo M et al (2019) Serotonergic pathology and disease burden in the premotor and motor phase of A53T α-synuclein parkinsonism: a cross-sectional study. Lancet Neurol 18(8):748–775. https://doi.org/10.1016/S1474-4422(19)30140-1

Winer JR, Maass A, Pressman P, Stiver J, Schonhaut DR, Baker SL et al (2017) Associations between tau, β-amyloid, and cognition in Parkinson disease. JAMA Neurol 94702:1–9. https://doi.org/10.1001/jamaneurol.2017.3713

Wu L, Liu F-T, Ge J-J, Zhao J, Tang Y-L, Yu W-B et al (2018) Clinical characteristics of cognitive impairment in patients with Parkinson's disease and its related pattern in 18F-FDG PET imaging. Hum Brain Mapp 39(12):4652–4662. https://doi.org/10.1002/hbm.24311

Yarnall A, Rochester L, Burn DJ (2011) The interplay of cholinergic function, attention, and falls in Parkinson's disease. Mov Disord 26(14):2496–2503. https://doi.org/10.1002/mds.23932

Yoshita M, Hayashi M, Hirai S (1998) Decreased myocardial accumulation of 123I-meta-iodobenzyl guanidine in Parkinson's disease. Nucl Med Commun 19(2):137–142

Computer-Aided Diagnosis of Parkinson's Disease, Based on SPECT Scans of the Dopamine Transporter

25

Francisco P. M. Oliveira and Durval C. Costa

Contents

Abstract

Computer-aided diagnosis (CAD) tools have been, more and more frequently, proposed as a complement to the visual evaluation of dopamine transporter (DaT) single-photon emission computed tomography (SPECT) scans. Classification accuracies up to 98% have been reported in the differentiation between healthy control (HC) subjects and patients with Parkinson's disease (PD) based on DaT SPECT. CAD systems have also been used to differentiate between different types of Parkinsonism, but the accuracies are not as high as for the classification of PD patients versus HC subjects. When compared with cutoff-based classification techniques or visual classification, the CAD originated higher accuracy. The works reported in the literature on CAD systems of DaT SPECT have some limitations, with the lack of postmortem diagnosis the most

F. P. M. Oliveira (✉) · D. C. Costa
Nuclear Medicine – Radiopharmacology, Champalimaud Centre for the Unknown, Champalimaud Foundation, Lisbon, Portugal
e-mail: francisco.oliveira@fundacaochampalimaud.pt; durval.costa@fundacaochampalimaud.pt

R. A. J. O. Dierckx et al. (eds.), *PET and SPECT in Neurology*,
https://doi.org/10.1007/978-3-030-53168-3_25

important of them. The lack of consistency in the definition of the groups of patients and overlap of datasets used are also significant limitations. Despite all limitations and inconsistencies found in the published works, there is evidence that CAD based on DaT SPECT can effectively help in the clinics and is surely a better solution than the cutoff-based techniques only. Therefore, we believe CAD should be used in clinics as a complement to the visual and quantitative evaluation.

25.1 Introduction

Parkinson's disease is a progressive neurological disorder characterized by tremor, rigidity, and bradykinesia associated with progressive dopaminergic neuronal loss projecting into the striatum originated from the substantia nigra and other brain structures (Tolosa et al. 2006). DaT integrity assessment is frequently done using ^{123}I-FP-CIT (DaTscan™, GE Healthcare) with SPECT. Besides the visual evaluation, quantitative analysis is recommended (Darcourt et al. 2010).

Other radiopharmaceuticals have been developed for DaT integrity assessment with SPECT, namely, ^{123}I-β-CIT and ^{99m}Tc-TRODAT-1 (Van Laere et al. 2004). For positron emission tomography (PET), ^{11}C-FE-CIT (Antonini et al. 2001) and ^{11}C-PE2I (Appel et al. 2015) have been reported as successful with similar sensitivity and specificity values.

CAD has been emerging in different areas of medicine with increasing utility. Basically, it takes a set of features or characteristics of the subject, organ, tumor, exam, etc., and based on that and a previously built model, an output is obtained, usually claiming a binary decision or probability.

The idea of classifying a new case based on a previously built model is the oldest in medicine. The physician takes his/her decision based on a mental or written model or set of rules he/she has learned with experience. In the simplest CAD systems, the classification model may be similar to the rule or set of rules the clinicians use, taking advantage of the automated computation and therefore hopefully reducing the probability of error and increasing performance.

The CAD systems used in DaT SPECT can be broadly divided in two types: hypothesis driven and data driven. In the first case, the features or data extracted from the subjects are predefined based on the knowledge about the disease and how the disease is represented in the scan. Frequently, in the particular case of DaT SPECT, the features are related to the uptake in the striatum. Fully data-driven methods make no assumption on the features. Frequently, the selection of the features and the building of the model are optimized simultaneously.

Several different machine learning algorithms have been used for the classification task. In the literature survey done in the scope of this work, support vector machines (SVM) were the most often used. But decision trees, artificial neural networks (ANN), convolutional neural networks (CNN), k-nearest neighbors (k-NN), nearest mean classifier (NMC), logistic regression, and discriminant analysis techniques were also employed.

The construction of well-documented and validated databases has given a boost in the development of CAD systems for DaT SPECT. The most frequently referred and utilized in the literature, regarding this subject, is the Parkinson's Progression Markers Initiative (PPMI) (Marek et al. 2011, 2018).

25.2 ^{123}I-FP-CIT SPECT

^{123}I-FP-CIT is an analogue of cocaine and therefore binds selectively to the dopamine (and catecholamine) presynaptic transporter. Used with SPECT technology, ^{123}I-FP-CIT imaging is the most popular imaging method to confirm dopaminergic neuronal degeneration in vivo, mainly of the nigrostriatal pathway. It is therefore used in clinics to confirm the diagnosis of neurodegenerative Parkinsonism distinguishing bilateral from mainly unilateral disease. It is also of value in clearly distinguishing patients with drug-induced Parkinsonism (DIP) and essential tremor (ET), where there is no significant dopaminergic degeneration, from those with true Parkinsonism due to dopaminergic degeneration. Although envisaged as difficult and frequently doubtful, in some occasions, it is possible to demonstrate more cortico-striatal degeneration than nigrostriatal degeneration, in particular in patients with corticobasal ganglionic degeneration whose SPECT data with ^{123}I-FP-CIT reveal more often reduced uptake in the caudate nucleus compared to reduced putaminal uptake. Asymmetrical putaminal uptake reduction is the most frequent characteristic found in patients with PD of the idiopathic type. This is associated with less marked volumetric reduction as measured with high-resolution X-ray computed tomography (CT) and/or magnetic resonance imaging (MRI). In patients with very early signs of PD, the uptake reduction is so asymmetric that one of the striata (and particularly the putamen) appears with normal or almost normal uptake, either visually or quantitatively. Patients with other Parkinsonism types, such as multiple system atrophy (MSA) and progressive supranuclear palsy (PSP), frequently show clearly bilateral (symmetrical or slightly asymmetrical) reduced uptake from early stages of the disease.

The majority of data available for disease classification are based on clinical diagnosis and patient follow-up. However, the work of Walker et al. (2002) on correlation of clinical diagnosis with ^{123}I-FP-CIT SPECT imaging results and autopsy confirmatory diagnosis emphasizes shortcomings in the accuracy of the clinical diagnostic criteria that show a tendency to overdiagnose dementia with Lewy bodies (DLB). Consequently, the semiquantitative binding measures for the DLB group were all made somewhat narrower, after autopsy diagnosis, and more importantly the separation of the DLB group from the Alzheimer's disease (AD) group became larger. Due to difficulties inherent to the time it takes to obtain autopsy data from AD, DLB, PD patients, and also normal volunteers, this work is still ongoing to try and obtain a larger cohort possible of postmortem data.

It is clear that inaccuracies concerning clinical criteria in the final (autopsy data) diagnosis may be reduced with time and longitudinal clinical follow-up. However, it is highly likely that relatively early quantitative DaT SPECT will be able to tease out AD from DLB and PD, in addition to normal volunteer controls. Autopsy confirmatory diagnosis will improve group separation and therefore diagnostic classification.

We think that it is paramount to try and emphasize the importance of DaT SPECT data quantification by promoting several types of data extraction as described in this chapter.

25.3 Striatal Uptake Indices and Shape Extraction

Striatal uptake indices are frequently based on ratios between the counts in the striatal regions of interest and the counts in the reference region (a region without specific uptake). Striatal regions are computed separately for the left and right hemisphere and frequently are divided into whole striatum, caudate, and putamen (sometimes divided into two or three regions). The common reference regions are situated in the occipital lobe with possible partial inclusion of the cerebellum or other regions of the brain excluding the striatum and neighbor regions (Costa et al. 1988; Habraken et al. 1999; Tossici-Bolt et al. 2006; Oliveira et al. 2018). Ratios between the caudate and putamen uptake and left-right asymmetry coefficient are also occasionally used (Morton et al. 2005; Prashanth et al. 2016; Oliveira et al. 2018).

Geometric features extracted from the shape of the striatal uptake have been used in recent works (Augimeri et al. 2016; Prashanth et al. 2016; Oliveira et al. 2018). These features are assessed only in the striatal region with high uptake, at least higher than the background. They do not measure the real shape of the striatum. Examples of shape features are striatal volume, length (anterior-posterior), width (left-right), thickness (inferior-superior), and orientation-related features (Augimeri et al. 2016; Oliveira et al. 2018).

Nowadays, there are several software solutions to extract striatal uptake indices or shape descriptors. In many cases, it is possible to compare the measures with a database of normal scans. Examples are, for instance:

- BasGan software (Calvini et al. 2007) starts by a manual rigid preregistration, followed by an automatic affine registration with a template. Then, the uptake in the left and right caudate and putamen is extracted independently and automatically. Uptake in an occipital region is also extracted to be used as reference region.
- Hermes Brass™ is a commercial software that has a tool for automatic ^{123}I-FP-CIT analysis. It automatically quantifies uptake in the striatum and compares it with a normal database.
- PMOD software is a commercial tool that has been used in many research works found in the literature. It is a general tool but with some adaptation can be used for the quantification of DaT SPECT.

As some other groups, our group has its own solution to extract relevant features from the DaT SPECT (Oliveira et al. 2014, 2018). Our solution starts by automatic rigid or affine registration with a template. Then, predefined striatal regions of interest are optimally positioned. From that, uptake in the left and right caudate and putamen is extracted independently and automatically. The reference region is automatically defined. It can be an occipital region or whole brain except a region around the basal ganglia and ventricles. Volume, length, width, and thickness of left and right striatal regions with normal uptake are also automatically measured.

25.4 How Classifiers Work

To build a classifier, two fundamental things are necessary: a dataset of observations (or measurements or features), labeled by class, and a theoretical classification model. The features are the independent variables, and the known classification labels are the dependent variable. Then, in most of the classifiers, an optimization algorithm is used to optimize the parameters of the model, i.e., the parameters that make the model as accurate as possible in predicting the classification. This optimization step is usually known as training or learning. After optimizing the model, it can be used to predict the classification of new cases. To assess the accuracy of the model, a dataset of cases not used in the training process are classified by the model, and the output is compared with the known gold standard classification.

There are several conceptually different models that can be used, each one with several variants. Here, we briefly explain the foundation of the models found in the literature regarding the classification of patients with Parkinsonism based on DaT SPECT. As previously referred, in all cases, the input is a set of features describing the case. These may be discrete or continuous variables or even the images themselves. The final output is always a discrete variable, i.e., the predicted label.

A SVM classifier is a linear model, like linear regression, i.e., the output is a linear combination of the input variables. The main difference is the goal of the optimization. In linear regression, the goal is to fit the model to the data, while in the SVM the goal is to find the optimal model (usually a hyperplane) that best separates the two classes of the training data. With adequate transformation of the input variables, nonlinear behavior of the input variables may be modulated to a linear one. The output of the SVM model is a continuous variable that needs to be binarized. If it is higher than zero, the case is classified in one way (positive, for instance); otherwise, it is classified in the other way.

Logistic regression is a well-known technique used in statistics. The output is the probability of a case to be positive, for instance. Thus, defining a threshold, usually 0.5, the output is binarized. The classification model is obtained by optimizing the parameters of the model (a logistic function) with the goal to fit the model to the training data.

Naive Bayes is other technique to build classifiers. It assumes the features are independent of each other, regardless if possible correlations between the features may exist. The idea is to compute the probability of an observation that occurs assuming that observation belongs to a predefined class (Bayes theorem). Using, for instance, the method of maximum likelihood, the optimal parameters of the model can be estimated. Usually, the decision rule is based on the hypothesis that is most probable (maximum a posterior rule).

Decision tree is a conceptually simple classifier. In its basic formulation, it starts by the feature that best separates the cases. It splits "optimally" the cases in two groups based on that feature, creating two branches. Then, for each branch, a new split is done based on other feature and so on. The optimal cutoffs are optimally defined during the training process. The final classification model is the rule with the cutoffs that optimally classify the training dataset.

The ANN classifiers are based on the idea of the connections between neurons. It may have several neurons and layers. In the basic implementation, all neurons of the first layer have as inputs the original features. Then, each neuron computes an output measure, usually a real number, based on the features and a specific mathematical model for that neuron. The outputs of the neurons of the first layer are then passed as inputs to the neurons of the second layer and so on till the last layer. The neurons and the connections between neurons ("synapses") have weights that are optimized in the training process. By reducing or increasing the weight of a synapse, that synapse may be reinforced or eliminated. The same happens with neurons.

The CNN is a type of ANN. In very short, the input is the image or a patch of the image. The first layer is a convolutional layer, i.e., a set of convolution filters are applied to the image. The kernels of the filters are not static; they are optimized/learned during the process. Next layers may be convolutional or not. In a CNN, there is no need for feature extraction, since this process is incorporated in the convolution layers.

Discriminant analysis is a classical statistics technique. It assumes the distribution of the features is normally distributed in each class. It tries to find a linear combination of the features that best describe or separate the classes of objects based on some threshold. It is related to regression analysis.

The NMC is very simple. The training dataset is used to compute the mean feature vector of each class (centroid of each class). Then, a new case gets the classification of the nearest centroid.

The k-NN classifier is almost as simple as the NMC. A case is classified based on its k most "closed" cases in the training dataset by voting of closeness. The distance is taken from the values of the features extracted from the cases. This is the only classifier here presented that always needs the full training dataset. The other classifiers here presented only need the training dataset to optimize the classification model or to obtain the centroids of the classes, and then only the model or the centroids are needed.

There are several measures that can be used to report the quality of a binary classifier. In this work, we opted to use the simplest measures for a nonexpert in classification/statistics area. The simplest one is the accuracy (Acc), which is defined by the ratio of number of correct classifications (true positive plus true negative) and the number of cases (see Fig. 25.1). The sensitivity and specificity are also very useful, the first being the ratio of the number of true positive and the number of positives and the second being the ratio between the number of true negative and the

		Gold standard	
		Positive	Negative
Classifier outcome	Predicted positive	True positive (TP)	False positive (FP)
	Predicted negative	False negative (FN)	True negative (TN)

Fig. 25.1 General binary confusion matrix

number of negatives. The balanced accuracy (BAcc) is the mean of the sensitivity and specificity, which makes it very suitable as a measure of the classifier quality. Besides that, the balanced accuracy is more informative in unbalanced datasets than the accuracy. For this reason, in this work, whenever possible, we use the balanced accuracy.

For multiclass classifiers, i.e., more than two classes, the accuracy can always be computed. The sensitivity and specificity may also be computed for the classification of each class against all the others together.

25.5 Classification Methods Based Only on DaT SPECT

As referred before, the PD pathology hallmark is characterized by a progressive dopaminergic neuronal loss projecting into the striatum originated from the substantia nigra and other brain structures. This causes a decrease of the DaT ligand uptake in the striatum, mostly in the putamen in the initial stages of the disease. This uptake pattern led to the appearing of classification techniques based on cutoffs. If a single measure is taken from the striatum, there is no need for a computer to assess if the measure is above or below the cutoff. This type of classification has been used for a long time. For instance, Costa et al. (1988) defined a striatal binding index (SBI) related to the uptake in whole striatum. Then, the patients that had an SBI inferior to the cutoff at least in one side of the striatum were considered as having striatal DaT degeneration. The cutoff-based approaches are still very common and used in many clinical sites.

Nowadays, most common uptake indices are computed separately in the caudate and putamen. Figure 25.2 shows two examples of the delineation of the caudate and putamen nucleus on a transaxial slice. The indices may be simply the ratio of the mean counts per voxel in the specific region and the mean counts per voxel in the reference region or the binding potential (BP) in the specific regions:

$$\left(\text{BP} = \frac{\text{Mean counts per voxel in the specific region}}{\text{Mean counts per voxel in the reference region}} - 1 \right)$$

Other four uptake indices frequently used in quantification and classification problems are shown in Fig. 25.3 with their distribution in the differential diagnosis between healthy controls and patients with PD. They are the specific binding ratio

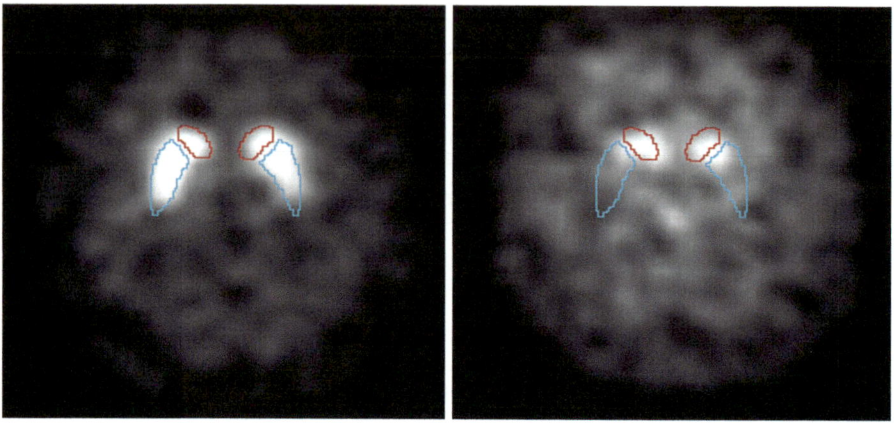

Fig. 25.2 Two transaxial slice images taken from two DaT SPECT examinations of two different patients. On the left, there is a typical normal uptake distribution throughout the striatum (including caudate and putamen) from a patient with no dopaminergic degeneration. On the right, very abnormal uptake is demonstrated within both striata of a patient (more intensely reduced in the putamen) with bilateral nigrostriatal degeneration. The red and blue contours delineate the caudate and putamen, respectively

(SBR) (Tossici-Bolt et al. 2006), caudate binding potential (CBP), putamen binding potential (PBP), and striatum binding potential (SBP) (Oliveira et al. 2018). Data represented were obtained from the analysis of 209 HC subjects and 443 PD patients based on the work of Oliveira et al. (2018). It is clear that all indices separate well, but not perfectly, the PD patients from the HC subjects.

Many research works found in the literature measured the discriminative power of a feature based on the area under the receiver operating characteristic (ROC) curve. The ROC curve is a graphical representation of the false positive rate (1 − specificity) versus the true positive rate (sensitivity) for different cutoffs of the feature. If there is a cutoff value that separates perfectly the cases in two classes, then the area under the ROC curve is 1. This technique allows obtaining a measure of the feature classification discriminative power (area under the ROC curve) on the training dataset. It does not give the expected classification accuracy if the "optimal" cutoff chosen were applied to a different dataset. It does not involve validation. Yet, it was frequently used in many works (Staff et al. 2009; Skanjeti et al. 2014, 2015; Iwabuchi et al. 2018). Figure 25.4 shows four ROC curves obtained from the same data as in Fig. 25.3.

Currently, several uptake indices can be extracted from the scans. Thus, establishing a cutoff for each one is not the ideal solution because frequently there are disagreements among them, especially for the borderline cases. A better solution is using optimization to build a classification model based on all known relevant features available. This is the fundamental idea behind the hypothesis-driven classifiers.

In the next subsections, a compilation of published papers that use a CAD strategy on DaT SPECT images for differential diagnosis of Parkinsonism is presented.

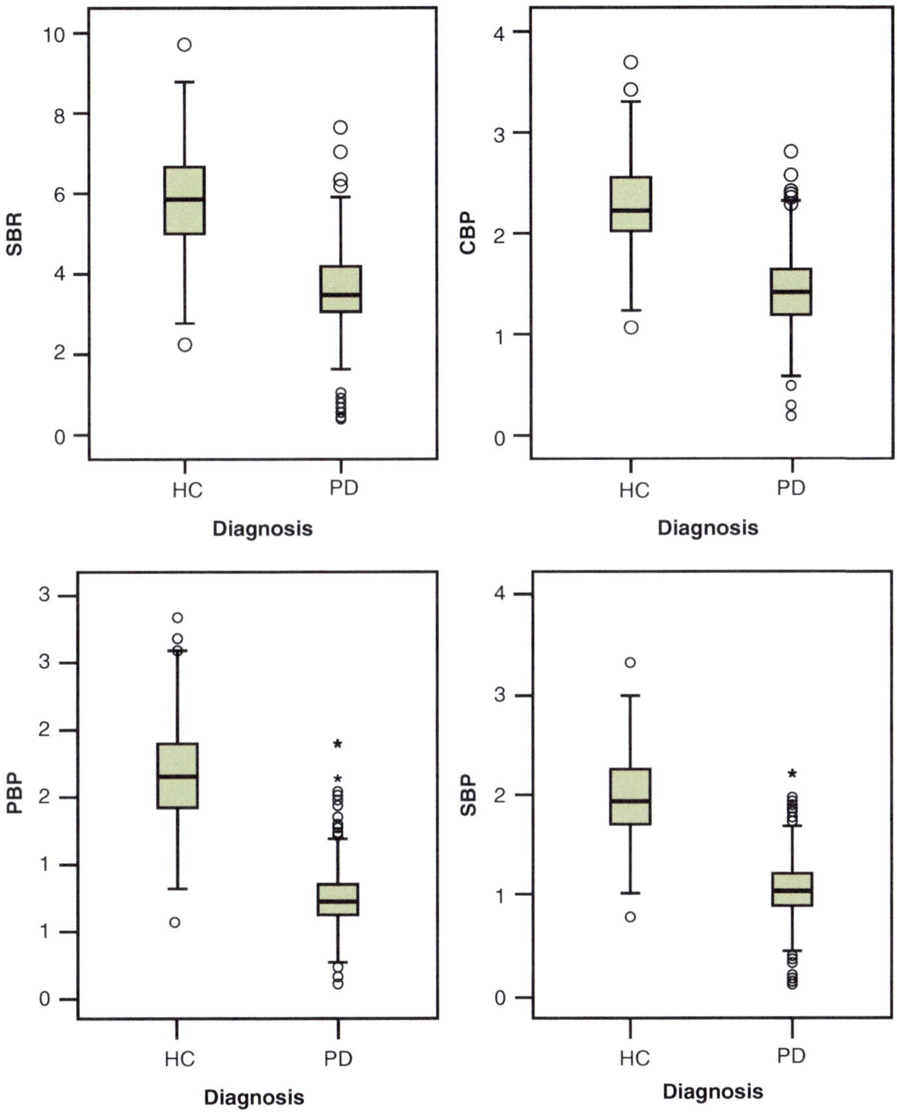

Fig. 25.3 Four boxplots representing the distribution of the SBR, CBP, PBP, and SBP when analyzing 209 HC subjects and 443 PD patients based on the work of Oliveira et al. (2018). For each subject, only the minimum value of both hemispheres was considered

Most common classifiers classify PD patients versus HC subjects; however, groups of patients with ET, corticobasal degeneration (CBD), DLB, DIP, PSP, MSA, and vascular Parkinsonism (VP) were also included in some works. In addition, some research works divided the PD patients into early PD (ePD) and advanced PD (aPD). In some works, the authors defined a Parkinsonian syndrome (PS) group

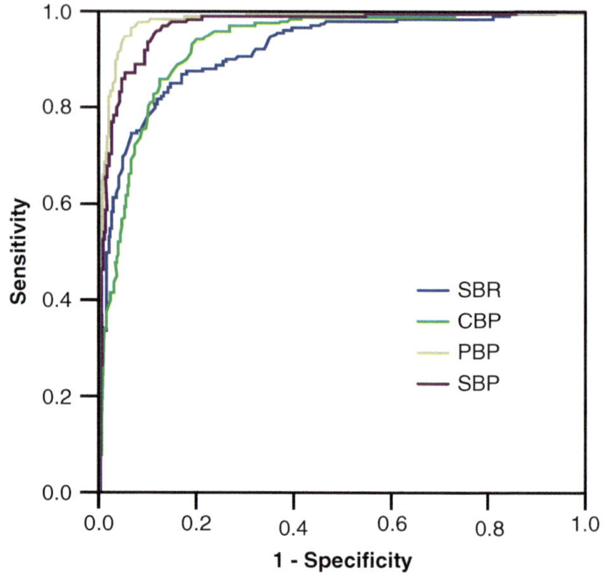

Fig. 25.4 Four ROC curves from the analysis of 209 HC subjects and 443 PD patients based on the work of Oliveira et al. (2018). The ROC curves are shown for the uptake indices SBR, CBP, PBP, and SBP. For each subject/patient, only the minimum value of both hemispheres was considered. Areas under the curves are 0.922, 0.933, 0.982, and 0.971 for the SBR, CBP, PBP, and SBP, respectively. Based on these values, the PBP index can separate better the HC subjects from the PD patients than the other indices

including all Parkinsonism cases with evidence of dopaminergic deficit. Other works did not have a class of healthy controls; instead, they included a category of controls containing the scans without evidence of dopaminergic deficit (SWEDD).

Only works that used cross-validation or an independent dataset for validation and described the dataset used are here presented. There are works that have tested different classifiers and/or different sets of features. In these cases, only the best result per classifier is presented.

Based on the survey done, there are works that also compared the classification accuracy obtained with the CAD systems against the cutoff-based techniques. In all cases, the CAD gave higher accuracy (see, for instance, Taylor and Fenner (2017) and Oliveira et al. (2018)).

25.5.1 Hypothesis-Driven Classification Methods

A compilation of the works found in the literature survey that used hypothesis-driven CAD based only on DaT SPECT images for differential diagnosis of Parkinsonism is presented in Table 25.1. ^{123}I-FP-CIT was the radiopharmaceutical used in all studies, except one that reports to have used ^{99m}Tc-TRODAT-1 instead. The extraction of the indices was fully automated in some of them and observer dependent in others. Examples of both cases are included. At least two uptake indices were used in all the works, one related to the uptake in the caudate and the other in the putamen.

Table 25.1 Papers found in the literature using hypothesis-driven classifiers based on DaT SPECT

Paper	Features used	Groups of subjects or images (total including training and validation)	Type of classifier	Main results
Van Laere et al. (2004)	Striatal uptake indices	PD ($n = 47$), controls ($n = 10$)	Discriminant analysis	BAcc: 91% (PD vs. controls)
	Striatal uptake indices (^{99m}Tc-TRODAT-1)	PD ($n = 47$), controls ($n = 10$)	Discriminant analysis	BAcc: 81% (PD vs. controls)
Van Laere et al. (2006)	Striatal uptake indices	PD ($n = 58$), ET ($n = 27$), MSA ($n = 24$), PSP ($n = 12$), DLB ($n = 8$)	Discriminant analysis	BAcc: 93% (PD + MSA + PSP + DLB vs. ET)
Hamilton et al. (2006)	Striatal uptake indices	PD ($n = 13$), ET ($n = 5$)	ANN	BAcc: 100% (PD vs. ET)
Palumbo et al. (2010)	Striatal uptake indices	ET ($n = 89$), ePD ($n = 64$), aPD ($n = 63$)	ANN	Acc: 82% ePD, 79% aPD, 97% ET (ePD vs. aPD vs. ET)
Palumbo et al. (2014)	Striatal uptake indices	PD ($n = 56$), ET + DIP ($n = 34$)	SVM	BAcc: 90% (PD vs. DIP)
Prashanth et al. (2014)	Striatal uptake indices	PD ($n = 396$), HC ($n = 179$)	SVM	BAcc: 96% (PD vs. HC)
			Logistic regression	BAacc: 87% (PD vs. HC) (no cross-validation reported)
Huertas-Fernández et al. (2015)	Striatal uptake indices	PD ($n = 164$), VP ($n = 80$)	SVM	BAcc: 87% (PD vs. VP)
			Discriminant analysis	BAcc: 87% (PD vs. VP)
			Logistic regression	BAcc: 87% (PD vs. VP)
Prashanth et al. (2016)	Striatal uptake indices and uptake shape	PD ($n = 427$), HC ($n = 208$), SWEDD ($n = 80$)	SVM	BAcc: 97% (PD vs. HC + SWEDD)
			Boosted trees (a type of decision trees)	BAcc: 97% (PD vs. HC + SWEDD)
			Random forest (a multitude of decision trees)	BAcc: 97% (PD vs. HC + SWEDD)
			Naive Bayes	BAcc: 96% (PD vs. HC + SWEDD)

(continued)

Table 25.1 (continued)

Paper	Features used	Groups of subjects or images (total including training and validation)	Type of classifier	Main results
Taylor and Fenner (2017))	Striatal uptake indices	PPMI dataset: PD ($n = 448$), HC ($n = 209$)	SVM	BAcc: 97% (PD vs. HC)
		Local dataset: PD ($n = 191$), non-PD patients ($n = 191$)	SVM	BAcc: 91% (PD vs. non-PD)
Oliveira et al. (2018)	Striatal uptake indices and uptake shape	PD ($n = 443$), HC ($n = 209$)	SVM	BAcc: 98% (PD vs. HC)
			Logistic regression	BAcc: 96% (PD vs. HC)
			KNN	BAcc: 97% (PD vs. HC)
Nicastro et al. (2019)	Striatal uptake indices	PD ($n = 280$), CBD ($n = 28$), MSA-P ($n = 21$), PSP ($n = 41$), HC ($n = 208$)	SVM	BAcc: 93% (HC vs. CBD + MSA-P + PSP)
			SVM	BAcc: range from 61% (PD vs. MSA-P) to 84% (CBD vs. MSA-P)
Wenzel et al. (2019))	Specific binding ratio	PPMI dataset: PD ($n = 438$), HC ($n = 207$)	Based on optimal cutoff	BAcc: 97% (PD vs. HC)
		Local dataset: PS ($n = 149$), controls ($n = 149$)	Based on optimal cutoff	BAcc: 97% (PS vs. controls)

25.5.2 Data-Driven Classification Methods

In Table 25.2, a compilation of published papers that used a data-driven approach to classify patients based on DaT SPECT is presented. By definition, data-driven methods do not make any assumption on the uptake pattern of the scan. They should use all image content to search for the features and/or regions that best separate the cases. In some works, as are, for instance, Martínez-Murcia et al. (2014) and Oliveira and Castelo-Branco (2015), only a striatal region was used to feed the classifier. Illán et al. (2012) also assumed previous knowledge on the DaT SPECT, in this case to do the intensity normalization of the scans. Even though these types of methods are not truly data driven because they assume that the relevant information is in the striatum, they are included in Table 25.2.

The simpler approach for the data-driven methods is the voxel-as-feature (VAF) approach, i.e., each voxel is an independent feature. However, as for other approaches, this method may not be robust if the number of cases is not much higher than the number of features, ideally at least 6–12 times higher. Thus, a

Table 25.2 Papers found in the literature using data-driven classifiers based on DaT SPECT. In all cases, the ^{123}I-FP-CIT radiopharmaceutical was used

Paper	Features and reduction strategy	Groups of subjects or images (total including training and validation)	Type of classifier	Main results
Towey et al. (2011)	All voxels followed by SVD	PS ($n = 79$), controls ($n = 37$)	Naive Bayes	BAcc: 96% (PS vs. controls)
			NMC	BAcc: 94% (PS vs. controls)
Illán et al. (2012)	Voxels in a striatal region	PS ($n = 100$), controls ($n = 108$)	SVM	BAcc: 91% (PS vs. controls)
			KNN	BAcc: 86% (PS vs. controls)
			NMC	BAcc: 87% (PS vs. controls)
Segovia et al. (2012)	Voxels in a striatal region followed by PLS	PS ($n = 95$), controls ($n = 94$)	SVM	BAcc: 93% (PD vs. controls)
Rojas et al. (2013)	Voxels in a striatal region followed by PCA or ICA	PS ($n = 41$), controls ($n = 39$)	SVM	BAcc: 95% (PS vs. controls)
Martínez-Murcia et al. (2014)	Voxels in a striatal region followed by PCA	PD ($n = 222$), controls ($n = 275$)	SVM	BAcc: 91% to 95% (PD vs. controls)
Oliveira and Castelo-Branco (2015)	Voxels in a striatal region	PD ($n = 445$), HC ($n = 209$)	SVM	BAcc: 98% (PD vs. HC)
Brahim et al. (2015)	Voxels in a striatal region	PS ($n = 95$), controls ($n = 94$)	SVM	BAcc: 91% (PS vs. controls)
	Voxels in a striatal region followed by PCA		SVM	BAcc: 93% (PS vs. controls)
Huertas-Fernández et al. (2015)	Voxels in a striatal region	PD ($n = 164$), VP ($n = 80$)	SVM	BAcc: 88% (PD vs. VP)
			Discriminant analysis	BAcc: 86% (PD vs. VP)
			Logistic regression	BAcc: 84% (PD vs. VP)
Tagare et al. (2017)	Voxels in a striatal region; feature selection was done together with the optimization	PD ($n = 448$), HC ($n = 210$)	Logistic regression	BAcc: 97% (PD vs. HC)
Zhang and Kagen (2017))	All voxels	PD ($n = 1171$), HC ($n = 211$), SWEDD ($n = 131$)	ANN	BAcc: 90% (PD vs. HC + SWEDD)

(continued)

Table 25.2 (continued)

Paper	Features and reduction strategy	Groups of subjects or images (total including training and validation)	Type of classifier	Main results
Taylor and Fenner (2017)	All voxels followed by PCA	PPMI dataset: PD ($n = 448$), HC ($n = 209$)	SVM	BAcc: 98% (PD vs. HC)
		Local dataset: PD ($n = 191$), non-PD patients ($n = 191$)	SVM	BAcc: 91% (PD vs. non-PD)
Choi et al. (2017)	All voxels	PD ($n = 431$), HC ($n = 193$)	CNN	BAcc: 97% (PD vs. HC)
Martinez-Murcia et al. (2018)	All voxels	PD ($n = 448$), HC ($n = 194$)	CNN	BAcc: 95% (PD vs. HC)
Wenzel et al. (2019)	Voxels of the slices containing the striatum	PPMI dataset: PD ($n = 438$), HC ($n = 207$)	CNN	BAcc: 97% (PD vs. HC)
		Local dataset: PS ($n = 149$), controls ($n = 149$)	CNN	BAcc: 98% (PS vs. controls)

technique of feature reduction should be used. Singular value decomposition (SVD), principal component analysis (PCA), or partial least squares (PLS) are used in some works. These three techniques are similar; they try to explain a set of variables by a smaller number of variables that explain as much as possible the total variability contained in the original variables. Feature reduction based on independent component analysis (ICA) was also found.

25.6 Classification Methods Combining DaT SPECT and Other Data

The DaT SPECT is a valuable tool to assist on the differential diagnosis of neurodegenerative and non-neurodegenerative Parkinsonism. However, DaT SPECT may not be conclusive regarding the type of neurodegenerative Parkinsonism. In the survey done, two works were found that developed CAD systems using perfusion SPECT as complement to DaT SPECT. They are presented in Table 25.3.

25.7 Discussion and Conclusions

Several CAD strategies and classifiers have been implemented to classify any single DaT SPECT examination. SVM classifiers have been the most frequent choice for hypothesis-driven classification methodologies, giving also the best results.

Table 25.3 Papers found in the literature combining features from DaT SPECT and features from other SPECT scans

Paper	Features and reduction strategy	Groups of subjects or images (total including training and validation)	Type of classifier	Main results
Van Laere et al. (2006))	^{123}I-FP-CIT—striatal uptake indices ^{99m}Tc-Ethylcysteinate dimer SPECT (perfusion imaging)—cortical regions	PD ($n = 58$), ET ($n = 27$), MSA ($n = 24$), PSP ($n = 12$), DLB ($n = 8$)	Discriminant analysis	Acc: 98% (PD + MSA + PSP + DLB vs. ET), 82% (PD vs. MSA vs. PSP vs. DLB)
Takaya et al. (2018)	^{123}I-FP-CIT—several brain regions [^{123}I] Iodoamphetamine SPECT (perfusion imaging)—several brain regions	PD ($n = 44$), DLB ($n = 2$), PSP ($n = 10$), CBD ($n = 8$), MSA ($n = 15$)	Logistic regression	Acc: 86% (PD + DLB vs. PSP + CBD + MSA), 95% (DLB vs. PSP), 87% (DLB vs. CBD), 80% (DLB vs. MSA), 91% (CBD vs. MSA), 88% (MSA vs. PSP)

Balanced accuracy in the binary classification of PD patients versus HC subjects has reached 98% based on a PPMI cohort.

CAD of different types of neurodegenerative Parkinsonism has also been tested. However, the accuracies are lower, and the inconsistencies among studies are much higher than those found during the distinction between PD patients and HC. This is mainly because the datasets used in these cases are small and the confirmatory clinical diagnosis is harder to find than for the PD patients. Thus, there are no conclusive results.

Based on DaT SPECT, data-driven methods are less frequently used than hypothesis-driven methods. Both of them achieve similar accuracies according to what can be encountered in the published literature. Most of the classifiers here identified as data-driven methods are, in reality, mixed methods, since they assume a priori the striatum to be the relevant area, and for this reason only the voxels inside and in its vicinity are included. Fully data-driven methods have an apparent advantage over the others since feature extraction is already incorporated within themselves. However, if they do not support their classification results with understandable language and characteristics for the physician, their implementation must be considered with extreme caution.

The works found in the literature on CAD systems of DaT SPECT have a fundamental limitation: the gold standard diagnoses are clinical; thus, they are not true gold standard. Besides that, the DaT SPECT has been used to aid the clinical diagnosis. Another issue is related to the definition of the control group. In the papers based on PPMI database, there is a clear healthy control group. However, in other works, the control group is sometimes made of patients with a visually normal DaT SPECT.

In our survey, we only included works where an independent dataset or cross-validation technique had been used to assess the classification accuracy. However, in most of the selected work, the authors tested different approaches for the feature selection and classification. This increases the risk of obtaining high accuracies by chance.

Some research works reported classification results obtained using simultaneous features extracted from DaT SPECT and clinical or demographic features to build the classifiers. These results were not included because they diverge from the main focus of this work.

Other limitation of the results found in the literature survey is the overlap of datasets used. Most commonly, there is a partial overlap of datasets extracted from PPMI database, but there is also overlap in some non-PPMI-based works. In addition, some PPMI dataset-based works included more than one DaT SPECT of the same patients, in particular follow-up examinations.

Only one work tested the robustness of the CAD systems according to the reconstruction protocols/parameters/algorithms (Wenzel et al. 2019). Authors conclude the CNN classifier is more robust than the SBR optimal cutoff. This result was expected since the SBR optimal cutoff is influenced by the reconstruction protocol. Besides that, in the CNN classifier, authors optimized approximately 2.87 million parameters, which obviously may have more potential to separate two classes than a single uptake index. These issues need to be better addressed in future work; otherwise, each classifier may only be valid for a specific protocol or a specific setting.

Despite all limitations and inconsistencies found in the published works related to CAD of DaT SPECT, there is evidence that CAD can effectively help in the clinics. Irrespective of the author, when comparing the classification accuracy obtained with the CAD systems against the cutoff techniques based on uptake indices, the CAD gave always higher accuracy that is on its own better than the accuracy based on qualitative visual evaluation (Badiavas et al. 2011).

In conclusion, CAD of DaT SPECT has been increasingly used in research. We believe it is now mature enough to be used in clinics as a complement to the visual and quantitative evaluation. It should, at least, serve as quality control and guide for experienced clinicians from now on. In addition, it may also be used to help train less experienced clinicians.

References

Antonini A, Moresco RM, Gobbo C, De Notaris R et al (2001) The status of dopamine nerve terminals in Parkinson's disease and essential tremor: a PET study with the tracer [11-C]FE-CIT. Neurol Sci 22(1):47–48. https://doi.org/10.1007/s100720170040

Appel L, Jonasson M, Danfors T, Nyholm D et al (2015) Use of ^{11}C-PE2I PET in differential diagnosis of Parkinsonian disorders. J Nucl Med 56(2):234–242. https://doi.org/10.2967/jnumed.114.148619

Augimeri A, Cherubini A, Cascini GL, Galea D et al (2016) CADA-computer-aided DaTSCAN analysis. EJNMMI Phys 3(1):4–4. https://doi.org/10.1186/s40658-016-0140-9

Badiavas K, Molyvda E, Iakovou I, Tsolaki M et al (2011) SPECT imaging evaluation in movement disorders: far beyond visual assessment. Eur J Nucl Med Mol Imaging 38(4):764–773. https://doi.org/10.1007/s00259-010-1664-1

Brahim A, Ramírez J, Górriz JM, Khedher L, Salas-Gonzalez D (2015) Comparison between different intensity normalization methods in ^{123}I-ioflupane imaging for the automatic detection of Parkinsonism. PLoS One 10(6):e0130274–e0130274. https://doi.org/10.1371/journal.pone.0130274

Calvini P, Rodriguez G, Inguglia F, Mignone A et al (2007) The basal ganglia matching tools package for striatal uptake semi-quantification: description and validation. Eur J Nucl Med Mol Imaging 34(8):1240–1253. https://doi.org/10.1007/s00259-006-0357-2

Choi H, Ha S, Im HJ, Paek SH, Lee DS (2017) Refining diagnosis of Parkinson's disease with deep learning-based interpretation of dopamine transporter imaging. NeuroImage Clin 16:586–594. https://doi.org/10.1016/j.nicl.2017.09.010

Costa DC, Walker Z, Dizdarevic S, Ionnides C et al (1988) Striatal binding of FP-CIT: a simple method to separate Parkinson's disease patients and normal controls. Paper presented at the Joint Congress of the European Association of Nuclear Medicine and the World Federation of Nuclear Medicine and Biology, Berlin, Germany, 30 Aug to 4 Sep

Darcourt J, Booij J, Tatsch K, Varrone A et al (2010) EANM procedure guidelines for brain neurotransmission SPECT using ^{123}I-labelled dopamine transporter ligands, version 2. Eur J Nucl Med Mol Imaging 37(2):443–450. https://doi.org/10.1007/s00259-009-1267-x

Habraken JBA, Booij J, Slomka P, Sokole EB, Royen EAV (1999) Quantification and visualization of defects of the functional dopaminergic system using an automatic algorithm. J Nucl Med 40:1091–1097

Hamilton D, List A, Butler T, Hogg S, Cawley M (2006) Discrimination between parkinsonian syndrome and essential tremor using artificial neural network classification of quantified DaTSCAN data. Nucl Med Commun 27(12):939–944. https://doi.org/10.1097/01.mnm.0000243369.80765.24

Huertas-Fernández I, García-Gómez FJ, García-Solís D, Benítez-Rivero S et al (2015) Machine learning models for the differential diagnosis of vascular parkinsonism and Parkinson's disease using [^{123}I]FP-CIT SPECT. [journal article]. Eur J Nucl Med Mol Imaging 42(1):112–119. https://doi.org/10.1007/s00259-014-2882-8

Illán IA, Górriz JM, Ramírez J, Segovia F et al (2012) Automatic assistance to Parkinson's disease diagnosis in DaTSCAN SPECT imaging. Med Phys 39(10):5971–5980. https://doi.org/10.1118/1.4742055

Iwabuchi Y, Nakahara T, Kameyama M, Yamada Y et al (2018) Quantitative evaluation of the tracer distribution in dopamine transporter SPECT for objective interpretation. Ann Nucl Med 32(5):363–371. https://doi.org/10.1007/s12149-018-1256-x

Marek K, Jennings D, Lasch S, Siderowf A et al (2011) The Parkinson progression marker initiative (PPMI). Prog Neurobiol 95(4):629–635. https://doi.org/10.1016/j.pneurobio.2011.09.005

Marek K, Chowdhury S, Siderowf A, Lasch S et al (2018) The Parkinson's progression markers initiative (PPMI) – establishing a PD biomarker cohort. Ann Clin Transl Neurol 5(12):1460–1477. https://doi.org/10.1002/acn3.644

Martínez-Murcia FJ, Górriz JM, Ramírez J, Illán IA et al (2014) Automatic detection of Parkinsonism using significance measures and component analysis in DaTSCAN imaging. Neurocomputing 126:58–70. https://doi.org/10.1016/j.neucom.2013.01.054

Martinez-Murcia FJ, Górriz JM, Ramírez J, Ortiz A (2018) Convolutional neural networks for neuroimaging in Parkinson's disease: is preprocessing needed? Int J Neural Syst 28(10):1850035. https://doi.org/10.1142/s0129065718500351

Morton RJ, Guy MJ, Clauss R, Hinton PJ et al (2005) Comparison of different methods of DatSCAN quantification. Nucl Med Commun 26(12):1139–1146

Nicastro N, Wegrzyk J, Preti MG, Fleury V et al (2019) Classification of degenerative parkinsonism subtypes by support-vector-machine analysis and striatal ^{123}I-FP-CIT indices. J Neurol 266(7):1771–1781. https://doi.org/10.1007/s00415-019-09330-z

Oliveira FPM, Castelo-Branco M (2015) Computer-aided diagnosis of Parkinson's disease based on [^{123}I]FP-CIT SPECT binding potential images, using the voxels-as-features approach and support vector machines. J Neural Eng 12(2):026008. https://doi.org/10.1088/1741-2560/12/2/026008

Oliveira FPM, Faria DB, Costa DC, Tavares JMRS (2014) A robust computational solution for automated quantification of a specific binding ratio based on [^{123}I]FP-CIT SPECT images. Q J Nucl Med Mol Imaging 58(1):74–84

Oliveira FPM, Faria DB, Costa DC, Castelo-Branco M, Tavares JMRS (2018) Extraction, selection and comparison of features for an effective automated computer-aided diagnosis of Parkinson's disease based on [^{123}I]FP-CIT SPECT images. Eur J Nucl Med Mol Imaging 45(6):1052–1062. https://doi.org/10.1007/s00259-017-3918-7

Palumbo B, Fravolini ML, Nuvoli S, Spanu A et al (2010) Comparison of two neural network classifiers in the differential diagnosis of essential tremor and Parkinson's disease by ^{123}I-FP-CIT brain SPECT. Eur J Nucl Med Mol Imaging 37(11):2146–2153. https://doi.org/10.1007/s00259-010-1481-6

Palumbo B, Fravolini ML, Buresta T, Pompili F et al (2014) Diagnostic accuracy of Parkinson disease by support vector machine (SVM) analysis of ^{123}I-FP-CIT brain SPECT data: implications of putaminal findings and age. Medicine 93(27):e228–e228. https://doi.org/10.1097/md.0000000000000228

Prashanth R, Roy SD, Mandal PK, Ghosh S (2014) Automatic classification and prediction models for early Parkinson's disease diagnosis from SPECT imaging. Expert Syst Appl 41(7):3333–3342. https://doi.org/10.1016/j.eswa.2013.11.031

Prashanth R, Roy SD, Mandal PK, Ghosh S (2016) High accuracy classification of Parkinson's disease through shape analysis and surface fitting in ^{123}I-Ioflupane SPECT imaging. IEEE J Biomed Health Inform. https://doi.org/10.1109/JBHI.2016.2547901

Rojas A, Górriz JM, Ramírez J, Illán IA et al (2013) Application of empirical mode decomposition (EMD) on DaTSCAN SPECT images to explore Parkinson disease. Expert Syst Appl 40(7):2756–2766. https://doi.org/10.1016/j.eswa.2012.11.017

Segovia F, Górriz JM, Ramírez J, Álvarez I et al (2012) Improved Parkinsonism diagnosis using a partial least squares based approach. Med Phys 39(7):4395–4403. https://doi.org/10.1118/1.4730289

Skanjeti A, Angusti T, Iudicello M, Dazzara F et al (2014) Assessing the accuracy and reproducibility of computer-assisted analysis of ^{123}I-FP-CIT SPECT using BasGan (V2). J Neuroimaging 24(3):257–265. https://doi.org/10.1111/jon.12008

Skanjeti A, Castellano G, Elia BO, Zotta M et al (2015) Multicenter semiquantitative evaluation of ^{123}I-FP-CIT brain SPECT. J Neuroimaging 25(6):1023–1029. https://doi.org/10.1111/jon.12242

Staff R, Ahearn T, Wilson K, Counsell C et al (2009) Shape analysis of ^{123}I-N-omega-fluoropropyl-2-beta-carbomethoxy-3beta-(4-iodophenyl) nortropane single-photon emission computed tomography images in the assessment of patients with parkinsonian syndromes. Nucl Med Commun 30(3):194–201. https://doi.org/10.1097/MNM.0b013e328314b863

Tagare HD, DeLorenzo C, Chelikani S, Saperstein L, Fulbright RK (2017) Voxel-based logistic analysis of PPMI control and Parkinson's disease DaTscans. NeuroImage 152:299–311. https://doi.org/10.1016/j.neuroimage.2017.02.067

Takaya S, Sawamoto N, Okada T, Okubo G et al (2018) Differential diagnosis of parkinsonian syndromes using dopamine transporter and perfusion SPECT. Parkinsonism Relat Disord 47:15–21. https://doi.org/10.1016/j.parkreldis.2017.11.333

Taylor JC, Fenner JW (2017) Comparison of machine learning and semi-quantification algorithms for (I123)FP-CIT classification: the beginning of the end for semi-quantification? EJNMMI Phys 4(1):29. https://doi.org/10.1186/s40658-017-0196-1

Tolosa E, Wenning G, Poewe W (2006) The diagnosis of Parkinson's disease. Lancet Neurol 5:75–86. https://doi.org/10.1016/S1474-4422(05)70285-4

Tossici-Bolt L, Hoffmann SMA, Kemp PM, Mehta RL, Fleming JS (2006) Quantification of [^{123}I]FP-CIT SPECT brain images: an accurate technique for measurement of the specific binding ratio. Eur J Nucl Med Mol Imaging 33(12):1491–1499. https://doi.org/10.1007/s00259-006-0155-x

Towey DJ, Bain PG, Nijran KS (2011) Automatic classification of ^{123}I-FP-CIT (DaTSCAN) SPECT images. Nucl Med Commun 32(8):699–707. https://doi.org/10.1097/MNM.0b013e328347cd09

Van Laere K, De Ceuninck L, Dom R, Van den Eynden J et al (2004) Dopamine transporter SPECT using fast kinetic ligands: ^{123}I-FP-β-CIT versus ^{99m}Tc-TRODAT-1. Eur J Nucl Med Mol Imaging 31(8):1119–1127. https://doi.org/10.1007/s00259-004-1480-6

Van Laere K, Casteels C, Ceuninck LD, Vanbilloen B et al (2006) Dual-tracer dopamine transporter and perfusion SPECT in differential diagnosis of Parkinsonism using template-based discriminant analysis. J Nucl Med 47(3):384–392

Walker Z, Costa DC, Walker RWH, Shaw K et al (2002) Differentiation of dementia with Lewy bodies from Alzheimer's disease using a dopaminergic presynaptic ligand. J Neurol Neurosurg Psychiatry 73(2):134–140. https://doi.org/10.1136/jnnp.73.2.134

Wenzel M, Milletari F, Krüger J, Lange C et al (2019) Automatic classification of dopamine transporter SPECT: deep convolutional neural networks can be trained to be robust with respect to variable image characteristics. Eur J Nucl Med Mol Imaging. https://doi.org/10.1007/s00259-019-04502-5

Zhang YC, Kagen AC (2017) Machine learning interface for medical image analysis. J Digit Imaging 30(5):615–621. https://doi.org/10.1007/s10278-016-9910-0

PET and SPECT Imaging in Atypical Parkinsonian Syndromes

26

Martin Niethammer, Yoon Young Choi, Chris C. Tang, and David Eidelberg

Contents

Abstract

Parkinson's disease and parkinsonian disorders can present with a variety of symptoms, and there is often a significant overlap between the different disorders. Diagnosis typically relies on clinical examination, especially at follow-up visits, which has limitations. Neuroimaging has played a major role in the eluci-

M. Niethammer · D. Eidelberg (✉)
Center for Neurosciences, The Feinstein Institutes for Medical Research, Manhasset, NY, USA

Department of Neurology, North Shore University Hospital, Northwell Health, Manhasset, NY, USA
e-mail: mniethamme@northwell.edu; deidelbe@northwell.edu

Y. Y. Choi · C. C. Tang
Center for Neurosciences, The Feinstein Institutes for Medical Research, Manhasset, NY, USA
e-mail: ychoi3@northwell.edu; ctang@northwell.edu

R. A. J. O. Dierckx et al. (eds.), *PET and SPECT in Neurology*,
https://doi.org/10.1007/978-3-030-53168-3_26

dation of anatomical and functional abnormalities in different parkinsonian disorders. Various imaging techniques have been investigated for their potential to aid in diagnosis during routine clinical practice. In this chapter, we describe the use of functional imaging with PET and SPECT in the research of atypical parkinsonian syndromes (APS), including multiple system atrophy, progressive supranuclear palsy, and corticobasal degeneration. We focus on the utility of these imaging techniques to facilitate differential diagnosis and assess disease progression in patients with APS, especially in the early stages of disease.

Abbreviations

^{11}C-(R)-PK11195	^{11}C(R)-1-(2-Chlorophenyl)-N-methyl-N-(1-methylpropyl)-3-isoquinolinecarboxamide
^{11}C-DPA713	(N,N-Diethyl-2-[2-(4-methoxyphenyl)-5,7-dimethylpyrazolo[1,5-a]pyrimidin-3-yl]acetamide
^{11}C-PBR28	*N*-Acetyl-N-(2-[11C]methoxybenzyl)-2-phenoxy-5-pyridinamine
^{123}I-IBF	^{123}I-Iodolisuride
^{123}I-IBZM	^{123}I-Iodobenzamide
6-OHDA	6-Hydroxydopamine
^{99m}Tc-ECD	Technetium-99m ethyl cysteinate dimer
ADRP	Alzheimer's disease-related pattern
APS	Atypical parkinsonian syndromes
CBD	Corticobasal degeneration
CBDRP	Corticobasal degeneration-related pattern
CIT	Carboxymethyoxy-3-β-(4-iodophenyl) tropane
COX-2	Cyclooxygenase-2
CVLT	California Verbal Learning Test
DAT	Dopamine transporter
DLB	Dementia with Lewy bodies
DWI	Diffusion-weighted imaging
FDG	^{18}F-Fluorodeoxyglucose
FP	Fluoropropyl
HVLT	Hooper Verbal Learning Test
MCI	Mild cognitive impairment
MIBG	Meta-^{123}I-iodobenzylguanidine
MR	Magnetic resonance
MRI	Magnetic resonance imaging
MSA	Multiple system atrophy
MSA-C	Multiple system atrophy—cerebellar
MSA-P	Multiple system atrophy—parkinsonian
MSARP	Multiple system atrophy-related pattern
PAGF	Pure akinesia with gait freezing

PBBS	Peripheral benzodiazepine binding site
PCA	Principal component analysis
PD	Parkinson's disease
PDCP	Parkinson's disease-related cognitive pattern
PDRP	Parkinson's disease-related motor pattern
PDTP	Parkinson's disease tremor-related pattern
PET	Positron emission tomography
PPV	Positive predictive value
PSP	Progressive supranuclear palsy
PSPRP	Progressive supranuclear palsy-related pattern
RVM	Relevance vector machine analysis
SPECT	Single-photon emission computed tomography
TCS	Transcranial sonography
TSPO	Translocator protein 18 kDa
UPDRS	Unified Parkinson's Disease Rating Scale

26.1 Atypical Parkinsonian Syndromes (APS)

26.1.1 Clinical Features

Parkinsonism is characterized clinically by a combination of features that include tremor, bradykinesia, rigidity, and postural instability. Syndromes with parkinsonism can be divided into neurodegenerative (sporadic and hereditary) and secondary parkinsonism. Idiopathic Parkinson's disease (PD) is the most common cause of neurodegenerative parkinsonism. Additionally, multiple system atrophy (MSA), progressive supranuclear palsy (PSP), and corticobasal degeneration (CBD) represent as much as 15% of parkinsonian syndromes seen in specialty practice.

MSA is characterized by a combination of autonomic dysfunction and varying degrees of parkinsonism or cerebellar symptoms (Gilman et al. 2008). Historically, patients with these symptoms were classified as having Shy-Drager syndrome, striatonigral degeneration, or spontaneous olivopontocerebellar atrophy, depending on the predominant symptomatology. Once a common underlying pathology was identified, these syndromes were grouped as MSA and later subdivided by the predominant motor symptoms into cerebellar (MSA-C, 20% of cases) and parkinsonian (MSA-P, 80% of cases) subtypes (Gilman et al. 2008; Papp et al. 1989; Wenning and Stefanova 2009).

Similar to PD, MSA is characterized pathologically by intracytoplasmic α-synuclein inclusions, albeit in oligodendroglia. In contrast, the pathology of both PSP and CBD involves tau filaments. Clinically, PSP is characterized by marked postural instability with early falls, coupled with vertical supranuclear gaze palsy, frontal subcortical dementia, and levodopa unresponsiveness (Williams and Lees 2009). In addition to this constellation of symptoms, termed Richardson's syndrome, clinical variants have recently been identified. These include PSP-parkinsonism, which includes patients with asymmetric onset, limited response to levodopa, and pure akinesia with gait freezing (PAGF) (Williams et al. 2005, 2007). Asymmetry is the principal feature of CBD, in addition to rigidity, bradykinesia, limb apraxia, and stimulus-induced myoclonus (Litvan et al. 1997; Boeve et al. 2003), though cognitive dysfunction can also predominate early in the disease and may confound the diagnosis (Litvan 2003; Mahapatra et al. 2004; Hu et al. 2009; Boeve 2011).

Diagnosis of these atypical parkinsonian syndromes (APS) and differentiation from PD is made following clinical examination and is based on established consensus criteria (Gilman et al. 2008; Armstrong et al. 2013; Postuma et al. 2015; Hoglinger et al. 2017). Nevertheless, postmortem studies show only 76–80% accuracy in the diagnosis of PD at initial presentation (Hughes et al. 2002; Rizzo et al. 2016). Though this accuracy does increase with longer follow-up and evaluations by movement disorders specialists, it remains under 90% for PD and significantly lower for atypical syndromes (Hughes et al. 2002; Rizzo et al. 2016; Josephs and Dickson 2003).

Thus, one important aim of neuroimaging is to provide increased diagnostic accuracy, which would allow for better selection of appropriate treatments and a more accurate prognosis. Multiple imaging modalities have been investigated in this regard, though the majority of studies to date have utilized patient cohorts with established diagnoses, i.e., later in the disease course.

26.1.2 Structural Imaging

Magnetic resonance imaging (MRI) has been a standard imaging technique in neurology for nearly 30 years. Perhaps the most important role of conventional MRI is the identification of cases of secondary parkinsonism that result from structural lesions, including neoplasms, multiple sclerosis, hydrocephalus, and vascular parkinsonism (Benamer and Grosset 2009; Winikates and Jankovic 1999). The role of conventional MRI in the diagnosis of neurodegenerative parkinsonism continues to evolve. Atrophy in the substantia nigra may be evident, but these findings do not rise to a level of specificity that allows for differentiation of PD from other forms of neurodegeneration or even from healthy controls, especially early in the disease (Linder et al. 2009; Jesse et al. 2012). In patients with MSA, PSP, or CBD, several characteristic findings have been described, though practical application is often hampered by the need for quantitative measurements that are not readily available in clinical practice (Schott et al. 2007; Paviour et al. 2005; Watanabe et al. 2002; Soliveri et al. 1999). Other MR modalities such as morphometric MR, diffusion-weighted imaging (DWI), or MR spectroscopy have shown promise in the differentiation of these parkinsonian syndromes (Minnerop et al. 2007; Seppi and Schocke 2005; Nicoletti et al. 2006; Kanazawa et al. 2004; Quattrone et al. 2008; Paviour et al. 2006, 2007; Albrecht et al. 2017, 2019; Sako et al. 2019). While these measures can distinguish APS and PD, they often are of low sensitivity (Mueller et al. 2018), and most have not been applied prospectively to patients in the early stages of disease (Holtbernd and Eidelberg 2014; Heim et al. 2018).

Transcranial sonography (TCS) is another imaging technique that is widely available and does not require radiotracers. TCS has the potential to aid in the diagnosis of PD and to distinguish APS from PD. Hyperechogenicity is detected in the substantia nigra (SN) in most PD patients (Berg et al. 2001, 2011; Richter et al. 2017), with normal echogenicity being more suggestive of MSA (Behnke et al. 2005; Walter et al. 2007), whereas hyperechogenicity of the lentiform nucleus (LN) is identified in the majority of patients with MSA, PSP, or CBD (Walter et al. 2004, 2003), albeit with low sensitivity or specificity (Gaenslen et al. 2008). Overall, the literature suggests that the diagnostic accuracy of TCS is high for differentiating PD from patients with essential tremor (ET) or APS but relatively low for the different types of APS in early parkinsonian patients (Tao et al. 2019).

26.2 Functional Imaging

Functional imaging techniques with single-photon emission computed tomography (SPECT) and positron emission tomography (PET) use different radioligands or radiotracers to quantitatively measure brain glucose metabolism, blood perfusion, and functional changes in neural pathways in neurodegenerative disorders. PET provides higher resolution than SPECT but at a higher cost. Both SPECT and PET are commonly applied in clinical diagnosis of parkinsonian patients as well as in the study of functional abnormalities in these disorders. These imaging techniques have proven to be particularly useful in investigating the underlying disease processes and improving the diagnostic accuracy for MSA, PSP, and CBD.

26.2.1 Dopaminergic Imaging

Radioligands for SPECT imaging, such as ^{123}I-β-CIT and ^{123}I-FP-CIT, are typically derivatives of cocaine that bind to the dopamine transporter (DAT) for measurement of dopamine reuptake. SPECT imaging with these radiotracers for DAT is used to detect presynaptic neural degeneration. In comparison, SPECT imaging with radiotracers for the dopamine D_2 receptor, such as ^{123}I-iodobenzamide (^{123}I-IBZM) and ^{123}I-iodolisuride (^{123}I-IBF), assesses the density of postsynaptic neuronal loss in the brain, particularly in the basal ganglia where these radiotracers are highly concentrated. Using PET, ^{18}F-DOPA provides measures of dopa-decarboxylase activity and integrity of presynaptic terminals, while ^{11}C-raclopride is used as a postsynaptic dopaminergic radiotracer.

SPECT imaging is a useful method for assessing nigrostriatal degeneration in patients with parkinsonism (Benamer et al. 2003; Marshall et al. 2009). In the striatum of PD patient, there is a marked decrease in DAT binding, which correlates with clinical measures of disease severity (Benamer et al. 2000; Spiegel et al. 2005), as well as an upregulation of postsynaptic D_2 receptors in this region (Ichise et al. 1999). The SPECT technique is particularly sensitive in detecting subtle functional abnormalities in PD, contributing to a better assessment of disease progression and more accurate diagnosis in early-stage patients (Pirker et al. 2002). SPECT has also proven useful in differentiating PD patients from healthy controls (Eshuis et al. 2006), vascular parkinsonism (Gerschlager et al. 2002), or between early and advanced PD patients (Eshuis et al. 2009).

Likewise, DAT SPECT imaging has proven to be a useful tool to study the progression and differential diagnosis of patients with APS. In a longitudinal ^{123}I-β-CIT SPECT study, baseline striatal binding was found to be less reduced in APS patients (−36% of age-corrected normal values) than in PD patients with short (−42%) or long (−51%) disease duration (Pirker et al. 2002). However, striatal binding declined significantly over time in APS (14.9% per year) at a faster rate than for both short- (7.1% per year) and long-duration (no significant change) PD. These results suggest that striatal ^{123}I-β-CIT binding may be more sensitive in measuring the progression of APS than PD (Pirker et al. 2002). In cases of CBD, initial SPECT imaging may be normal early in the disease, only to become abnormal on follow-up scan, suggesting delayed substantia nigra neuronal loss compared to other APS (Ceravolo et al. 2013; O'Sullivan et al. 2008).

While there is general consensus that presynaptic dopaminergic imaging (SPECT or PET) cannot reliably distinguish between PD and APS or between the different APS (Bajaj et al. 2013; Thobois et al. 2019), regional differences can be seen with DAT imaging. Unlike PD, ^{123}I-β-CIT SPECT studies have further shown reduced and symmetrical DAT binding in the striatum in patients with MSA.

A study comparing 26 MSA patients with 157 PD patients found that there was a substantial reduction of striatal DAT binding in both PD and MSA groups (Varrone et al. 2001). Likewise, studying 51 subjects with PD and 127 with APS, Ko et al. (2017) found significant reductions of putaminal DAT binding in all subjects except those with MSA-C. In all patient groups with the exception of MSA-C and CBD, DAT binding correlated with disease duration and severity measures.

Although the magnitude of DAT loss does differentiate between the MSA and PD, MSA patients may exhibit less asymmetric loss in the striatum relative to the PD patients, thought to be compatible with the less asymmetric symptoms in MSA (Varrone et al. 2001). These findings were substantiated in another ^{123}I-β-CIT SPECT study (Knudsen et al. 2004), in which MSA patients were also found to have less asymmetry in striatal binding than PD patients (with the exception of one MSA patient who had high asymmetry). Furthermore, a 15% hemispheric difference in binding value was suggested as the cutoff for differentiating PD (>15%) from MSA (5–15%), relative to healthy controls (<5%) (Knudsen et al. 2004). Nevertheless, other SPECT studies have reported that the asymmetry in striatal binding was either not significantly different between MSA and PD (Pirker et al. 2000) or even greater in patients with MSA (Perju-Dumbrava et al. 2012). Indeed, Perju-Dumbrava and colleagues found that there was a trend of greater asymmetry of striatal DAT binding in MSA compared with PD. Among the six MSA cases studied, two patients had been misdiagnosed during their lifetime; in particular, one patient with pronounced asymmetry in striatal DAT binding and clear asymmetry of clinical symptoms had been misdiagnosed as CBD. Based on these data and the relatively low accuracy of clinical diagnosis in MSA reported in literature (Hughes et al. 2002), the authors pointed out that because MSA patients with clear clinical asymmetry were more likely to have been misdiagnosed or excluded from prior imaging studies, the striatal binding asymmetry could have been underestimated for MSA resulting in a possible bias of patient selection. Thus, they concluded that individual MSA and PD patients cannot be differentiated accurately by subregional analysis of striatal DAT binding (Perju-Dumbrava et al. 2012).

DAT reduction has also been observed in the midbrain of MSA patients. In an ^{123}I-β-CIT SPECT study of 15 patients with early-stage MSA, 15 early PD patients, and 13 healthy control subjects, both MSA and PD patients showed significant loss of striatal DAT binding, while only MSA patients had binding loss in the midbrain. More interestingly, binding values in the caudate and midbrain together provided an accurate classification (95.2%) of subjects as MSA, PD, or normal controls. Although it is perhaps more clinically relevant to exclude the normal controls from this discriminant analysis, the data underscore the potential importance of applying midbrain DAT binding to the differential diagnosis of patients with uncertain parkinsonism (Scherfler et al. 2005). Other extrastriatal regions may also prove to be useful in the differential diagnosis of parkinsonism. Employing a region-of-interest (ROI) approach to parkinsonian patients (30 PD, 9 MSA-P, 7 MSA-C, 13 PSP), extrastriatal ^{123}I-FP-CIT SPECT binding ratios in the hypothalamus (presumed to be to serotonin transporters) were found to be significantly lower in PSP than MSA-C subjects (Joling et al. 2017). Furthermore, binding ratios in the caudate nucleus of PSP patients were lower than those of both PD and MSA-C patients, and in the posterior putamen, binding ratios were significantly lower in MSA-P, PSP, and PD than MSA-C patients. Thus, striatal ^{123}I-FP-CIT binding and hypothalamic ^{123}I-FP-CIT binding are significantly lower in MSA-P and PSP than in PD and MSA-C patients and might therefore be of interest for differential diagnosis (Joling et al. 2017).

More recently, Badoud and colleagues applied voxel-wise univariate statistical parametric mapping and multivariate pattern recognition to the DAT scans of 392 consecutive patients with degenerative parkinsonism (Badoud et al. 2016). MSA and PSP showed less tracer uptake in the head of caudate nucleus relative to PD and CBD, and CBD had higher uptake in both putamen relative to PD, MSA, and PSP. Classification was significant for PD versus APS ($p < 0.05$) and between APS subtypes (MSA vs. CBD, $p < 0.05$; MSA vs. PSP, $p < 0.05$; CBD vs. PSP, $p < 0.05$). While both striatal and extrastriatal regions contained classification information, the combination of both regions did not significantly improve classification accuracy (Badoud et al. 2016). Building on this, support-vector-machine analysis applied to DAT scans from 370 patients with degenerative parkinsonism was able to reliably distinguish parkinsonism from controls, as well as between different parkinsonian syndromes with sensitivities and specificities between 60% and 80%, with particularly good separation of CBD from other parkinsonian syndromes (Nicastro et al. 2019).

In general, metabolic imaging has proven to be more useful in the differentiation of APS (see below) than dopaminergic imaging. However, cerebral perfusion and metabolism generally are linked, and early phase dopaminergic imaging does contain information related to perfusion (Koeppe et al. 2005). Using dynamic PET data acquired during the first 10 minutes after ^{18}F-FP-CIT administration in 67 subjects with parkinsonism (23 PD, 27 MSA-C, 12 MSA-P, 5 PSP), Jin et al. were able to show correlation between the CIT images and FDG PET images from the same subjects (Jin et al. 2017). Visual concordance between the two modalities was high (86.2–93.1% diagnostic), and both MSA subtypes showed different regional uptake patterns compared to PD. Thus, it may be possible to use images acquired in the first 10 minutes of CIT imaging in the differential diagnosis of APS, though this will need to be confirmed in further studies, as well as with ^{123}I-β-CIT SPECT imaging for greater clinical utility.

In addition, SPECT imaging with dopamine D_2 receptor radioligands (e.g., ^{123}I-IBZM) has been used to study postsynaptic cell loss in patients with APS. In contrast to upregulated binding in the striatum of early PD (Kaasinen et al. 2000; Leenders 2003), striatal D_2 binding was found to be markedly reduced in MSA and PSP (Knudsen et al. 2004; Kim et al. 2002) while relatively preserved in CBD (Klaffke et al. 2006; Plotkin et al. 2005). Nonetheless, the role of ^{123}I-IBZM SPECT on differential diagnosis of parkinsonism remains controversial. In a ^{123}I-IBZM SPECT study, Vlaar et al. reported a low accuracy in differentiating between PD and APS (Vlaar et al. 2008). This result is in contrast with another SPECT study suggesting that a combination of ^{123}I-FP-CIT, ^{123}I-IBZM, and meta-^{123}I-iodobenzylguanidine (MIBG) scintigraphy resulted in high accuracy of 94% sensitivity and 94% specificity in differentiating PD from APS (Sudmeyer et al. 2011). More studies are needed to investigate the utility of these imaging tracers in the diagnosis of APS.

26.2.2 Perfusion Imaging

Technetium-99m ethyl cysteinate dimer (^{99m}Tc-ECD) perfusion SPECT has also been used in the differentiation of PD and MSA. One study found that the putamen was the only region where there was a significant difference in uptake between MSA and PD (Bosman et al. 2003). Using the putamen uptake value as the discriminating factor, an accuracy of 83.6% was achieved in classifying MSA patients against a combined group of PD and healthy controls but decreased to 67% in a three-group analysis of MSA, PD, and healthy volunteers. Furthermore, dual-tracer brain SPECT with ^{99m}Tc-ECD/^{123}I-FP-CIT, which allows for simultaneous assessment of blood perfusion and dopamine transporter function in parkinsonian patients, was applied to the differential diagnosis of parkinsonism, allowing for differentiation of PD and MSA, as well as PSP and CBD (El Fakhri et al. 2006; El Fakhri and Ouyang 2011). There was significantly lower perfusion in the striatum in MSA compared to PD, while striatal DAT binding was higher in MSA than PD (El Fakhri et al. 2006). Using statistical parametric mapping in ECD SPECT scans of PD and MSA patients, Van Laere et al. (2004) were able to separate PD from MSA and healthy controls, finding symmetric hypoperfusion in the thalamus and putamen of MSA subjects, whereas PD patients had additional cortical hypoperfusion. In a second study, discriminant analysis revealed that the two imaging measures together improved the overall classification accuracy to 82.4% in differentiating patients with PD, MSA, PSP, or dementia with Lewy bodies (DLB) over either imaging measure alone (DAT, 58.8%; perfusion, 67.6%) (Van Laere et al. 2006). After excluding PD subjects from the analysis, a striking 100% separation was achieved among MSA, PSP, and DLB (Van Laere et al. 2006). Although these results require rigorous validation in independent patient populations, dual-tracer DAT and perfusion SPECT may be a potentially useful approach for accurate differentiation between the most common APS in clinically uncertain cases.

26.2.3 Metabolic Imaging

26.2.3.1 Metabolic Imaging Networks

Functional imaging with ^{18}F-fluorodeoxyglucose (FDG) positron emission tomography (PET) can be applied to measure glucose utilization of neurons, which in turn provides an estimate of rest-state regional and global metabolism in the brain. Prior PET studies have shown hypometabolism in the striatum and cerebellum with increased metabolism in the frontal cortex in MSA (Eckert et al. 2005), while in PSP, hypometabolism was present in the supplementary motor area (SMA), anterior cingulate, thalamus, and striatum (Eckert et al. 2005; Bartels et al. 2006; Park et al. 2009; Teune et al. 2010). Moreover, regional hypometabolism in the striatum was found to be a common feature in both MSA and PSP (Ghaemi et al. 2002), in contrast to the increased metabolic activity in this region in PD (Bosman et al. 2003; Eckert et al. 2005; Eidelberg et al. 1993). In addition, profound asymmetric hypometabolism in the frontal and parietal areas is a unique feature in CBD (Eckert et al. 2005; Teune et al. 2010).

The use of spatial covariance analysis on FDG PET imaging data has led to the discovery of abnormal brain metabolic networks specifically related to neurodegenerative diseases such as PD and APS (Eckert et al. 2005; Eidelberg 2009; Poston and Eidelberg 2009; Schindlbeck and Eidelberg 2018). The technical details of the spatial covariance analysis (or network analysis) have been previously described in detail (Eidelberg 2009; Spetsieris et al. 2013). Briefly, a multivariate method utilizing principal component analysis (PCA) is employed to analyze voxel-wise metabolic imaging data in FDG PET scans from a combined group of patients and healthy subjects. This approach allows for the identification of spatial covariance patterns of brain regions in which metabolic abnormalities can be quantified as subject scores, used to differentiate between the patient and healthy control groups (Feigin et al. 2007; Habeck et al. 2008; Ma et al. 2007). After a disease-related metabolic pattern is identified in the original derivation cohort, the expression of this pattern (i.e., subject score) can be computed prospectively in individual scans of new subjects. In each individual scan, the subject score of the disease-related pattern can be viewed as a quantitative representation of the whole-brain metabolic abnormality for this subject at the time of imaging. Because of their quantitative nature, subject scores can be used to examine group separation, disease progression, treatment responses, and even individual correlations of imaging changes with clinical or neuropsychological measures in neurodegenerative disorders.

26.2.3.2 PD-Related Networks

In PD, FDG PET with network analysis has proven useful in identifying abnormal metabolic networks associated with motor and cognitive manifestations in PD. The motor-related pattern, termed PDRP, is characterized by pallido-thalamic metabolic increases and concurrent metabolic decreases in the premotor cortex, supplementary motor area, and parietal association areas (Nicastro et al. 2019; Schindlbeck and Eidelberg 2018; Niethammer et al. 2012).

PDRP has been extensively studied in numerous independent populations around the world. It has proven to be highly reproducible and stable, both at a single imaging center (Ma et al. 2007) and in independent PD populations scanned with different scanners. Indeed, in six independent cohorts, individual PDRP expression was consistently elevated in PD patients compared to healthy controls, when scanned at rest at least 12 hours after their last medication dose (i.e., in the off-state) (Eidelberg 2009; Wu et al. 2013; Holtbernd et al. 2015; Teune et al. 2013; Tripathi et al. 2016).

Individual PDRP expression scores reliably correlate with the Unified Parkinson's Disease Rating Scale (UPDRS) motor ratings (Asanuma et al. 2006; Lozza et al. 2004; Eidelberg et al. 1994, 1995; Niethammer and Eidelberg 2012), and PDRP expression declines (i.e., normalizes) with treatment, either dopaminergic medication or deep brain stimulation (DBS) (Asanuma et al. 2006; Pourfar et al. 2009).

Additional distinct PD-related patterns that correlate with tremor (PDTP; Mure et al. 2011) and cognition (PDCP; Huang et al. 2007) have also been identified. PDTP is characterized by increased metabolic activity of the cerebellum/dentate nucleus and primary motor cortex and, to a lesser degree, the caudate/putamen (Mure et al. 2011). At baseline, PDTP expression was abnormally elevated in PD patients with DBS implanted electrodes. When tremor was effectively improved by stimulation, this led to reductions of PDTP expression.

PDCP is characterized by metabolic reductions in the rostral supplementary motor area (pre-SMA), prefrontal cortex, precuneus, and parietal association regions, with metabolic increases in the cerebellar vermis and dentate nuclei. PDCP expression was correlated with performance on neuropsychological tests of executive functioning, such as the California and Hopkins Verbal Learning Tests (CVLT/HVLT), in the original derivation and in prospective groups of non-demented PD patients with or without mild cognitive impairment (MCI) (Huang et al. 2008). Importantly, PDCP does not simply reflect cognitive decline regardless of the cause and is specific to cognitive dysfunction in PD, as its topography is distinct from the independently characterized Alzheimer's disease-related patterns (ADRP) (Ma et al. 2003; Mattis et al. 2016; Teune et al. 2014).

Compared to PDRP, PDCP is expressed later in the disease course. In a 4-year longitudinal study of early PD patients (Huang et al. 2007; Tang et al. 2010a), both PDRP and PDCP expressions were found to increase with disease progression over time in the whole brain and in the two hemispheres independently, although PDCP expression reached abnormal levels approximately 4 years later than PDRP expression.

26.2.3.3 Networks Related to APS

This network-based approach has also been employed to identify specific disease-related metabolic patterns for MSA, PSP, and CBD. The MSA-related pattern (MSARP) is characterized by metabolic decreases in the putamen and cerebellum (Fig. 26.1a); the PSP-related pattern (PSPRP) is characterized by metabolic reductions in the upper brainstem, medial prefrontal cortex, and medial thalamus (Fig. 26.1b); and the CBD-related pattern (CBDRP) is characterized by bilateral, asymmetric metabolic reductions involving frontal and parietal cortex, thalamus, and caudate nucleus (Fig. 26.1c) (Eckert et al. 2008; Spetsieris et al. 2009; Poston et al. 2012; Ge et al. 2018; Niethammer et al. 2014). In accordance with the clinical picture of these disorders, MSARP and PSPRP were relatively symmetric, while in CDBRP, these pattern-related changes were greater in magnitude in the cerebral hemisphere opposite the more clinically affected body side (reflecting the marked asymmetry seen in CBD (Poston 2010)). CBDRP and PSPRP are not abnormally elevated in MSA patients, whereas the expression of both patterns is abnormally elevated in both PSP and CBD cohorts, and there is overlap (~24%) in the topography of the two patterns (Niethammer et al. 2014). Pathologically, PSP and CBD are distinct, but both diseases are classified as tauopathies (Dickson et al. 2007), suggesting that these patterns capture regional overlap in the pathologies of these diseases. Nevertheless, CBDRP is more asymmetric than PSPRP, a feature that may be helpful in using PSPRP and CBDRP for clinical diagnosis (see Sect. 2.3.4).

MSARP and PSPRP have recently been reproduced and validated in independent cohorts of MSA and PSP patients from the Netherlands (Teune et al. 2013). Like PDRP, the expression of each of these patterns accurately discriminated between patients and healthy controls on an individual basis in the original pattern derivation cohort. These data demonstrated that the atypical parkinsonian syndromes are indeed associated with distinct patterns of abnormal metabolic activity.

Additionally, MSARP, but not PDRP expression, is correlated with clinical severity and disease duration in MSA patients (Fig. 26.2) (Poston et al. 2012). In this study, two MSA patients who were clinically followed for up to 7 years exhibited continuous increases in MSARP expression over time, while their PDRP scores fluctuated within the normal range over the same time period (Poston et al. 2012). Clinically, MSA is further subdivided into cerebellar (MSA-C) and parkinsonian (MSA-P) subtypes. Remarkably, while patients in the two subgroups displayed some difference in regional metabolism, MSARP elevations were remarkably similar. Thus, these covariance networks provide descriptors based on underlying disease pathology rather than specific clinical features (Poston et al. 2012).

Moreover, the correlation between MSARP scores and disease duration suggests that these metabolic networks may also be used as potential imaging biomarkers for disease progression in APS (Poston et al. 2012). Although this potential association between pattern expression and disease progression needs to be further examined in prospective longitudinal studies of larger populations, especially for early-stage patients, the present findings suggest that the MSARP could be a sensitive biomarker for disease severity and progression in patients with MSA. Likewise, the investigation of progressive changes of metabolic networks in other parkinsonian syndromes will need to be the focus of future PET studies.

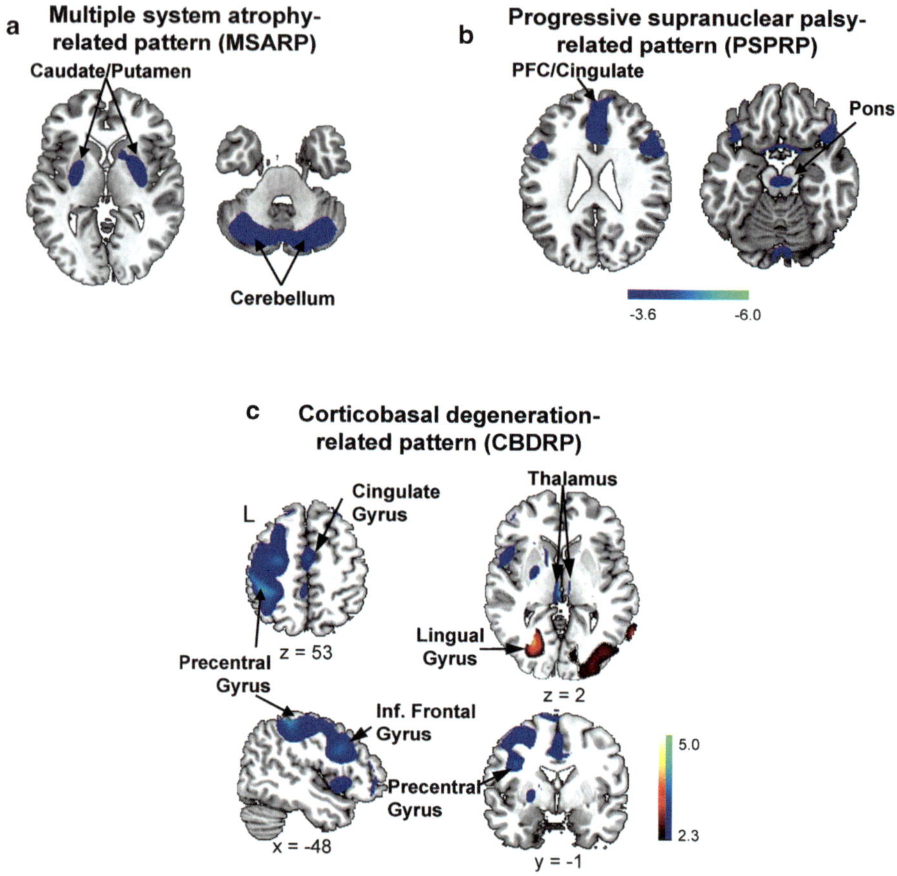

Fig. 26.1 Abnormal networks in atypical parkinsonian disorders. (**a**) Multiple system atrophy-related metabolic pattern (MSARP) identified by spatial covariance analysis of FDG PET scans from ten MSA patients and ten healthy volunteer subjects (Eckert et al. 2008; Poston et al. 2012). (Adapted from *Mov Disord*, 23, Eckert T, Tang C, Ma Y, Brown N, Lin T, Frucht S, Feigin A, Eidelberg D, Abnormal metabolic networks in atypical parkinsonism, pp. 727–733, Copyright (2008), with permission from John Wiley and Sons.) (**b**) Progressive supranuclear palsy-related metabolic pattern (PSPRP) identified by spatial covariance analysis of FDG PET scans from ten PSP patients and ten healthy volunteer subjects (Eckert et al. 2008). (Adapted from *Mov Disord*, 23, Eckert T, Tang C, Ma Y, Brown N, Lin T, Frucht S, Feigin A, Eidelberg D, Abnormal metabolic networks in atypical parkinsonism, pp. 727–733, Copyright (2008), with permission from John Wiley and Sons.) (**c**) Corticobasal degeneration-related pattern (CBDRP) identified by spatial covariance analysis of FDG PET scans from a derivation cohort of ten patients with CBD and ten healthy volunteer subjects scanned at the North Shore University Hospital (eight CBD and ten control subjects) and Stanford University (two CBD subjects) (Niethammer et al. 2014). (Displays of the MSARP and PSPRP covariance maps are thresholded at $Z = 3.61$, $p < 0.001$, and overlaid on T1-weighted magnetic resonance template images. The display of CBDRP represents regions that contributed significantly to the network thresholded at $Z = 2.33$ ($p < 0.01$). Voxels with positive region weights (metabolic increases) are color-coded red, and those with negative region weights (metabolic decreases) are color-coded blue. Left hemisphere is labeled as "L.") (From Niethammer M, Tang CC, Feigin A, Allen PJ, Heinen L, Hellwig S, Amtage F, Hanspal E, Vonsattel JP, Poston KL, Meyer PT, Leenders KL, Eidelberg D, A disease-specific metabolic brain network associated with corticobasal degeneration, *Brain*, 2014, 137, pp. 3036–46, by permission of Oxford University Press.)

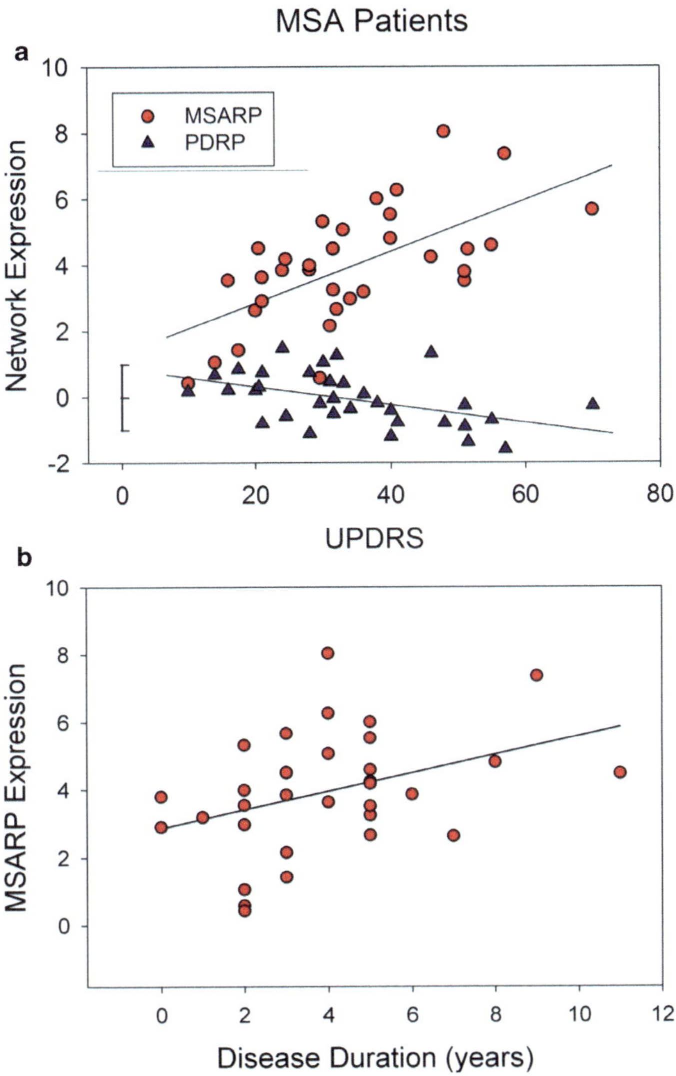

Fig. 26.2 MSARP expression correlates with disease severity and duration. (**a**) In MSA patients, increased MSARP expression (*red circles*) correlated with greater clinical disability as measured by increased Unified Parkinson's Disease Rating Scale (UPDRS) motor ratings ($r = 0.57$, $p < 0.001$). In contrast, increased motor disability in these subjects was associated with lower PDRP expression values (*blue triangles*; $r = 0.53$, $p < 0.002$). (**b**) In the MSA patients, there was a linear correlation between MSARP expression and symptom duration ($r = 0.38$, $p = 0.03$). (Reprinted with permission from Poston KL, Tang CC, Eckert T, Dhawan V, Frucht S, Vonsattel JP, Fahn S, Eidelberg D, Network correlates of disease severity in multiple system atrophy, *Neurology*, 2012, 78, pp.1237–1244.)

Potentially, metabolic networks may also be of use in the premotor stages of parkinsonian disorders. While REM sleep behavior disorder (RBD) can occur in isolation, many individuals develop a neurodegenerative syndrome within 5 years of diagnosis, and it is considered a strong risk factor for the future development of PD (Berg et al. 2015; Postuma et al. 2012). Most often, phenoconversion is a manifestation of underlying synuclein pathology as seen in idiopathic PD, DLB, and MSA (Boeve 2010). Indeed, PDRP expression is elevated in many RBD patients. However, in a longitudinal study of RBD subjects, those with low PDRP scores appeared more likely to phenoconvert to MSA, though this finding will need to be confirmed in larger cohorts and with inclusion of MSARP (Holtbernd et al. 2014).

26.2.3.4 Differential Diagnosis

As mentioned above, the diagnosis of PD and parkinsonian disorders can be challenging, especially early in the disease course. This uncertainty necessitates better diagnostic criteria, especially in the clinical trial setting when participant numbers may be small or subjects early in the diseases are being enrolled. In addition to providing unique information on disease progression, metabolic imaging and network analysis may be valuable in facilitating differential diagnosis in patients with APS.

Visual inspection of FDG PET images, aided by standard templates based on statistical parametric mapping, has typically been used to facilitate clinical diagnosis in patients with parkinsonism (Eckert et al. 2005) and is superior to DAT imaging, though the two measures may provide complementary information (Ko et al. 2017). In a study of 78 patients with APS, the area under the receiver-operating-characteristic (ROC) curve for discrimination between APS and Lewy body disease (PD and DLB) was significantly larger for FDG PET (0.94) than for IBZM SPECT (0.74; $p < 0.001$), with a sensitivity and specificity of 86% and 91%, respectively, for diagnosing APS with FDG PET (Hellwig et al. 2012). However, this approach may be difficult to scale due to the need for trained readers and does not yield quantifiable measures.

To automate the differential diagnosis procedure, a computerized algorithm was developed based on network analysis of FDG PET scans of 167 patients with uncertain parkinsonism who were referred for PET (Tang et al. 2010b). These patients were then followed by movement disorders specialists for over 2 years to obtain a final clinical diagnosis. For each patient, subject scores of different metabolic patterns related to PD, MSA, and PSP were computed and used to calculate the probability of each disease. The algorithm is a fully automated two-level classification procedure. At the first level, a logistic regression model was utilized to discriminate between the PD group and a combined group of MSA and PSP patients and to compute the probabilities of having PD and APS for each subject. At the second level, logistic regression analysis was also used to further discriminate MSA and PSP patients by computing the probabilities of these two diseases for each subject. At both levels, image-based classification was determined for individual patients based on each subject's disease probabilities with reference to the diagnostic criteria that were established from the ROC curve analysis of the probabilities of all subjects.

Finally, the image-based classifications of individual patients were compared to their follow-up clinical diagnosis. It was found that the image-based algorithm achieved highly accurate classification results (91–98% positive predictive value (PPV), 94–96% specificity, and 84–88% of sensitivity) for differential diagnosis of PD, MSA, and PSP. In addition, the classification results remained accurate in a subset of early patients with very short symptom durations (i.e., <2 years) at the time of PET as well as in a small subgroup of subjects whose clinical diagnoses were confirmed at autopsy.

This approach was recently validated in an independent cohort of 129 parkinsonian patients with uncertain diagnosis (Fig. 26.3) (Tripathi et al. 2016, 2012). Of

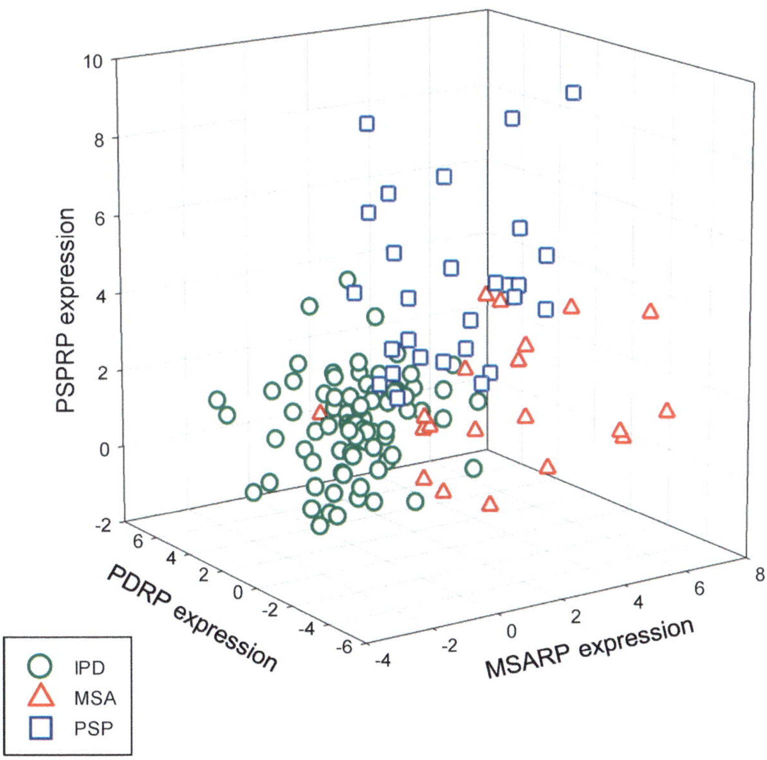

Fig. 26.3 Using network analysis for differential diagnosis. Three-dimensional plot of pattern expression. Expression values for PDRP (x-axis), MSARP (y-axis), and PSPRP (z-axis) topographies are shown for Indian validation cohort (Tripathi et al. 2016). This group comprised 129 parkinsonian patients with uncertain clinical diagnosis. On the basis of serial clinical examinations by movement disorders specialists blind to scan data, 81 of these subjects were subsequently diagnosed with idiopathic PD (IPD) and 48 subjects with APS (20 with MSA and 28 with PSP). Pattern expression values were computed in FDG PET scans from these subjects acquired 2.2 ± 0.4 years (mean ± SD) before final clinical diagnosis. (Reprinted from Tripathi M, Tang CC, Feigin A, De Lucia I, Nazem A, Dhawan V, Eidelberg D, Automated differential diagnosis of early parkinsonism using metabolic brain networks: A validation study, *J Nucl Med*, 2016, 57, pp. 60–66.)

these patients, 60% had disease duration of under 2 years. Nevertheless, idiopathic PD subjects were distinguished from APS with 94% specificity and 96% PPV. The algorithm achieved 90% specificity and 85% PPV for MSA and 94% specificity and 94% PPV for PSP. Diagnostic accuracy was similarly high (specificity and PPV > 90%) for parkinsonian subjects with short symptom duration, underlining the possible utility of this approach early in the disease course.

It is worthwhile to point out that in the study by Tang et al. (2010b), a small proportion (14%) of subjects could not be definitively classified as having either PD or APS and were classified into an indeterminate parkinsonism category. These indeterminate cases may not have developed sufficient metabolic abnormalities at the time of PET, thus requiring clinical follow-up to reach a definitive diagnosis, or they may have had other atypical parkinsonian syndromes such as CBD. Indeed, based on a small study, a similar approach can be used to distinguish patients with CBD from those with other APS (Niethammer et al. 2014). However, an additional step was required in this case. While increased PDRP and MSARP values are seen predominantly in their respective diseases, CBDRP and PSPRP are both abnormally elevated in both CBD and PSP cohorts (Ko et al. 2017; Niethammer et al. 2014). In order to differentiate the two diseases, the algorithm used expression of PSPRP, as well as an index of asymmetry in CBDRP expression. Of note, preliminary results did not find elevated CBDRP expression in patients with AD, which has a different tau pathology. To date, CBDRP has not been incorporated into the larger algorithm for PD and APS, and it is not clear which (if any) pattern would be elevated in patients with pathologically proven CBD who have a different clinical syndrome in life (Litvan et al. 1997; Hu et al. 2009; Boeve 2011; Hassan et al. 2011). Though these preliminary results are promising, this pattern was derived from a small group of patients and has not been validated in independent patient cohorts. Nonetheless, once a specific network for CBD is confirmed, it can be incorporated into the present automated algorithm for differential diagnosis of this disease.

Other automated methods for the differential diagnosis of PD and APS have been reported, such as relevance vector machine analysis (RVM) (Garraux et al. 2013) and decision trees applied to covariance patterns (Mudali et al. 2015), with promising results (Fig. 26.4). Using RVM on 120 FDG PET scans from patients with parkinsonism (42 PD, 31 MSA, 26 PSP, 21 CBD), classification sensitivity, specificity, and positive and negative predictive values for PD were 93%, 83%, 75%, and 96%, respectively, for distinguishing PD from APS (Garraux et al. 2013). Multiclass RVM achieved 45%, 55%, and 62% classification accuracy for, MSA, PSP, and CBS, respectively. The decision tree method employed by Mudali et al. on FDG PET scans from parkinsonian patients (20 PD, 21 MSA, 17 PSP) and 18 healthy controls was able to separate MSA and PSP relatively well from healthy controls, but PD less well from healthy controls (Mudali et al. 2015). Differentiation between the different parkinsonian syndromes was promising, but larger subject numbers are needed to further refine this approach. Likewise, prospective validation studies, preferably comparing multiple methods in larger cohorts, will be needed before the relative utility of these methods can be determined.

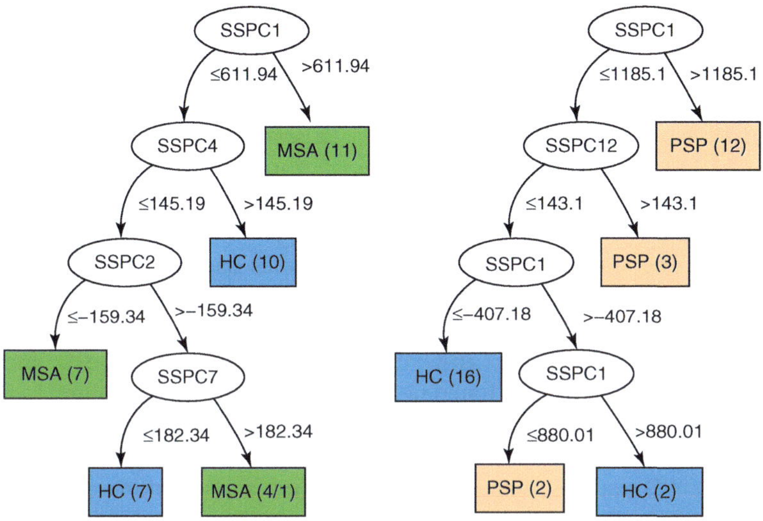

Fig. 26.4 Classification of APS using decision tree analysis. Example of discrimination tree applied to FDG PET scan between MSA subjects ($n = 21$) and healthy controls (HC, $n = 18$) (*left*) and between PSP ($n = 17$) and HC ($n = 18$) (*right*) (Mudali et al. 2015). The subject scores derived from 38 principal components are the attributes on which decisions are made and are represented as oval-shaped nodes in the tree. The threshold values used to split the dataset are shown next to the arrows. The leaf nodes are represented as rectangles and show the final class or decision made at that level of the tree. The numbers in the rectangles show the total number of cases classified at that leaf. Additionally, the number after the slash (if present) represents the number of misclassified cases at that leaf. (Reprinted from Mudali M, Teune LK, Renken RJ, Leenders KL, Roerdink JBTM, Classification of parkinsonian syndromes from FDG-PET brain data using decision trees with SSM/PCA features, *Comput Math Methods Med*, 2015, 136921.)

These data have demonstrated that the imaging classification approach based on disease-related metabolic networks can assist in accurate differential diagnosis for parkinsonian patients several years before a final diagnosis is made. Before its application to clinical cases, the automated differential diagnosis algorithm needs to be prospectively tested in independent patient populations with rigorously ascertained follow-up diagnosis in multicenter longitudinal studies. The algorithm may also prove useful as a screening test for the recruitment of participants in clinical trials for APS. The identification of misdiagnosed subjects and even "indeterminate" cases before enrollment provides a distinct advantage of the image-based classification procedure for identifying appropriate candidates in clinical studies.

26.2.4 Microglial Imaging

Neuropathological studies have demonstrated that neuroinflammation associated with increased microglial activation is present in PD (Imamura et al. 2003, 2005), MSA (Ishizawa et al. 2004), and PSP and CBD (Ishizawa and Dickson 2001), suggesting that activated microglia play a role in the pathogenesis of these neurodegenerative disorders. ^{11}C-(R)-PK11195 is a specific ligand for the mitochondrial translocator protein 18 kDa (TSPO, previously also known as the peripheral benzodiazepine binding site, PBBS) which is highly expressed in activated microglial cells (Papadopoulos et al. 2006). While specific for TSPO, ^{11}C-(R)-PK11195 exhibits low signal-to-noise ratio; accordingly, several newer TSPO radioligands with improved signal have been developed, including ^{11}C-PBR28, ^{11}C-DPA713, ^{18}F-FEPPA, and ^{11}C-DAA1106 (Venneti et al. 2006; Varnas et al. 2019). The majority of TSPO imaging studies have been performed in PD patients, though ^{11}C-(R)-PK11195 has been utilized to investigate microglial activation in APS.

In a 6-hydroxydopamine (6-OHDA)-induced PD rat model, increased ^{11}C-(R)-PK11195 binding was found in the substantia nigra and striatum, indicating marked microglial activation in these areas, further confirmed by postmortem immunohistochemical evidence of regional neuroinflammatory responses (Cicchetti et al. 2002). PD patients with established diagnosis also exhibited significantly increased ^{11}C-(R)-PK11195 binding in the basal ganglia, as well as in the pons and frontal/temporal cortical regions. The binding levels, however, were not correlated with clinical severity and remain stable over time (Gerhard et al. 2006a). Using a second-generation TSPO radioligand, ^{11}C-PBR28, Real and colleagues reported increased tracer uptake in the striatum 10 days after 6-OHDA injection, though this increase reversed by 30 days, perhaps suggesting that the microglial activation is an acute process accompanying nigral neurodegeneration (Real et al. 2019). In early drug-naïve PD patients, microglial activation in the midbrain has been found to be correlated with clinical severity and dopamine loss in the putamen (Ouchi et al. 2005). Likewise, in PD patients with and without dementia, ^{11}C-(R)-PK11195 binding correlates with lower cognitive scores and cortical metabolism (Edison et al. 2013; Fan et al. 2015).

It has been postulated that neuroinflammation with microglial activation contributes to the early neurodegenerative process of the disease and that, theoretically, early treatment with anti-inflammatory or neuroprotective drugs may be beneficial to patients with PD (Bartels and Leenders 2007). This hypothesis was explored in a small pilot study of ^{11}C-(R)-PK11195 PET imaging in five PD patients treated with celecoxib—a cyclooxygenase-2 (COX-2) inhibitor (Bartels et al. 2010). COX-2 inhibition did not result in significant posttreatment changes in the putamen and midbrain binding levels in this small sample, suggesting that the neuroinflammation is likely to be a persistent neuropathological process in PD that is not easily altered by the conventional anti-inflammatory therapy.

However, at least one study with ^{11}C-PBR28 of 16 PD patients could not demonstrate increased TSPO binding or any relationship between TSPO binding and DAT binding (Varnas et al. 2019). Indeed, studies with both ^{11}C-PBR28 and ^{18}F-FEPPA suggest that TSPO polymorphisms strongly influence ligand binding, which may affect the utility of these tracers as biomarkers in PD and parkinsonism (Ghadery et al. 2017; Koshimori et al. 2015; Owen et al. 2012; Mizrahi et al. 2012).

Only a small number of studies have focused on investigating neuroinflammatory changes with [11]C-(R)-PK11195 PET in APS patients. In MSA, compared to healthy controls, increased binding has been found in the substantia nigra, putamen, pallidum, pons, and dorsolateral prefrontal cortex in one study (Gerhard et al. 2003), with another reporting widespread increased binding in the caudate nucleus, putamen, pallidum, precentral gyrus, orbitofrontal cortex, pre-subgenual anterior cingulate cortex, and the superior parietal gyrus (Fig. 26.5) (Kubler et al. 2019). However, this increased binding did not correlate with clinical measures such as age, disease duration, motor scores, and Schwab and England Scale (Kubler et al. 2019). In a clinical trial on MSA patients treated with minocycline, a second-generation tetracycline that has anti-inflammatory effects, two of the three patients scanned with [11]C-(R)-PK11195 PET showed decreased binding at 24 weeks after the treatment, in contrast to a longitudinal increase in binding in the placebo group (Dodel et al. 2010).

Increased binding and microglial activation was also evident in the basal ganglia and cortical/subcortical regions in patients with PSP (Gerhard et al. 2006b) or CBD

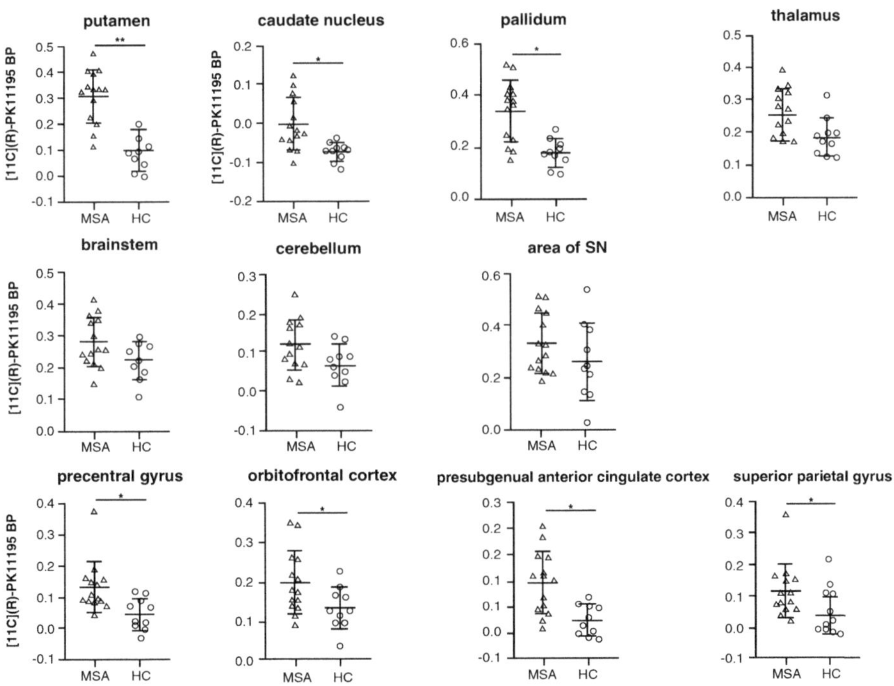

Fig. 26.5 Microglial activation in multiple system atrophy. Comparison of [11]C-(R)-PK11195 binding potential (BP) values of MSA patients (n = 14) and healthy controls (HC, n = 10) in selected volumes of interest (VOI) (Kubler et al. 2019). Horizontal bars indicate mean and standard deviation. $^{*}p < 0.01$, $^{**}p \leq 0.001$ (Reprinted from Kubler D, Wachter T, Cabanel N, Su Z, Turkheimer FE, Dodel R, Brooks DJ, Oertel WH, Gerhard A, Widespread microglial activation in multiple system atrophy, *Mov Disord*, 2019, 34, pp. 564–568.)

(Gerhard et al. 2004; Henkel et al. 2004), in accordance with the neuropathological changes in these disorders. In a study of patients with Alzheimer's disease (AD) or PSP, Passamonti et al. found increased ^{11}C-(R)-PK11195 binding in the medial temporal lobe and occipital, temporal, and parietal cortices in AD patients, relative both to patients with PSP and to controls (Passamonti et al. 2018). In PSP patients, compared to controls, there was elevated ^{11}C-(R)-PK11195 binding in the thalamus, putamen, and pallidum. ^{11}C-(R)-PK11195 binding in the cuneus/precuneus correlated with episodic memory impairment in AD, while ^{11}C-(R)-PK11195 binding in the pallidum, midbrain, and pons correlated with disease severity in PSP.

Kobylecki and colleagues studied the relation between microglial activation (measured by ^{11}C-(R)-PK11195 binding) and regional microstructural changes (measured by regional apparent diffusion coefficient, rADC) in patients with PD or APS (MSA and PSP) (Kobylecki et al. 2013). In APS, ^{11}C-(R)-PK11195 binding correlated with rADC in the pons, but not the basal ganglia, suggesting the microglial activation does not contribute to microstructural damage in all regions.

These findings, though based on studies of small patient cohorts, support the notion that neuroinflammation and associated microglial activation contribute to the pathogenesis of APS, regardless of the underlying pathology. Large-scale studies on APS patients and healthy controls are needed to confirm these results and, importantly, examine the relationship between changes in microglial activation and disease progression. Whether anti-inflammatory therapy is an effective strategy for APS is also a topic of further investigation.

26.3 Future Directions

In this chapter, we have briefly reviewed recent advances in SPECT and PET imaging in the study of the progression and differential diagnosis of APS. We discussed the use of various presynaptic and postsynaptic radioligands with SPECT in the research of MSA, PSP, and CBD, as well as the latest FDG PET findings of brain metabolic networks associated with these disorders. A distinct advantage of network analysis over conventional imaging analytical techniques, such as group-mean-based statistical parametric mapping analysis, is its prospective application on individual subjects. That is, once a disease-specific pattern has been identified and validated, the expression of this pattern in a given subject can be computed prospectively from that individual's scan. The resulting pattern expression values for individual subjects can be used to discriminate between groups, assess the progression of the disease, or correlate with other measures/biomarkers in cross-sectional or longitudinal datasets (Eidelberg 2009; Schindlbeck and Eidelberg 2018).

Although the disease-specific patterns identified were derived originally from FDG PET scans using spatial covariance analysis, the application of these patterns is not limited to metabolic imaging. Eckert et al. have demonstrated that the expression of the disease-related metabolic pattern (i.e., PDRP) derived from FDG PET scans can be quantified prospectively in ECD SPECT or early phase CIT SPECT images (Jin et al. 2017; Eckert et al. 2007). This proof-of-principle study indicates that network analysis can be applied to SPECT scans of parkinsonian patients and that the disease-related brain networks represent the underlying pathology of respective disorders rather than the imaging modality per se. Thus, it is conceivable that spatial covariance analysis may be utilized in future SPECT imaging studies to identify abnormal functional networks specific to each parkinsonian disorder.

For differential diagnosis of APS, we focused on the development and application of an automated algorithm integrating multiple disease-related networks for accurate classification of individual patients with PD, MSA, or PSP at early disease stages when the clinical diagnosis is still uncertain. This algorithm for differential diagnosis can be further developed to include other less common APS, such as CBD, after the disease-related patterns for these disorders are validated. Needless to say, this method may have a profound impact on the research of parkinsonism as it can be used as an objective screening tool that, in addition to improving clinical diagnosis, can identify ideal candidates in clinical trials of APS. It may also help general neurologists and even the specialists to achieve higher accuracy in recognizing and diagnosing APS in routine clinical practice.

References

Albrecht F, Bisenius S, Morales Schaack R, Neumann J, Schroeter ML (2017) Disentangling the neural correlates of corticobasal syndrome and corticobasal degeneration with systematic and quantitative ALE meta-analyses. NPJ Parkinsons Dis 3:12

Albrecht F, Bisenius S, Neumann J, Whitwell J, Schroeter ML (2019) Atrophy in midbrain & cerebral/cerebellar pedunculi is characteristic for progressive supranuclear palsy – a double-validation whole-brain meta-analysis. Neuroimage Clin 22:101722

Armstrong MJ, Litvan I, Lang AE, Bak TH, Bhatia KP, Borroni B et al (2013) Criteria for the diagnosis of corticobasal degeneration. Neurology 80(5):496–503

Asanuma K, Tang C, Ma Y, Dhawan V, Mattis P, Edwards C et al (2006) Network modulation in the treatment of Parkinson's disease. Brain 129(Pt 10):2667–2678

Badoud S, Van De Ville D, Nicastro N, Garibotto V, Burkhard PR, Haller S (2016) Discriminating among degenerative parkinsonisms using advanced (123)I-ioflupane SPECT analyses. Neuroimage Clin 12:234–240

Bajaj N, Hauser RA, Grachev ID (2013) Clinical utility of dopamine transporter single photon emission CT (DaT-SPECT) with (123I) ioflupane in diagnosis of parkinsonian syndromes. J Neurol Neurosurg Psychiatry 84(11):1288–1295

Bartels AL, Leenders KL (2007) Neuroinflammation in the pathophysiology of Parkinson's disease: evidence from animal models to human in vivo studies with [11C]-PK11195 PET. Mov Disord 22(13):1852–1856

Bartels AL, de Jong BM, Giladi N, Schaafsma JD, Maguire RP, Veenma L et al (2006) Striatal dopa and glucose metabolism in PD patients with freezing of gait. Mov Disord 21(9):1326–1332

Bartels AL, Willemsen AT, Doorduin J, de Vries EF, Dierckx RA, Leenders KL (2010) [11C]-PK11195 PET: quantification of neuroinflammation and a monitor of anti-inflammatory treatment in Parkinson's disease? Parkinsonism Relat Disord 16(1):57–59

Behnke S, Berg D, Naumann M, Becker G (2005) Differentiation of Parkinson's disease and atypical parkinsonian syndromes by transcranial ultrasound. J Neurol Neurosurg Psychiatry 76(3):423–425

Benamer H, Grosset D (2009) Vascular parkinsonism: a clinical review. Eur Neurol 61(1):11–15

Benamer HT, Patterson J, Wyper DJ, Hadley DM, Macphee GJ, Grosset DG (2000) Correlation of Parkinson's disease severity and duration with 123I-FP-CIT SPECT striatal uptake. Mov Disord 15(4):692–698

Benamer HT, Oertel WH, Patterson J, Hadley DM, Pogarell O, Hoffken H et al (2003) Prospective study of presynaptic dopaminergic imaging in patients with mild parkinsonism and tremor disorders: part 1. Baseline and 3-month observations. Mov Disord 18(9):977–984

Berg D, Siefker C, Becker G (2001) Echogenicity of the substantia nigra in Parkinson's disease and its relation to clinical findings. J Neurol 248(8):684–689

Berg D, Seppi K, Behnke S, Liepelt I, Schweitzer K, Stockner H et al (2011) Enlarged substantia nigra hyperechogenicity and risk for Parkinson disease: a 37-month 3-center study of 1847 older persons. Arch Neurol 68(7):932–937

Berg D, Postuma RB, Adler CH, Bloem BR, Chan P, Dubois B et al (2015) MDS research criteria for prodromal Parkinson's disease. Mov Disord 30(12):1600–1611

Boeve BF (2010) REM sleep behavior disorder: updated review of the core features, the REM sleep behavior disorder-neurodegenerative disease association, evolving concepts, controversies, and future directions. Ann N Y Acad Sci 1184:15–54

Boeve BF (2011) The multiple phenotypes of corticobasal syndrome and corticobasal degeneration: implications for further study. J Mol Neurosci 45(3):350–353

Boeve BF, Lang AE, Litvan I (2003) Corticobasal degeneration and its relationship to progressive supranuclear palsy and frontotemporal dementia. Ann Neurol 54(Suppl 5):S15–S19

Bosman T, Van Laere K, Santens P (2003) Anatomically standardised 99mTc-ECD brain perfusion SPET allows accurate differentiation between healthy volunteers, multiple system atrophy and idiopathic Parkinson's disease. Eur J Nucl Med Mol Imaging 30(1):16–24

Ceravolo R, Rossi C, Cilia R, Tognoni G, Antonini A, Volterrani D et al (2013) Evidence of delayed nigrostriatal dysfunction in corticobasal syndrome: a SPECT follow-up study. Parkinsonism Relat Disord 19(5):557–559

Cicchetti F, Brownell AL, Williams K, Chen YI, Livni E, Isacson O (2002) Neuroinflammation of the nigrostriatal pathway during progressive 6-OHDA dopamine degeneration in rats monitored by immunohistochemistry and PET imaging. Eur J Neurosci 15(6):991–998

Dickson DW, Rademakers R, Hutton ML (2007) Progressive supranuclear palsy: pathology and genetics. Brain Pathol 17(1):74–82

Dodel R, Spottke A, Gerhard A, Reuss A, Reinecker S, Schimke N et al (2010) Minocycline 1-year therapy in multiple-system-atrophy: effect on clinical symptoms and [(11)C] (R)-PK11195 PET (MEMSA-trial). Mov Disord 25(1):97–107

Eckert T, Barnes A, Dhawan V, Frucht S, Gordon MF, Feigin AS et al (2005) FDG PET in the differential diagnosis of parkinsonian disorders. NeuroImage 26(3):912–921

Eckert T, Van Laere K, Tang C, Lewis DE, Edwards C, Santens P et al (2007) Quantification of Parkinson's disease-related network expression with ECD SPECT. Eur J Nucl Med Mol Imaging 34(4):496–501

Eckert T, Tang C, Ma Y, Brown N, Lin T, Frucht S et al (2008) Abnormal metabolic networks in atypical parkinsonism. Mov Disord 23(5):727–733

Edison P, Ahmed I, Fan Z, Hinz R, Gelosa G, Ray Chaudhuri K et al (2013) Microglia, amyloid, and glucose metabolism in Parkinson's disease with and without dementia. Neuropsychopharmacology 38(6):938–949

Eidelberg D (2009) Metabolic brain networks in neurodegenerative disorders: a functional imaging approach. Trends Neurosci 32(10):548–557

Eidelberg D, Takikawa S, Moeller JR, Dhawan V, Redington K, Chaly T et al (1993) Striatal hypometabolism distinguishes striatonigral degeneration from Parkinson's disease. Ann Neurol 33(5):518–527

Eidelberg D, Moeller J, Dhawan V, Spetsieris P, Takikawa S, Ishikawa T et al (1994) The metabolic topography of parkinsonism. J Cereb Blood Flow Metab 14(5):783–801

Eidelberg D, Moeller JR, Ishikawa T, Dhawan V, Spetsieris P, Chaly T et al (1995) Assessment of disease severity in parkinsonism with fluorine-18-fluorodeoxyglucose and PET. J Nucl Med 36(3):378–383

El Fakhri G, Ouyang J (2011) Dual-radionuclide brain SPECT for the differential diagnosis of parkinsonism. Methods Mol Biol 680:237–246
El Fakhri G, Habert MO, Maksud P, Kas A, Malek Z, Kijewski MF et al (2006) Quantitative simultaneous (99m)Tc-ECD/123I-FP-CIT SPECT in Parkinson's disease and multiple system atrophy. Eur J Nucl Med Mol Imaging 33(1):87–92
Eshuis SA, Maguire RP, Leenders KL, Jonkman S, Jager PL (2006) Comparison of FP-CIT SPECT with F-DOPA PET in patients with de novo and advanced Parkinson's disease. Eur J Nucl Med Mol Imaging 33(2):200–209
Eshuis SA, Jager PL, Maguire RP, Jonkman S, Dierckx RA, Leenders KL (2009) Direct comparison of FP-CIT SPECT and F-DOPA PET in patients with Parkinson's disease and healthy controls. Eur J Nucl Med Mol Imaging 36(3):454–462
Fan Z, Aman Y, Ahmed I, Chetelat G, Landeau B, Ray Chaudhuri K et al (2015) Influence of microglial activation on neuronal function in Alzheimer's and Parkinson's disease dementia. Alzheimers Dement 11(6):608–21.e7
Feigin A, Tang C, Ma Y, Mattis P, Zgaljardic D, Guttman M et al (2007) Thalamic metabolism and symptom onset in preclinical Huntington's disease. Brain 130(Pt 11):2858–2867
Gaenslen A, Unmuth B, Godau J, Liepelt I, Di Santo A, Schweitzer KJ et al (2008) The specificity and sensitivity of transcranial ultrasound in the differential diagnosis of Parkinson's disease: a prospective blinded study. Lancet Neurol 7(5):417–424
Garraux G, Phillips C, Schrouff J, Kreisler A, Lemaire C, Degueldre C et al (2013) Multiclass classification of FDG PET scans for the distinction between Parkinson's disease and atypical parkinsonian syndromes. Neuroimage Clin 2:883–893
Ge J, Wu J, Peng S, Wu P, Wang J, Zhang H et al (2018) Reproducible network and regional topographies of abnormal glucose metabolism associated with progressive supranuclear palsy: multivariate and univariate analyses in American and Chinese patient cohorts. Hum Brain Mapp 39(7):2842–2858
Gerhard A, Banati RB, Goerres GB, Cagnin A, Myers R, Gunn RN et al (2003) [11C](R)-PK11195 PET imaging of microglial activation in multiple system atrophy. Neurology 61(5):686–689
Gerhard A, Watts J, Trender-Gerhard I, Turkheimer F, Banati RB, Bhatia K et al (2004) In vivo imaging of microglial activation with [11C](R)-PK11195 PET in corticobasal degeneration. Mov Disord 19(10):1221–1226
Gerhard A, Pavese N, Hotton G, Turkheimer F, Es M, Hammers A et al (2006a) In vivo imaging of microglial activation with [11C](R)-PK11195 PET in idiopathic Parkinson's disease. Neurobiol Dis 21(2):404–412
Gerhard A, Trender-Gerhard I, Turkheimer F, Quinn NP, Bhatia KP, Brooks DJ (2006b) In vivo imaging of microglial activation with [11C](R)-PK11195 PET in progressive supranuclear palsy. Mov Disord 21(1):89–93
Gerschlager W, Bencsits G, Pirker W, Bloem BR, Asenbaum S, Prayer D et al (2002) [123I]beta-CIT SPECT distinguishes vascular parkinsonism from Parkinson's disease. Mov Disord 17(3):518–523
Ghadery C, Koshimori Y, Coakeley S, Harris M, Rusjan P, Kim J et al (2017) Microglial activation in Parkinson's disease using [(18)F]-FEPPA. J Neuroinflammation 14(1):8
Ghaemi M, Hilker R, Rudolf J, Sobesky J, Heiss WD (2002) Differentiating multiple system atrophy from Parkinson's disease: contribution of striatal and midbrain MRI volumetry and multi-tracer PET imaging. J Neurol Neurosurg Psychiatry 73(5):517–523
Gilman S, Wenning G, Low P, Brooks D, Mathias C, Trojanowski J et al (2008) Second consensus statement on the diagnosis of multiple system atrophy. Neurology 71(9):670–676
Habeck C, Foster N, Perneczky R, Kurz A, Alexopoulos P, Koeppe R et al (2008) Multivariate and univariate neuroimaging biomarkers of Alzheimer's disease. NeuroImage 40(4):1503–1515
Hassan A, Whitwell JL, Josephs KA (2011) The corticobasal syndrome-Alzheimer's disease conundrum. Expert Rev Neurother 11(11):1569–1578
Heim B, Krismer F, Seppi K (2018) Structural imaging in atypical parkinsonism. Int Rev Neurobiol 142:67–148

Hellwig S, Amtage F, Kreft A, Buchert R, Winz OH, Vach W et al (2012) [(1)(8)F]FDG-PET is superior to [(1)(2)(3)I]IBZM-SPECT for the differential diagnosis of parkinsonism. Neurology 79(13):1314–1322

Henkel K, Karitzky J, Schmid M, Mader I, Glatting G, Unger JW et al (2004) Imaging of activated microglia with PET and [11C]PK 11195 in corticobasal degeneration. Mov Disord 19(7):817–821

Hoglinger GU, Respondek G, Stamelou M, Kurz C, Josephs KA, Lang AE et al (2017) Clinical diagnosis of progressive supranuclear palsy: the movement disorder society criteria. Mov Disord 32(6):853–864

Holtbernd F, Eidelberg D (2014) The utility of neuroimaging in the differential diagnosis of parkinsonian syndromes. Semin Neurol 34(2):202–209

Holtbernd F, Gagnon JF, Postuma RB, Ma Y, Tang CC, Feigin A et al (2014) Abnormal metabolic network activity in REM sleep behavior disorder. Neurology 82(7):620–627

Holtbernd F, Ma Y, Peng S, Schwartz F, Timmermann L, Kracht L et al (2015) Dopaminergic correlates of metabolic network activity in Parkinson's disease. Hum Brain Mapp 36(9):3575–3585

Hu WT, Rippon GW, Boeve BF, Knopman DS, Petersen RC, Parisi JE et al (2009) Alzheimer's disease and corticobasal degeneration presenting as corticobasal syndrome. Mov Disord 24(9):1375–1379

Huang C, Mattis P, Tang C, Perrine K, Carbon M, Eidelberg D (2007) Metabolic brain networks associated with cognitive function in Parkinson's disease. NeuroImage 34(2):714–723

Huang C, Mattis P, Perrine K, Brown N, Dhawan V, Eidelberg D (2008) Metabolic abnormalities associated with mild cognitive impairment in Parkinson disease. Neurology 70(16 Pt 2):1470–1477

Hughes A, Daniel S, Ben-Shlomo Y, Lees A (2002) The accuracy of diagnosis of parkinsonian syndromes in a specialist movement disorder service. Brain 125(Pt 4):861–870

Ichise M, Kim YJ, Ballinger JR, Vines D, Erami SS, Tanaka F et al (1999) SPECT imaging of pre- and postsynaptic dopaminergic alterations in L-dopa-untreated PD. Neurology 52(6):1206–1214

Imamura K, Hishikawa N, Sawada M, Nagatsu T, Yoshida M, Hashizume Y (2003) Distribution of major histocompatibility complex class II-positive microglia and cytokine profile of Parkinson's disease brains. Acta Neuropathol 106(6):518–526

Imamura K, Hishikawa N, Ono K, Suzuki H, Sawada M, Nagatsu T et al (2005) Cytokine production of activated microglia and decrease in neurotrophic factors of neurons in the hippocampus of Lewy body disease brains. Acta Neuropathol 109(2):141–150

Ishizawa K, Dickson DW (2001) Microglial activation parallels system degeneration in progressive supranuclear palsy and corticobasal degeneration. J Neuropathol Exp Neurol 60(6):647–657

Ishizawa K, Komori T, Sasaki S, Arai N, Mizutani T, Hirose T (2004) Microglial activation parallels system degeneration in multiple system atrophy. J Neuropathol Exp Neurol 63(1):43–52

Jesse S, Kassubek J, Muller HP, Ludolph AC, Unrath A (2012) Signal alterations of the basal ganglia in the differential diagnosis of Parkinson's disease: a retrospective case-controlled MRI data bank analysis. BMC Neurol 12:163

Jin S, Oh M, Oh SJ, Oh JS, Lee SJ, Chung SJ et al (2017) Additional value of early-phase 18F-FP-CIT PET image for differential diagnosis of atypical parkinsonism. Clin Nucl Med 42(2):e80–ee7

Joling M, Vriend C, van den Heuvel OA, Raijmakers P, Jones PA, Berendse HW et al (2017) Analysis of extrastriatal (123)I-FP-CIT binding contributes to the differential diagnosis of parkinsonian diseases. J Nucl Med 58(7):1117–1123

Josephs K, Dickson D (2003) Diagnostic accuracy of progressive supranuclear palsy in the Society for Progressive Supranuclear Palsy brain bank. Mov Disord 18(9):1018–1026

Kaasinen V, Ruottinen HM, Nagren K, Lehikoinen P, Oikonen V, Rinne JO (2000) Upregulation of putaminal dopamine D2 receptors in early Parkinson's disease: a comparative PET study with [11C] raclopride and [11C]N-methylspiperone. J Nucl Med 41(1):65–70

Kanazawa M, Shimohata T, Terajima K, Onodera O, Tanaka K, Tsuji S et al (2004) Quantitative evaluation of brainstem involvement in multiple system atrophy by diffusion-weighted MR imaging. J Neurol 251(9):1121–1124
Kim YJ, Ichise M, Ballinger JR, Vines D, Erami SS, Tatschida T et al (2002) Combination of dopamine transporter and D2 receptor SPECT in the diagnostic evaluation of PD, MSA, and PSP. Mov Disord 17(2):303–312
Klaffke S, Kuhn AA, Plotkin M, Amthauer H, Harnack D, Felix R et al (2006) Dopamine transporters, D2 receptors, and glucose metabolism in corticobasal degeneration. Mov Disord 21(10):1724–1727
Knudsen GM, Karlsborg M, Thomsen G, Krabbe K, Regeur L, Nygaard T et al (2004) Imaging of dopamine transporters and D2 receptors in patients with Parkinson's disease and multiple system atrophy. Eur J Nucl Med Mol Imaging 31(12):1631–1638
Ko JH, Lee CS, Eidelberg D (2017) Metabolic network expression in parkinsonism: clinical and dopaminergic correlations. J Cereb Blood Flow Metab 37(2):683–693
Kobylecki C, Counsell SJ, Cabanel N, Wachter T, Turkheimer FE, Eggert K et al (2013) Diffusion-weighted imaging and its relationship to microglial activation in parkinsonian syndromes. Parkinsonism Relat Disord 19(5):527–532
Koeppe RA, Gilman S, Joshi A, Liu S, Little R, Junck L et al (2005) 11C-DTBZ and 18F-FDG PET measures in differentiating dementias. J Nucl Med 46(6):936–944
Koshimori Y, Ko JH, Mizrahi R, Rusjan P, Mabrouk R, Jacobs MF et al (2015) Imaging striatal microglial activation in patients with Parkinson's disease. PLoS One 10(9):e0138721
Kubler D, Wachter T, Cabanel N, Su Z, Turkheimer FE, Dodel R et al (2019) Widespread microglial activation in multiple system atrophy. Mov Disord 34(4):564–568
Leenders KL (2003) Significance of non-presynaptic SPECT tracer methods in Parkinson's disease. Mov Disord 18(Suppl 7):S39–S42
Linder J, Birgander R, Olsson I, Riklund K, Larsson A, Edstrom M et al (2009) Degenerative changes were common in brain magnetic resonance imaging in patients with newly diagnosed Parkinson's disease in a population-based cohort. J Neurol 256(10):1671–1680
Litvan I (2003) Update on epidemiological aspects of progressive supranuclear palsy. Mov Disord 18(Suppl 6):S43–S50
Litvan I, Agid Y, Goetz C, Jankovic J, Wenning GK, Brandel JP et al (1997) Accuracy of the clinical diagnosis of corticobasal degeneration: a clinicopathologic study. Neurology 48(1):119–125
Lozza C, Baron JC, Eidelberg D, Mentis MJ, Carbon M, Marie RM (2004) Executive processes in Parkinson's disease: FDG-PET and network analysis. Hum Brain Mapp 22(3):236–245
Ma Y, Feigin A, Okulski J, Dhawan V, Chaly T, Eidelberg D (2003) Implementation of atrophy correction in metabolic mapping studies of presymptomatic Huntington's disease. J Cereb Blood Flow Metab 2003:S629
Ma Y, Tang C, Spetsieris P, Dhawan V, Eidelberg D (2007) Abnormal metabolic network activity in Parkinson's disease: test-retest reproducibility. J Cereb Blood Flow Metab 27(3):597–605
Mahapatra RK, Edwards MJ, Schott JM, Bhatia KP (2004) Corticobasal degeneration. Lancet Neurol 3(12):736–743
Marshall VL, Reininger CB, Marquardt M, Patterson J, Hadley DM, Oertel WH et al (2009) Parkinson's disease is overdiagnosed clinically at baseline in diagnostically uncertain cases: a 3-year European multicenter study with repeat [123I]FP-CIT SPECT. Mov Disord 24(4):500–508
Mattis PJ, Niethammer M, Sako W, Tang CC, Nazem A, Gordon ML et al (2016) Distinct brain networks underlie cognitive dysfunction in Parkinson and Alzheimer diseases. Neurology 87(18):1925–1933
Minnerop M, Specht K, Ruhlmann J, Schimke N, Abele M, Weyer A et al (2007) Voxel-based morphometry and voxel-based relaxometry in multiple system atrophy-a comparison between clinical subtypes and correlations with clinical parameters. NeuroImage 36(4):1086–1095
Mizrahi R, Rusjan PM, Kennedy J, Pollock B, Mulsant B, Suridjan I et al (2012) Translocator protein (18 kDa) polymorphism (rs6971) explains in-vivo brain binding affinity of the PET radioligand [(18)F]-FEPPA. J Cereb Blood Flow Metab 32(6):968–972

Mudali D, Teune LK, Renken RJ, Leenders KL, Roerdink JB (2015) Classification of Parkinsonian syndromes from FDG-PET brain data using decision trees with SSM/PCA features. Comput Math Methods Med 2015:136921

Mueller C, Hussl A, Krismer F, Heim B, Mahlknecht P, Nocker M et al (2018) The diagnostic accuracy of the hummingbird and morning glory sign in patients with neurodegenerative parkinsonism. Parkinsonism Relat Disord 54:90–94

Mure H, Hirano S, Tang CC, Isaias IU, Antonini A, Ma Y et al (2011) Parkinson's disease tremor-related metabolic network: characterization, progression, and treatment effects. NeuroImage 54(2):1244–1253

Nicastro N, Wegrzyk J, Preti MG, Fleury V, Van de Ville D, Garibotto V et al (2019) Classification of degenerative parkinsonism subtypes by support-vector-machine analysis and striatal (123) I-FP-CIT indices. J Neurol 266(7):1771–1781

Nicoletti G, Lodi R, Condino F, Tonon C, Fera F, Malucelli E et al (2006) Apparent diffusion coefficient measurements of the middle cerebellar peduncle differentiate the Parkinson variant of MSA from Parkinson's disease and progressive supranuclear palsy. Brain 129(Pt 10):2679–2687

Niethammer M, Eidelberg D (2012) Metabolic brain networks in translational neurology: concepts and applications. Ann Neurol 72(5):635–647

Niethammer M, Feigin A, Eidelberg D (2012) Functional neuroimaging in Parkinson's disease. Cold Spring Harb Perspect Med 2(5):a009274

Niethammer M, Tang CC, Feigin A, Allen PJ, Heinen L, Hellwig S et al (2014) A disease-specific metabolic brain network associated with corticobasal degeneration. Brain 137(Pt 11):3036–3046

O'Sullivan SS, Burn DJ, Holton JL, Lees AJ (2008) Normal dopamine transporter single photon-emission CT scan in corticobasal degeneration. Mov Disord 23(16):2424–2426

Ouchi Y, Yoshikawa E, Sekine Y, Futatsubashi M, Kanno T, Ogusu T et al (2005) Microglial activation and dopamine terminal loss in early Parkinson's disease. Ann Neurol 57(2):168–175

Owen DR, Yeo AJ, Gunn RN, Song K, Wadsworth G, Lewis A et al (2012) An 18-kDa translocator protein (TSPO) polymorphism explains differences in binding affinity of the PET radioligand PBR28. J Cereb Blood Flow Metab 32(1):1–5

Papadopoulos V, Baraldi M, Guilarte TR, Knudsen TB, Lacapere JJ, Lindemann P et al (2006) Translocator protein (18kDa): new nomenclature for the peripheral-type benzodiazepine receptor based on its structure and molecular function. Trends Pharmacol Sci 27(8):402–409

Papp M, Kahn J, Lantos P (1989) Glial cytoplasmic inclusions in the CNS of patients with multiple system atrophy (striatonigral degeneration, olivopontocerebellar atrophy and Shy-Drager syndrome). J Neurol Sci 94(1–3):79–100

Park HK, Kim JS, Im KC, Oh SJ, Kim MJ, Lee JH et al (2009) Functional brain imaging in pure akinesia with gait freezing: [18F] FDG PET and [18F] FP-CIT PET analyses. Mov Disord 24(2):237–245

Passamonti L, Rodriguez PV, Hong YT, Allinson KSJ, Bevan-Jones WR, Williamson D et al (2018) [(11)C]PK11195 binding in Alzheimer disease and progressive supranuclear palsy. Neurology 90(22):e1989–e1e96

Paviour D, Price S, Stevens J, Lees A, Fox N (2005) Quantitative MRI measurement of superior cerebellar peduncle in progressive supranuclear palsy. Neurology 64(4):675–679

Paviour DC, Price SL, Jahanshahi M, Lees AJ, Fox NC (2006) Regional brain volumes distinguish PSP, MSA-P, and PD: MRI-based clinico-radiological correlations. Mov Disord 21(7):989–996

Paviour DC, Thornton JS, Lees AJ, Jager HR (2007) Diffusion-weighted magnetic resonance imaging differentiates Parkinsonian variant of multiple-system atrophy from progressive supranuclear palsy. Mov Disord 22(1):68–74

Perju-Dumbrava LD, Kovacs GG, Pirker S, Jellinger K, Hoffmann M, Asenbaum S et al (2012) Dopamine transporter imaging in autopsy-confirmed Parkinson's disease and multiple system atrophy. Mov Disord 27(1):65–71

Pirker W, Asenbaum S, Bencsits G, Prayer D, Gerschlager W, Deecke L et al (2000) [123I]beta-CIT SPECT in multiple system atrophy, progressive supranuclear palsy, and corticobasal degeneration. Mov Disord 15(6):1158–1167

Pirker W, Djamshidian S, Asenbaum S, Gerschlager W, Tribl G, Hoffmann M et al (2002) Progression of dopaminergic degeneration in Parkinson's disease and atypical parkinsonism: a longitudinal beta-CIT SPECT study. Mov Disord 17(1):45–53

Plotkin M, Amthauer H, Klaffke S, Kuhn A, Ludemann L, Arnold G et al (2005) Combined 123I-FP-CIT and 123I-IBZM SPECT for the diagnosis of parkinsonian syndromes: study on 72 patients. J Neural Transm (Vienna) 112(5):677–692

Poston KL (2010) Overview of rare movement disorders. Continuum (Minneap Minn) 16(1 Movement Disorders):49–76

Poston KL, Eidelberg D (2009) Network biomarkers for the diagnosis and treatment of movement disorders. Neurobiol Dis 35(2):141–147

Poston K, Tang C, Eckert T, Dhawan V, Frucht S, Vonsattel J et al (2012) Network correlates of disease severity in multiple system atrophy. Neurology 78(16):1237–1244

Postuma RB, Gagnon JF, Montplaisir JY (2012) REM sleep behavior disorder: from dreams to neurodegeneration. Neurobiol Dis 46:553–558

Postuma RB, Berg D, Stern M, Poewe W, Olanow CW, Oertel W et al (2015) MDS clinical diagnostic criteria for Parkinson's disease. Mov Disord 30(12):1591–1601

Pourfar M, Tang C, Lin T, Dhawan V, Kaplitt MG, Eidelberg D (2009) Assessing the microlesion effect of subthalamic deep brain stimulation surgery with FDG PET. J Neurosurg 110(6):1278–1282

Quattrone A, Nicoletti G, Messina D, Fera F, Condino F, Pugliese P et al (2008) MR imaging index for differentiation of progressive supranuclear palsy from Parkinson disease and the Parkinson variant of multiple system atrophy. Radiology 246(1):214–221

Real CC, Doorduin J, Kopschina Feltes P, Vallez Garcia D, de Paula FD, Britto LR et al (2019) Evaluation of exercise-induced modulation of glial activation and dopaminergic damage in a rat model of Parkinson's disease using [(11)C]PBR28 and [(18)F]FDOPA PET. J Cereb Blood Flow Metab 39(6):989–1004

Richter D, Woitalla D, Muhlack S, Gold R, Tonges L, Krogias C (2017) Coronal transcranial sonography and M-mode tremor frequency determination in Parkinson's disease and essential tremor. J Neuroimaging 27(5):524–530

Rizzo G, Copetti M, Arcuti S, Martino D, Fontana A, Logroscino G (2016) Accuracy of clinical diagnosis of Parkinson disease: a systematic review and meta-analysis. Neurology 86(6):566–576

Sako W, Abe T, Haji S, Murakami N, Osaki Y, Izumi Y et al (2019) "One line": a method for differential diagnosis of parkinsonian syndromes. Acta Neurol Scand 140(3):229–235

Scherfler C, Seppi K, Donnemiller E, Goebel G, Brenneis C, Virgolini I et al (2005) Voxel-wise analysis of [123I]beta-CIT SPECT differentiates the Parkinson variant of multiple system atrophy from idiopathic Parkinson's disease. Brain 128(Pt 7):1605–1612

Schindlbeck KA, Eidelberg D (2018) Network imaging biomarkers: insights and clinical applications in Parkinson's disease. Lancet Neurol 17(7):629–640

Schott J, Williams D, Butterworth R, Janssen J, Larner A, Holton J et al (2007) Shunt responsive progressive supranuclear palsy? Mov Disord 22(6):902–903

Seppi K, Schocke M (2005) An update on conventional and advanced magnetic resonance imaging techniques in the differential diagnosis of neurodegenerative parkinsonism. Curr Opin Neurol 18(4):370–375

Soliveri P, Monza D, Paridi D, Radice D, Grisoli M, Testa D et al (1999) Cognitive and magnetic resonance imaging aspects of corticobasal degeneration and progressive supranuclear palsy. Neurology 53(3):502–507

Spetsieris P, Ma Y, Dhawan V, Eidelberg D (2009) Differential diagnosis of parkinsonian syndromes using PCA-based functional imaging features. NeuroImage 45(4):1241–1252

Spetsieris P, Ma Y, Peng S, Ko JH, Dhawan V, Tang CC et al (2013) Identification of disease-related spatial covariance patterns using neuroimaging data. J Vis Exp 76:e50319

Spiegel J, Mollers MO, Jost WH, Fuss G, Samnick S, Dillmann U et al (2005) FP-CIT and MIBG scintigraphy in early Parkinson's disease. Mov Disord 20(5):552–561

Sudmeyer M, Antke C, Zizek T, Beu M, Nikolaus S, Wojtecki L et al (2011) Diagnostic accuracy of combined FP-CIT, IBZM, and MIBG scintigraphy in the differential diagnosis of degenerative parkinsonism: a multidimensional statistical approach. J Nucl Med 52(5):733–740

Tang CC, Poston KL, Dhawan V, Eidelberg D (2010a) Abnormalities in metabolic network activity precede the onset of motor symptoms in Parkinson's disease. J Neurosci 30(3):1049–1056

Tang CC, Poston KL, Eckert T, Feigin A, Frucht S, Gudesblatt M et al (2010b) Differential diagnosis of parkinsonism: a metabolic imaging study using pattern analysis. Lancet Neurol 9(2):149–158

Tao A, Chen G, Deng Y, Xu R (2019) Accuracy of transcranial sonography of the substantia nigra for detection of Parkinson's disease: a systematic review and meta-analysis. Ultrasound Med Biol 45(3):628–641

Teune LK, Bartels AL, de Jong BM, Willemsen AT, Eshuis SA, de Vries JJ et al (2010) Typical cerebral metabolic patterns in neurodegenerative brain diseases. Mov Disord 25(14):2395–2404

Teune LK, Renken RJ, Mudali D, De Jong BM, Dierckx RA, Roerdink JB et al (2013) Validation of parkinsonian disease-related metabolic brain patterns. Mov Disord 28(4):547–551

Teune LK, Strijkert F, Renken RJ, Izaks GJ, de Vries JJ, Segbers M et al (2014) The Alzheimer's disease-related glucose metabolic brain pattern. Curr Alzheimer Res 11(8):725–732

Thobois S, Prange S, Scheiber C, Broussolle E (2019) What a neurologist should know about PET and SPECT functional imaging for parkinsonism: a practical perspective. Parkinsonism Relat Disord 59:93–100

Tripathi M, Tang C, Peng S, Dhawan V, Sharma R, Jaimini A et al (2012) Metabolic image-based algorithm for accurate differential diagnosis of parkinsonism: prospective validation in Indian patient population. J Nucl Med 53(Suppl 1):1974

Tripathi M, Tang CC, Feigin A, De Lucia I, Nazem A, Dhawan V et al (2016) Automated differential diagnosis of early parkinsonism using metabolic brain networks: a validation study. J Nucl Med 57(1):60–66

Van Laere K, Santens P, Bosman T, De Reuck J, Mortelmans L, Dierckx R (2004) Statistical parametric mapping of (99m)Tc-ECD SPECT in idiopathic Parkinson's disease and multiple system atrophy with predominant parkinsonian features: correlation with clinical parameters. J Nucl Med 45(6):933–942

Van Laere K, Casteels C, De Ceuninck L, Vanbilloen B, Maes A, Mortelmans L et al (2006) Dual-tracer dopamine transporter and perfusion SPECT in differential diagnosis of parkinsonism using template-based discriminant analysis. J Nucl Med 47(3):384–392

Varnas K, Cselenyi Z, Jucaite A, Halldin C, Svenningsson P, Farde L et al (2019) PET imaging of [(11)C]PBR28 in Parkinson's disease patients does not indicate increased binding to TSPO despite reduced dopamine transporter binding. Eur J Nucl Med Mol Imaging 46(2):367–375

Varrone A, Marek KL, Jennings D, Innis RB, Seibyl JP (2001) [(123)I]beta-CIT SPECT imaging demonstrates reduced density of striatal dopamine transporters in Parkinson's disease and multiple system atrophy. Mov Disord 16(6):1023–1032

Venneti S, Lopresti BJ, Wiley CA (2006) The peripheral benzodiazepine receptor (translocator protein 18 kDa) in microglia: from pathology to imaging. Prog Neurobiol 80(6):308–322

Vlaar AM, de Nijs T, Kessels AG, Vreeling FW, Winogrodzka A, Mess WH et al (2008) Diagnostic value of 123I-ioflupane and 123I-iodobenzamide SPECT scans in 248 patients with parkinsonian syndromes. Eur Neurol 59(5):258–266

Walter U, Niehaus L, Probst T, Benecke R, Meyer BU, Dressler D (2003) Brain parenchyma sonography discriminates Parkinson's disease and atypical parkinsonian syndromes. Neurology 60(1):74–77

Walter U, Dressler D, Wolters A, Probst T, Grossmann A, Benecke R (2004) Sonographic discrimination of corticobasal degeneration vs progressive supranuclear palsy. Neurology 63(3):504–509

Walter U, Dressler D, Probst T, Wolters A, Abu-Mugheisib M, Wittstock M et al (2007) Transcranial brain sonography findings in discriminating between parkinsonism and idiopathic Parkinson disease. Arch Neurol 64(11):1635–1640

Watanabe H, Saito Y, Terao S, Ando T, Kachi T, Mukai E et al (2002) Progression and prognosis in multiple system atrophy: an analysis of 230 Japanese patients. Brain 125(Pt 5):1070–1083

Wenning G, Stefanova N (2009) Recent developments in multiple system atrophy. J Neurol 256(11):1791–1808

Williams D, Lees A (2009) Progressive supranuclear palsy: clinicopathological concepts and diagnostic challenges. Lancet Neurol 8(3):270–279

Williams D, de Silva R, Paviour D, Pittman A, Watt H, Kilford L et al (2005) Characteristics of two distinct clinical phenotypes in pathologically proven progressive supranuclear palsy: Richardson's syndrome and PSP-parkinsonism. Brain 128(6):1247–1258

Williams D, Holton J, Strand K, Revesz T, Lees A (2007) Pure akinesia with gait freezing: a third clinical phenotype of progressive supranuclear palsy. Mov Disord 22(15):2235–2241

Winikates J, Jankovic J (1999) Clinical correlates of vascular parkinsonism. Arch Neurol 56(1):98–102

Wu P, Wang J, Peng S, Ma Y, Zhang H, Guan Y et al (2013) Metabolic brain network in the Chinese patients with Parkinson's disease based on 18F-FDG PET imaging. Parkinsonism Relat Disord 19(6):622–627

Amyotrophic Lateral Sclerosis

27

Martin R. Turner and Marco Pagani

Contents

Abstract

The core of the clinical syndrome of amyotrophic lateral sclerosis (ALS) is a progressive and typically rapid and uniformly fatal disintegration of the motor system, comprising upper motor neurons (UMNs) of the primary motor cortex and corticospinal tract (CST), brainstem nuclei and the lower motor neurons (LMNs) arising from the anterior horns of the spinal cord. While the spinal anterior horns and corticospinal tract superficially appear to bear the brunt of histopathology in ALS, it is clear that neurodegeneration extends to involve the extra-motor brain, preferentially involving the frontal and temporal lobes having clinical, histopathological and genetic overlap with frontotemporal dementia

M. R. Turner (✉)
Nuffield Department of Clinical Neurosciences, John Radcliffe Hospital, Oxford University, Oxford, UK
e-mail: martin.turner@ndcn.ox.ac.uk

M. Pagani
Institute of Cognitive Sciences and Technologies, CNR, Rome, Italy

Medical Radiation Physics and Nuclear Medicine, Karolinska University Hospital, Stockholm, Sweden
e-mail: marco.pagani@istc.cnr.it

R. A. J. O. Dierckx et al. (eds.), *PET and SPECT in Neurology*,
https://doi.org/10.1007/978-3-030-53168-3_27

(FTD). There is a profound microglial and astrocytic component to pathology, with cortical hyperexcitability thought to be underpinned by changes in the balance of cortical inhibitory interneuronal influences. The marked clinical heterogeneity of the ALS-FTD spectrum, frequent diagnostic delay and reliance of therapeutic trials on survival as the primary outcome measure have made biomarker development a research priority. PET, in particular, continues to provide key mechanistic insights into pathogenesis at a unique systems level.

Abbreviations

5-HT	5-Hydroxytriptamine (serotonin)
ALS	Amyotrophic lateral sclerosis
ALSFRS-R	Revised amyotrophic lateral sclerosis functional rating scale
ATSM	Diacetyl-bis(N4-methylthiosemicarbazone)
CBF	Cerebral blood flow
CST	Corticospinal tract
DA	Discriminant analysis
DLPFC	Dorsolateral prefrontal cortex
ECD	Ethyl cysteinate dimer
FA	Fractional anisotropy
fALS	Familial ALS
FDG	Fluorodeoxyglucose
FMZ	Flumazenil
FTD	Frontotemporal dementia
FU	Follow-up
GABA	γ-Aminobutyric acid
HC	Healthy controls
HMPAO	Hexamethylpropyleneamine oxime
IMP	Iodoamphetamine
KD	Kennedy's disease
LMN	Lower motor neuron
mI/Cr	Myoinositol-creatinine ratio
MMSE	Mini-mental state examination
NAA/Cr	N-Acetylaspartate-creatinine ratio
PBB3	2-([1E,3E]-4-[6-([11C]Methylamino)pyridin-3-yl]buta-1,3-dienyl) benzo[d]thiazol-6-ol
PBR	Peripheral benzodiazepine receptor
PLS	Primary lateral sclerosis
PMA	Progressive muscular atrophy
PMC	Primary motor cortex
SOD1	Superoxide dismutase (ps, presymptomatic; hom, homozygous)
SVM	Support vector machine
TARDBP	Transactive region DNA-binding protein
UMN	Upper motor neuron
UMNB	Upper motor neuron burden

27.1 Introduction

The core of the clinical syndrome of amyotrophic lateral sclerosis (ALS) is a progressive and typically rapid degeneration of a previously normally functioning motor system, comprising upper motor neurons (UMNs) of the primary motor cortex and corticospinal tract (CST), brainstem nuclei and the lower motor neurons (LMNs) arising from the anterior horns of the spinal cord. Weakness, with variable wasting, of the musculature of the limbs and of speech and swallowing ensues, with involvement of the diaphragm resulting in respiratory insufficiency and a median survival of 3 years (van Es et al. 2017). The marked clinical heterogeneity, frequent diagnostic delay and reliance of therapeutic trials on survival as the primary outcome measure have made the discovery of biomarkers across the ALS-FTD spectrum a research priority (Turner et al. 2009).

While the spinal anterior horns and corticospinal tract superficially appear to bear the brunt of histopathology in ALS, it has been known for several decades that neurodegeneration extends to involve the extra-motor brain (Smith 1960), preferentially involving areas of the frontal and temporal lobes having clinical (Phukan et al. 2007) and genetic (DeJesus-Hernandez et al. 2011; Renton et al. 2011) overlap with some forms of frontotemporal dementia (FTD) (Giordana et al. 2011). Variable motor and extra-motor neuronal cytoplasmic inclusions of the transactive region DNA-binding protein TDP-43 are the unifying pathological feature (Neumann et al. 2006). Thus, involvement of the central nervous system has become a core feature of ALS pathogenesis, even in those with no clinical signs of UMN pathology (cases sometimes termed progressive muscular atrophy, PMA) (Brownell et al. 1970; Ince et al. 2003). The development of neuroimaging has revealed a range of novel aspects of ALS pathogenesis (Turner and Verstraete 2015). SPECT and particularly PET were the first tools to demonstrate this wider extra-motor involvement in vivo and to lay the foundation for the modern understanding of ALS as a broad system failure, revealing extra-motor involvement (and related cognitive impairment) in patients unable to comply with standard neuropsychological testing because of physical disability. The individual studies in ALS (and related clinical subtypes) are listed in Table 27.1.

27.2 Single-Photon Emission Computed Tomography

Early SPECT in ALS used the tracer N-isopropyl-p-^{123}I-iodoamphetamine (^{123}I-IMP). This revealed widespread cortical reductions, pronounced in those with longer disease duration (Ludolph et al. 1989) (Fig. 27.1). Soon afterwards, ^{99m}Tc-HMPAO (hexamethylpropyleneamine oxime) SPECT revealed frontotemporal changes in four ALS cases with dementia (Neary et al. 1990), the same group proffering the now accepted concept of a continuum between ALS and FTD (Talbot et al. 1995). A comparative study involving patients with a slowly progressive LMN 'mimic' of ALS, Kennedy's disease (KD, X-linked spinobulbar muscular atrophy), showed no equivalent decreases in cerebral blood flow (CBF) observed in the

Table 27.1 Radionuclide studies in ALS and related disorders

Scan type	Radiotracer	Participants	Main findings	Reference
SPECT	^{123}I-IMP	1 ALS-FTD 1 HC	Marked loss of frontotemporal uptake	Sawada et al. (1988)
		17 ALS (1 FU after 9 months); 15 disease controls	Widespread uptake reduction, correlated with disease severity and duration	Ludolph et al. (1989)
		1 ALS (16-month FU)	Extension of uptake reduction from PMC to frontal lobes over scan interval	Waragai et al. (1997)
	^{99m}Tc-HMPAO	4 ALS-dementia	Reduced frontal lobe uptake (*postmortem* details included)	Neary et al. (1990)
		14 ALS; 14 HC	8/14 prominently reduced frontal lobe uptake (3 with dementia, 1 with aphasia)	Waldemar et al. (1992)
		18 ALS; 8 disease controls	Categorisation into four groups by reduced uptake: frontal + motor, mainly motor, just motor and no reductions, which then correlated with the spectrum of cognitive impairment	Abe et al. (1993)
		19 ALS; 8 ALS-dementia; 29 FTD; 10 HC	Frontal and anterior temporal reduced uptake in all groups, greater in those with ALS-dementia and FTD	Talbot et al. (1995)
		26 ALS; 26 HC	Reduced frontal uptake in those with cognitive impairment (*postmortem* details included)	Abe et al. (1997)
	^{99m}Tc-ECD	35 ALS; 12 KD; 88 HC	Reduced frontal uptake in those with progressive bulbar palsy (correlated with bulbar functional scores); no change in KD patients compared with controls	Morimoto et al. (2012)
		1 *C9ORF72* fALS-FTD; 3 FTD	Hypoperfusion in regions overlapping with the resting-state functional MRI-derived 'salience network'	Boeve et al. (2012)

Table 27.1 (continued)

Scan type	Radiotracer	Participants	Main findings	Reference
PET blood flow/ metabolism	^{18}FDG	12 ALS (5 FU); 3 poliomyelitis; 11 HC	Widespread and progressively reduced cerebral metabolism (not cerebellum) in those with clinical UMN signs	Dalakas et al. (1987)
		3 PLS	Reduced uptake in pericentral cortex	Garnett et al. (1990)
		18 ALS	Reduced glucose metabolism over entire cortex and frontal lobes. Some correlation with neuropsychological impairments	Ludolph et al. (1992)
		3 PLS	Reduced uptake in pericentral cortex in 2/3 patients	Pringle et al. (1992)
		7 ALS (3 FU); 1 PMA; 11 HC	No overall group difference. Progressive decrease in glucose metabolism in precentral gyrus but *increase* in middle frontal gyrus with progression	Hoffman et al. (1992)
		3 PLS with parkinsonian signs; control database	Precentral, prefrontal and cingulate uptake reductions	Mabuchi et al. (2004)
		3 *TARDBP* fALS-FTD	Hypometabolism in frontal associative areas	Chio et al. (2010)
		3 PLS	Focal hypometabolism in the precentral gyri—the 'stripe sign'	Claassen et al. (2010)
		32 ALS 22 HC	*Increased* metabolism in brainstem, amygdalae and cerebellum in all patients. Decreased metabolism in frontal and parietal regions in bulbar versus spinal onset	Cistaro et al. (2012)
		6 ALS; 4 ALS-FTD	More extensive hypometabolism in ALS, including orbitofrontal cortex; relative *preservation* of anterolateral frontal metabolism in ALS patients and perirolandic region in ALS-FTD	Renard et al. (2012)

(continued)

Table 27.1 (continued)

Scan type	Radiotracer	Participants	Main findings	Reference
		1 ALS-dementia	FTD-like hypometabolism despite clinical Alzheimer-like dementia; *C9ORF72* hexanucleotide expansion later identified	Adeli et al. (2014)
		9 ALS;4 ALS-dementia; 13 HC	Hypoperfusion and hypometabolism in anterior cerebral hemispheres (and cerebellar hypoperfusion) in ALS-dementia	Tanaka et al. (1993)
		30 ALS; 12 ALS-FTD; 15 C9ORF72-ALS; 40 HC	Hypometabolism in *C9ORF72*-ALS in anterior and posterior cingulate cortex, insula, caudate and thalamus more widespread than in ALS-FTD	Cistaro et al. (2014)
		70 ALS; 7 PLS; 4 PMA; 20 HC	Perirolandic and prefrontal hypometabolism in ALS and PLS patients. DA correctly classified 95% of ALS cases	Van Laere et al. (2014)
		195 ALS; 40 HC	Hypometabolism in frontal, motor and occipital cortex. Hypermetabolism in midbrain, temporal pole and CST in ALS patients. DA correctly classified 95% of ALS cases	Pagani et al. (2014)
		175 ALS; 10 PLS; 4 PMA; 20 HC	Frontal hypometabolism and cerebellar-occipital hypermetabolism in ALS and PLS patients. SVM approach predicted 100% of the new ALS cases. Extensive frontotemporal hypometabolism was predictive for a lower survival	Van Weehaeghe et al. (2016)

Table 27.1 (continued)

Scan type	Radiotracer	Participants	Main findings	Reference
		259 ALS; 40 HC	Eight independent components discriminated ALS patients with 99.0% accuracy. Bilateral cerebellum/midbrain alone discriminated 96.3% of ALS patients	Pagani et al. (2016)
		94 ALS-Cn; 20 ALS-FTD; 37 ALS-Ci	Frontal and prefrontal hypometabolism and cerebellar, midbrain and CST hypermetabolism progressively more severe proportionally with cognitive impairment	Canosa et al. (2016)
		30 ALS; 30 HC	Spinal cord hypermetabolism in ALS patients	Marini et al. (2016)
		10 ALS; 10 HC	Spinal cord hypermetabolism correlated in ALS patients with the progression of the ALS FRS. No changes in 11C-FMZ uptake	Yamashita et al. (2017)
		10 ALS	The extent of hypometabolism in primary motor cortex correlated with symptom duration	Endo et al. (2017)
		SET 1: 175 ALS 20 HC; SET 2: 195 ALS 40 HC	ALS pattern consistency between the two sets. Frontal hypometabolism in HC of SET 2 as compared to HC SET 1	D'hulst et al. (2018)
		70 ALS; 33 PP; 29 HC	DA correctly classified 82% of ALS and PP, 85% for disease-specific pattern expression scores	Devrome et al. (2018)
		44 ALS; 44 HC	Cervical and dorsal spinal cord hypermetabolism and frontal-dorsolateral cortex hypometabolism in ALS patients	Marini et al. (2018)
		265 ALS; 60 HC	Good evidence for FDG-PET utility to support the diagnosis also if not justified as a routine investigation	Agosta et al. (2018)

(continued)

Table 27.1 (continued)

Scan type	Radiotracer	Participants	Main findings	Reference
		95 ALS (60 spinal-onset, 35 bulbar-onset); 112 HC	Hypometabolism in primary motor cortex and hypermetabolism in cerebellum discriminated spinal versus bulbar symptom onset with 63% accuracy	Sala et al. (2019)
		159 ALS	Positive correlation in prefrontal and anterior cingulate cortex between metabolism and *APOE* with lower metabolism towards the ε2/ε2 extreme	Canosa et al. (2019)
	$^{15}O_2$ and $C^{15}O_2$	12 ALS; 6 HC	Widespread impairment of activation, with expanded region of activation in response to movement task	Kew et al. (1993b)
		10 ALS; 5 HC	Widespread reductions in blood flow in response to motor task, greatest in those with cognitive impairment (reduced verbal fluency)	Kew et al. (1993a)
		12 ALS; 6 HC	Those with cognitive impairment (reduced verbal fluency) showed reduced frontal (insula and thalamic) reductions in rCBF in response to cognitive task	Abrahams et al. (1995)
	$H_2{}^{15}O$	17 ALS; 17 HC	Widespread reductions in cortical binding	Lloyd et al. (2000)
PET ligand	^{11}C-Flumazenil ($GABA_A$ receptor)	5 PLS	Regional cerebral blood flow reductions in fronto-opercular region, mainly precentral gyrus, extending to ventrolateral prefrontal region and anterior cingulate cortex	Le Forestier et al. (2001)
		24 ALS; 10 homozygous 'D90' *SOD1* fALS; 2 presymptomatic homozygous 'D90' *SOD1* carriers; 24 HC	Distinct less motor, more frontal reductions in binding in more slowly progressive 'D90A' (including two presymptomatics) compared with sporadic ALS patients	Turner et al. (2005b)

Table 27.1 (continued)

Scan type	Radiotracer	Participants	Main findings	Reference
		4 PLS; 24 ALS; 10 hom 'D90' *SOD1* fALS 24 HC	Similar pattern of reduced binding in PLS and sporadic ALS patients. Preserved orbitofrontal binding in PLS versus both ALS groups	Turner et al. (2007a)
		12 ALS	Reduced binding in right inferior frontal and superior temporal gyri plus insula with poorer verbal fluency. Reduced left middle frontal gyrus and left cuneus with poorer confrontation naming	Wicks et al. (2008)
		10 ALS	Reduced binding in anterior cingulate gyrus related to writing errors	Yabe et al. (2012)
		10 ALS 10 HC	Widespread binding, including CST, DLPFC, thalamus (linked to clinical UMN signs)	Turner et al. (2004)
	11C-PK11195 (peripheral BZP receptor on activated microglia)	5 FTD 8 HC	Increased binding in frontotemporal regions	Cagnin et al. (2004)
		1 PLS and 1 Mills' syndrome patient with predominant right hemiparesis	Binding predominantly in left hemisphere	Turner et al. (2005a)
	18F-DPA-714 (TSPO ligand expressed on activated microglia)	10 ALS 10 HC	Significantly increased binding in primary motor, supplementary motor and temporal lobe cortices	Corcia et al. (2012)
	11C-WAY100635 (5-HT1A receptor)	21 ALS (nondepressed); 19 HC	Marked frontotemporal reductions in binding	Turner et al. (2005c)
		21 ALS (nondepressed); 11 homozygous (nondepressed) 'D90A' fALS; 19 HC	Proportionately increased regional binding in more slowly progressive familial ALS patients	Turner et al. (2007b)
		4 FTD (nondepressed); 8 HC	Marked frontotemporal reductions in binding	Lanctot et al. (2007)

(continued)

Table 27.1 (continued)

Scan type	Radiotracer	Participants	Main findings	Reference
	18F-6-Fluorodopa (presynaptic dopamine receptor)	12 ALS-parkinsonism-dementia complex of Guam; 7 HC	Intermediate presynaptic dopaminergic deficit in ALS-predominant patients ($n = 4$)	Snow et al. (1990)
		16 ALS; 13 HC	Progressive decline in dopaminergic function with disease duration	Takahashi et al. (1993)
	11C-Raclopride (postsynaptic dopamine receptor)	1 *FUS* fALS; HC	Decreased putamenal binding (no clinical parkinsonian features)	Kono et al. (2012)
	11C-PBR28 (peripheral benzodiazepine receptors)	10 ALS; 10 HC	Higher uptake in precentral gyrus positively correlated with UMNB scores and negatively with ALSFRS-R	Zürcher et al. (2015)
		10 ALS; 10 HC	Higher uptake in motor cortex colocalised and correlated negatively with reduced FA and cortical thinning. All correlated with UMNB	Alshikho et al. (2016)
		40 ALS	In precentral gyrus, positive correlation with mI/Cr and UMNB and negative correlations with NAA/Cr and FA	Ratai et al. (2018)
		10 ALS; 10 HC	Higher uptake in motor regions colocalises with reduced cortical thickness and FA	Paganoni et al. (2018)
	62Cu-ATSM (over-reductive mitochondrial state)	12 ALS; 9 HC	Increased uptake in bilateral motor cortex negatively correlated with ALSFRS-R	Ikawa et al. (2015)
	11C PBB (Tau protein tracer)	5 ALS/Parkinson; 13 HC	Deposition of 11C PBB in cerebral cortex, white matter and CST correlating in frontal, temporal and parietal cortex with MMSE	Shinotoh et al. (2019)
	18F-Fluorbetaben (amyloid tracer); 18F-FDG	18 ALS; 24 HC	Three ALS patients were 18F-fluorbetaben positive. Hypometabolism in frontal cortex and hypermetabolism in cerebellum	Matías-Guiu et al. (2016)

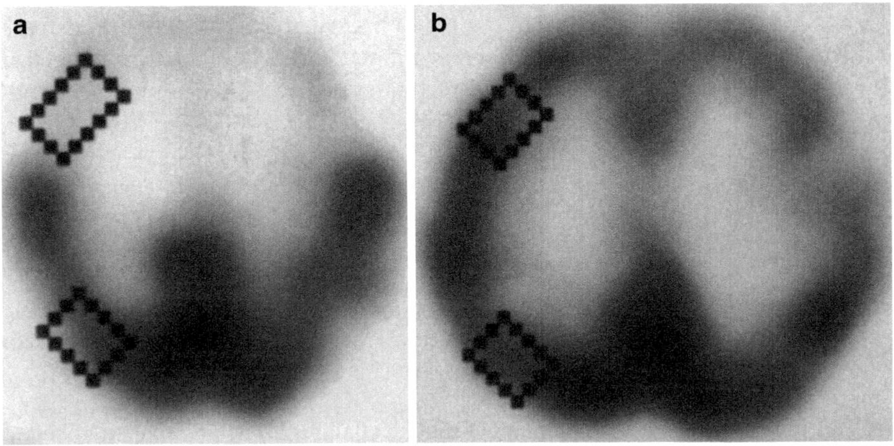

Fig. 27.1 ^{123}I-IMP SPECT in an ALS patient with dementia (**a**) compared to a healthy control (**b**). There is a clear loss of frontotemporal uptake in keeping with the understanding of extra-motor spread of pathology (Adapted from Sawada et al. (1988) with kind permission of Springer Science+Business Media; superimposed boxes show quantitative sampling regions)

frontal lobes of the larger ALS patient group (when compared to healthy controls) (Morimoto et al. 2012).

At least one third of cases with a family history of ALS are linked to an intronic hexanucleotide repeat expansion within *C9ORF72*, and carriers within the same pedigree may manifest 'pure' (usually behavioural variant) FTD, ALS or mixed ALS-FTD (Majounie et al. 2012). A SPECT study in affected gene carriers showed a similar frontal hypometabolism in the single ALS-FTD subject to those with pure FTD, with the overall pattern showing overlap with the 'salience network' as defined by resting-state functional MRI (Boeve et al. 2012).

27.3 PET

27.3.1 Blood Flow and Metabolism

The initial application of PET to ALS was in studies of cerebral blood flow and metabolism, though superseded by noninvasive functional MRI (Turner et al. 2012). Early and longitudinal studies with PET in ALS using ^{18}F-fluorodeoxyglucose (FDG) as a surrogate for cerebral metabolism (regional cerebral metabolic rate for glucose—rCMRGIc) confirmed widespread and progressive reductions in those ALS patients with clinical UMN signs (Dalakas et al. 1987). This was linked to neuropsychological deficits of a frontal lobe nature in ALS patients, particularly verbal fluency (Ludolph et al. 1992), in keeping with the predilection of ALS to cause a dysexecutive syndrome (Phukan et al. 2012). Alternative tracers $H_2{}^{15}O$ and $C^{15}O_2$ were used to measure similar reductions in regional cerebral blood flow

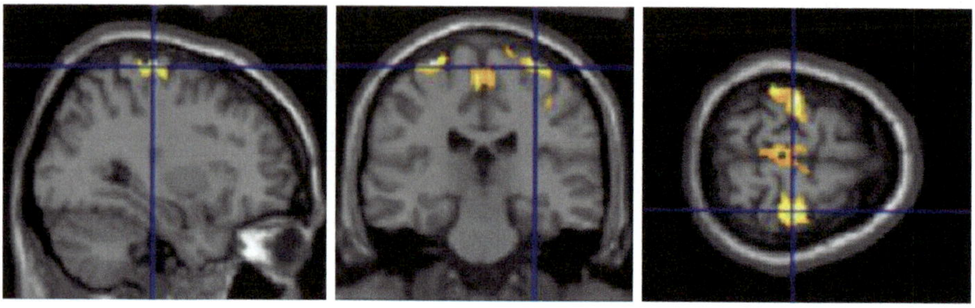

Fig. 27.2 FDG-PET findings in an ALS patient with spinal onset compared with 40 control subjects. Statistically significant hypometabolic clusters (SPM8, $p < 0.05$ $FDR_{corrected}$) are highlighted on a MRI T1 template. Left sagittal view; middle, coronal view; right, transverse view

(rCBF) in ALS patients with dementia (Tanaka et al. 1993) and were also linked to abnormalities of verbal fluency in ALS patients without overt dementia (Kew et al. 1993a). Some studies of patients with the UMN-only, consistently slowly progressive and related disorder primary lateral sclerosis (PLS) have demonstrated a strikingly focal, though inconsistent, hypometabolism of the precentral gyri (the 'stripe sign'), in keeping with the frequent observation of atrophy in this region (Pringle et al. 1992; Claassen et al. 2010).

The increasing availability and low cost of FDG-PET have increased its application to both research and clinical practice in ALS (Fig. 27.2). Studies in which the number of recruited ALS patients dramatically increased were able to delineate metabolic patterns of patients with spinal versus bulbar onset to symptoms (Cistaro et al. 2012) and between patients carrying the *C9ORF72* expansion mutation and apparently sporadic cases (Cistaro et al. 2014). Two studies recruiting a very large number of patients set a well-defined metabolic pattern for ALS. Frontal, prefrontal and pre- and post-central hypometabolism coupled to cerebellar, midbrain and corticospinal tract hypermetabolism, the latter originating by extensive astrocytosis in these areas, characterised ALS patients and allowed up to a 95% discrimination at the single patient level (Van Laere et al. 2014; Pagani et al. 2014). Further studies underscored the impact of frontal hypometabolism on survival (Van Weehaeghe et al. 2016), identified independent components able to discriminate ALS patients with an accuracy of 99% (Pagani et al. 2016) and cross-validated these findings comparing the respective datasets (D'hulst et al. 2018). Further FDG-PET studies have investigated metabolic differences between ALS patients and Parkinson-plus syndromes (Devrome et al. 2018), the association between hypometabolism extension and disease progression (Endo et al. 2017) and the correlation between metabolism and *APOE* genotypes, strengthening the role for ε2 as a risk factor for cognitive impairment in ALS (Canosa et al. 2019).

With potential for more routine clinical applications, FDG-PET focused on the detection of cognitive impairment in ALS patients and spinal cord pathology. Using a much higher sample size than the original investigations, the cerebral hypometabolic pattern was noted to progressively spread towards the prefrontal cortex in relation to executive cognitive impairment and frontotemporal dementia (Canosa et al. (2016). Spinal cord hypermetabolism in ALS has been noted in three FDG-PET investigations (Yamashita et al. 2017; Marini et al. 2016, 2018), though univariate analysis failed to discriminate ALS patients with spinal versus bulbar onset to symptoms (Sala et al. 2019). The overall clinical value of FDG-PET in ALS was evaluated by a panel of expert neurologists and nuclear medicine physicians, concluding that although the methodology has a good utility to support the diagnosis, it is not yet justified as a routine investigation (Agosta et al. 2018).

27.3.2 Ligand Studies

PET ligands have probed specific molecular pathways and provided unique in vivo insight into ALS pathogenesis (Fig. 27.3).

27.3.2.1 An Inhibitory Interneuronal Deficit

A variety of clinical and pathological evidence supports a potentially fundamental loss of cortical inhibitory influence with or without concomitant cortical hyperexcitability in the pathogenesis of ALS (Turner and Douaud 2012; Turner and Kiernan 2012). Cortical hyperexcitability is a consistent feature of ALS, across phenotypes (Van den Bos et al. 2018). The 'boundary shift' in cortical activation seen in response to a joystick task led to the initial hypothesis of a loss of cortical inhibitory interneuronal circuits (Kew et al. 1993b) (Fig. 27.4). Widespread extra-motor cortical changes were then seen using the inhibitory neurotransmitter γ-aminobutyric acid $(GABA)_A$ receptor ligand ^{11}C-flumazenil, providing further evidence for loss of inhibitory influences (Lloyd et al. 2000).

Subsequent comparative ^{11}C-flumazenil PET studies were carried out in familial cases associated with a rare recessive mutation in the superoxide dismutase-1 gene (*SOD1*) linked to a consistently slowly progressive form of ALS. These demonstrated relative preservation of tracer binding in motor regions, in patients matched for disability and UMN signs, supporting the view that preservation of inhibitory influence might have prognostic significance (Turner et al. 2005b).

Comparative studies in PLS revealed preservation of inhibitory influences frontally (Turner et al. 2007a), in keeping with the generally lower incidence of overt cognitive impairment in this group.

27.3.2.2 Neuroinflammation

A key role for neuroinflammatory mechanisms in the pathogenesis of ALS remains the subject of active research (Philips and Robberecht 2011; Evans et al. 2013). The PET ligand ^{11}C-PK11195 binds to the peripheral benzodiazepine receptor expressed by activated microglia. A study in ALS patients provided in vivo evidence of widespread corticospinal tract and extra-motor microglial activation (Turner et al. 2004). A particularly tight correlation between thalamic ^{11}C-PK11195 binding and clinical UMN burden scores in this study may reflect the widespread connectivity of this structure and its disease-related disconnection in ALS. Cortical binding was notably

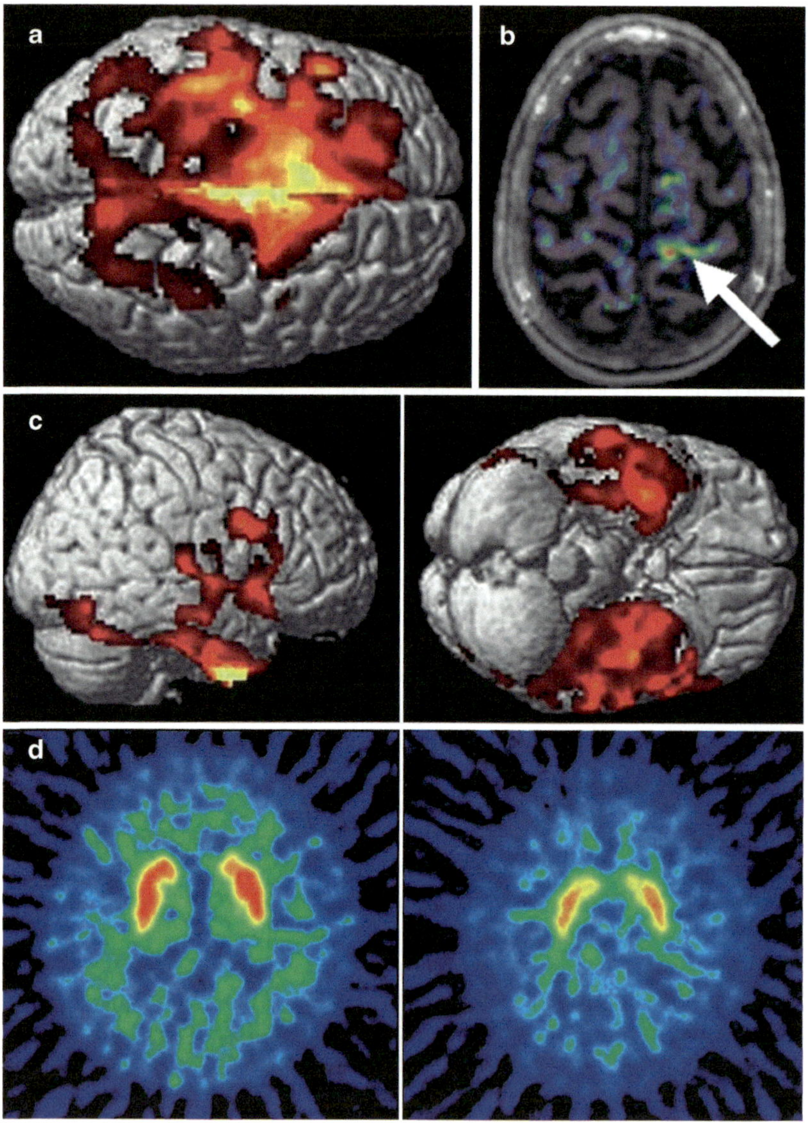

Fig. 27.3 Composite image from ligand PET studies in ALS, revealing different aspects of pathogenesis. A large area of motor and premotor cortex with reduced binding of the $GABA_A$ receptor ligand ^{11}C-flumazenil in ALS patients compared with healthy controls (**a**) supporting a loss of interneuronal inhibitory influence. Evidence of activated microglia, as demonstrated by binding of the peripheral benzodiazepine receptor ^{11}C-PK11195 (**b**), was localised to the left motor cortex (*arrow*) of a patient with weakness lateralised to the right-sided limbs. Right and inferior views of the brain show strikingly frontotemporal localisation of reduced binding of the serotonin 5-HT_{1A} receptor ligand ^{11}C-WAY100635 (**c**) in keeping with the pathological links between ALS and FTD. Reduced ^{11}C-raclopride binding to the striatal postsynaptic dopamine D2 receptor (**d**) (control subject on *left*, *FUS* fALS patient on the *right*) may reflect the occasional observation of parkinsonian signs in those with ALS (Adapted from Turner et al. (2012) with permission of Future Medicine Ltd., and Kono et al. (2012), with kind permission of Springer Science+Business Media)

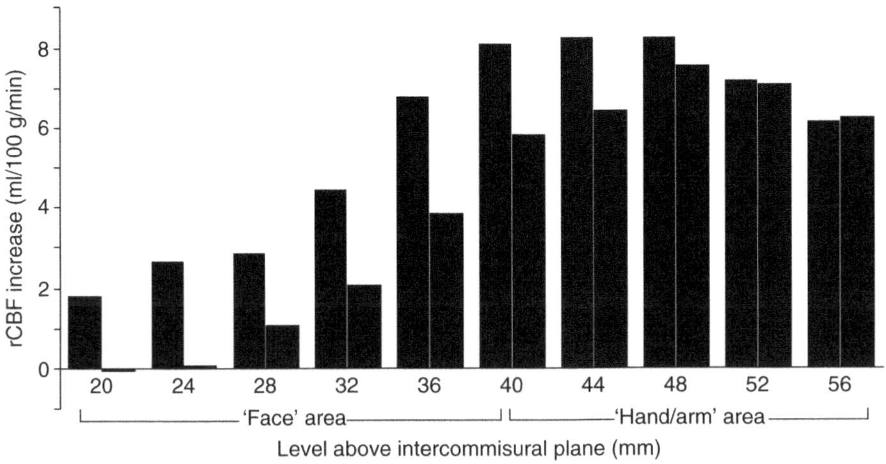

Fig. 27.4 Paired histogram showing mean regional CBF increases at ten points along the motor cortex in ALS (left column of each pair) and healthy controls (right column of each pair) in response to a motor task using hand-held joystick. The ALS patients demonstrated a 'boundary shift' in activation spreading to involve the face as well as hand motor areas. Loss of local inhibitory neuronal circuits was hypothesised (Adapted from Kew et al. (1993b), with permission of Oxford University Press)

lateralised within the hemisphere contralateral to the most affected body side in individuals with rare forms of motor neuron disease (Turner et al. 2005a). Immunohistochemistry studies have subsequently confirmed extensive microglial activation in the CST (Brettschneider et al. 2012). A new ligand for the translocator protein (TSPO) expressed by activated microglia—^{18}F-DPA-714—shows promise for future human ALS studies, with significantly increased binding in primary motor, supplementary motor and temporal lobe cortices, though with marked overlap between healthy control and patient distribution volume ratios (Corcia et al. 2012).

Previous ALS studies have described a significant proliferation and activation of astrocytes as well as activated microglia, in pyramidal cells of the motor cortex and in their projections to the spinal cord (Barbeito et al. 2004). Such reactive proliferation has been investigated by ^{11}C-PBR28, a radiotracer with 80 times greater binding specificity than ^{11}C-PK11195 for peripheral benzodiazepine receptors in the outer mitochondrial membrane of microglia and astrocytes. Increase of ^{11}C-PBR28 intensity in motor cortex and corticospinal tracts was similarly correlated with the clinical UMN burden scores (Zürcher et al. 2015, Fig. 27.5), and additionally reported to colocalise with cortical thinning and decreased fractional anisotropy (Alshikho et al. 2016; Paganoni et al. 2017), and correlated with precentral gyrus with markers of gliosis as detected by magnetic resonance spectroscopy (Ratai et al. 2018).

A PET oxidative stress marker, ^{62}Cu-ATSM, was found to accumulate in regions around the central sulcus in proportion to decreased motor function, underscoring a role of mitochondrial dysfunction in motor neuron degeneration (Ikawa et al. 2015).

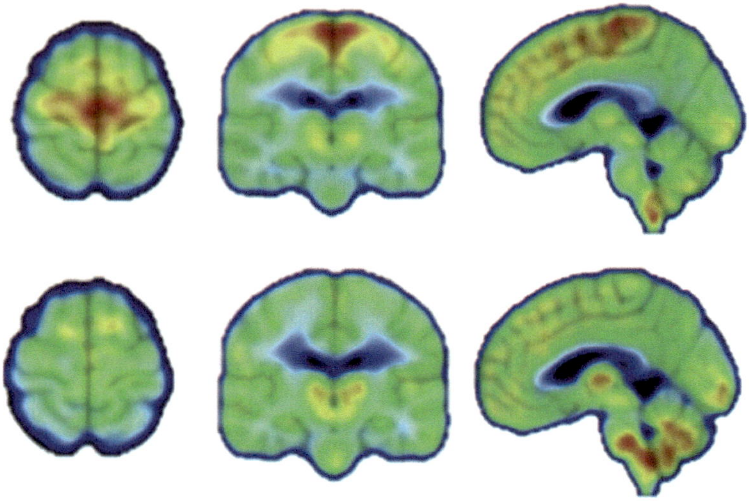

Fig. 27.5 [^{11}C]-PBR28 PET images from ALS patients showing areas of microglial activation (binding potential shown as a heat map). The top row is based on a group of ALS patients with limb onset to symptoms, with the signal predominantly located in motor cortex. The bottom row shows a group of bulbar-onset patients where there is signal more concentrated in the pons and cerebellum. Figure adapted from Zürcher et al. 2015

Finally, deposits of fibrillar amyloid were found in some ALS patients suggesting comorbid Alzheimer's disease (Matías-Guiu et al. 2016).

27.3.2.3 Serotonergic Neuronal Involvement

A serotonin 5-HT$_{1A}$ receptor PET ligand ^{11}C-WAY100635 revealed unexpectedly marked reductions in binding in a group of (importantly) nondepressed ALS patients (Turner et al. 2005c), with proportionately greater regional binding seen in those with a more slowly progressive form of familial ALS (Turner et al. 2007b). Loss of binding was located mainly in frontotemporal regions and was strikingly similar in distribution to a subsequent study in patients with pure FTD (Lanctot et al. 2007), later also confirmed histologically (Bowen et al. 2008). Ostensibly assumed to be a surrogate marker of cerebral pyramidal cell loss in ALS (DeFelipe et al. 2001), this transmitter system has a number of other potential roles in ALS pathogenesis (Sandyk 2006), including the regulation of motoneuronal excitability, neurotrophic actions and spasticity (Dentel et al. 2013), and warrants further study.

27.3.2.4 Parkinsonian Overlap

With the emerging theme of a multisystem cerebral degeneration, and the long-standing observation of extrapyramidal signs among some ALS patients (Hudson 1981), PET studies using ligands previously applied to Parkinson's disease (PD) patients have been applied to ALS. Both pre- and postsynaptic dopamine receptors, namely, ^{18}F-6-fluorodopa and ^{11}C-raclopride, have provided evidence for involvement of the dopaminergic system in cases of ALS, even in the absence of clinical signs (Takahashi et al. 1993; Kono et al. 2012). In contrast, cases of PLS with marked parkinsonian features clinically showed no changes in nigrostriatal regions with either ligand but hypometabolism in the precentral gyrus, extending to prefrontal and cingulate regions using FDG PET (Mabuchi et al. 2004). The same held true for ALS patients with parkinsonian signs in which 123I-ioflupane SPECT was normal in 17/19 patients but metabolism relatively decreased in left cerebellum and increased in right insula and frontal regions (Calvo et al. 2019). Tau protein imaging in patients with the ALS-PD-dementia complex found in inhabitants of the Kii Peninsula, using ^{11}C-PBB3 PET, revealed (unsurprisingly) widespread grey and white matter distribution, including corticospinal tracts, pons and cerebellum (Shinotoh et al. 2019).

27.3.3 The Future

Cerebral radionuclide studies in ALS were prescient of the current era in which ALS and FTD are accepted to have fundamental overlap. Advanced MRI-based techniques, including resting-state functional and network-based analysis of whole-brain structural connectivity, may ultimately offer greater specificity but currently lack application at the individual patient level (Menke et al. 2017).

Ligand PET offers great potential to explore disease mechanisms, particularly with advances in statistical methods for whole-brain analysis that are not reliant on a priori region-of-interest definition, which may be difficult to define in early disease. However, this has typically required short-lived radionuclides to date, entailing a local cyclotron, and so access has been restricted to a few centres with appropriate experience. Moreover, the precise pharmacodynamic properties required for a successful radioligand lie within a narrow range, so that an active radiochemistry research and development programme, including quality control processes, places further restrictions on the availability of this kind of PET research.

It seems likely that, as for other neurodegenerative disorders, the emergence of symptoms in ALS occurs years, perhaps decades, after the earliest cellular changes. There is a consistent diagnostic delay of up to 1 year after symptom onset in ALS, and studies of individuals soon after symptoms are all too rare as a result. The identification of familial ALS cases (~5%) with common and highly penetrant genetic mutations such as those in *SOD1* gene and the *C9ORF72* repeat expansion offers a potential window on such events, through the study of presymptomatic carriers (Benatar and Wuu 2012). Flumazenil PET was one of the first applications of this approach, in which two presymptomatic individuals showed some evidence for an early deficit in $GABA_A$ receptor function in the left operculum region (Turner et al. 2005b). Novel $GABA_A$ receptor radioligands with longer half-lives may offer broader applicability of PET to study at least one potentially important pathogenic mechanism (Jackson et al. 2013). Re-evaluation of the serotonergic system using PET in the post-FTD-linked era of ALS, as well as the application of novel neuroinflammatory target ligands, might also identify novel therapeutic targets. PET ligands might then serve as pharmacodynamic markers for drug discovery, providing proof of mechanism in the early stages of drug development. Finally, with the accumulation of aggregated protein as a common theme across neurodegenerative disorders, the development of PET ligands for *intracellular* targets has been anticipated. Tau imaging is the exemplar, which has made a major contribution to advancing Alzheimer's disease research (Wang and Edison 2019). It has been interesting to note that the tau ligand 18F-AV-1451 has shown increased binding in areas associated with TDP-43 pathology (Bevan-Jones et al. 2018a, b), suggesting it may have wider potential in ALS. The challenges of detecting TDP-43 as a biomarker in biofluid studies are already recognised (Feneberg et al. 2018). Significant technical challenges notwithstanding (Skotland 2012), TDP-43 PET imaging would have the potential to detect many more presymptomatic individuals and provide a readout for the neuroprotective therapies of the future.

References

Abe K, Fujimura H, Toyooka K, Hazama T, Hirono N, Yorifuji S, Yanagihara T (1993) Single-photon emission computed tomographic investigation of patients with motor neuron disease. Neurology 43:1569–1573

Abe K, Fujimura H, Toyooka K, Sakoda S, Yorifuji S, Yanagihara T (1997) Cognitive function in amyotrophic lateral sclerosis. J Neurol Sci 148:95–100

Abrahams S, Leigh PN, Kew JJ, Goldstein LH, Lloyd CM, Brooks DJ (1995) A positron emission tomography study of frontal lobe function (verbal fluency) in amyotrophic lateral sclerosis. J Neurol Sci 129(Suppl):44–46

Adeli A, Savica R, Lowe VJ, Vemuri P, Knopman DS, Dejesus-Hernandez M, Rademakers R, Fields JA, Crum BA, Jack CR, Petersen RC, Boeve BF (2014) The GGGGCC repeat expansion in C9ORF72 in a case with discordant clinical and FDG-PET findings: PET trumps syndrome. Neurocase 20:110–120

Agosta F, Altomare D, Festari C et al (2018) Clinical utility of FDG-PET in amyotrophic lateral sclerosis and Huntington's disease. Eur J Nucl Med Mol Imaging 45:1546–1556

Alshikho MJ, Zürcher NR, Loggia ML et al (2016) Glial activation colocalizes with structural abnormalities in amyotrophic lateral sclerosis. Neurology 87:2554–2561

Barbeito LH, Pehar M, Cassina P, Vargas MR, Peluffo H, Viera L et al (2004) A role for astrocytes in motor neuron loss in amyotrophic lateral sclerosis. Brain Res Rev 47(1–3):263–274

Benatar M, Wuu J (2012) Presymptomatic studies in ALS: rationale, challenges, and approach. Neurology 79:1732–1739

Bevan-Jones RW, Cope TE, Jones SP, Passamonti L, Hong YT, Fryer T et al (2018a) [(18) F]AV-1451 binding is increased in frontotemporal dementia due to C9orf72 expansion. Ann Clin Transl Neurol 5(10):1292–1296

Bevan-Jones WR, Cope TE, Jones PS, Passamonti L, Hong YT, Fryer TD et al (2018b) [(18) F]AV-1451 binding in vivo mirrors the expected distribution of TDP-43 pathology in the semantic variant of primary progressive aphasia. J Neurol Neurosurg Psychiatry 89(10):1032–1037

Boeve BF, Boylan KB, Graff-Radford NR, DeJesus-Hernandez M, Knopman DS, Pedraza O, Vemuri P, Jones D, Lowe V, Murray ME, Dickson DW, Josephs KA, Rush BK, Machulda MM, Fields JA, Ferman TJ, Baker M, Rutherford NJ, Adamson J, Wszolek ZK, Adeli A, Savica R, Boot B, Kuntz KM, Gavrilova R, Reeves A, Whitwell J, Kantarci K, Jack CR Jr, Parisi JE, Lucas JA, Petersen RC, Rademakers R (2012) Characterization of frontotemporal dementia and/or amyotrophic lateral sclerosis associated with the GGGGCC repeat expansion in C9ORF72. Brain 135:765–783

Bowen DM, Procter AW, Mann DM, Snowden JS, Esiri MM, Neary D, Francis PT (2008) Imbalance of a serotonergic system in frontotemporal dementia: implication for pharmacotherapy. Psychopharmacology 196:603–610

Brettschneider J, Toledo JB, Van Deerlin VM, Elman L, McCluskey L, Lee VM, Trojanowski JQ (2012) Microglial activation correlates with disease progression and upper motor neuron clinical symptoms in amyotrophic lateral sclerosis. PLoS One 7:e39216

Brownell B, Oppenheimer DR, Hughes JT (1970) The central nervous system in motor neurone disease. J Neurol Neurosurg Psychiatry 33:338–357

Cagnin A, Rossor M, Sampson EL, Mackinnon T, Banati RB (2004) In vivo detection of microglial activation in frontotemporal dementia. Ann Neurol 56:894–897

Calvo A, Chiò A, Pagani M et al (2019) Parkinsonian traits in amyotrophic lateral sclerosis (ALS): a prospective population-based study. J Neurol 266:1633–1642

Canosa A, Pagani M, Cistaro A et al (2016) 18F-FDG-PET correlates of cognitive impairment in ALS. Neurology 86:44–49

Canosa A, Pagani M, Brunetti M et al (2019) Correlation between apolipoprotein E genotype and brain metabolism in amyotrophic lateral sclerosis. Eur J Neurol 26:306–312

Chio A, Calvo A, Moglia C, Restagno G, Ossola I, Brunetti M, Montuschi A, Cistaro A, Ticca A, Traynor BJ, Schymick JC, Mutani R, Marrosu MG, Murru MR, Borghero G (2010) Amyotrophic lateral sclerosis-frontotemporal lobar dementia in 3 families with p. Ala382Thr TARDBP mutations. Arch Neurol 67:1002–1009

Cistaro A, Valentini MC, Chio A, Nobili F, Calvo A, Moglia C, Montuschi A, Morbelli S, Salmaso D, Fania P, Carrara G, Pagani M (2012) Brain hypermetabolism in amyotrophic lateral sclerosis: a FDG PET study in ALS of spinal and bulbar onset. Eur J Nucl Med Mol Imaging 39:251–259

Cistaro A, Pagani M, Montuschi A, Calvo A, Moglia C, Canosa A, Restagno G, Traynor BJ, Nobili F, Carrara G, Fania PC, Lopiano L, Valentini MC, Chiò A (2014) The metabolic signature of C9ORF72-related ALS, compared to non-mutated patients: a FDG PET study. Eur J Nucl Med Mol Imaging 41:844–852

Claassen DO, Josephs KA, Peller PJ (2010) The stripe of primary lateral sclerosis: focal primary motor cortex hypometabolism seen on fluorodeoxyglucose F18 positron emission tomography. Arch Neurol 67:122–125

Corcia P, Tauber C, Vercoullie J, Arlicot N, Prunier C, Praline J, Nicolas G, Venel Y, Hommet C, Baulieu JL, Cottier JP, Roussel C, Kassiou M, Guilloteau D, Ribeiro MJ (2012) Molecular imaging of microglial activation in amyotrophic lateral sclerosis. PLoS One 7:e52941

D'hulst L, Van Weehaeghe D, Chiò A et al (2018) Multicenter validation of [18F]-FDG PET and support-vector machine discriminant analysis in automatically classifying patients with amyotrophic lateral sclerosis versus controls. Amyotroph Lateral Scler Frontotemporal Degener 2018:1–8. https://doi.org/10.1080/21678421.2018.1476548

Dalakas MC, Hatazawa J, Brooks RA, Di Chiro G (1987) Lowered cerebral glucose utilization in amyotrophic lateral sclerosis. Ann Neurol 22:580–586

DeFelipe J, Arellano JI, Gomez A, Azmitia EC, Munoz A (2001) Pyramidal cell axons show a local specialization for GABA and 5-HT inputs in monkey and human cerebral cortex. J Comp Neurol 433:148–155

DeJesus-Hernandez M, Mackenzie IR, Boeve BF, Boxer AL, Baker M, Rutherford NJ, Nicholson AM, Finch NA, Flynn H, Adamson J, Kouri N, Wojtas A, Sengdy P, Hsiung GY, Karydas A, Seeley WW, Josephs KA, Coppola G, Geschwind DH, Wszolek ZK, Feldman H, Knopman DS, Petersen RC, Miller BL, Dickson DW, Boylan KB, Graff-Radford NR, Rademakers R (2011) Expanded GGGGCC hexanucleotide repeat in noncoding region of C9ORF72 causes chromosome 9p-linked FTD and ALS. Neuron 72:245–256

Dentel C, Palamiuc L, Henriques A, Lannes B, Spreux-Varoquaux O, Gutknecht L, Rene F, Echaniz-Laguna A, Gonzalez de Aguilar JL, Lesch KP, Meininger V, Loeffler JP, Dupuis L (2013) Degeneration of serotonergic neurons in amyotrophic lateral sclerosis: a link to spasticity. Brain 136:483–493

Devrome M, Van Weehaeghe D, De Vocht J et al (2018) Glucose metabolic brain patterns to discriminate amyotrophic lateral sclerosis from Parkinson plus syndromes. EJNMMI Res 8:110

Endo H, Sekiguchi K, Ueda T et al (2017) Regional glucose hypometabolic spread within the primary motor cortex is associated with amyotrophic lateral sclerosis disease progression: a fluoro-deoxyglucose positron emission tomography study. eNeurol Sci 6:74–79

Evans MC, Couch Y, Sibson N, Turner MR (2013) Inflammation and neurovascular changes in amyotrophic lateral sclerosis. Mol Cell Neurosci 53:34–41

Feneberg E, Gray E, Ansorge O, Talbot K, Turner MR (2018) Towards a TDP-43-Based Biomarker for ALS and FTLD. Mol Neurobiol 55(10):7789–7801

Garnett ES, Chirakal R, Firnau G, Nahmias C, Hudson AJ (1990) Recent developments in PET scanning related to amyotrophic lateral sclerosis and primary lateral sclerosis. In: Hudson AJ (ed) Amyotrophic lateral sclerosis: concepts in pathogenesis and etiology. University of Toronto Press, Toronto, ON, pp 358–370

Giordana MT, Ferrero P, Grifoni S, Pellerino A, Naldi A, Montuschi A (2011) Dementia and cognitive impairment in amyotrophic lateral sclerosis: a review. Neurol Sci 32:9–16

Hoffman JM, Mazziotta JC, Hawk TC, Sumida R (1992) Cerebral glucose utilization in motor neuron disease. Arch Neurol 49:849–854

Hudson AJ (1981) Amyotrophic lateral sclerosis and its association with dementia, parkinsonism and other neurological disorders: a review. Brain 104:217–247

Ikawa M, Okazawa H, Tsujikawa T et al (2015) Increased oxidative stress is related to disease severity in the ALS motor cortex: a PET study. Neurology 84:2033–2039

Ince PG, Evans J, Knopp M, Forster G, Hamdalla HH, Wharton SB, Shaw PJ (2003) Corticospinal tract degeneration in the progressive muscular atrophy variant of ALS. Neurology 60:1252–1258

Jackson A, Guilbert BB, Plant SD, Goggi J, Battle MR, Woodcraft JL, Gaeta A, Jones CL, Bouvet DR, Jones PA, O'Shea DM, Zheng PH, Brown SL, Ewan AL, Trigg W (2013) The development of potential new fluorine-18 labelled radiotracers for imaging the GABA (A) receptor. Bioorg Med Chem Lett 23:821–826

Kew JJ, Goldstein LH, Leigh PN, Abrahams S, Cosgrave N, Passingham RE, Frackowiak RS, Brooks DJ (1993a) The relationship between abnormalities of cognitive function and cerebral activation in amyotrophic lateral sclerosis. A neuropsychological and positron emission tomography study. Brain 116(Pt 6):1399–1423

Kew JJ, Leigh PN, Playford ED, Passingham RE, Goldstein LH, Frackowiak RS, Brooks DJ (1993b) Cortical function in amyotrophic lateral sclerosis. A positron emission tomography study. Brain 116(Pt 3):655–680

Kono S, Ouchi Y, Terada T, Suzuki M, Yagi S, Miyajima H (2012) Combined FDG and raclopride PET study in a case of ALS with the R521C FUS gene mutation. J Neurol 259:367–369

Lanctot KL, Herrmann N, Ganjavi H, Black SE, Rusjan PM, Houle S, Wilson AA (2007) Serotonin-1A receptors in frontotemporal dementia compared with controls. Psychiatry Res 156:247–250

Le Forestier N, Maisonobe T, Spelle L, Lesort A, Salachas F, Lacomblez L, Samson Y, Bouche P, Meininger V (2001) Primary lateral sclerosis: further clarification. J Neurol Sci 185:95–100

Lloyd CM, Richardson MP, Brooks DJ, Al Chalabi A, Leigh PN (2000) Extramotor involvement in ALS: PET studies with the GABA (A) ligand [(11) C] flumazenil. Brain 123(Pt 11):2289–2296

Ludolph AC, Elger CE, Bottger IW, Kuttig AG, Lottes G, Brune GG (1989) N-isopropyl-p-123I-amphetamine single photon emission computer tomography in motor neuron disease. Eur Neurol 29:255–260

Ludolph AC, Langen KJ, Regard M, Herzog H, Kemper B, Kuwert T, Bottger IG, Feinendegen L (1992) Frontal lobe function in amyotrophic lateral sclerosis: a neuropsychologic and positron emission tomography study. Acta Neurol Scand 85:81–89

Mabuchi N, Watanabe H, Atsuta N, Hirayama M, Ito H, Fukatsu H, Kato T, Ito K, Sobue G (2004) Primary lateral sclerosis presenting parkinsonian symptoms without nigrostriatal involvement. J Neurol Neurosurg Psychiatry 75:1768–1771

Majounie E, Renton AE, Mok K, Dopper EG, Waite A, Rollinson S, Chio A, Restagno G, Nicolaou N, Simon-Sanchez J, van Swieten JC, Abramzon Y, Johnson JO, Sendtner M, Pamphlett R, Orrell RW, Mead S, Sidle KC, Houlden H, Rohrer JD, Morrison KE, Pall H, Talbot K, Ansorge O, Hernandez DG, Arepalli S, Sabatelli M, Mora G, Corbo M, Giannini F, Calvo A, Englund

E, Borghero G, Floris GL, Remes AM, Laaksovirta H, McCluskey L, Trojanowski JQ, Van Deerlin VM, Schellenberg GD, Nalls MA, Drory VE, Lu CS, Yeh TH, Ishiura H, Takahashi Y, Tsuji S, Le Ber I, Brice A, Drepper C, Williams N, Kirby J, Shaw P, Hardy J, Tienari PJ, Heutink P, Morris HR, Pickering-Brown S, Traynor BJ (2012) Frequency of the C9orf72 hexanucleotide repeat expansion in patients with amyotrophic lateral sclerosis and frontotemporal dementia: a cross-sectional study. Lancet Neurol 11:323–330

Marini C, Cistaro A, Campi C et al (2016) A PET/CT approach to spinal cord metabolism in amyotrophic lateral sclerosis. Eur J Nucl Med Mol Imaging 43:2061–2071

Marini C, Morbelli S, Cistaro A et al (2018) Interplay between spinal cord and cerebral cortex metabolism in amyotrophic lateral sclerosis. Brain 141:2272–2279

Matías-Guiu JA, Pytel V, Cabrera-Martín MN, Galán L, Valles-Salgado M, Guerrero A, Moreno-Ramos T, Matías-Guiu J, Carreras JL (2016) Amyloid- and FDG-PET imaging in amyotrophic lateral sclerosis. Eur J Nucl Med Mol Imaging 43:2050–2060

Menke RA, Agosta F, Grosskreutz J, Filippi M, Turner MR (2017) Neuroimaging endpoints in amyotrophic lateral sclerosis. Neurotherapeutics 14(1):11–23

Morimoto N, Kurata T, Sato K, Ikeda Y, Sato S, Abe K (2012) Frontal dysfunctions of ALS-PBP patients in relation to their bulbar symptoms and rCBF decline. J Neurol Sci 319:96–101

Neary D, Snowden JS, Mann DM, Northen B, Goulding PJ, Macdermott N (1990) Frontal lobe dementia and motor neuron disease. J Neurol Neurosurg Psychiatry 53:23–32

Neumann M, Sampathu DM, Kwong LK, Truax AC, Micsenyi MC, Chou TT, Bruce J, Schuck T, Grossman M, Clark CM, McCluskey LF, Miller BL, Masliah E, Mackenzie IR, Feldman H, Feiden W, Kretzschmar HA, Trojanowski JQ, Lee VM (2006) Ubiquitinated TDP-43 in frontotemporal lobar degeneration and amyotrophic lateral sclerosis. Science 314:130–133

Pagani M, Chiò A, Valentini MC et al (2014) Functional pattern of brain FDG-PET in amyotrophic lateral sclerosis. Neurology 83:1067–1074

Pagani M, Öberg J, De Carli F et al (2016) Metabolic connectivity in amyotrophic lateral sclerosis as revealed by independent component analysis. Hum Brain Mapp 37:942–953

Paganoni S, Alshikho MJ, Zürcher NR, Cernasov P, Babu S, Loggia ML, Chan J, Chonde DB, Garcia DI, Catana C, Mainero C, Rosen BR, Cudkowicz ME, Hooker JM, Atassi N (2017) Imaging of glia activation in people with primary lateral sclerosis. Neuroimage Clin 17:347–353

Philips T, Robberecht W (2011) Neuroinflammation in amyotrophic lateral sclerosis: role of glial activation in motor neuron disease. Lancet Neurol 10:253–263

Phukan J, Pender NP, Hardiman O (2007) Cognitive impairment in amyotrophic lateral sclerosis. Lancet Neurol 6:994–1003

Phukan J, Elamin M, Bede P, Jordan N, Gallagher L, Byrne S, Lynch C, Pender N, Hardiman O (2012) The syndrome of cognitive impairment in amyotrophic lateral sclerosis: a population-based study. J Neurol Neurosurg Psychiatry 83:102–108

Pringle CE, Hudson AJ, Munoz DG, Kiernan JA, Brown WF, Ebers GC (1992) Primary lateral sclerosis. Clinical features, neuropathology and diagnostic criteria. Brain 115(Pt 2):495–520

Ratai EM, Alshikho MJ, Zürcher NR et al (2018) Integrated imaging of [11C]-PBR28 PET, MR diffusion and magnetic resonance spectroscopy 1H-MRS in amyotrophic lateral sclerosis. Neuroimage Clin 20:357–364

Renard D, Collombier L, Castelnovo G, Fourcade G, Kotzki PO, LaBauge P (2012) Brain FDG-PET changes in ALS and ALS-FTD. Acta Neurol Belg 111:306–309

Renton AE, Majounie E, Waite A, Simon-Sanchez J, Rollinson S, Gibbs JR, Schymick JC, Laaksovirta H, van Swieten JC, Myllykangas L, Kalimo H, Paetau A, Abramzon Y, Remes AM, Kaganovich A, Scholz SW, Duckworth J, Ding J, Harmer DW, Hernandez DG, Johnson JO, Mok K, Ryten M, Trabzuni D, Guerreiro RJ, Orrell RW, Neal J, Murray A, Pearson J, Jansen IE, Sondervan D, Seelaar H, Blake D, Young K, Halliwell N, Callister JB, Toulson G, Richardson A, Gerhard A, Snowden J, Mann D, Neary D, Nalls MA, Peuralinna T, Jansson L, Isoviita VM, Kaivorinne AL, Holtta-Vuori M, Ikonen E, Sulkava R, Benatar M, Wuu J, Chio A, Restagno G, Borghero G, Sabatelli M, Heckerman D, Rogaeva E, Zinman L, Rothstein JD, Sendtner M, Drepper C, Eichler EE, Alkan C, Abdullaev Z, Pack SD, Dutra A, Pak E, Hardy J, Singleton A, Williams NM, Heutink P, Pickering-Brown S, Morris HR, Tienari PJ, Traynor

BJ (2011) A hexanucleotide repeat expansion in C9ORF72 is the cause of chromosome 9p21-linked ALS-FTD. Neuron 72:257–268

Sala A, Iaccarino L, Fania PC et al (2019) Testing the diagnostic accuracy of [18F]FDG-PET in discriminating spinal- and bulbar-onset amyotrophic lateral sclerosis. Eur J Nucl Med Mol Imaging 46:1117–1131

Sandyk R (2006) Serotonergic mechanisms in amyotrophic lateral sclerosis. Int J Neurosci 116:775–826

Sawada H, Udaka F, Kishi Y, Seriu N, Mezaki T, Kameyama M, Honda M, Tomonobu M (1988) Single photon emission computed tomography in motor neuron disease with dementia. Neuroradiology 30:577–578

Shinotoh H, Shimada H, Kokubo Y et al (2019) Tau imaging detects distinctive distribution of tau pathology in ALS/PDC on the Kii Peninsula. Neurology 92:e136–e147

Skotland T (2012) Molecular imaging: challenges of bringing imaging of intracellular targets into common clinical use. Contrast Media Mol Imaging 7:1–6

Smith MC (1960) Nerve fibre degeneration in the brain in amyotrophic lateral sclerosis. J Neurol Neurosurg Psychiatry 23:269–282

Snow BJ, Peppard RF, Guttman M, Okada J, Martin WR, Steele J, Eisen A, Carr G, Schoenberg B, Calne D (1990) Positron emission tomographic scanning demonstrates a presynaptic dopaminergic lesion in Lytico-Bodig. The amyotrophic lateral sclerosis-parkinsonism-dementia complex of Guam. Arch Neurol 47:870–874

Takahashi H, Snow BJ, Bhatt MH, Peppard R, Eisen A, Calne DB (1993) Evidence for a dopaminergic deficit in sporadic amyotrophic lateral sclerosis on positron emission scanning. Lancet 342:1016–1018

Talbot PR, Goulding PJ, Lloyd JJ, Snowden JS, Neary D, Testa HJ (1995) Inter-relation between "classic" motor neuron disease and frontotemporal dementia: neuropsychological and single photon emission computed tomography study. J Neurol Neurosurg Psychiatry 58:541–547

Tanaka M, Kondo S, Hirai S, Sun X, Yamagishi T, Okamoto K (1993) Cerebral blood flow and oxygen metabolism in progressive dementia associated with amyotrophic lateral sclerosis. J Neurol Sci 120:22–28

Turner MR, Douaud G (2012) Faulty brakes: an inhibitory neuronal deficit in the pathogenesis of motor neuron disease. Adv Clin Neurosci Rehabil 12:10–11

Turner MR, Kiernan MC (2012) Does interneuronal dysfunction contribute to neurodegeneration in amyotrophic lateral sclerosis? Amyotroph Lateral Scler 13:245–250

Turner MR, Verstraete E (2015) What does imaging reveal about the pathology of amyotrophic lateral sclerosis? Curr Neurol Neurosci Rep 15(7):569

Turner MR, Cagnin A, Turkheimer FE, Miller CC, Shaw CE, Brooks DJ, Leigh PN, Banati RB (2004) Evidence of widespread cerebral microglial activation in amyotrophic lateral sclerosis: an [(11) C]®-PK11195 positron emission tomography study. Neurobiol Dis 15:601–609

Turner MR, Gerhard A, Al-Chalabi A, Shaw CE, Hughes RAC, Banati RB, Brooks DJ, Leigh PN (2005a) Mills' and other isolated upper motor neuron syndromes: in vivo study with [11C]-PK11195 PET. J Neurol Neurosurg Psychiatry 76:871–874

Turner MR, Hammers A, Al-Chalabi A, Shaw CE, Andersen PM, Brooks DJ, Leigh PN (2005b) Distinct cerebral lesions in sporadic and 'D90A' SOD1 ALS: studies with [11C] flumazenil PET. Brain 128:1323–1329

Turner MR, Rabiner EA, Hammers A, Al-Chalabi A, Grasby PM, Shaw CE, Brooks DJ, Leigh PN (2005c) [11C]-WAY100635 PET demonstrates marked 5-HT1A receptor changes in sporadic ALS. Brain 128:896–905

Turner MR, Hammers A, Al-Chalabi A, Shaw CE, Andersen PM, Brooks DJ, Leigh PN (2007a) Cortical involvement in four cases of primary lateral sclerosis using [(11) C]-flumazenil PET. J Neurol 254:1033–1036

Turner MR, Rabiner EA, Al-Chalabi A, Shaw CE, Brooks DJ, Leigh PN, Andersen PM (2007b) Cortical 5-HT1A receptor binding in patients with homozygous D90A SOD1 vs sporadic ALS. Neurology 68:1233–1235

Turner MR, Kiernan MC, Leigh PN, Talbot K (2009) Biomarkers in amyotrophic lateral sclerosis. Lancet Neurol 8:94–109

Turner MR, Agosta F, Bede P, Govind V, Lule D, Verstraete E (2012) Neuroimaging in amyotrophic lateral sclerosis. Biomark Med 6:319–337

Van den Bos MAJ, Higashihara M, Geevasinga N, Menon P, Kiernan MC, Vucic S (2018) Imbalance of cortical facilitatory and inhibitory circuits underlies hyperexcitability in ALS. Neurology 91(18):e1669–e1e76

van Es MA, Hardiman O, Chio A, Al-Chalabi A, Pasterkamp RJ, Veldink JH et al (2017) Amyotrophic lateral sclerosis. Lancet 390(10107):2084–2098

Van Laere K, Vanhee A, Verschueren J et al (2014) Value of 18fluorodeoxyglucose-positron-emission tomography in amyotrophic lateral sclerosis: a prospective study. JAMA Neurol 71:553–561

Van Weehaeghe D, Ceccarini J, Delva A et al (2016) Prospective validation of 18F-FDG brain PET discriminant analysis methods in the diagnosis of amyotrophic lateral sclerosis. J Nucl Med 57:1238–1243

Waldemar G, Vorstrup S, Jensen TS, Johnsen A, Boysen G (1992) Focal reductions of cerebral blood flow in amyotrophic lateral sclerosis: a [99mTc]-d, l-HMPAO SPECT study. J Neurol Sci 107:19–28

Wang YT, Edison P (2019) Tau imaging in neurodegenerative diseases using positron emission tomography. Curr Neurol Neurosci Rep 19(7):45

Waragai M, Takaya Y, Hayashi M (1997) Serial MRI and SPECT in amyotrophic lateral sclerosis: a case report. J Neurol Sci 148:117–120

Wicks P, Turner MR, Abrahams S, Hammers A, Brooks DJ, Leigh PN, Goldstein LH (2008) Neuronal loss associated with cognitive performance in amyotrophic lateral sclerosis: an (11C)-flumazenil PET study. Amyotroph Lateral Scler 9:43–49

Yabe I, Tsuji-Akimoto S, Shiga T, Hamada S, Hirata K, Otsuki M, Kuge Y, Tamaki N, Sasaki H (2012) Writing errors in ALS related to loss of neuronal integrity in the anterior cingulate gyrus. J Neurol Sci 315:55–59

Yamashita T, Hatakeyama T, Sato K et al (2017) Flow-metabolism uncoupling in the cervical spinal cord of ALS patients. Neurol Sci 38:659–665

Zürcher NR, Loggia ML, Lawson R et al (2015) Increased in vivo glial activation in patients with amyotrophic lateral sclerosis: assessed with [(11)C]-PBR28. Neuroimage Clin 7:409–414

PET in Huntington's Disease

28

H. P. H. (Berry) Kremer

Contents

Abstract

From the 1980s onward, PET molecular imaging has yielded a wealth of information on the molecular and structural biology of neurodegeneration in patients with Huntington's disease. While currently not in use for day-to-day diagnostic or predictive clinical purposes in patients, it may acquire new relevance. In this review, I will outline its applications to the study of human preclinical and clinical disease, to our understanding of the neurobiology of Huntington's, as well as in the field of experimental therapeutics.

H. P. H. (Berry) Kremer (✉)
Department of Neurology AB51, University Medical Center Groningen,
University of Groningen, Groningen, The Netherlands
e-mail: h.p.h.kremer@umcg.nl

R. A. J. O. Dierckx et al. (eds.), *PET and SPECT in Neurology*,
https://doi.org/10.1007/978-3-030-53168-3_28

28.1 Introduction

PET imaging has contributed considerably to our understanding of the biology of Huntington's disease (HD). It did confirm *in vivo*—in patients—molecular observations that had been made previously in human postmortem brains, and it has introduced novel concepts regarding the pathophysiology of the clinical manifestations as well as the neurodegenerative process itself. Moreover, PET imaging has been developed as a valuable biomarker that can be used in experimental therapeutics.

This chapter reviews how PET molecular imaging has been used in HD research. It focuses on how it has helped to delineate the extent of the neuropathology, on how molecular changes underlie the disease, and on how this has helped to better understand the clinical disease phenotype. Then, the role of PET in experimental therapeutics will be addressed. A discussion of how PET can be used in HD (dys) functional network analysis and how it has been used in animal models of the disease will be omitted, as will a consideration of differences and similarities between PET and SPECT molecular imaging.

28.2 Clinical Features and Neuropathology of HD

Huntington's disease is a hereditary autosomal dominant neurodegenerative disorder that was first described by George Huntington in 1872. The end of his now classical three-page paper in *The Medical and Surgical Reporter*, "On Chorea," still summarizes, almost in passing, concisely the core clinical features of the disease: motor, cognitive, and behavioral impairment (Lanska 2000). In George Huntington's own and sometimes dramatic words:

> The hereditary chorea as I shall call it is confined to certain and fortunately few families and has been transmitted to them as an heirloom from generations way back in the dim past. It is spoken of by those in whose veins the seeds of the disease are known to exist with a kind of horror and not at all alluded to except through dire necessity with it being mentioned as 'that disorder.' It is attended generally by all the symptoms of common chorea only in an aggravated degree, hardly ever manifesting itself until adult or middle life and then coming on gradually but surely, increasing by degrees and often occupying years in its development until the hapless sufferer is but a quivering wreck of his former self. There are three marked peculiarities in this disease; (1) its hereditary nature, (2) a tendency to insanity and suicide, and (3) its manifesting itself as a grave disease only in adult life.

The best known motor feature is chorea, but dystonia, myoclonus, bradykinesia, general clumsiness, and motor impairment can all be observed in various stages in various patients. Cognitive impairment initially manifests in attentional and executive deficits—primarily a frontal type of dysfunction. Over the course of the disease, more global and massive deficits develop. As to the behavioral or psychiatric alterations, mood disorders, apathy, and loss of impulse control are among the most common manifestations. Rarely, psychosis, mania, and paranoid delusions develop late in the disease. These neuropsychiatric impairments lead to the gradual and surprisingly linear decrease over time of total functional capacity. From a genetic point of view, HD is the archetypical autosomal dominant adult-onset disease with complete penetrance. Each child of an affected parent has 50% chance of developing the disease, irrespective of sex. Patients who are homozygous (i.e., have two mutated alleles instead of one) have a disease that cannot be differentiated from the heterozygous state (one mutated allele), although they may experience a more severe disease course (Squitieri et al. 2003).

In 1983, the gene for HD was found to be linked to a locus on the short arm of chromosome 4. In 1993, the actual gene and its causative mutation were identified (Gusella et al. 1983; MacDonald et al. 1993). This mutation turned out to be an expanded CAG trinucleotide repeat in what is now called the *Huntingtin* gene. The repeat in this gene is highly polymorphic in the normal population, varying between 10 and 29 repeats. In HD patients, the repeat contains 36 or more CAG trinucleotides (Kremer et al. 1994). CAG size correlates strongly (typically $r = 0.7$) with age at onset of the disease (Andrew et al. 1993). Thus, CAG repeat length assessment not only allows the establishment of an unambiguous diagnosis but also an estimate of the time when the motor manifestations will occur (Kremer et al. 1994; Langbehn et al. 2004).

The function of the gene is still unknown, although in its mutated, CAG expanded form, it may interfere with such diverse cellular processes as energy metabolism, transcriptional regulation, intracellular transport, vesicular trafficking, proteasome function, or excitatory amino acid toxicity (Landles and Bates 2004; Lieberman et al. 2018). These toxic effects are mediated by protein fragments derived from the full-length Huntingtin that contain an expanded polyglutamine stretch encoded by the genomic expanded CAG triplet repeat stretch.

Whatever the exact effects of Huntingtin in its wild-type and mutated forms, on a neuropathological level, the effects are quite specific and can be summarized as follows: early and profound loss of striatal (caudate nuclear and putaminal) GABA-ergic medium-sized spiny projection neurons, followed by cortical neurons in layers 3, 5, and 6, as well as neuronal loss in various subcortical areas such as the thalamus and the hypothalamus (Vonsattel et al. 1985; Rüb et al. 2016). Intraneuronal inclusions consist of Huntingtin-derived protein aggregates that are found in the nucleus and the cytoplasm, sometimes extending into the axonal and dendritic tree (Vonsattel and Keller 2011). The macroscopic alterations such as striatal and cortical atrophy can also be observed with structural imaging such as MRI (Tabrizi et al. 2012).

The pattern of neurodegeneration in HD is commonly considered "regionally selective," but this implies temporal selectivity, more so than "many regions not being affected." Different regions pursue different temporal neurodegenerative trajectories. Moreover, while specific neuronal populations degenerate earlier and faster than others, at any time in the course of the disease, complex changes in neuronal structure and molecular makeup should be expected. Neuronal markers such as glucose metabolism, neurotransmitters, their pre- and postsynaptic receptors, and inflammation-associated markers will change over time in a complex pattern that reflects the interwoven and interdependent molecular networks. PET imaging of these changes may teach us a lot about the underlying neurobiology.

28.3 Structural Defects Are Associated with Metabolic Defects

The first studies of dynamic and quantitative (Kuwert et al. 1993) FDG-PET in HD patients were published in the early 1980s. They described a strong and consistent reduction in glucose utilization in the caudate nucleus and the putamen, not only in more or less advanced symptomatic patients but also in some persons who were at 50% risk for the disease but did not (yet) display any signs. (At that time, an unambiguous molecular diagnosis was not yet possible.) Moreover, this local hypometabolism might precede striatal shrinkage as revealed by CT or MRI. This led to the concept of a regional metabolic defect that precedes actual structural changes (Kuhl et al. 1982; Hayden et al. 1986; Young et al. 1986; Mazziotta et al. 1987).

Based on these findings, it was proposed to use dynamic (Kuwert et al. 1993) FDG-PET as a way to identify very early or even preclinical disease and to identify the carriers of the mutated gene (Hayden et al. 1986; Mazziotta et al. 1987; Kuwert et al. 1993). This last application has become obsolete since the identification of the HD gene itself in 1993 (MacDonald et al. 1993), which allowed direct molecular testing.

In subsequent (Kuwert et al. 1993) FDG-PET studies of presymptomatic mutation carriers, as identified by CAG repeat analysis, it turned out that such definitely presymptomatic individuals may have normal striatal glucose utilization during an extended period before becoming symptomatic. A few years prior to converting from presymptomatic to symptomatic, the striatal glucose metabolism goes down (Mazziotta et al. 1992; Antonini et al. 1996). This transition may probably occur as early as 10 years prior to onset of the movement disorder (López-Mora et al. 2016). Repeat examinations of initially asymptomatic persons after follow-up of 58–83 months suggested that in those who converted to the symptomatic state, initial striatal glucose metabolism may be a predictor of time to conversion, independent from CAG size (Ciarmiello et al. 2012).

Basal ganglia local metabolic rates correlated surprisingly strong with total functional capacity; with measures of motor performance, such as chorea, bradykinesia, and rigidity, fine motor control, and oculomotor impairment; and with neuropsychological performance on tests for verbal learning and memory (Young et al. 1986; Berent et al. 1988).

Not only the basal ganglia but also various cortical areas showed a decline of local metabolic rates of glucose consumption in HD patients (Kuwert et al. 1990). The application of network analysis, for example, by establishing metabolic covariance pattern models, has further refined our understanding of large-scale alterations in (early or pre-) symptomatic patients. Thus, medial temporal hypometabolism and occipital hypermetabolism could be defined in relation to the striatal hypometabolism (Feigin et al. 2001). Network analysis also revealed that in presymptomatic gene carriers, thalamic metabolism may initially be somewhat increased but will decline later, concurrent with clinical progression (Feigin et al. 2007). Spatial covariance network analysis of FDG data from presymptomatic gene carriers, acquired at baseline, after follow-up of 1.5 years, 4 years, and in some after 7 years, revealed a distinct and linear, monotonous metabolic progression pattern that could be confirmed in an independent group of premanifest subjects (Tang et al. 2013). Regions in which metabolism declined were the caudate/putamen, the mediodorsal thalamus, and the posterior cingulate, prefrontal, insular, and medial occipital cortices. Metabolic activity was found increased in the pons, the cerebellum, the hippocampus, and temporal, orbitofrontal, and lateral occipital cortices (Tang et al. 2013).

Although these findings and resulting applications were considered to be completely in line with what was known from neuropathology, conceptual problems remained. Particularly, the question what the decrease in metabolism really represents—intrinsic neuronal loss or loss of synapses of neurons that project into the striatum—was never definitely answered. Moreover, it has always been an issue which part of the metabolic signal decrease should be attributed to concurrent nerve cell loss and which part is due to a true metabolic defect that precedes neuronal fallout. It should also be pointed out that the way to analyze these FDG measurements has mostly been through delineation of "regions of interest" (ROIs) or later "voxels of interest" (VOIs). Presenting single ROI/VOI values for regional cerebral metabolic rates of glucose consumption—rCMRglc—introduced methodological issues of local tissue inhomogeneities, partial volume effects, and the effects of ROI size (Kuwert et al. 1992a, b). However, reliable partial volume correction algorithms have been established using co-registered MRI data, and they were applied in studies since the late 1990s (Rousset et al. 1998; Müller-Gärtner et al. 1992). Using such methods, the view has gradually emerged that both regional structural loss and regional metabolic decline are indeed very early features in the brains of HD gene carriers who do not yet display clinical signs of the disease (Ciarmiello et al. 2006).

Results consistent with the concept of basal ganglia and cortical hypometabolism, and similar to FDG-PET results, have been obtained with 99mTc-HMPAO SPECT perfusion imaging in HD patients, but the method, due to its limited quantifiability, as well as its likely inferiority to FDG-PET, has never gained wide acceptance as a diagnostic or disease-monitoring biomarker (Botsch et al. 1987; Reid et al. 1988; Hasselbalch et al. 1992; Kuwert et al. 1993; Boecker et al. 1994; Harris et al. 1996).

From a clinical point of view, neither PET nor SPECT is currently of any use for routine clinical care in terms of early demonstration of decreased metabolism. Making a definite diagnosis can be done by DNA testing of individuals with specific clinical manifestations, and the same applies for predictive testing of at-risk individuals. Tracking progress of the disease is primarily done by using standardized clinical assessments, while MRI structural imaging may be gaining increasing significance (Tabrizi et al. 2012). On the other hand, measurements of local metabolic rates may turn out to be useful as a specific biomarker for disease-modifying intervention trials, e.g., in drug trials that aim at stimulation of mitochondrial function (discussed below). It should be mentioned here that FDG-PET has also been used as a way to unravel the functional connectivity of cognitive performance in (pre)clinical HD patients. As this subject is outside the scope of this chapter, with results to be discussed in relation to many subsequent fMRI studies, I refer to a slightly older but still excellent review (Paulsen 2009).

28.4 Dopamine Receptor Imaging: A Way to Establish Neuronal Integrity?

A second approach to reveal neuronal damage, and one that attempts to measure structural neuronal integrity as opposed to metabolic impairment, has been post- and presynaptic receptor imaging. The implicit assumption is that a measured loss of receptors is related to a loss of receptor carrying structures such as neurites or neurons. The problem here is that receptor up- or downregulation may occur in structurally intact neurons, either as a result of molecular pathology in the neuron itself, as a result of altered input from connected systems, or as a result of general factors such as drugs. Despite these caveats, receptor imaging in HD patients has provided a wealth of biological and clinical insights.

Most work has been done on postsynaptic dopamine receptor imaging, particularly using D1 and D2 ligands as tracers. These two receptors are highly enriched in the mammalian caudate and putamen and therefore of particular interest as markers of HD pathology. The first attempt at dopaminergic molecular imaging in HD was made using IBZM-SPECT. This already allowed the visualization of a decrease in striatal receptor binding (Brucke et al. 1991). ^{123}I-epidepride turned out to be an alternative for SPECT studies (Leslie et al. 1996, 1999; Pirker et al. 1997).

But PET allows for better quantification of this phenomenon. The first published PET study used the D1-receptor benzazepine PET ligand C-SCH 23390. A decrease in both calculated receptor density and total number of D1 receptors was found that equaled (for density) or exceeded (for total number) the magnitude of the 50% striatal volume loss as measured by MRI (Sedvall et al. 1994; Rüb et al. 2016).

The most widely used D2-receptor tracer has been ^{11}C-raclopride (which has also high affinity for D3 receptors, e.g., those localized in the nucleus accumbens). Binding studies, sometimes combining multiple ligands, have revealed a consistent and strong decrease in striatal D2-receptor binding of 50% or more, similar to D1 binding reduction, in all symptomatic and some but not in all presymptomatic subjects (Turjanski et al. 1995; Andrews et al. 1999). Their decline was related to the duration of the disease, with disease progression over the years being accompanied by a progressive receptor binding decline in both symptomatic patients and presymptomatic individuals who converted to symptomatic status (Antonini et al. 1996; Andrews et al. 1999; Ginovart et al. 1997; Pavese et al. 2003; Van Oostrom et al. 2005, 2009). Reduced striatal metabolism as revealed by FDG correlated with reduced raclopride binding (Antonini et al. 1996), but D2 binding may be a more sensitive and earlier marker of striatal damage in presymptomatic patients (Van Oostrom et al. 2005).

In statistical models that used D2-receptor density as a dependent variable, in both presymptomatic and symptomatic patients, CAG size was found to be an independent explanatory variable among others such as measures of tissue atrophy (Van Oostrom et al. 2005; Antonini et al. 1998).

Dopamine receptors can also be detected in the human cortex. Decreases in temporal cortical D1 binding and in temporal, frontal, and amygdalar D2 binding in HD patients suggest that D1 and D2 ligands may be markers for cortical neuronal damage (Ginovart et al. 1997; Pavese et al. 2003, 2010). No such decrease in cortical nor thalamic binding could be demonstrated in one study with the D2/D3 ligand ^{11}C-FLB 457 (Esmaeilzadeh et al. 2011a). Dopamine receptor binding correlates with clinical symptoms. Strong correlations between performance in cognitive tasks that assessed executive function and aspects of visuospatial ability, episodic memory, verbal fluency, perceptual speed, and reasoning on the one hand and D1, D2, and dopamine transporter (DAT) tracer binding on the other hand were found (Bäckman et al. 1997; Lawrence et al. 1998). This was not only true for symptomatic individuals but also for presymptomatic gene carries near their estimated age of onset (Lawrence et al. 1998). Similar correlations between neuropsychological performance and striatal D2 binding were confirmed by some but not by others (Pavese et al. 2003; Sanchez-Pernaute et al. 2000).

In symptomatic patients, a decrease in cortical raclopride binding correlated with measures of impaired executive functions and attention, apparently independent of striatal D2 binding reduction (Pavese et al. 2010). An important additional and significantly contributing covariable in these studies, however, was striatal volume as assessed by MRI.

All these data are consistent with the hypothesis that D1- and D2-receptor densities offer a measure of local neuronal loss. In general, it can be summarized that all HD symptomatic patients have decreased striatal D2-receptor densities, while a variable portion of presymptomatic gene carriers—depending on the number of years prior to projected onset—display a similar biomarker pattern.

Moreover, many correlations between motor and cognitive performance on the one hand with receptor binding have been reported. But before inferring neurobiological conclusions from correlations between such regional receptor binding changes (or, for that part, FDG changes) with specific neuropsychological alterations, one should be aware of the huge collinearity in the data. HD is a generalized brain disease, and over the course of the disease, everything goes down.

Presynaptic nigrostriatal dopamine transporter density has been studied using ^{11}C-βCIT SPECT or α-^{11}C-dihydrotetrabenazine (DTBZ) PET. These ligands reflect nigrostriatal terminal integrity; their derived transporter densities were also found to be decreased in patients, either as a consequence of loss of nerve terminals or as a result of downregulated expression (Ginovart et al. 1997; Gamez et al. 2010; Kiferle et al. 2013). Nigrostriatal integrity may be particularly compromised in akinetic-rigid (often juvenile) HD patients (Bohnen et al. 2000). Thus, not only the striatum itself is affected but also, as in Parkinson's disease, the nigrostriatal dopaminergic projections. Anatomical correlates have been reported in postmortem brain samples of HD patients (Yohrling et al. 2003).

28.5 Imaging of Other Neurotransmitter Receptors

GABA is the main neurotransmitter of many striatal efferents, while GABA receptors can be found in high density in most basal ganglia components. Cannabinoid CB1 and adenosine A2A receptors are abundant as well, the latter colocalizing with dopamine receptors in the striatum (Jamwal and Kumar 2018; Glass et al. 2000). These properties have invited *in vivo* ligand-receptor interaction studies in HD patients using either PET or SPECT.

^{11}C-Flumazenil, a non-subtype-selective central benzodiazepine/GABA-receptor ligand, binds with strong regional specificity to neurons in the basal ganglia and the thalamus. Decreased ^{11}C-flumazenil binding has been found in the caudate nucleus of HD patients but not in the putamen (Holthoff et al. 1993; Künig et al. 2000). An inverse correlation between putaminal D2-receptor density and flumazenil binding has been described and interpreted as indicating GABA-receptor upregulation in early disease (Künig et al. 2000). The results of a SPECT study using ^{123}I-iomazenil to calculate flumazenil affinity constants (K_d) demonstrated distribution volumes in the unblocked state that were in line with the degree of basal ganglia degeneration, while flumazenil K_d was similar in the patients and controls. The study concluded that the benzodiazepine receptor must be functionally intact (Pinborg et al. 2001).

Imaging of cannabinoid CB1 receptors was performed in 20 symptomatic HD patients and 14 healthy controls, using a novel highly selective high-affinity CB1 radioligand ^{18}F-MK-9470 (Casteels et al. 2010). A significant decrease in CB1 availability was found in many regions. This decrease occurred also in regions that were macroscopically intact and affected early HD patients and more advanced patients equally (Van Laere et al. 2010).

28.6 Other Intraneuronal Markers of Neurodegeneration

Any intraneuronal structural molecule or neuronal membrane-bound molecule that can be targeted by a radiotracer may potentially be used to evaluate neurodegeneration. Tracers that measure intraneuronal enzymatic activity may demonstrate either structural neuronal demise or metabolic alterations that precede actual structural changes. FDG is the prime example of this principle in *in vivo* PET studies.

Phosphodiesterase10A offers another example. The enzyme's substrates are cyclic adenosine and guanosine monophosphate (cAMP, cGMP). PDE10A is highly enriched in the brain, particularly in the striatum, where it plays an important role in intracellular cyclic nucleotide-mediated signaling and thus in many downstream signaling cascades that are involved in gene transcription, growth, differentiation, and neurotransmitter-mediated signaling (Wilson and Brandon 2014). Striatal PDE10A levels were found significantly reduced in R6/1 and R6/2 mice, which are accepted transgenic models for HD (Hebb et al. 2004). Mutations in the PDE10A gene have been found associated with childhood-onset chorea with striatal abnormalities (Mencacci et al. 2016; Narayanan et al. 2018).

The first study in five HD patients and 11 controls, using ^{18}F-JNJ42259152 in dynamic scans, found 60–70% reduction in striatal ligand binding potential in all patients, even in two patients who were only mildly affected (Ahmad et al. 2014). A similar magnitude of basal ganglia binding potential decrease, using the ligand ^{18}F-MNI-659, was replicated in eight affected individuals with early motor manifestations. Three premanifest gene carriers showed decreased binding that was intermediate between affected and controls (Russell et al. 2014). A second scan in 8 of these 11 individuals, 1 year later, revealed 5–6% deterioration in binding potential (Russell et al. 2016). Significant changes in PDE10A binding up to 34% could even be detected in gene carriers who were estimated to be 17–43 years before onset, with a decrease in basal ganglia binding but an increase in motor thalamus binding (Niccolini et al. 2015). It should be noted that such individuals have no discernable macroscopic striatal volume loss on MRI, which argues in favor of a very early neuronal dysfunction signal. PDE10A expression was also found decreased in the insular and occipital fusiform cortex of early presymptomatic gene carriers (Wilson et al. 2016).

The adenosine A_1A receptor (A_1AR) was visualized with ^{18}F-CPFPX in a cross-sectional study of 13 presymptomatic mutation carriers and eight symptomatic persons. A decrease in striatal and orbitofrontal cortical binding potential was observed from those who were >10 years from estimated disease onset to those who had symptomatic disease. Presymptomatic individuals far away from disease onset displayed 13% higher whole brain binding than controls; those who were close to symptom onset had binding similar to controls, while symptomatic subjects had lowest values, particularly in the striatum (up to 19%). Regional differences were quite outspoken. Considering that the magnitude of these changes is smaller than that of, for example, dopamine receptor binding and that A_1AR regulation is complex, with various molecular signaling systems being involved, the current role of A_1AR imaging may be primarily in experimental pharmacotherapy (Matusch et al. 2014).

28.7 Inflammation as an Indicator of Neurodegeneration

A true challenge is imaging the mechanisms of the neurodegenerative process itself. Several theories consider neuro-inflammation as a key component of neurodegeneration, not only in Alzheimer's and in Parkinson's disease but also in Huntington's disease (Crotti and Glass 2015). This hypothesis was examined by PET imaging using ^{11}C-PK11195 as an intracerebral microglial marker. Formerly known as the peripheral benzodiazepine receptor ligand, PK11195 is now considered to bind to a translocator protein (TSPO) that is expressed by the mitochondria of activated microglia, indicating the transition of microglia from a resting to an activated state. PK11195 binding was found to be increased in the striatum of HD patients, as well as in the prefrontal and anterior cingulate cortex (Pavese et al. 2006). Moreover, the binding correlated with disease severity as indicated by clinical measures and decreased raclopride binding (Tomasi et al. 2011).

PK11195 binding was found to be also increased in both the striatum and the cortex of presymptomatic gene carriers, in whom it correlated inversely with striatal raclopride D2 binding (Tai et al. 2007). In the hypothalamus, one of the affected extrastriatal areas, similar changes appear to present very early in the disease (Politis et al. 2008). A more detailed study in 32 subjects was able to demonstrate very early increases in PK11195 binding in cortical and subcortical areas that are involved in various motor, cognitive, and behavioral functions (Politis et al. 2011).

28.8 PET Imaging as a Biomarker in Experimental Therapeutics

Perhaps the greatest contribution of PET imaging to HD research and care may turn out to be in the field of experimental therapeutics (Kuwert et al. 1993). FDG imaging has proven to be valid as a biomarker of disease progression. It was used in a drug trial which assessed the efficacy of lamotrigine (a sodium-channel blocker with glutamate release-inhibiting properties) in retarding disease progression. No outcome differences were found in the two treatment groups, but over the 30-month treatment period of the study, FDG metabolic rates declined detectably. Significant decreases were found in the basal ganglia, the frontal cortex, the temporal cortex, and the thalamus. In contrast, neither the parietal nor the cerebellar metabolic rates decreased over this time span. The most profound decrease in metabolic rates occurred in the basal ganglia, with a decrease of approximately 7% per year (Kremer et al. 1999).

In a later small trial using riluzole as a potential neuroprotective agent, FDG-PET in combination with MRI was used in a similar way to assess neuroprotective efficacy (Squitieri et al. 2009). Although this study claimed a more rapid decline for the placebo-treated group, potential clinical efficacy of riluzole had previously already been excluded in a very large European multicenter trial (Landwehrmeyer et al. 2007).

In an open-label trial with pridopidine (ACR16), a compound that can both enhance and counteract ("stabilize") central dopamine functions, eight treated HD patients were examined by two successive FDG scans at a 2-week interval. An increase in metabolic activity in the precuneus bilaterally, the left superior temporal gyrus and the left middle frontal gyrus, and the left mediodorsal thalamic nucleus was found. The relevance of this finding, however, is currently unknown (Esmaeilzadeh et al. 2011b).

Yet another application of ^{18}FDG-PET has been in the field of experimental neuronal grafting in the striatum of animal models and human HD patients. The first animal models were obtained by intrastriatal injection of excitotoxins in rodents and nonhuman primates. Grafting of intra- or cross-species fetal striatal cells into the lesioned areas was able to partially restore resulting motor and behavioral abnormalities. FDG-PET was able to demonstrate local graft metabolism, as well as graft rejection (Schumacher et al. 1992).

The most remarkable results of this approach were demonstrated in a French trial in which five patients received fetal striatoneuronal allografts. After 1–2-year follow-up, increased metabolism in functioning grafts in three patients could be contrasted with hypometabolism in presumably nonfunctioning grafts in two patients, and these assessments correlated with clinical improvement in the motor, cognitive, and general functional domains (Bachoud-Lévi et al. 2000). Functioning striatal grafts did not only improve striatal hypometabolism but also cortical hypometabolism, thus demonstrating improvement of striatocortical connections (Gaura et al. 2004). In an Italian study in which four patients were grafted and followed up for 2 years, similar FDG-PET results of patients with either metabolically active or inactive grafts were reported (Paganini et al. 2010). In this study, D2-receptor imaging was done by IBZM-SPECT. An initial increase in D2 binding was interpreted as indicating newly generated tissue. In a North American study of seven patients who were examined at a 2-year follow-up after intrastriatal fetal neuronal grafts, lack of clinical benefit was associated with persisting and unaltered striatal glucose hypometabolism. D1-receptor density (SCH23390) was unchanged after 2 years, but D2-receptor density (raclopride) had decreased significantly. This was interpreted as either loss of graft viability or disease progression (Furtado et al. 2005).

28.9 Conclusions

These data illustrate several points. Both metabolic FDG studies and dopamine receptor-binding studies and PDEA10 are sensitive in detecting neurodegeneration in vivo in HD patients. They are able to track the progression of the disease, from the truly presymptomatic to the clearly affected stages. They provide correlations with clinical measures of neurological impairment, and they may be used as surrogate outcome measures in experimental therapeutics. Moreover, basic aspects of the neurodegenerative process, e.g., inflammation, are not beyond reach of in vivo imaging. But perhaps the most remarkable point is how much has *not* yet been accomplished in HD PET research. Many receptor systems, e.g., serotoninergic or noradrenergic, have remained untouched. Examining the relation of neurotransmitter alterations with psychiatric and behavioral symptoms is an area largely unexplored. The visualization and measurement of the massive corticostriatal glutamatergic projections remain a daunting challenge (Gruber and Ametamey 2017). Also the molecular imaging of the underlying intracellular Huntingtin aggregation is a highly desirable target—probably not out of reach (Mestre and Sampaio 2017). Thus, many opportunities for novel PET molecular imaging applications exist.

References

Ahmad R, Bourgeois S, Postnov A, Schmidt ME, Bormans G, Van Laere K et al (2014) PET imaging shows loss of striatal PDE10A in patients with Huntington disease. Neurology 82:279–281

Andrew SE, Goldberg YP, Kremer B, Telenius H, Theilmann J, Adam S et al (1993) The relationship between trinucleotide (CAG) repeat length and clinical features of Huntington's disease. Nat Genet 4:398–403

Andrews TC, Weeks RA, Turjanski N, Gunn RN, Watkins LHA, Sahakian B et al (1999) Huntington's disease progression. PET and clinical observations. Brain 122:2353–2363

Antonini A, Leenders KL, Spiegel R, Meier D, Vontobel P, Weigell-Weber M et al (1996) Striatal glucose metabolism and dopamine D2 receptor binding in asymptomatic gene carriers and patients with Huntington's disease. Brain 119:2085–2095

Antonini A, Leenders KL, Eidelberg D (1998) [11C]Raclopride-PET studies of the Huntington's disease rate of progression: relevance of the trinucleotide repeat length. Ann Neurol 43:253–255

Bachoud-Lévi AC, Rémy P, Nǵuyen JP, Brugières P, Lefaucheur JP, Bourdet C et al (2000) Motor and cognitive improvements in patients with Huntington's disease after neural transplantation. Lancet 356:1975–1979

Bäckman L, Robins-Wahlin TB, Lundin A, Ginovart N, Farde L (1997) Cognitive deficits in Huntington's disease are predicted by dopaminergic PET markers and brain volumes. Brain 120:2207–2217

Berent S, Giordani B, Lehtinen S, Markel D, Penney JB, Buchtel HA et al (1988) Positron emission tomographic scan investigations of Huntington's disease: cerebral metabolic correlates of cognitive function. Ann Neurol 23:541–546

Boecker H, Kuwert T, Langen KJ, Lange HW, Czech N, Ziemons K et al (1994) SPECT with HMPAO compared to PET with FDG in Huntington disease. J Comput Assist Tomogr 18:542–548

Bohnen NI, Koeppe RA, Meyer P, Ficaro E, Wernette K, Kilbourn MR et al (2000) Decreased striatal monoaminergic terminals in huntington disease. Neurology 54:1753–1759

Botsch H, Oepen G, Deuschl G, Wolff G (1987) SPECT-Untersuchungen mit 99m Tc-HMPAO bei Patienten mit Huntingtonscher Chorea. RöFo Fortschritte auf dem Gebiet der Röntgenstrahlen und der Bildgeb Verfahren 147:666–668

Brucke T, Podreka I, Angelberger P, Wenger S, Topitz A, Kufferle B et al (1991) Dopamine D2 receptor imaging with SPECT: studies in different neuropsychiatric disorders. J Cereb Blood Flow Metab 11:220–228

Casteels C, Martinez E, Bormans G, Camon L, De Vera N, Baekelandt V et al (2010) Type 1 cannabinoid receptor mapping with [18F]MK-9470 PET in the rat brain after quinolinic acid lesion: a comparison to dopamine receptors and glucose metabolism. Eur J Nucl Med Mol Imaging 37:2354–2363

Ciarmiello A, Cannella M, Lastoria S, Simonelli M, Frati L, Rubinsztein DC et al (2006) Brain white-matter volume loss and glucose hypometabolism precede the clinical symptoms of Huntington's disease. J Nucl Med 47:215–222

Ciarmiello A, Giovacchini G, Orobello S, Bruselli L, Elifani F, Squitieri F (2012) 18F-FDG PET uptake in the pre-Huntington disease caudate affects the time-to-onset independently of CAG expansion size. Eur J Nucl Med Mol Imaging 39:1030–1036

Crotti A, Glass CK (2015) The choreography of neuroinflammation in Huntington's disease. Trends Immunol 36:364–373

Esmaeilzadeh M, Farde L, Karlsson P, Varrone A, Halldin C, Waters S et al (2011a) Extrastriatal dopamine D 2 receptor binding in Huntington's disease. Hum Brain Mapp 32:1626–1636

Esmaeilzadeh M, Kullingsjö J, Ullman H, Varrone A, Tedroff J (2011b) Regional cerebral glucose metabolism after pridopidine (ACR16) treatment in patients with huntington disease. Clin Neuropharmacol 34:95–100

Feigin A, Leenders KL, Moeller JR, Missimer J, Kuenig G, Spetsieris P et al (2001) Metabolic network abnormalities in early Huntington's disease: an [(18)F]FDG PET study. J Nucl Med 42:1591–1595

Feigin A, Tang C, Ma Y, Mattis P, Zgaljardic D, Guttman M et al (2007) Thalamic metabolism and symptom onset in preclinical Huntington's disease. Brain 130:2858–2867

Furtado S, Sossi V, Hauser RA, Samii A, Schulzer M, Murphy CB et al (2005) Positron emission tomography after fetal transplantation in Huntington's disease. Ann Neurol 58:331–337

Gallina P, Paganini M, Lombardini L, Mascalchi M, Porfirio B, Gadda D et al (2010) Human striatal neuroblasts develop and build a striatal-like structure into the brain of Huntington's disease patients after transplantation. Exp Neurol 222:30–41

Gamez J, Lorenzo-Bosquet C, Cuberas-Borrós G, Carmona F, Hernández-Vara J, Castilló J et al (2010) Does reduced [123I]-FP-CIT binding in Huntington's disease suggest pre-synaptic dopaminergic involvement? Clin Neurol Neurosurg 112:870–875

Gaura V, Bachoud-Lévi AC, Ribeiro MJ, Nguyen JP, Frouin V, Baudic S et al (2004) Striatal neural grafting improves cortical metabolism in Huntington's disease patients. Brain 127:65–72

Ginovart N, Lundin A, Farde L, Halldin C, Bäckman L, Swahn CG et al (1997) PET study of the pre- and post-synaptic dopaminergic markers for the neurodegenerative process in Huntington's disease. Brain 120:503–514

Glass M, Dragunow M, Faull RLM (2000) The pattern of neurodegeneration in Huntington's disease: a comparative study of cannabinoid, dopamine, adenosine and GABA(A) receptor alterations in the human basal ganglia in Huntington's disease. Neuroscience 97:505–519

Gruber S, Ametamey SM (2017) Imaging the glutamate receptor subtypes—much achieved, and still much to do. Drug Discov Today Technol 25:27–36

Gusella JF, Wexler NS, Conneally PM, Naylor SL, Anderson MA, Tanzi RE et al (1983) A polymorphic DNA marker genetically linked to Huntington's disease. Nature 306:234–238

Harris GJ, Aylward EH, Peyser CE, Pearlson GD, Brandt J, Roberts-Twillie JV et al (1996) Single photon emission computed tomographic blood flow and magnetic resonance volume imaging of basal ganglia in Huntington's disease. Arch Neurol 53:316–324

Hasselbalch SG, Øberg G, Sørensen SA, Andersen AR, Waldemar G, Schmidt JF et al (1992) Reduced regional cerebral blood flow in Huntington's disease studied by SPECT. J Neurol Neurosurg Psychiatry 55:1018–1023

Hayden MR, Martin WRW, Stoessl AJ, Clark C, Hollenberg S, Adam MJ et al (1986) Positron emission tomography in the early diagnosis of Huntington's disease. Neurology 36:888–894

Hebb ALO, Robertson HA, Denovan-Wright EM (2004) Striatal phosphodiesterase mRNA and protein levels are reduced in Huntington's disease transgenic mice prior to the onset of motor symptoms. Neuroscience 123:967–981

Holthoff VA, Koeppe RA, Frey KA, Penney JB, Markel DS, Kuhl DE et al (1993) Positron emission tomography measures of benzodiazepine receptors in Huntington's disease. Ann Neurol 34:76–81

Jamwal S, Kumar P (2018) Insight into the emerging role of striatal neurotransmitters in the pathophysiology of Parkinson's disease and Huntington's disease: a review. Curr Neuropharmacol 17:165–175

Kiferle L, Mazzucchi S, Unti E, Pesaresi I, Fabbri S, Nicoletti V et al (2013) Nigral involvement and nigrostriatal dysfunction in Huntington's disease: evidences from an MRI and SPECT study. Parkinsonism Relat Disord 19:800–805

Kremer B, Goldberg P, Andrew SE, Theilmann J, Telenius H, Zeisler J et al (1994) A worldwide study of the Huntington's disease mutation: the sensitivity and specificity of measuring CAG repeats. N Engl J Med 330:1401–1406

Kremer B, Clark CM, Almqvist EW, Raymond LA, Graf P, Jacova C et al (1999) Influence of lamotrigine on progression of early Huntington disease: a randomized clinical trial. Neurology 53:1000–1011

Kuhl DE, Phelps ME, Markham CH, Metter EJ, Riege WH, Winter J (1982) Cerebral metabolism and atrophy in Huntington's disease determined by 18FDG and computed tomographic scan. Ann Neurol 12:425–434

Künig G, Leenders KL, Sanchez-Pernaute R, Antonini A, Vontobel P, Verhagen A et al (2000) Benzodiazepine receptor binding in Huntington's disease: [11C]flumazenil uptake measured using positron emission tomography. Ann Neurol 47:644–648

Kuwert T, Lange HW, Langen KJ, Herzog H, Aulich A, Feinendegen LE (1990) Cortical and subcortical glucose consumption measured by pet in patients with Huntington's disease. Brain 113:1405–1423

Kuwert T, Sures T, Herzog H, Loken M, Hennerici M, Langen KJ et al (1992a) On the influence of spatial resolution and of the size and form of regions of interest on the measurement of regional cerebral metabolic rates by positron emission tomography. J Neural Transm Suppl 37:53–66

Kuwert T, Ganslandt T, Jansen P, Jülicher F, Lange H, Herzog H et al (1992b) Influence of size of regions of interest on PET evaluation of caudate glucose consumption. J Comput Assist Tomogr 16:789–794

Kuwert T, Lange HW, Boecker H, Titz H, Herzog H, Aulich A et al (1993) Striatal glucose consumption in chorea-free subjects at risk of Huntington's disease. J Neurol 241:31–36

Landles C, Bates GP (2004) Huntingtin and the molecular pathogenesis of Huntington's disease. EMBO Rep 5:958–963

Landwehrmeyer GB, Dubois B, De Yébenes JG, Kremer B, Gaus W, Kraus PH et al (2007) Riluzole in Huntington's disease: a 3-year, randomized controlled study. Ann Neurol 62:262–272
Langbehn DR, Brinkman RR, Falush D, Paulsen JS, Hayden MR (2004) A new model for prediction of the age of onset and penetrance for Huntington's disease based on CAG length. Clin Genet 65:267–277
Lanska DJ (2000) George Huntington (1850–1916) and hereditary chorea. J Hist Neurosci 2000:76–89
Lawrence AD, Weeks RA, Brooks DJ, Andrews TC, Watkins LHA, Harding AE et al (1998) The relationship between striatal dopamine receptor binding and cognitive performance in Huntington's disease. Brain 121:1343–1355
Leslie WD, Abrams DN, Greenberg CR, Hobson D (1996) Comparison of iodine-123-epidepride and iodine-123-IBZM for dopamine D2 receptor imaging. J Nucl Med 37:1589–1591
Leslie WD, Greenberg CR, Abrams DN, Hobson D (1999) Clinical deficits in Huntington disease correlate with reduced striatal uptake on iodine-123 epidepride single-photon emission tomography. Eur J Nucl Med 26:1458–1464
Lieberman AP, Shakkottai VG, Albin RL (2018) Polyglutamine repeats in neurodegenerative diseases. Annu Rev Pathol Mech Dis 14:1–27
López-Mora DA, Camacho V, Pérez-Pérez J, Martínez-Horta S, Fernández A, Sampedro F et al (2016) Striatal hypometabolism in premanifest and manifest Huntington's disease patients. Eur J Nucl Med Mol Imaging 43:2183–2189
MacDonald ME, Ambrose CM, Duyao MP, Myers RH, Lin C, Srinidhi L et al (1993) A novel gene containing a trinucleotide repeat that is expanded and unstable on Huntington's disease chromosomes. Cell 72:971–983
Matusch A, Saft C, Elmenhorst D, Kraus PH, Gold R, Hartung HP et al (2014) Cross sectional PET study of cerebral adenosine A1 receptors in premanifest and manifest Huntington's disease. Eur J Nucl Med Mol Imaging 41:1210–1220
Mazziotta JC, Phelps ME, Pahl JJ, Huang S-C, Baxter LR, Riege WH et al (1987) Reduced Cerebral glucose metabolism in asymptomatic subjects at risk for Huntington's disease. N Engl J Med 316:357–362
Mazziotta JC, Baxter LR, Phelps ME, Haines JL, Gusella J, Grafton ST et al (1992) Serial changes of cerebral glucose metabolism and caudate size in persons at risk for Huntington's disease. Arch Neurol 49:1161–1167
Mencacci NE, Kamsteeg EJ, Nakashima K, R'Bibo L, Lynch DS, Balint B et al (2016) De novo mutations in PDE10A cause childhood-onset chorea with bilateral striatal lesions. Am J Hum Genet 98:763–771
Mestre TA, Sampaio C (2017) Huntington disease: linking pathogenesis to the development of experimental therapeutics. Curr Neurol Neurosci Rep 17:18
Müller-Gärtner HW, Links JM, Prince JL, Bryan RN, McVeigh E, Leal JP et al (1992) Measurement of radiotracer concentration in brain gray matter using positron emission tomography: MRI-based correction for partial volume effects. J Cereb Blood Flow Metab 12:571–583
Narayanan DL, Deshpande D, Das Bhowmik A, Varma DR, Dalal A (2018) Familial choreoathetosis due to novel heterozygous mutation in PDE10A. Am J Med Genet Part A 176:146–150
Niccolini F, Haider S, Reis Marques T, Muhlert N, Tziortzi AC, Searle GE et al (2015) Altered PDE10A expression detectable early before symptomatic onset in Huntington's disease. Brain 138:3016–3029
Paulsen JS (2009) Functional imaging in Huntington's disease. Exp Neurol 216:272–277
Pavese N, Andrews TC, Brooks DJ, Ho AK, Rosser AE, Barker RA et al (2003) Progressive striatal and cortical dopamine receptor dysfunction in Huntington's disease: a PET study. Brain 126:1127–1135
Pavese N, Gerhard A, Tai YF, Ho AK, Turkheimer F, Barker RA et al (2006) Microglial activation correlates with severity in Huntington disease: a clinical and PET study. Neurology 66:1638–1643

Pavese N, Politis M, Tai YF, Barker RA, Tabrizi SJ, Mason SL et al (2010) Cortical dopamine dysfunction in symptomatic and premanifest Huntington's disease gene carriers. Neurobiol Dis 37:356–361
Pinborg LH, Videbæk C, Hasselbalch SG, Paulson OB, Knudsen GM, Sørensen SA et al (2001) Benzodiazepine receptor quantification in Huntington's disease with [123I]iomazenil and SPECT. J Neurol Neurosurg Psychiatry 70:657–661
Pirker W, Asenbaum S, Wenger S, Kornhuber J, Angelberger P, Deecke L et al (1997) Iodine-123-epidepride-SPECT: studies in Parkinson's disease, multiple system atrophy and Huntington's disease. J Nucl Med 38:1711–1717
Politis M, Pavese N, Tai YF, Tabrizi SJ, Barker RA, Piccini P (2008) Hypothalamic involvement in Huntington's disease: an in vivo PET study. Brain 131:2860–2869
Politis M, Pavese N, Tai YF, Kiferle L, Mason SL, Brooks DJ et al (2011) Microglial activation in regions related to cognitive function predicts disease onset in Huntington's disease: a multimodal imaging study. Hum Brain Mapp 32:258–270
Reid IC, Besson JAO, Best PV, Sharp PF, Gemmell HG, Smith FW (1988) Imaging of cerebral blood flow markers in Huntington's disease using single photon emission computed tomography. J Neurol Neurosurg Psychiatry 51:1264–1268
Rousset OG, Ma Y, Evans AC (1998) Correction for partial volume effects in PET: principle and validation. J Nucl Med 39:904–911
Rüb U, Seidel K, Heinsen H, Vonsattel JP, den Dunnen WF, Korf HW (2016) Huntington's disease (HD): the neuropathology of a multisystem neurodegenerative disorder of the human brain. Brain Pathol 26:726–740
Russell DS, Barret O, Jennings DL, Friedman JH, Tamagnan GD, Thomae D et al (2014) The phosphodiesterase 10 positron emission tomography tracer, [18F]MNI-659, as a novel biomarker for early Huntington disease. JAMA Neurol 71:1520–1528
Russell DS, Jennings DL, Barret O, Tamagnan GD, Carroll VM, Caillé F et al (2016) Change in PDE10 across early Huntington disease assessed by [18 F]MNI-659 and PET imaging. Neurology 86:748–754
Sanchez-Pernaute R, Kunig G, del Barrio AA, de Yebenes JG, Vontobel P, Leenders KL (2000) Bradykinesia in early Huntington's disease. Neurology 54:119–125
Schumacher JM, Hantraye P, Brownell AL, Riche D, Madras BK, Davenport PD et al (1992) A primate model of Huntington's disease: functional neural transplantation and CT-guided stereotactic procedures. Cell Transplant 1:313–322
Sedvall G, Karlsson P, Lundin A, Anvret M, Suhara T, Halldin C et al (1994) Dopamine D1 receptor number—a sensitive PET marker for early brain degeneration in Huntington's disease. Eur Arch Psychiatry Clin Neurosci 243:249–255
Squitieri F, Gellera C, Cannella M, Mariotti C, Cislaghi G, Rubinsztein DC et al (2003) Homozygosity for CAG mutation in Huntington disease is associated with a more severe clinical course. Brain 126:946–955
Squitieri F, Orobello S, Cannella M, Martino T, Romanelli P, Giovacchini G et al (2009) Riluzole protects Huntington disease patients from brain glucose hypometabolism and grey matter volume loss and increases production of neurotrophins. Eur J Nucl Med Mol Imaging 36:1113–1120
Tabrizi SJ, Reilmann R, Roos RAC, Durr A, Leavitt B, Owen G et al (2012) Potential endpoints for clinical trials in premanifest and early Huntington's disease in the TRACK-HD study: analysis of 24 month observational data. Lancet Neurol 11:42–53
Tai YF, Pavese N, Gerhard A, Tabrizi SJ, Barker RA, Brooks DJ et al (2007) Microglial activation in presymptomatic Huntington's disease gene carriers. Brain 130:1759–1766
Tang CC, Feigin A, Ma Y, Habeck C, Paulsen JS, Leenders KL et al (2013) Metabolic network as a progression biomarker of premanifest Huntington's disease. J Clin Invest 123:4076–4088
Tomasi G, Bertoldo A, Cobelli C, Pavese N, Tai YF, Hammers A et al (2011) Global-two-stage filtering of clinical PET parametric maps: application to [11 C]-(R)-PK11195. Neuroimage 55:942–953

Turjanski N, Weeks R, Dolan R, Harding AE, Brooks DJ (1995) Striatal D1 and D2 receptor binding in patients with Huntington's disease and other choreas A PET study. Brain 118:689–696
Van Laere K, Casteels C, Dhollander I, Goffin K, Grachev I, Bormans G et al (2010) Widespread decrease of type 1 cannabinoid receptor availability in Huntington disease in vivo. J Nucl Med 51:1413–1417
Van Oostrom JCH, Maguire RP, Verschuuren-Bemelmans CC, Veenma-Van Der Duin L, Pruim J, RAC R et al (2005) Striatal dopamine D2 receptors, metabolism, and volume in preclinical Huntington disease. Neurology 65:941–943
Van Oostrom JCH, Dekker M, Willemsen ATM, De Jong BM, Roos RAC, Leenders KL (2009) Changes in striatal dopamine D2 receptor binding in pre-clinical Huntington's disease. Eur J Neurol 16:226–231
Vonsattel JP, Myers RH, Stevens TJ, Ferrante RJ, Bird ED, Richardson EP (1985) Neuropathological classification of Huntington's disease. J Neuropathol Exp Neurol 44:559–577
Vonsattel JPG, Keller C, Cortes Ramirez EP (2011) Huntington's disease – neuropathology. In: William J, Weiner ET (eds) Handbook on clinical neurology, vol 100. Elsevier, Amsterdam, pp 83–100
Wilson L, Brandon N (2014) Emerging biology of PDE10A. Curr Pharm Des 21:378–388
Wilson H, Niccolini F, Haider S, Marques TR, Pagano G, Coello C et al (2016) Loss of extra-striatal phosphodiesterase 10A expression in early premanifest Huntington's disease gene carriers. J Neurol Sci 368:243–248
Yohrling GJ, Jiang GC-T, DeJohn MM, Miller DW, Young AB, Vrana KE et al (2003) Analysis of cellular, transgenic and human models of Huntington's disease reveals tyrosine hydroxylase alterations and substantia nigra neuropathology. Brain Res Mol Brain Res 119:28–36
Young AB, Penney JB, Starosta-Rubinstein S, Markel DS, Berent S, Giordani B et al (1986) PET scan investigations of Huntington's disease: cerebral metabolic correlates of neurological features and functional decline. Ann Neurol 20:296–303

PET and SPECT Imaging in Dystonia

29

Evelien Zoons, Jan Booij, Bauke de Jong, and Marina A. J. Tijssen

Contents

E. Zoons
Department of Neurology, Zaans Medisch Centrum, Zaandam, The Netherlands
e-mail: zoons.e@zaansmc.nl

J. Booij
Department of Radiology and Nuclear Medicine, Academic Medical Center, Amsterdam, The Netherlands
e-mail: j.booij@amsterdamumc.nl

B. de Jong · M. A. J. Tijssen (✉)
Department of Neurology, University Medical Center Groningen, Groningen, The Netherlands
e-mail: b.de.jong@umcg.nl; m.a.j.de.koning-tijssen@umcg.nl

R. A. J. O. Dierckx et al. (eds.), *PET and SPECT in Neurology*,
https://doi.org/10.1007/978-3-030-53168-3_29

Abstract

Dystonia is a syndrome characterized by involuntary, sustained muscle contractions causing twisting movements and abnormal postures. It is a common movement disorder with different forms that can be classified based on different clinical characteristics. Idiopathic focal dystonia (dystonia in one body part with no known cause) is the most common form. The more generalized (throughout the body) forms of dystonia have a younger age of onset and usually an underlying genetic defect. The mode of inheritance is usually autosomal dominant. Of these, the most common are DYT-TOR1A and DYT-THAP1 dystonia. In combined dystonia syndromes, also autosomal dominantly inherited disorders, dystonia patients have additional neurological symptoms (e.g., parkinsonism or myoclonus). This group includes dopamine-responsive dystonia, myoclonus-dystonia, rapid-onset dystonia-parkinsonism, and paroxysmal dystonia. In this chapter, we describe results from positron emission tomography (PET) and single-photon emission computed tomography (SPECT) studies in the different forms of dystonia.

Three different kinds of PET and SPECT techniques have been used in patients with dystonia: glucose metabolism scans, regional cerebral blood flow studies, and receptor imaging. Increased glucose metabolism was found in the basal ganglia, thalamus, and cerebellum of patients with different forms of focal dystonia and in DYT1 dystonia. Patients with DYT6 dystonia showed decreased glucose metabolism in the putamen. Results from regional cerebral blood flow (rCBF)-activation studies differed extensively among different studies and different patient groups, mainly because of study design. Overall, the primary and secondary motor and sensory cortices were found to be abnormal in almost all forms of dystonia, although the direction of the abnormalities differed. Dopamine was found to play a role in dystonia reflected by decreased dopamine D2/3 receptor binding in the striatum of patients with almost all forms of dystonia. In recent years, it has been established that other neurotransmitter systems, such as serotonin and gamma aminobutyric acid (GABA) also play a role in dystonia. In conclusion, dystonia is likely to be a network disorder with abnormalities in a large number of cortical and subcortical areas. There might be a central role for the basal ganglia with abnormalities in dopamine receptor binding, as well as other neurotransmitter systems.

29.1 General Introduction

29.1.1 Historical Background

Dystonia was first described in 1911 by Hermann Oppenheim, a renowned German neurologist, as a disorder causing variable muscle tone and recurrent muscle spasm and was initially called "dystonia musculorum deformans." Two neurologists from Poland, Flatau and Sterling, objected to the term dystonia, since they did not consider the varying muscle tone to be the clinical hallmark. They proposed the term "progressive torsion spasm," as patients showed torsion spasms of unknown origin. The two terms were combined and the term "primary torsion dystonia" became widely accepted (Grundmann 2005; Tarsy and Simon 2006). The etiology has been a matter of debate over the years. Especially in the time of Sigmund Freud, several patients with dystonia were described and considered to suffer from hysteria. In 1959, the hereditary nature of primary torsion dystonia was demonstrated. Since then, dystonia is considered to be a neurologic condition, although case reports of psychogenic dystonia have been published over the years (Munts and Koehler 2010).

29.1.2 Epidemiology

Dystonia is the third most common movement disorder (annual incidence: 15–25 per 100,000; ESDE 2000; Le et al. 2003) after Parkinson's disease (PD; von Campenhausen et al. 2005) and tremor (Louis and Ferreira 2010). Idiopathic cervical dystonia (CD; dystonia of the neck) is the most common form of dystonia. The estimated prevalence of CD in the Netherlands (total population: 16.9 million) is 8000 patients, although less than half of these patients are regularly seen by a neurologist (ESDE 2000; Le et al. 2003).

29.1.3 Classification, Clinical Features, and Etiology

Dystonia is a syndrome characterized by involuntary, sustained muscle contractions causing twisting movements and abnormal postures (Tarsy and Simon 2006). Dystonia can be classified based on different characteristics. A frequently used classification is based on topographic distribution, including focal dystonia (one body region), segmental dystonia (two or more adjacent regions), multifocal dystonia (two or more nonadjacent regions), hemidystonia (ipsilateral arm and leg), and generalized dystonia (Tarsy and Simon 2006). Another important division is made in associated features: isolated dystonia, combined dystonia (dystonia with another movement disorder), and dystonia associated with other neurological and systemic manifestations. The third commonly used classification is based on etiology:

nervous system pathology (neurodegenerative disorders and structural lesions), inherited dystonia, acquired dystonia, and idiopathic dystonia. In idiopathic dystonia, there is no underlying disorder recognized causing the dystonia (Albanese et al. 2013). A small proportion of these patients has an inherited form of dystonia. Combined dystonia syndromes are genetic syndromes with dystonia and another movement disorder, for example myoclonus (jerks) or parkinsonism. Acquired dystonia can be caused by a large number of neurological and other conditions, medication, and intoxications. Imaging today has a small role in clinical practice and is mainly used to exclude acquired dystonia in young patients or patients with an atypical disease course (Tarsy and Simon 2006). For an overview and classification of the different forms of dystonia, see Table 29.1.

Idiopathic focal dystonia is dystonia of unknown origin in one body part. The most common form of focal dystonia is CD. Other forms are for example blepharospasm (BLS; dystonia of the eyelids), writer's cramp (WC) or focal hand dystonia, oromandibular dystonia (dystonia of the jaw), and spasmodic dysphonia (dystonia of the vocal cords). Most forms of focal dystonia debut around the age of 50 years. One of the most extraordinary features of focal dystonia is that it can be action specific, a feature that is often used in imaging studies. The most well-known form of action-specific dystonia is WC where patients get a dystonic posture of the hand while trying to write, but not in rest or during other hand movements. Action-specific dystonia has been described in other body parts than the hands as well, for example in the mouth in musicians playing a wind instrument (embouchure dystonia). There usually is no identifiable genetic cause in focal dystonia, although in 20–30% of patients the family history is positive for dystonia (Tarsy and Simon 2006; Lohmann and Klein 2017). Over the years, many loci have been linked to dystonia; however, the precise role of these genetic risk factors remains to be determined (Lohmann and Klein 2017).

Patients with generalized dystonia usually develop dystonia in childhood or during adolescence. These patients frequently have a genetic cause for dystonia and most of these familial syndromes have been allocated a DYT number based on clinical characteristics. The combined dystonia syndromes are included in the DYT numbering as well (Muller 2009). Over the years, it has become clear that several DYT syndromes were caused by one gene, while in other DYT syndromes multiple genes were responsible for one phenotype. Recently, the DYT classification has therefore been changed to a system where DYT is now followed by the causative gene. For example, DYT1 is now named DYT-TOR1A (Lohmann and Klein 2017).

Two forms of generalized dystonia that have been well studied are DYT-TOR1A (formerly DYT1) and DYT-THAP1 (formerly DYT6) dystonia. Onset of dystonia in DYT-TOR1A is usually in childhood and first symptoms are typically in the limbs. Dystonia generalizes over the course of a few years in most cases. DYT-TOR1A dystonia is caused by a mutation in the TorsinA gene. The penetrance of the mutation is 30% meaning that only 30% of gene carriers develop dystonia during their lifetime (Muller 2009).

DYT-THAP1 is the second most common genetic cause of inherited dystonia. Age at onset is more variable than in DYT-TOR1A dystonia, varying from onset in

Table 29.1 Classification of dystonia

Type of dystonia	Prominent symptoms	Etiology
Focal dystonia		
Cervical	Dystonia of the neck muscles	Mostly idiopathic, some cases due to DYT-ANO3
Blepharospasm	Dystonia of the eyelids	Unknown
Writer's cramp	Action-specific dystonia of the hands	Unknown
Focal hand dystonia	Nonaction-specific dystonia of the hands	Unknown
Oromandibular dystonia	Dystonia of the jaw and tongue	Unknown
Spasmodic dysphonia	Dystonia of the vocal cords	Unknown
Segmental dystonia		
Meige syndrome	Blepharospasm with dystonia of the jaw or lower face muscles	Unknown
Inherited form of adult-onset segmental dystonia	Craniocervical dystonia with or without dystonia of one arm	DYT-GNAL
Multifocal dystonia		
Hemidystonia		
Post-stroke dystonia	Dystonia of the arm and leg on one side of the body	Usually post-stroke
Generalized dystonia		
Acquired	Generalized dystonia	Usually post-anoxia, e.g., birth trauma
DYT-TOR1A	Generalized dystonia starting in the limbs	TorsinA gene mutation
DYT-THAP1	Focal or generalized dystonia starting in the cranial or cervical muscles	THAP1 gene mutation
Combined dystonia		
Dopamine-responsive dystonia	Generalized dystonia starting in one leg that responds to levodopa	GCH1 gene or SRG gene mutation
Myoclonus-dystonia	Myoclonus, dystonia, and psychiatric symptoms	SGCE gene mutation
Rapid-onset dystonia-parkinsonism	Acute-onset dystonia and parkinsonism	ATP1A3 gene mutation
Paroxysmal dystonia		
Paroxysmal kinesigenic dystonia	Attacks of generalized dystonia triggered by sudden movements	Most commonly PRRT2 gene mutation, however several other genes described
Paroxysmal non-kinesigenic dystonia (DYT8 and 20)	Spontaneous attacks of generalized dystonia	Most commonly PNKD1 gene mutation
Paroxysmal exercise-induced dystonia (DYT18)	Attacks of generalized dystonia triggered by prolonged exercise	GLUT1 gene mutation

childhood to adult onset. Dystonia typically starts in cranial or cervical muscles after which it slowly progresses. Dysphonia is a common symptom in DYT-THAP1 dystonia. DYT-THAP1 dystonia is caused by a mutation in the THAP1 gene. This mutation also has reduced penetrance: 60% of gene carriers develop dystonia (Muller 2009).

The combined dystonia dopamine-responsive dystonia (DRD, also known as Segawa syndrome) has been named DYT-GCH1 dystonia (formerly DYT5). DRD usually starts in childhood with dystonia of a leg. After this, dystonia usually progresses and patients also develop parkinsonian features. Typical features of DRD are worsening of symptoms after sustained action and reduction of symptoms after rest or sleep (Muller 2009). DRD is most commonly (~80% of cases) caused by a mutation in the GCH1 gene encoding GTP-cyclohydrolase-1, an enzyme necessary for the production of dopamine. This mutation is transmitted in an autosomal dominant fashion with a penetrance of ~30%. The second most commonly affected gene is the sepiapterine reductase gene (SRG), another enzyme used in the production of dopamine. Both mutations lead to reduced production of endogenous dopamine (Muller 2009).

Myoclonus-dystonia (MD; DYT-SCGE formerly DYT11) is a form of combined dystonia. Patients exhibit both dystonia and myoclonic jerks. Onset is usually in childhood or adolescence with myoclonic jerks, later followed by a relatively mild form of dystonia. Patients with MD often also exhibit psychiatric symptoms, mainly depression, anxiety, and obsessive-compulsive syndrome. Motor symptoms in MD are highly responsive to alcohol. MD is caused by a mutation in the epsilon-sarcoglycan gene (SGCE gene) and is transmitted in an autosomal dominant matter with reduced penetrance and maternal imprinting. The latter means that only gene carriers inheriting the gene from their father can get the disease. This is largely true, but a small percentage of patients inheriting the gene from their mother also has (mild) symptoms (Muller 2009).

Rapid-onset dystonia-parkinsonism (RDP; DYT-ATP1A3 formerly DYT12) is an autosomal dominant disease with abrupt onset of dystonia and parkinsonism over days to weeks, followed by little or no improvement. Permanent and disabling dystonia presents acutely after physical or psychological stress, fever, or alcohol excess. RDP is caused by mutations in the α3 subunit of the Na/K-ATPase, the ATP1A3 gene (Muller 2009).

Paroxysmal dystonia is a group of disorders that is characterized by attacks of dystonic movements and postures with sometimes chorea or myoclonus. The disorders that can be distinguished are paroxysmal kinesigenic dystonia (PKD; attacks of several seconds triggered by sudden movements), paroxysmal non-kinesigenic dystonia (PNKD; spontaneous attacks lasting minutes to several hours), and exercise-induced dystonia (PED; Muller 2009). The most common form, PKD, was shown to be caused by mutations in the *PRRT2* gene (Wang et al. 2011). Exercise-induced dystonia is found to be caused by a mutation in the *GLUT1* gene, encoding a glucose transporter in the blood-brain barrier. Due to the mutation in this gene, there is reduced glucose transport to the brain (Muller 2009). Recent studies suggest that the phenotypes of the different genes are overlapping and there are even nongenetic disorders that can present with paroxysmal dystonia (Erro and Bhatia 2019).

29.1.4 Pathophysiology

The pathophysiology of dystonia is still largely unknown even for the inherited forms of dystonia. In the last few years, evidence has been gathered that suggests that TorsinA is needed for neuronal cell membrane stability and architecture, nuclear export, and protein trafficking (Gonzalez-Alegre 2019). It is still unclear what the function of the THAP1, GCH, SRG, and SGCE gene is and what happens at a cellular level when these genes are mutated. For focal dystonia, a combination of genetic and environmental factors is hypothesized to play a role (Tarsy and Simon 2006). Imaging studies with positron emission tomography (PET) and single-photon emission computed tomography (SPECT), though also with varying magnetic resonance imaging (MRI) techniques, have been performed over the years to try to unravel the pathophysiology of dystonia. Dopamine is believed to play an important role in the pathophysiology of all forms of dystonia and has been one of the points of focus in PET and SPECT imaging. One argument for the role of dopamine is DRD, which can successfully be treated with levodopa (Naumann et al. 1997). Other important arguments are the coexistence of dystonia in patients with Parkinson's disease, especially in patients who develop PD at a young age and patients who have been treated with levodopa for longer periods (Wickremaratchi et al. 2009) and the possibility of developing dystonia after use of antipsychotics (dopamine $D_{2/3}$ receptor blockers; Haddad and Dursun 2008). We will collaborate more on results from PET and SPECT studies below.

29.1.5 Treatment

Treatment differs for the different types of dystonia. Most forms of focal dystonia are treated locally with intramuscular botulinum toxin (BTX) injections (Zoons et al. 2012). BTX can also be used in patients with generalized dystonia or MD in the body part that is most affected or causes most disability. Usually patients with generalized dystonia are treated with drugs, for example, trihexyphenidyl (Artane), benzodiazepines, or baclofen, or with deep brain stimulation (DBS). Patients with DRD are treated with small amounts of levodopa with dramatic treatment response. The treatment for paroxysmal dystonia consists of anti-epileptics, for example, carbamazepine (Tarsy and Simon 2006).

29.2 Imaging with PET and SPECT in Different Forms of Dystonia

PET and SPECT studies have been performed in patients with different forms of dystonia. The studies that have been performed can roughly be divided into three types: PET studies for glucose metabolism, PET studies for regional cerebral blood flow (rCBF-activation studies), and PET and SPECT studies for receptor imaging, mainly dopamine; however, the serotonin, gamma aminobutyric acid (GABA), and opioid systems have also been studied. The information in this chapter is divided by forms of dystonia, starting with focal dystonia and followed by generalized dystonia and combined dystonia: DRD, MD, RDP, and paroxysmal dystonia. We will not discuss the results in acquired dystonia. As mentioned above, the causes for acquired dystonia are numerous and the abnormalities found with imaging are usually a result of the underlying condition and not of dystonia per se. A general overview of findings is presented in Table 29.2.

29.3 Focal Dystonia

Several PET and SPECT studies have been performed over the years trying to unravel the pathophysiology of focal dystonia (for a review, see Zoons et al. 2011)

29.3.1 Glucose Metabolism PET

Using [18F]-fluorodeoxyglucose (FDG) PET, increases and decreases in FDG uptake have been found in the basal ganglia, cerebellum, and sensorimotor cortex (SMC) of patients with focal dystonia. A bilateral increase in glucose metabolism in the basal ganglia, thalamus, lentiform nucleus, premotor-motor cortex, and cerebellum has been found in patients with CD compared to controls (Galardi et al. 1996; Magyar-Lehmann et al. 1997). There was an increase in glucose metabolism in the striatum and thalamus of patients with BLS and Meige syndrome (combined dystonia of the eyes and mouth/jaw) compared to controls (Esmaeli-Gutstein et al. 1999) and in the cerebellum and pons in patients with BLS compared to controls (Hutchinson et al. 2000). During induced sleep, patients with BLS showed glucose hypometabolism in the superior-medial aspect of Brodmann area 8 compared to controls. This region is associated with supranuclear control of eyelid opening (Hutchinson et al. 2000). The glucose hypermetabolism in the cerebellum and the pons has been replicated in a study that examined patients with BLS after treatment with BTX. A bilateral glucose hypermetabolism in the thalamus and the pons of patients with BLS was found compared to controls as well as a trend toward glucose hypermetabolism in the putamen bilaterally. Patients with incomplete suppression of BLS on BTX had glucose hypermetabolism in the cerebellum and the pons compared to patients with complete suppression (Suzuki et al. 2007). Furthermore, a complex network of cortical and subcortical regions with increased and decreased metabolism was found in patients with BLS compared to controls. There was increased metabolism in the inferior frontal gyri, right posterior cingulated gyrus, left middle occipital gyrus, fusiform gyrus of the right temporal lobe, left anterior cingulate gyrus, and the caudate nucleus. Decreased glucose metabolism was found in the inferior frontal gyri, left cerebellar hemisphere, and thalamus. Lateralization of activation of the frontal and temporal cortex to the right with contralateral deactivation of the left cerebellum suggests a connection mediated by the corticoponto-cerebellar pathway (Kerrison et al. 2003). One study compared untreated patients with various forms of isolated focal dystonia (mainly CD and WC) to patients with

Table 29.2 Results of PET and SPECT imaging in dystonia

Type of dystonia	Glucose metabolism	Regional cerebral blood flow	Receptor imaging
Focal			
Cervical	↑ Basal ganglia, thalamus, lentiform nucleus, premotor-motor cortex, cerebellum ↓ Caudate nucleus, thalamus, lentiform nucleus, and temporal, frontal, prefrontal, and parietal cortices	↓ SMA, precentral gyrus, SMC and ↑ ipsilateral parietal cortex, and bilateral occipital cortex (during sensory trick)	↓ Striatal D2/3R binding = DAT binding ↓ Striatal VAChT binding ↓ Midbrain SERT binding (SPECT) = SERT binding (PET) ↑ GABA right precentral gyrus, left parahippocampal gyrus
Blepharospasm	↑ Striatum, thalamus, cerebellum, pons ↓ Brodmann area 8 (supranuclear control of eyelid opening; during induced sleep) *Network*: ↑ inf frontal gyri, r post-cingulated gyrus, l mid-occipital gyrus, fusiform gyrus of the r temp lobe, l ant cingulated gyrus and caudate nucleus and ↓ inf frontal gyri, l cerebellar hemisphere and thalamus	↓ PMC (in response to facial vibration; patients with OMD were also included)	↓ D2/3R binding
Writer's cramp/ focal hand dystonia	↓ Caudate nucleus, thalamus, lentiform nucleus, and temporal, frontal, prefrontal, and parietal cortices	↓ PMC, ↑ frontal and parietal association areas, PSC, SMA (while writing) ↓ SMC and premotor structures (during tasks) ↑ Inferior prefrontal cortex (rest) ↑ Contralateral thalamus, SMC and premotor cortex, and ipsilateral cerebellum (while writing)	↓ D2/3R binding ↓ GABA right cerebellum, left sensorimotor cortex ↑ GABA inferior prefrontal cortex
Segmental dystonia			
Meige syndrome	↑ striatum, thalamus	ND	ND

(continued)

Table 29.2 (continued)

Type of dystonia	Glucose metabolism	Regional cerebral blood flow	Receptor imaging
Inherited generalized dystonia			
DYT-TOR1A	↑ Sup frontal gyrus (incl pre-SMA), precuneus, inf parietal cortex ↑ Putamen ↑ Cerebellum	↑ l premotor area, SMA, ant cingulate cortex, l DLPFC, cerebellum, putamen, gyrus frontalis medialis, sup frontal gyrus, fronto-orbital cortex, and thalamus (during right-hand movements)	↓ D2/3R binding ↓ GABAa receptor binding in PMC, premotor cortex, PSC, SSC, posterior insula, l ant cingulate gyrus = Opioid receptor binding
DYT-THAP1	↑ Sup frontal gyrus (incl pre-SMA), precuneus, inf parietal cortex ↓ Putamen = Cerebellum	ND	↓ D2/3R binding
Combined dystonia			
Dopamine-responsive dystonia	ND	ND	↑ D2/3R binding = DAT binding = D1R binding ↑ VMAT2 binding
Myoclonus-dystonia	ND	ND	↓ D2/3R binding (stabilizes after GPi DBS)
Rapid-onset dystonia-parkinsonism	ND	=	↑ DAT binding = DAT binding ↓ DAT binding
Paroxysmal dystonia			
Paroxysmal kinesigenic dystonia (DYT9 and 10)	ND	↓ Basal ganglia and thalamus	ND
Paroxysmal non-kinesigenic dystonia (DYT8 and 20)	ND	ND	= VMAT2 binding
Paroxysmal exercise-induced dystonia (DYT18)	ND	↓ Cerebellum	ND

↑ increase, ↓ decrease; = no abnormalities, *ant* anterior, *D2/3R* dopamine D2/3 receptors, *DAT* dopamine transporter, *DBS* deep brain stimulation, *DLPFC* dorsolateral prefrontal cortex, *GPi* globus pallidus interna, *incl* including, *inf* inferior, *l* left, *mid* middle, *ND* not done, *OMD* oromandibular dystonia, *PET* positron emission tomography, *PMC* primary motor cortex, *post* posterior, *PSC* primary sensory cortex, *r* right, *SMA* supplementary motor area, *SMC* sensorimotor cortex, *SPECT* single-photon emission computed tomography, *SSC* secondary sensory cortex, *sup* superior, *VAChT* vesicular acetylcholine transporter, *VMAT2* vesicular monoamine transporter type 2 essential tremor (ET) and found that both groups show hypometabolism in the caudate nucleus, thalamus, lentiform nucleus, and temporal, frontal, prefrontal, and parietal cortices. There was a significant difference in the extent of decrease in glucose metabolism between these two groups in the left thalamus, right lentiform nucleus, cingulate gyrus, and pons. The authors propose that quantification of glucose metabolism in these areas can be used to differentiate between the two disorders; however, these results have not been replicated yet (Belenky et al. 2018).

In summary, both patients with CD and BLS showed hypermetabolism in basal ganglia, thalamus, and cerebellum. A network of other cortical and subcortical areas could also be affected in patients with BLS. There could be a difference in glucose metabolism between isolated focal dystonia and ET.

29.3.2 Regional Cerebral Blood Flow PET

Where the above-described studies using [18F]-FDG found abnormalities in glucose metabolism mainly in the basal ganglia, the abnormalities in regional cerebral blood flow-activation studies (rCBF-activation studies) as measured with [15O]-H_2O are mainly cortically localized. [15O]-H_2O PET is often used in task-related studies on WC patients. Due to the short half-life of [15O] (2 min), repeated studies can be performed in a short time period. rCBF-activation PET is essentially the prelude of functional MRI (fMRI) and can still be used in research especially in patients in whom movement artifacts are a problem, for example, dystonia patients (Mishina 2008).

One study showed impaired activation of the primary motor cortex (PMC) and greater activation in frontal and parietal association areas in WC patients compared to controls while writing. BTX treatment failed to normalize the impaired activation of primary motor cortex, but did enhance activation of parietal cortex and accessory motor areas (Ceballos-Baumann et al. 1997). Patients with WC also showed reduced rCBF-activation in sensorimotor and premotor structures in different tasks compared to controls. Certain regions were significantly abnormal for specific tasks. Patients showed significantly less rCBF-activation in the contralateral versus ipsilateral primary sensorimotor cortex, during sustained flexion or extension of the wrist. There was a significant decrease in rCBF-activation in the left premotor cortex with writing, but there were no differences during tapping (Ibanez et al. 1999). A significant increase was found in rCBF-activation of the primary sensory cortex and decrease in rCBF-activation of the supplementary motor area (SMA) in patients with WC during writing and tapping compared to controls. Increased activation of the primary sensory cortex found in this study might reflect more intense processing of the sensory information or possibly expanded cortical representation of the hand area. The investigators also found increased activation of the right cerebellum of patients with WC compared to controls (Lerner et al. 2004). In patients with CD using a sensory trick, a significant decrease in motor cortical activation contralateral to the side toward which the head tends to rotate was found. This modulation includes the SMA (anterior part), part of the precentral gyrus, and the primary sensorimotor cortex (SMC). In addition, the sensory trick leads to an increased activation of the parietal cortex ipsilateral to the direction of dystonic head rotation and bilateral occipital cortex (Naumann et al. 2000). A study of patients with facial dystonia (blepharospasm and oromandibular dystonia) showed a significantly reduced primary sensorimotor area (PSA) activation response to vibration of the lower face in patients with facial dystonia compared to healthy controls. The peak activations the authors observed in this study were centered in the precentral gyrus, adjacent to the central sulcus, consistent with the primary motor cortex (Feiwell et al. 1999). The only study using [15O]-butanol in patients with WC found increased blood flow in the contralateral thalamus and primary sensorimotor and premotor cortical areas, though also in the ipsilateral cerebellum as the patients with WC invoked progressively greater dysfunction by a longer duration of writing (Odergren et al. 1998). Concluding, abnormalities in rCBF-activation were less consistent than those in glucose metabolism. The most consistent findings included a decreased rCBF-activation in the PMC, SMC, SMA, and PSA and an increase in rCBF-activation in frontal and parietal association areas.

29.3.3 Dopamine Receptor Imaging with PET and SPECT

Two PET studies looked at $D_{2/3}$ receptor (D2/3R) availability in patients with focal dystonia. Leenders and coworkers found no difference in striatal [11C]-*N*-methylspiperone (NMSP) binding to D2-like receptors in patients with mainly CD when compared to healthy controls. A trend was observed regarding the side to side differences: specific binding of the tracer tended to be higher in the striatum contralateral to the side to which the head was turning to (Leenders et al. 1993). Another study showed decreased [18F]-spiperone (SP; another D2-like receptor tracer) binding in the putamen of patients with hand and facial dystonia. There was no significant difference between patients with hand and facial dystonia (Perlmutter et al. 1997).

In patients with CD, the average specific striatal binding to D2/3Rs, measured with [123I]-iodobenzamide ([123I]-IBZM) SPECT, was not significantly different from a group of healthy controls. However, patients exhibited a more asymmetric striatal binding compared to controls and 50% of the patient group did show a higher receptor binding in the striatum contralateral to the direction of head rotation. The difference in binding was statistically significant for this patient group (Hierholzer et al. 1994). This is in accordance with the increased dopamine receptor binding in the contralateral striatum found in the PET study in patients with CD mentioned above and has also been found in other SPECT studies (Leenders et al. 1993). For example, a tendency for a reduced iodobenzamide (IBZM) binding in the dorsal portion and an increase in the ventral parts of the striatum contralateral to the side of head rotation was found by Becker et al. (1997) in CD patients, but these results did not reach statistical significance, probably because of small study size ($n = 10$). The low IBZM binding contralateral to the side of head deviation may indicate a reduced postsynaptic D2/3R density within the lentiform nucleus. These findings may point toward the medial lentiform nucleus or pallidothalamic pathway as the site of pathology in CD (Becker et al. 1997). Another study evaluated both the pre- and postsynaptic dopaminergic system in patients with CD, using [123I]-epidepride (a tracer for D2/3R) and [123I]-β-CIT (a tracer for the presynaptic dopamine transporter, DAT). Striatal D2/3R binding was bilaterally significantly reduced in patients compared to controls, but there was no difference in striatal DAT binding (Naumann et al. 1998). A similar design has been used in a more recent study using [123I]-IBZM and [123I]-FP-CIT (DAT tracer) in 27 patients with CD and 15 controls. This study found no difference in striatal DAT binding overall and only a trend toward lower striatal IBZM binding. However, both striatal DAT and D2/3R binding correlated significantly with depressive symptoms, which are common in CD. Both striatal DAT and D2/3R binding were significantly lower in depressed CD patients compared to nondepressed CD patients (Zoons et al. 2017a). Previous dopamine imaging studies in patients with CD and other forms of focal dystonia did not correct for depressive symptoms, which could have caused the difference in results.

In a study evaluating patients with WC, the striatal D2/3R binding was bilaterally decreased in patients compared to controls (Horstink et al. 1997). Another SPECT study evaluated patients with WC pre- and post-biofeedback-based sensorimotor training with [123I]-IBZM SPECT and also found decreased striatal binding. The training made patients more confident to write with a relaxed limb, writing improved, and striatal D2R-binding restored to nearly normal levels (Berger et al. 2007).

In summary, the findings in PET and SPECT studies implicate a role for the striatal dopaminergic system and the basal ganglia in the pathophysiology of focal dystonia. However, it can be debated whether dopamine plays a more important role in the pathophysiology of motor or non-motor symptoms in patients with focal dystonia.

29.3.4 Receptor Imaging of Other Neurotransmitter Systems with PET and SPECT

Recently, other neurotransmitter systems than the dopamine systems have received more attention. One study evaluated the integrity of cholinergic nerve terminals in patients with CD using [123I]-iodobenzavesamicol ([123I]-IBVM), a SPECT tracer that binds to the vesicular acetylcholine transporter (VAChT). They found a reduced IBVM binding in the putamen as well as in the whole striatum in patients with CD compared to controls (Albin et al. 2003).

One PET and one SPECT study have evaluated the presynaptic serotonin transporter (SERT) in patients with CD. In the SPECT study, the nonselective tracer [123I], FP-CIT (this tracer binds predominantly to the DAT in the striatum, and to the SERT in extrastriatal brain areas; Booij et al. 2007) was used and consequently only SERT binding in the diencephalon/midbrain area could be evaluated in patients with CD. A clear trend toward lower SERT binding in CD patients with psychiatric symptoms (mainly depression and anxiety) was found compared to controls.

Furthermore, in CD patients with head jerks or tremor, there was a significant positive correlation between extrastriatal SERT binding and striatal DAT binding that was absent in CD patients without head jerks or tremor (Zoons et al. 2017b). In the PET study, the selective SERT tracer [11C]-DASB was used that allowed a more extensive evaluation of SERT binding throughout the brain and more detailed imaging of small brain regions, which showed a completely different picture. No significant difference was found in SERT binding between CD patients and controls before or after correction for psychiatric symptoms. However, higher SERT binding in the dorsal raphe nucleus was statistically significantly correlated with motor symptom severity and to a lesser extent also to pain and sleep disturbances. There was also a significant relationship between SERT binding in the medial raphe nucleus and fatigue as well as a significant relationship between SERT binding in the caudate nucleus and sleep disturbances (Smit et al. 2018).

In two molecular imaging studies in patients with focal dystonia, the GABA system has been investigated. In a study in patients with CD, using the PET tracer [11C]-flumazenil (FMZ), increased $GABA_A$ availability was found in the right precentral gyrus and in the left parahippocampal gyrus. Furthermore, the side of head turning correlated to a specific pattern in $GABA_A$ availability in several motor regions. Disease severity positively correlated to $GABA_A$ availability in the cerebellar hemispheres and disease duration correlated negatively to several brain regions including cerebellum, thalamus, and basal ganglia (Berman et al. 2018). In a study in patients with focal hand dystonia using both [11C]-flumazenil and [15O]-H2O to measure perfusion, different results were found. In this study, a decreased GABA availability was found in the right cerebellum and left sensorimotor cortex. Increased GABA availability was found in the inferior prefrontal cortex, which also showed an increase in perfusion. These findings correlated negatively to disease duration (Gallea et al. 2018). Both PET studies hypothesize that the areas that show reduced GABA availability are a result of loss of inhibition.

Several studies have implicated a role for the acetylcholine, serotonin, and GABA systems. However, the number of studies is limited and the results vary too much to draw definitive conclusions about the precise role of these neurotransmitter systems.

29.4 Inherited Generalized Dystonia

The discovery of the DYT-TOR1A and DYT-THAP1 genes gave the opportunity to perform imaging studies in both manifesting gene carriers and non-manifesting gene carriers. It is believed that abnormalities found in non-manifesting gene carriers are related to genotype, whereas abnormalities found in patients but not in non-manifesting gene carriers are consistent with phenotype and are either caused by the dystonia or have been the trigger that caused dystonia. On the other hand, abnormalities that have only been found in non-manifesting gene carriers and not in patients or controls could be a physical protection system (Carbon et al. 2004a).

29.4.1 Glucose Metabolism and Regional Cerebral Blood Flow

Differences in glucose metabolism have been found between patients with DYT-TOR1A, DYT-THAP1, and controls. Both the DYT-TOR1A and the DYT-THAP1 patients showed a bilateral increase in glucose metabolism in the superior frontal gyrus, including the pre-SMA, precuneus, and the inferior parietal cortex compared to controls. This increase is a similarity between DYT-TOR1A and DYT-THAP1, but overall there are more differences between the two groups. When comparing DYT-TOR1A carriers, both manifesting and non-manifesting, to controls, there is an increased glucose metabolism in the putamen. In DYT-THAP1 carriers, there is a decreased glucose metabolism in the putamen compared to controls. This decrease is more pronounced in DYT-THAP1 patients than in non-manifesting carriers. Another difference between DYT-TOR1A and DYT-THAP1 is the activation of the cerebellum. In DYT-TOR1A carriers, there is an increased cerebellar glucose metabolism compared to controls; however, the metabolism in the cerebellum of DYT-THAP1 carriers is normal. These differences also become apparent when directly comparing DYT-TOR1A and DYT-THAP1 carriers. DYT-TOR1A carriers have a bilateral increased metabolism in the inferior cerebellum and putamen compared to DYT-THAP1 carriers. DYT-THAP1 carriers have an increased metabolism in the anterior cingulate cortex bilaterally including the subgenual region, the ventral prefrontal cortex, and the middle and superior temporal gyri compared to DYT-TOR1A carriers. Thus far, it is unclear why these patients have different activation patterns in the brain, while they have overlapping symptomatology (Carbon et al. 2004b). In an earlier FDG-PET study, there was no difference in global and regional metabolism between patients with idiopathic torsion dystonia with mainly right-sided symptoms (DYT-TOR1A phenotype) and controls. However, a brain network was identified consisting of increased metabolic activity in the lateral frontal and paracentral cortices, associated with relative covariate hypermetabolism of the contralateral lentiform nucleus, pons, and midbrain. The presence of this network was associated with severity of dystonia. These findings suggest that dystonia is a network disorder (Eidelberg et al. 1995).

In another PET study, rCBF-activation in patients with generalized torsion dystonia (mostly DYT-TOR1A) was compared to that of controls during rest and during a joystick task with their right hand. There was little or no dystonia during task execution. There were no differences in rCBF-activation during rest, but during right-hand movements patients showed more rCBF-activation in the left premotor area, SMA, anterior cingulate cortex, and left dorsolateral prefrontal cortex (DLPFC) compared to controls. Also, some subcortical areas were more active during the joystick task. There was an increase in rCBF-activation in cerebellum and putamen in patients compared to controls. There was a decrease in rCBF-activation in the sensorimotor cortex contralateral to the hand that was executing the task in patients compared to controls (Playford et al. 1998). The overactivation of the DLPFC has been replicated in patients with generalized dystonia and globus pallidus interna (GPi) DBS when they were OFF stimulation. In these patients, other areas that were overactivated were the gyrus frontalis medialis, superior frontal gyrus, fronto-orbital cortex, and thalamus. Turning the DBS stimulators ON reduced the activation in these areas, as well as in the putamen, but not to the level of controls (Detante et al. 2004).

Most abnormalities that have been found in patients with DYT-TOR1A dystonia have also been found in non-manifesting DYT-TOR1A carriers. In non-manifesting DYT-TOR1A carriers, there was reduced rCBF-activation during a sequence learning task bilateral in DLPFC, in the left dorsal premotor cortex, left ventral prefrontal cortex, and lateral cerebellum. DYT-TOR1A carriers deactivated their left cingulate cortex and activated the right inferotemporal areas during the task. This was opposite to the activation pattern in controls. In controls, there was activation of the left cingulate cortex and deactivation of the right inferotemporal areas (Carbon et al. 2011, 2008; Ghilardi et al. 2003). During a motor task with the right hand, non-manifesting DYT-TOR1A carriers showed increased activation of the left premotor cortex and right SMA and decreased activation of the posterior medial cerebellum compared to controls (Carbon et al. 2011, 2008; Ghilardi et al. 2003). As with FDG-PET, rCBF-activation PET has also been used to assess brain networks in generalized dystonia. A motor-related activation pattern was identified both in controls and DYT-TOR1A gene carriers consisting of covarying neural activity in the sensorimotor cortex, dorsal premotor cortex, SMA, and cerebellum. This network was hyperactive in manifesting DYT-TOR1A gene carriers compared to controls during movement, but not in asymptomatic gene carriers. In rest, there was increased activation of this network both in manifesting and non-manifesting DYT-TOR1A gene carriers compared to controls with the non-manifesting gene carriers showing activation levels between those of the patients and controls (Carbon et al. 2010).

In summary, glucose metabolism differs between patients with DYT-TOR1A and DYT-THAP1 dystonia, with increased metabolism in putamen and cerebellum in DYT-TOR1A dystonia and decreased metabolism in putamen and normal cerebellar metabolism in DYT-THAP1 dystonia. Large numbers of brain areas show abnormal rCBF-activation in patients with DYT-TOR1A, but the significance of these findings is uncertain. Both FDG-PET and rCBF-activation studies have indicated that DYT-TOR1A dystonia is likely to be a network disorder.

29.4.2 Receptor Imaging with PET

Different neurotransmitter systems have been imaged with PET in patients with inherited generalized dystonia. With [11C]-raclopride (RAC; a D2/3 receptor tracer), both manifesting and non-manifesting DYT-TOR1A and DYT-THAP1 carriers have been compared to healthy controls. Both DYT-TOR1A and DYT-THAP1 carriers had reduced RAC binding in the caudate nucleus, putamen, and right ventrolateral thalamus compared to controls (Asanuma et al. 2005; Carbon et al. 2009). In DYT-THAP1 carriers, RAC binding was more reduced than in DYT-TOR1A carriers. This finding combined with the abnormalities in glucose metabolism may indicate that DYT-THAP1 dystonia is associated with striatal receptor loss, while

DYT-TOR1A dystonia is associated with high levels of endogenous dopamine. Thus far, there is no clear evidence for this hypothesis (Carbon and Eidelberg 2009). Although the hypothesis was that RAC binding in non-manifesting carriers was between that of patients and controls, there were no differences in RAC binding between manifesting and non-manifesting carriers in either genotype (Asanuma et al. 2005; Carbon et al. 2009).

Besides dopamine, other neurotransmitters have been studied including GABA, since one hypothesis is that dystonia is a condition of disturbed inhibition. Patients with generalized dystonia (DYT-TOR1A carriers and sporadic cases) showed reduced binding of [11C]-flumazenil (FMZ), a selective $GABA_A$ receptor PET ligand, bilateral in the primary motor and premotor cortex compared to controls. FMZ binding was also reduced in the primary and secondary somatosensory cortex, posterior insula, and in the motor component of the left anterior cingulate gyrus of patients with generalized dystonia compared to controls (Garibotto et al. 2011).

The opioid system has also been investigated in patients with DYT-TOR1A dystonia with [11C]-diprenorphine and PET, but no differences were found cortically or subcortically in DYT-TOR1A patients compared to controls (Whone et al. 2004).

In summary, dopamine is likely to play a role in the pathophysiology of both DYT-TOR1A and DYT-THAP1 dystonia, as GABA in DYT-TOR1A dystonia.

29.5 Dopamine-Responsive Dystonia

Because of the extraordinary treatment effect of levodopa on DRD, molecular imaging studies have focused on dopaminergic neurotransmission.

One of the most consistent findings in DRD is an increased tracer binding to D2/3R in caudate nucleus and putamen measured with RAC (Kishore et al. 1998; Kunig et al. 1998; Rinne et al. 2004). This could be consistent with reduced endogenous dopamine or altered receptor characteristics due to chronic dopamine depletion (Kunig et al. 1998). Increased RAC binding has also been found in asymptomatic DYT-GCH1 carriers and is therefore probably a genotypic and not a phenotypic feature (Kishore et al. 1998). There are no abnormalities in tracer binding to the dopamine transporter (DAT) or dopamine D1 receptors between patients with DRD and controls (Rinne et al. 2004). However, one study using SPECT and the DAT tracer [99mTc]-TRODAT found that striatal uptake correlated to clinical heterogeneity. More specifically, in one family the family members with a predominant parkinsonian phenotype had reduced uptake compared to the family members with a predominant dystonia phenotype (Lin et al. 2018). Abnormalities have been found in [11C]-dihydrotetrabenazine (DTBZ) binding in DRD patients. DTBZ is a tracer that binds to the vesicular monoamine transporter type 2 (VMAT2). In the striatum, VMAT2 is believed to mainly transport dopamine. Patients with DRD showed an increased DTBZ binding compared to controls. This could have been caused by reduced competition because of low concentrations of intravesicular dopamine or by upregulation of VMAT2 (De La Fuente-Fernandez et al. 2003). Finally, one report on a case with DRD and a mutation in the SRG gene also showed no loss of striatal DAT and D2/3R (Abeling et al. 2006).

As expected from the levodopa response, dopamine plays an important role in the pathophysiology of DRD. This is characterized by increased tracer binding to D2R and VMAT2 and normal tracer binding to DAT and D1R.

29.6 Myoclonus-Dystonia

Imaging results in myoclonus-dystonia (MD) only consist of two SPECT studies with [123I]-iodobenzamide (IBZM), a selective D2/3R SPECT tracer. Both MD patients and asymptomatic DYT-SCGE carriers show reduced IBZM binding compared to controls. This is consistent with the theory that a high level of endogenous dopamine causes downregulation of D2 receptors and leads to more occupied receptors, limiting IBZM binding potential (Beukers et al. 2009). After globus pallidus interna (GPi) DBS, IBZM binding in MD patients remains stable over time, whereas in patients who did not receive DBS, IBZM binding decreased further over time. This may mean that DBS in the GPi stabilizes the dopaminergic system in these patients (Beukers et al. 2012).

29.7 Rapid-Onset Dystonia-Parkinsonism

Because of the relation between dystonia and parkinsonism in this rare form of combined dystonia, most studies evaluated the dopamine system, more specifically the DAT, and compared the results to normal controls and patients with idiopathic Parkinson's disease. Tracer binding to DAT in three reports in a total of five patients yielded different results. One study in three patients showed a slight increase in tracer binding to striatal DAT (Brashear et al. 1999), while two other case reports showed normal DAT binding (Svetel et al. 2010) and a slight reduction in DAT binding (Zanotti-Fregonara et al. 2008), respectively. A perfusion SPECT scan in one patient showed no abnormalities (Zanotti-Fregonara et al. 2008).

Overall, gross abnormalities in dopaminergic neurotransmission are unlikely in RDP.

29.8 Paroxysmal Dystonia

In PKD, interictal perfusion SPECT showed regional hypoperfusion of the basal ganglia and the thalamus (Tsai et al. 2005). In PNKD, no abnormalities were found in VMAT2 binding in the striatum (Bohnen et al. 1999). Patients with exercise-induced dystonia showed reduced perfusion to the frontal cortex and basal ganglia and increased perfusion to the cerebellum during an attack using [99mTc]-ethyl cysteinate dimer (ECD) and SPECT (Kluge et al. 1998).

29.9 Conclusion

PET and SPECT studies have been performed in different forms of dystonia. Surprisingly, found abnormalities are quite similar in patients with idiopathic focal dystonia and DYT-TOR1A inherited generalized dystonia. Both focal and DYT-TOR1A dystonia patients show increased glucose metabolism in the basal ganglia, the cerebellum, and premotor structures. The areas in which rCBF-activation is abnormal are also comparable in focal and DYT-TOR1A dystonia, with increased rCBF-activation in premotor structures, frontal areas including DLPFC and cerebellum, and decreased activation in sensorimotor cortex. The found abnormalities indicate that dystonia is a circuit disorder and that the underlying cause lies somewhere in the cortico-striato-thalamo-cortical loop. The dopamine system plays an important role in both focal and DYT-TOR1A dystonia, with decreased D2R binding in the striatum pointing toward a hyperdopaminergic system. The precise role of other neurotransmitter systems, such as acetylcholine, serotonin, and GABA, remains to be determined.

DYT-THAP1 dystonia seems to be a different condition, since the reported abnormalities are different from other forms of dystonia. Striking are the decreased rCBF-activation in the putamen and normal rCBF-activation in the cerebellum, in contrast to increased rCBF-activation in the putamen and cerebellum of patients with DYT-TOR1A dystonia. The only similarity between DYT-THAP1 dystonia and other forms of dystonia is the decreased D2/3R binding. Thus far, it is still unclear what causes the differences between DYT-THAP1 dystonia and other forms of dystonia.

D2/3R binding is also decreased in MD, but is increased in DRD. Patients with DRD have a problem with the synthesis of dopamine and are therefore hypodopaminergic. The studies in different forms of paroxysmal dystonia are too limited and diverse to draw any definite conclusions.

References

Abeling NG, Duran M, Bakker HD et al (2006) Sepiapterin reductase deficiency an autosomal recessive DOPA-responsive dystonia. Mol Genet Metab 89:116–120

Albanese A, Bhatia K, Bressman SB et al (2013) Phenomenology and classification of dystonia: a consensus update. Mov Disord 28:863–873

Albin RL, Cross D, Cornblath WT et al (2003) Diminished striatal [123I]iodobenzovesamicol binding in idiopathic cervical dystonia. Ann Neurol 53:528–532

Asanuma K, Ma Y, Okulski J et al (2005) Decreased striatal D2 receptor binding in non-manifesting carriers of the DYT1 dystonia mutation. Neurology 64:347–349

Becker G, Naumann M, Scheubeck M et al (1997) Comparison of transcranial sonography, magnetic resonance imaging, and single photon emission computed tomography findings in idiopathic spasmodic torticollis. Mov Disord 12:79–88

Belenky V, Stanzhevsky A, Klicenko O, Skoromets A (2018) Brain positron emission tomography with 2-(18)F-2-deoxi-D-glucose of patients with dystonia and essential tremor detects differences between these disorders. Neuroradiol J 31:60–68

Berger HJ, van der Werf SP, Horstink CA, Cools AR, Oyen WJ, Horstink MW (2007) Writer's cramp: restoration of striatal D2-binding after successful biofeedback-based sensorimotor training. Parkinsonism Relat Disord 13:170–173

Berman BD, Pollard RT, Shelton E, Karki R, Smith-Jones PM, Miao Y (2018) GABAA receptor availability changes underlie symptoms in isolated cervical dystonia. Front Neurol 9:188

Beukers RJ, Booij J, Weisscher N, Zijlstra F, van Amelsvoort TA, Tijssen MA (2009) Reduced striatal D2 receptor binding in myoclonus-dystonia. Eur J Nucl Med Mol Imaging 36:269–274

Beukers RJ, Contarino MF, Speelman JD, Schuurman PR, Booij J, Tijssen MA (2012) Deep brain stimulation of the pallidum is effective and might stabilize striatal D(2) receptor binding in myoclonus-dystonia. Front Neurol 3:22

Bohnen NI, Albin RL, Frey KA, Fink JK (1999) (+)-alpha-[11C]Dihydrotetrabenazine PET imaging in familial paroxysmal dystonic choreoathetosis. Neurology 52:1067–1069

Booij J, de Jong J, de Bruin K, Knol R, de Win MM, van Eck-Smit BL (2007) Quantification of striatal dopamine transporters with 123I-FP-CIT SPECT is influenced by the selective serotonin reuptake inhibitor paroxetine: a double-blind, placebo-controlled, crossover study in healthy control subjects. J Nucl Med 48:359–366

Brashear A, Mulholland GK, Zheng QH, Farlow MR, Siemers ER, Hutchins GD (1999) PET imaging of the pre-synaptic dopamine uptake sites in rapid-onset dystonia-parkinsonism (RDP). Mov Disord 14:132–137

Carbon M, Eidelberg D (2009) Abnormal structure-function relationships in hereditary dystonia. Neuroscience 164:220–229

Carbon M, Kingsley PB, Su S et al (2004a) Microstructural white matter changes in carriers of the DYT1 gene mutation. Ann Neurol 56:283–286

Carbon M, Su S, Dhawan V, Raymond D, Bressman S, Eidelberg D (2004b) Regional metabolism in primary torsion dystonia: effects of penetrance and genotype. Neurology 62:1384–1390

Carbon M, Ghilardi MF, Argyelan M, Dhawan V, Bressman SB, Eidelberg D (2008) Increased cerebellar activation during sequence learning in DYT1 carriers: an equiperformance study. Brain 131:146–154

Carbon M, Niethammer M, Peng S et al (2009) Abnormal striatal and thalamic dopamine neurotransmission: genotype-related features of dystonia. Neurology 72:2097–2103

Carbon M, Argyelan M, Habeck C et al (2010) Increased sensorimotor network activity in DYT1 dystonia: a functional imaging study. Brain 133:690–700

Carbon M, Argyelan M, Ghilardi MF et al (2011) Impaired sequence learning in dystonia mutation carriers: a genotypic effect. Brain 134:1416–1427

Ceballos-Baumann AO, Sheean G, Passingham RE, Marsden CD, Brooks DJ (1997) Botulinum toxin does not reverse the cortical dysfunction associated with writer's cramp. A PET study. Brain 120(Pt 4):571–582

De La Fuente-Fernandez R, Furtado S, Guttman M et al (2003) VMAT2 binding is elevated in dopa-responsive dystonia: visualizing empty vesicles by PET. Synapse 49:20–28

Detante O, Vercueil L, Thobois S et al (2004) Globus pallidus internus stimulation in primary generalized dystonia: a H215O PET study. Brain 127:1899–1908

Eidelberg D, Moeller JR, Ishikawa T et al (1995) The metabolic topography of idiopathic torsion dystonia. Brain 118(Pt 6):1473–1484

Erro R, Bhatia KP (2019) Unravelling of the paroxysmal dyskinesias. J Neurol Neurosurg Psychiatry 90:227–234

ESDE (2000) A prevalence study of primary dystonia in eight European countries. J Neurol 247:787–792

Esmaeli-Gutstein B, Nahmias C, Thompson M, Kazdan M, Harvey J (1999) Positron emission tomography in patients with benign essential blepharospasm. Ophthal Plast Reconstr Surg 15:23–27

Feiwell RJ, Black KJ, McGee-Minnich LA, Snyder AZ, MacLeod AM, Perlmutter JS (1999) Diminished regional cerebral blood flow response to vibration in patients with blepharospasm. Neurology 52:291–297

Galardi G, Perani D, Grassi F et al (1996) Basal ganglia and thalamo-cortical hypermetabolism in patients with spasmodic torticollis. Acta Neurol Scand 94:172–176
Gallea C, Herath P, Voon V et al (2018) Loss of inhibition in sensorimotor networks in focal hand dystonia. Neuroimage Clin 17:90–97
Garibotto V, Romito LM, Elia AE et al (2011) In vivo evidence for GABA(A) receptor changes in the sensorimotor system in primary dystonia. Mov Disord 26:852–857
Ghilardi MF, Carbon M, Silvestri G et al (2003) Impaired sequence learning in carriers of the DYT1 dystonia mutation. Ann Neurol 54:102–109
Gonzalez-Alegre P (2019) Advances in molecular and cell biology of dystonia: focus on torsinA. Neurobiol Dis 127:233–241
Grundmann K (2005) Primary torsion dystonia. Arch Neurol 62:682–685
Haddad PM, Dursun SM (2008) Neurological complications of psychiatric drugs: clinical features and management. Hum Psychopharmacol 23(Suppl 1):15–26
Hierholzer J, Cordes M, Schelosky L et al (1994) Dopamine D2 receptor imaging with iodine-123-iodobenzamide SPECT in idiopathic rotational torticollis. J Nucl Med 35:1921–1927
Horstink CA, Praamstra P, Horstink MW, Berger HJ, Booij J, van Royen EA (1997) Low striatal D2 receptor binding as assessed by [123I]IBZM SPECT in patients with writer's cramp. J Neurol Neurosurg Psychiatry 62:672–673
Hutchinson M, Nakamura T, Moeller JR et al (2000) The metabolic topography of essential blepharospasm: a focal dystonia with general implications. Neurology 55:673–677
Ibanez V, Sadato N, Karp B, Deiber MP, Hallett M (1999) Deficient activation of the motor cortical network in patients with writer's cramp. Neurology 53:96–105
Kerrison JB, Lancaster JL, Zamarripa FE et al (2003) Positron emission tomography scanning in essential blepharospasm. Am J Ophthalmol 136:846–852
Kishore A, Nygaard TG, de la Fuente-Fernandez R et al (1998) Striatal D2 receptors in symptomatic and asymptomatic carriers of dopa-responsive dystonia measured with [11C]-raclopride and positron-emission tomography. Neurology 50:1028–1032
Kluge A, Kettner B, Zschenderlein R et al (1998) Changes in perfusion pattern using ECD-SPECT indicate frontal lobe and cerebellar involvement in exercise-induced paroxysmal dystonia. Mov Disord 13:125–134
Kunig G, Leenders KL, Antonini A, Vontobel P, Weindl A, Meinck HM (1998) D2 receptor binding in dopa-responsive dystonia. Ann Neurol 44:758–762
Le KD, Nilsen B, Dietrichs E (2003) Prevalence of primary focal and segmental dystonia in Oslo. Neurology 61:1294–1296
Leenders K, Hartvig P, Forsgren L et al (1993) Striatal [11C]-N-methyl-spiperone binding in patients with focal dystonia (torticollis) using positron emission tomography. J Neural Transm Park Dis Dement Sect 5:79–87
Lerner A, Shill H, Hanakawa T, Bushara K, Goldfine A, Hallett M (2004) Regional cerebral blood flow correlates of the severity of writer's cramp symptoms. NeuroImage 21:904–913
Lin JJ, Lu CS, Tsai CH (2018) Variability of presynaptic nigrostriatal dopaminergic function and clinical heterogeneity in a dopa-responsive dystonia family with GCH-1 gene mutation. J Neurol 265:478–485
Lohmann K, Klein C (2017) Update on the genetics of dystonia. Curr Neurol Neurosci Rep 17:26
Louis ED, Ferreira JJ (2010) How common is the most common adult movement disorder? Update on the worldwide prevalence of essential tremor. Mov Disord 25:534–541
Magyar-Lehmann S, Antonini A, Roelcke U et al (1997) Cerebral glucose metabolism in patients with spasmodic torticollis. Mov Disord 12:704–708
Mishina M (2008) Positron emission tomography for brain research. J Nippon Med Sch 75:68–76
Muller U (2009) The monogenic primary dystonias. Brain 132:2005–2025
Munts AG, Koehler PJ (2010) How psychogenic is dystonia? Views from past to present. Brain 133:1552–1564
Naumann M, Pirker W, Reiners K, Lange K, Becker G, Brucke T (1997) [123I]beta-CIT single-photon emission tomography in DOPA-responsive dystonia. Mov Disord 12:448–451

Naumann M, Pirker W, Reiners K, Lange KW, Becker G, Brucke T (1998) Imaging the pre- and postsynaptic side of striatal dopaminergic synapses in idiopathic cervical dystonia: a SPECT study using [123I] epidepride and [123I] beta-CIT. Mov Disord 13:319–323
Naumann M, Magyar-Lehmann S, Reiners K, Erbguth F, Leenders KL (2000) Sensory tricks in cervical dystonia: perceptual dysbalance of parietal cortex modulates frontal motor programming. Ann Neurol 47:322–328
Odergren T, Stone-Elander S, Ingvar M (1998) Cerebral and cerebellar activation in correlation to the action-induced dystonia in writer's cramp. Mov Disord 13:497–508
Perlmutter JS, Stambuk MK, Markham J et al (1997) Decreased [18F]spiperone binding in putamen in idiopathic focal dystonia. J Neurosci 17:843–850
Playford ED, Passingham RE, Marsden CD, Brooks DJ (1998) Increased activation of frontal areas during arm movement in idiopathic torsion dystonia. Mov Disord 13:309–318
Rinne JO, Iivanainen M, Metsahonkala L et al (2004) Striatal dopaminergic system in dopa-responsive dystonia: a multi-tracer PET study shows increased D2 receptors. J Neural Transm (Vienna) 111:59–67
Smit M, Vallez Garcia D, de Jong BM et al (2018) Relationships between serotonin transporter binding in the raphe nuclei, basal ganglia, and hippocampus with clinical symptoms in cervical dystonia: a [(11)C]DASB Positron Emission Tomography Study. Front Neurol 9:88
Suzuki Y, Mizoguchi S, Kiyosawa M et al (2007) Glucose hypermetabolism in the thalamus of patients with essential blepharospasm. J Neurol 254:890–896
Svetel M, Ozelius LJ, Buckley A et al (2010) Rapid-onset dystonia-parkinsonism: case report. J Neurol 257:472–474
Tarsy D, Simon DK (2006) Dystonia. N Engl J Med 355:818–829
Tsai JD, Chou IC, Tsai FJ, Kuo HT, Tsai CH (2005) Clinical manifestation and carbamazepine treatment of patients with paroxysmal kinesigenic choreoathetosis. Acta Paediatr Taiwan 46:138–142
von Campenhausen S, Bornschein B, Wick R et al (2005) Prevalence and incidence of Parkinson's disease in Europe. Eur Neuropsychopharmacol 15:473–490
Wang JL, Cao L, Li XH et al (2011) Identification of PRRT2 as the causative gene of paroxysmal kinesigenic dyskinesias. Brain 134:3493–3501
Whone AL, Von Spiczak S, Edwards M et al (2004) Opioid binding in DYT1 primary torsion dystonia: an 11C-diprenorphine PET study. Mov Disord 19:1498–1503
Wickremaratchi MM, Ben-Shlomo Y, Morris HR (2009) The effect of onset age on the clinical features of Parkinson's disease. Eur J Neurol 16:450–456
Zanotti-Fregonara P, Vidailhet M, Kas A et al (2008) [123I]-FP-CIT and [99mTc]-HMPAO single photon emission computed tomography in a new sporadic case of rapid-onset dystonia-parkinsonism. J Neurol Sci 273:148–151
Zoons E, Booij J, Nederveen AJ, Dijk JM, Tijssen MA (2011) Structural, functional and molecular imaging of the brain in primary focal dystonia—a review. NeuroImage 56:1011–1020
Zoons E, Dijkgraaf MG, Dijk JM, van Schaik IN, Tijssen MA (2012) Botulinum toxin as treatment for focal dystonia: a systematic review of the pharmaco-therapeutic and pharmaco-economic value. J Neurol 259(12):2519–2526
Zoons E, Tijssen MA, Dreissen YE, Speelman JD, Smit M, Booij J (2017a) The relationship between the dopaminergic system and depressive symptoms in cervical dystonia. Eur J Nucl Med Mol Imaging 44:1375–1382
Zoons E, Booij J, Speelman JD, Dreissen YEM, Smit M, Tijssen MAJ (2017b) Lower serotonin transporter binding in patients with cervical dystonia is associated with psychiatric symptoms. EJNMMI Res 7:87

PET and SPECT Imaging in Hyperkinetic Movement Disorders

30

Evelien Zoons, Sarvi Sharifi, Jan Booij, Bauke de Jong, and Marina A. J. Tijssen

Contents

E. Zoons
Department of Neurology, Zaans Medisch Centrum, Zaandam, The Netherlands
e-mail: zoons.e@zaansmc.nl

S. Sharifi
Department of Neurology, Amsterdam University Medical Center, Amsterdam, The Netherlands
e-mail: s.sharifi@amsterdamumc.nl

J. Booij
Department of Radiology and Nuclear Medicine, Amsterdam University Medical Center, Amsterdam, The Netherlands
e-mail: j.booij@amsterdamumc.nl

B. de Jong · M. A. J. Tijssen (✉)
Department of Neurology, University Medical Center Groningen, Groningen, The Netherlands
e-mail: b.de.jong@umcg.nl; m.a.j.de.koning-tijssen@umcg.nl

R. A. J. O. Dierckx et al. (eds.), *PET and SPECT in Neurology*,
https://doi.org/10.1007/978-3-030-53168-3_30

Abstract

Movement disorders can be classified in hypokinetic (e.g., Parkinson's disease, PD) and hyperkinetic disorders (e.g., dystonia, chorea, tremor, tics, myoclonus, and restless legs syndrome). In this chapter, we will discuss results from positron emission tomography (PET) and single photon emission computed tomography (SPECT) imaging studies in patients with tremor, tics, myoclonus, and restless legs syndrome.

Most studies in patients with tremor included patients with essential tremor (ET): a bilateral, largely symmetric, postural or kinetic tremor mainly involving the upper limbs and sometimes the head. Other studies evaluated patients with orthostatic tremor (OT): an unusually high frequent tremor in the legs that mainly occurs when patients are standing still. Increased regional cerebral blood flow (rCBF) and increased glucose metabolism have been found in the cerebellum, sensorimotor cortex, and thalamus in both patients with ET and OT compared to controls. Both PET and SPECT studies have evaluated the dopamine system in patients with ET and OT. Most imaging studies in patients with ET showed no, or only subtle loss of striatal tracer binding to the dopamine transporter indicating that ET is not characterized by nigrostriatal cell loss. The serotonin and/or gamma-aminobutyric acid (GABA) systems may play a role in the pathophysiology of ET. PET and SPECT imaging of the dopamine and serotonin system in patients with OT showed no abnormalities.

Tics, the clinical hallmark of Gilles de la Tourette syndrome (TS), are relatively brief and intermittent involuntary movements (motor tic) and sounds (phonic tic). The essential features of tics are that (1) they can be temporarily suppressed; after suppression a rebound usually occurs with a flurry of tics; (2) the patient experiences an urge to tic, and (3) the tic is followed by a short moment of relief. Using ^{18}F-FDG PET, it was shown that TS is a network disorder where multiple brain areas are active or inactive at the same time. The exact composition of this network is yet to be determined. Using rCBF PET and SPECT many brain regions were found to be abnormal, however, tics mostly correlated with hypoperfusion of the caudate nucleus and cingulate cortex. Both dopamine and serotonin are likely to play a role in the pathophysiology of TS. It is hypothesized that TS is characterized by low serotonin levels that modulate increased phasic dopamine release.

Myoclonus is defined as a brief muscle jerk and occurs in many neurologic and non-neurologic disorders. Imaging with PET and SPECT in patients with myoclonus mainly showed abnormalities consistent with the underlying disorder. We described PET and SPECT imaging results in patients in which myoclonus was a prominent symptom. Hypoperfusion and/or hypometabolism of the frontoparietal cortex was found in patients with negative epileptic myoclonus, Alzheimer's disease, corticobasal degeneration, Creutzfeldt–Jakob disease, fatal familiar insomnia, and posthypoxic myoclonus. Other findings that were frequently reported were decreased rCBF and/or glucose metabolism in the cerebellum and thalamus and abnormalities in the dopamine system.

Restless legs syndrome (RLS) is defined as an urge to move the legs accompanied with an unpleasant sensation in the legs or in another body part that is especially present during the evening and night and that can be accompanied by periodic limb movements in sleep (PLMS). Imaging studies in these patients have mainly focused on the dopamine system. Most PET studies found decreased tracer binding to the dopamine transporter, although this was not found in SPECT studies. Both PET and SPECT studies showed conflicting results regarding dopamine $D_{2/3}$ receptor binding: both increased and decreased tracer binding was reported. Furthermore, it is likely that the serotonin and opioid systems also play a role in the pathophysiology of RLS.

30.1 General Introduction

Movement disorders can be classified in hypo- and hyperkinetic disorders. The hypokinetic movement disorders include Parkinson's disease and other syndromes with parkinsonian features, for example, bradykinesia (slowness of movements). The hyperkinetic movement disorders form a large group of disorders including dystonia, chorea, myoclonus, tremor, tics, restless legs syndrome, and other rarer movement disorders (Fahn 2011). PET and SPECT findings in dystonia and chorea are dealt with in separate chapters. In this chapter, we will discuss PET and SPECT imaging in the more jerky movement disorders: tremor, tics, myoclonus, and restless legs syndrome. Every section on a specific movement disorder will start with an introduction, including historical background, phenomenology and clinical features, epidemiology, etiology, pathophysiology, and treatment. After this, results from studies using PET and SPECT are discussed.

30.2 Tremor

30.2.1 Historical Background

The first comprehensive summary of different tremor syndromes was made as late as 1998 by the Movement Disorder Society (MDS) (Deuschl et al. 1998). It was recognized that many different disorders could cause tremor. In most patients, tremor is located in the upper limbs, present during posture and is not evidently associated with other neurological symptoms, so-called essential tremor (ET). In 1981, Marsden and co-workers separated postural hand tremor into four types based on its severity. Type 1 was defined as enhanced physiological tremor, and therefore not considered pathological. Type 4 was regarded an ET-like action tremor as a symptom of another disorder (e.g., Parkinson's disease, dystonic tremor, or neuropathic tremor). Types 2 and 3 were considered to be mild and severe "pure" ET, respectively. These two types are now considered to be one disorder, namely, ET. Several rare tremor syndromes, such as orthostatic tremor (OT) and palatal tremor, were not included in this classification, but are of interest (Elble and Deuschl 2011). In this chapter, we will discuss ET and OT.

30.2.2 Classification, Clinical Features, Etiology, and Pathophysiology

ET was defined in the 1998 MDS consensus statement as a bilateral, largely symmetric postural, or kinetic tremor involving the hands and forearms that are visible and persistent. An additional or isolated tremor of the head may occur in the absence of abnormal posturing and other causes for tremor must be excluded (Deuschl et al. 1998; Elble and Deuschl 2011). The overall prevalence of ET is estimated to be 0.4–0.9% in the general population, however, can be as high as 4.8% in patients over 60 years of age (Louis and Ferreira 2010). Most patients with ET have their first symptoms in early adulthood, and the disease is characterized by slow progression and usually does not lead to disability until older age (Elble and Deuschl 2011). The tremor is highly responsive to alcohol and tends to increase after alcohol withdrawal (Crawford and Zimmerman 2011). ET has always been thought to be a monogenic disorder inherited in an autosomal dominant manner. However, current thinking is that the pathophysiology is more complex. Besides monogenic forms of ET, which can have incomplete penetrance, there are also patients in which multiple genes in combination with environmental factors contribute to disease etiology (Louis 2018). So far, genetic studies have revealed three genes to be linked to ET. These include the FUS gene (16p11.2), one of the genes implicated in the pathophysiology of hereditary amyotrophic lateral sclerosis, which accounts for a small proportion of both familial and sporadic cases of ET (Merner et al. 2012). Furthermore, mutations in the LINGO1 and TENM4 gene have been linked to ET (Louis 2018). Most of the pathophysiology of ET is unclear. ET has been associated mainly with (GABAergic) cerebellar dysfunction and disturbance of cerebello-thalamo-cortical network (Zhang and Santaniello 2019). ET is probably not linked to neurodegeneration but to abnormalities of central oscillators arising within the olivocerebellar and thalamocortical loops (Deuschl et al. 2000; Jenkins and Frackowiak 1993). Case reports where ET disappears after a stroke in cerebellum, the pons, or the thalamus suggest that interruption in central neural networks affects this type of tremor (Duncan et al. 1988; Dupuis et al. 1989, 2010; Nagaratnam and Kalasabail 1997). Postmortem studies have mainly found cerebellar pathology, more specifically Purkinje cell changes regarding their number, dendritic fields, and axons in a large proportion of ET patients (Mavroudis et al. 2019; Louis et al. 2006; Louis and Vonsattel 2008). Other findings included increased number of Lewy bodies in the brainstem and cell loss in the locus ceruleus (Mavroudis et al. 2019).

OT is a tremor of unusual high frequency (13–18 Hz) that mainly occurs in the legs when patients are standing still (Elble and Deuschl 2011). Onset of complaints is mainly around 50 years of age (Gerschlager et al. 2004). Little is known of the epidemiology of this disorder. The tremor causes a feeling of discomfort and unsteadiness that is reduced by sitting or walking (Gerschlager et al. 2004). OT is palpable as a tremulous contraction of the muscle and is audible when a stethoscope is placed on the leg (Elble and Deuschl 2011). OT can be primary or occur as a symptom of another disorder (e.g., Parkinson's disease, RLS, tardive dyskinesias) (Gerschlager et al. 2004). In this chapter, we only describe studies in patients with primary OT. In OT, there is probably a common cerebral drive causing coherent tremor activity through widespread synchronous oscillation, but the location of this drive is unknown (Elble and Deuschl 2011).

30.2.3 Treatment

Several types of medication can be used for the treatment of ET. The nonselective beta-blocker propranolol and the antiepileptic drug primidone have proven to be efficient in reducing limb tremor and should therefore be considered treatment of first choice. Propranolol is probably also effective in reducing head tremor. If these therapies fail or yield too much side effects, other drugs (mainly other beta blockers, antiepileptics, or benzodiazepines) that are probably effective are alprazolam, atenolol, gabapentin, sotalol, or topiramate. In severe cases, where medication fails, deep brain stimulation (DBS) in the ventral intermediate nucleus (Vim) of the thalamus can be considered (Zesiewicz et al. 2011). There are a few treatment options in patients with OT, but most of them tend to be unsuccessful in the majority of patients. Drugs that can be tested are gabapentin, primidone, and clonazepam. Some patients have been treated with DBS in the thalamus (Elble and Deuschl 2011).

30.2.4 Imaging with PET and SPECT

PET and SPECT studies that have been performed in tremor syndromes can roughly be divided in three types: ^{18}F-fluorodeoxyglucose (FDG) PET studies to assess brain glucose metabolism, PET, and SPECT studies for regional cerebral blood flow (rCBF) and PET and SPECT studies for receptor imaging, mainly focusing on the dopamine and GABA systems.

30.2.4.1 Essential Tremor

Regional Cerebral Blood Flow and Glucose Metabolism

RCBF has been measured both with PET and SPECT in patients with ET. The most consistent finding was increased rCBF bilaterally in the cerebellum of patients with ET. This increased rCBF was seen when patients with ET were in rest as compared to healthy controls (Jenkins and Frackowiak 1993; Boecker et al. 1996; Czarnecki et al. 2011; Wills et al. 1994) as well as when patients were maintaining a posture that induced tremor compared to a resting condition (Jenkins and Frackowiak 1993; Boecker et al. 1996; Wills et al. 1994; Colebatch et al. 1990). After ethanol administration, rCBF in cerebellum reduces and the rCBF in the inferior olivary nucleus increases (Boecker et al. 1996). Other findings included increased rCBF in the sensorimotor cortex contralateral to the arm maintaining a tremor-inducing posture (Jenkins and Frackowiak 1993; Czarnecki et al. 2011; Colebatch et al. 1990) and in the thalamus (Jenkins and Frackowiak 1993; Wills et al. 1994). The thalamus was also found to be overactive at rest in patients with ET compared to controls (Wills et al. 1994). Furthermore, patients with ET showed increased rCBF in the contralateral primary motor cortex (Czarnecki et al. 2011; Colebatch et al. 1990), supplementary motor area (SMA) (Czarnecki et al. 2011), contralateral striatum (Jenkins and Frackowiak 1993), and midbrain (Wills et al. 1994) during the posture compared to resting state. The only decrease in rCBF was found in the inferior temporal and occipital areas in patients with ET during tremor compared to controls (Wills et al. 1994).

One study evaluated glucose metabolism with PET in patients with ET during rest and found increased metabolism in the inferior olivary nucleus and thalamus compared to controls (Hallett and Dubinsky 1993). A more recent study showed decreased glucose metabolism in the medial frontal lobe, medial temporal lobe, and the precuneus of the parietal lobe in 17 male ET patients compared to controls (Ha et al. 2015). No abnormalities in metabolism of the cerebellum were found in both studies. Another study did find decreased glucose metabolism in the cerebellum when comparing ET patients to healthy controls, as well as decreased glucose metabolism in the frontal, temporal and occipital lobes, and the precuneus of the right parietal lobe (Song et al. 2015). In the same study, ET patients with a good response to propranolol were compared to ET patients that did not respond to propranolol. The responders had lower tremor scores and decreased glucose metabolism in the left basal ganglia (Song et al. 2015).

In summary, results from perfusion and metabolism scans of a heterogeneous ET group implicate in rest and posture the cerebellum, sensorimotor cortex, and thalamus (implicating the cerebello-thalamo-cortical network) as well as other areas in the pathophysiology of ET.

Receptor Imaging

Receptor imaging has mainly focused on the dopamine system and in many studies patients with ET were compared to controls as well as to patients with Parkinson's disease (PD). Patients with PD also frequently suffer from tremor in the hands and the two disorders can be mistaken for each other early in the disease course.

Most studies found slightly diminished tracer binding to the dopamine transporter (DAT) in the striatum of patients with ET compared to controls (Gerasimou et al. 2012; Group PS 2000; Isaias et al. 2008a; Lee et al. 1999; Schwartz et al. 2004; Waln et al. 2015). Patients with PD in these studies had a far more distinct reduction in striatal DAT tracer binding and DAT SPECT and DOPA PET scans were able to distinguish patients with PD and ET (Gerasimou et al. 2012; Lee et al. 1999; Waln et al. 2015; Brooks et al. 1992; Isaias and Antonini 2010; Isaias et al. 2008b; Roselli et al. 2010). Three of these studies reporting reduced striatal DAT binding have not included "pure" ET patients, but patients with parkinsonism-like isolated rest tremor and visual-motor coordination failure (Lee et al. 1999; Schwartz et al. 2004; Waln et al. 2015). Other studies did not find any difference in tracer binding to DAT in patients with ET compared to controls (Brooks et al. 1992; Isaias and Antonini 2010; Roselli et al. 2010). Two of the largest studies including ET patients fulfilling official criteria without any parkinsonism showed normal DAT binding in ET (Asenbaum et al. 1998; Benamer et al. 2000). It is possible that the heterogeneity of the groups included is the cause that some studies found (slightly) reduced tracer binding and others did not. Overall, it can be concluded that ET is likely associated with normal DAT binding. One SPECT study using ^{123}I-FP-CIT as a radiotracer found increased tracer binding in the midbrain of patients with ET compared to controls as well as compared to patients with PD and other parkinsonian syndromes (progressive supranuclear palsy and dementia with Lewy bodies) (Roselli et al. 2010). FP-CIT binding in the midbrain area reflects predominant binding to the serotonin transporter (SERT) (Booij et al. 2007) but it is unclear if these finding reflect a disturbance in serotonergic neurotransmission (Roselli et al. 2010).

One study used ^{11}C-flumazenil and PET to evaluate GABAergic neurotransmission in patients with ET and found increased tracer binding in the cerebellum in patients with ET compared to controls. This may indicate reduced GABAergic function and therefore overactivity of cerebellothalamic circuits. These findings, however, await replication (Boecker et al. 2010).

Concluding, most imaging studies in pure ET showed no, or only subtle loss of striatal DAT binding/DOPA uptake, indicating that ET is not characterized by loss of nigrostriatal cells. However, preliminary results of imaging studies may indicate a possible role of disturbances of the serotonin and/or GABA systems in the pathophysiology of ET.

30.2.5 Orthostatic Tremor

As mentioned in the introductory section, the discussed studies included patients with primary OT. RCBF has been evaluated with PET in patients with OT both during rest and while maintaining a posture with the right arm that induced arm tremor. In comparison to rest state, during action there was increased rCBF in the cerebellum bilaterally and contralateral in the lentiform nucleus and thalamus. During rest, patients with OT had increased rCBF bilaterally in the cerebellum compared to controls. These findings are comparable to those in patients with other forms of tremor (Wills et al. 1996). In one patient with medication refractory OT, FDG PET scans were acquired before the implantation of deep brain stimulation in the Vim of the thalamus and afterward both OFF and ON stimulations. Scans were acquired after repeated periods of standing that induced OT. The FDG-PET scans before DBS and OFF stimulation showed hypermetabolism of the primary motor cortex and cerebellar vermis compared to the scan ON stimulation (Guridi et al. 2008). This study was later repeated in a group of ten OT patients compared to controls, where all subjects had to stand for 10 min prior to scanning. Patients showed an increase in glucose metabolism in the pontine brainstem tegmentum, bilateral posterior lobes of the cerebellum (dentate nuclei and paravermal areas), thalamus and bilateral primary motor cortex after resting (lying down). A decrease in glucose metabolism was found in the mesiofrontal cortex in OT patients after resting compared to controls. The same differences were found when comparing OT patients and controls after standing, with the only exception that a decrease in glucose metabolism was also found in the bilateral anterior insula and posterior cingulate cortex in OT (Schoberl et al. 2017).

Other studies have focused on (dopamine) receptor imaging with varying results. Some studies compared patients with OT not only with healthy controls, but also with patients with PD. Most studies found no differences in tracer binding to DAT or dopamine $D_{2/3}$ receptors (D2/3R) between patients with OT and healthy controls (Guridi et al. 2008; Raudino et al. 2009; Trocello et al. 2008; Wegner et al. 2008). Striatal DAT binding in patients with OT did also not show differences in caudate-to-putamen ratio or asymmetry index compared to controls. In contrast to most studies, 1 study in 11 patients with OT showed reduced DAT binding in the striatum compared to controls. Binding was equally reduced in the caudate nucleus and the putamen and was higher and more symmetrical compared to patients with PD. There was no correlation between tracer binding and age, severity of OT symptoms or disease duration (Katzenschlager et al. 2003). It is unclear why reduced DAT binding was found in this study and not in other studies, but it could be that some of the OT patients in the latter study had a premorbid form of PD. One study found no differences in SERT binding between patients with OT and healthy controls (Wegner et al. 2008).

Concluding, the cerebellum probably plays an important role in the pathophysiology of OT, as it does in other tremor syndromes. The results of molecular imaging studies may indicate that dopaminergic and serotonergic disturbances are unlikely to be important.

30.3 Gilles de la Tourette Syndrome and Tics

30.3.1 Historical Background

Tourette syndrome (TS) was defined in 1885 by Gilles de la Tourette (1885). This was probably not the first description of this syndrome, but it was the first clear and comprehensive overview. Gilles de la Tourette described his observations in nine patients with a condition that started in childhood. He suspected the disorder to be degenerative and caused by an inherited weakened nervous system. Since Gilles de la Tourette's description, little has changed in the definition of the syndrome that still bears his name (McNaught and Mink 2011).

30.3.2 Clinical Features and Etiology

TS is a neurodevelopmental disorder that starts in childhood. It is a hereditary condition characterized by motor and/or vocal tics. Motor tics are sudden, rapid, recurrent, nonrhythmic movements, while vocal tics are sounds or words. Both motor and vocal tics can be simple or complex. Simple tics involve only one group of muscles and occur rapidly and jerky (eye blinking, jerking of head, neck of limbs, throat clearing, and grunting) or slowly and dystonic. Where simple tics usually look involuntary, complex tics are more coordinated movements or verbalizations and seem intentional (bending, gyrating, echolalia (repeating someone else's words), palilalia (repeating one's own words), and coprolalia (saying obscene or socially offensive words)). The first symptoms in a patient with TS are usually simple motor tics and become apparent between the age of 4 and 6 years, after which they slowly become worse. Symptoms peak between the age of 10 and 12 years. Tics are usually preceded by a premonitory urge or inner tension and followed by a short period of relief. Most patients are able to suppress their tics for a short period of time, after which a worsening of tics occurs: rebound phenomenon. The diagnosis of TS can only be made when multiple motor tics and at least one vocal tic are present before the age of 18 years and last for more than 1 year from onset. The prevalence of TS in children is estimated to be between 0.3% and–0.8%. TS is present in every ethnic group, although African-American and sub-Saharan black African populations seem to be less affected. TS is three times more common in boys than it is in girls. Isolated tics are suggested to occur in up to 24% of children. In most children, simple isolated tics disappear in adolescence, but patients with TS will usually continue to have some tics (McNaught and Mink 2011). Next to motor and vocal tics, 50–90% of patients with TS suffer from psychiatric comorbidity, especially attention-deficit hyperactivity disorder (ADHD) and obsessive–compulsive disorder (OCD) (McNaught and Mink 2011). It is very likely that TS is a multifactorial disorder. It is clear that genetic variation plays a major role in the development of TS, considering its hereditary nature. The incidence of tics and TS is up to 100 times greater in first-degree relatives of a patient with TS compared to the general population. Recently, some vulnerability genes have been identified, but they are rare variants that only contribute to etiology in a small proportion of patients (Dale 2017). Next to genetic vulnerability, several environmental factors have been implicated in the development of TS, for example, tobacco smoking, stress, infections and autoimmune conditions prenatally, perinatally, or during early postnatal development. The exact role of these factors has not been determined yet (McNaught and Mink 2011).

30.3.3 Pathophysiology

The pathophysiology of TS is largely unclear and complex. The basal ganglia play an important role in the pathophysiology of TS. There is a reduction of ~60% of GABAergic and cholinergic neurons in the caudate nucleus and putamen of patients with TS at autopsy compared to control data. Studies also showed a decreased number of GABAergic neurons in the globus pallidus externa and an increased number of these neurons in the globus pallidus interna. These anatomic alterations could have been caused by disturbed neuronal cell migration in the central nervous system during development and could lead to reduced sensory and motor inhibition in turn leading to the urge to perform inappropriate or excessive vocal and motor activities. Furthermore, it is likely that dopaminergic neurotransmission plays an important role in the pathophysiology of TS. This is likely because dopamine blocking medication is effective on tics (see below), and dopaminergic medication, such as Levodopa, can aggravate tics. PET and SPECT studies have also shown alterations in the dopaminergic neurotransmission in these patients (see below) (McNaught and Mink 2011).

30.3.4 Treatment

Treatment in patients with TS consists of multiple options. Educating patients and surroundings about the nature of the syndrome is important and can lead to understanding and respect. Behavioral therapy is used quite often in patients with TS; teaching the patient how to modify the environmental factors that influence the severity of their tics, as well as optimizing the patients' management of his symptoms. Besides behavioral therapy, there are several pharmacologic options. First treatment choice usually consists of alpha-adrenergic agonists, such as clonidine. If ineffective, antipsychotics can be used. Antipsychotics are usually divided in typical antipsychotics that are dopamine D_2 receptor antagonists, such as haloperidol, and atypical antipsychotics that are dopamine and serotonin antagonists, such as risperidone. Atypical antipsychotics are preferred, since they have a lower risk on inducing extrapyramidal side effects. Other medications include benzodiazepines, injections with botulinum toxin, and tetrabenazine. If both behavioral and medical therapy fail, patients can sometimes receive deep brain stimulation. Thus far, it is unclear in which nucleus the stimulators have to be placed and how the stimulator settings should be for an optimal treatment effect, therefore DBS currently remains an experimental therapy (McNaught and Mink 2011).

30.3.5 Imaging with PET and SPECT

Many PET and SPECT studies have been performed in patients with tics and TS. We divided the information in PET studies investigating glucose metabolism, PET and

SPECT studies investigating regional cerebral blood flow, and PET and SPECT studies investigating receptor binding.

30.3.5.1 Glucose Metabolism

Using FDG-PET, patients with TS have been investigated. Global and regional metabolic rates were found to be normal in patients with TS compared to controls (Eidelberg et al. 1997). Later studies have mainly focused on brain networks: regions that simultaneously show an increase or decrease in metabolism in patients, but not in controls. Simultaneous increases in metabolism were found bilaterally in the premotor cortex, supplementary motor area (SMA), midbrain and cerebellum in patients with TS compared to controls (Eidelberg et al. 1997; Jeffries et al. 2002; Pourfar et al. 2011). Simultaneous decreases in metabolism were found in the striatum, primary motor cortex, somatosensory association areas, insula, orbitofrontal cortex, thalamus, lentiform nucleus, and hippocampus compared to controls (Eidelberg et al. 1997; Jeffries et al. 2002; Pourfar et al. 2011). All these brain regions have been implicated in other movement disorders as well, and are therefore considered as aspecific (Eidelberg et al. 1997). In both patients with TS and controls, there was a connection between the activity of the motor cortex and the lateral orbitofrontal cortex, but the interaction pattern between these areas may differ. In patients with TS, there was a positive interaction in these areas meaning they were both active or inactive at the same time, but in controls there was a negative interaction. In controls, either the motor cortex was active or the orbitofrontal cortex, but they were not active at the same time (Jeffries et al. 2002). In patients with TS and comorbid OCD, an additional network correlating with the severity of OCD consisted of reduced metabolic activity in the anterior cingulate cortex and dorsolateral prefrontal cortex (DLPFC) with increased activity in the primary motor cortex and precuneus (Pourfar et al. 2011).

In summary, TS is likely to be a network disorder, but the exact composition of the affected circuits is not clear yet.

30.3.5.2 Regional Cerebral Blood Flow

The first studies investigating rCBF in patients with tics and TS used [^{99m}Tc-D,L]-hexamethylpropyleneamine-oxime (HMPAO) and SPECT. Increased rCBF was found in the right frontal cortex in patients with TS, of which a part also had OCD, compared to controls. There was no difference between patients with and without OCD (George et al. 1992). Reduced rCBF was found in the right basal ganglia, orbitofrontal and medial frontal cortex, temporal lobes, left caudate nucleus, anterior cingulate cortex, and left DLPFC in patients with TS compared to controls (Klieger et al. 1997; Lampreave et al. 1998; Moriarty et al. 1995). The severity of tics was correlated to the hypoperfusion of the left caudate nucleus, anterior cingulate cortex, and a medial temporal region. Hypoperfusion of the DLPFC was correlated to mood in patients (Moriarty et al. 1995). The reduced rCBF in the orbitofrontal and medial frontal cortex and in the temporal lobes in patients increased after treatment with neuropsychotics, but not to the same level as controls (Lampreave et al. 1998).

A study with another SPECT tracer to assess rCBF, [^{99m}Tc]-ethylene cysteinate dimer (ECD), found comparable results in children with TS as the above-named studies. Children with TS had reduced rCBF in the left caudate nucleus, cingulate cortex, right cerebellum, left DLPFC, and left orbitofrontal cortex compared to controls. There was a correlation between the severity of the vocal tics and rCBF in cerebellum and bilateral DLPFC. Patients did not have psychiatric comorbidity, but scores on depression and OCD were negatively correlated to rCBF values, especially in temporal regions (Diler et al. 2002).

An event-related PET study with ^{15}O-H_2O showed activation of cerebellum, insula, SMA, motor cortex, thalamus, and putamen during tics (Lerner et al. 2007). In one study, five severely affected TS patients were compared to healthy controls and rescanned after implantation of DBS electrodes both in the globus pallidus pars interna (GPi) and the thalamus. After surgery, GPi, thalamus, and sham stimulation were applied in a random order each for 3 months and ECD SPECT was made at the end of each 3-month period. Preoperative TS patients had decreased rCBF in the right pre- and postcentral cortex, left paracentral cortex, bilateral SMA, bilateral superior frontal cortex, right middle frontal gyrus, and parietal cortex compared to healthy controls. rCBF was increased in the left temporal cortex and bilaterally in the cerebellum. After surgery, both GPi and thalamic stimulation resulted in significant decreases in rCBF in basal ganglia and cerebellum and increases in rCBF in the frontal cortex compared to sham stimulation. A relation to symptom improvement was not reported (Haense et al. 2016).

Concluding, the perfusion of many brain regions was found to be abnormal in patients with Tourette syndrome, but tics mostly correlated with hypoperfusion of the caudate nucleus and cingulate cortex. Treatment with medication and DBS can alter rCBF in TS patients.

30.3.5.3 Receptor Imaging

PET and SPECT studies investigating receptor binding in patients with tics and TS have mainly focused on the dopamine system, although some studies looked at the serotonin system.

One PET study found increased tracer binding to dopamine $D_{2/3}$ receptors (D2/3R) (Wong et al. 2008), where others did not (Abi-Jaoude et al. 2015; Turjanski et al. 1994; Wong et al. 1997). Increased dopamine release was found after administration of the dopamine releaser amphetamine or the neuroleptic haloperidol (Wong et al. 2008, 1997). There was a trend toward a correlation of D2/3R binding and severity of vocal tics (Wong et al. 1997). There were no differences in tracer binding to striatal DATs (Wong et al. 2008; Turjanski et al. 1994) or striatal vesicular monoamine transporters 2 (VMAT2) (Albin et al. 2009; Meyer et al. 1999). These results were confirmed by a large meta-analysis (Hienert et al. 2018). One study using ^{18}F-fallypride, a PET tracer which can be used to also assess extrastriatal dopamine D2/3R, found reduced binding in the orbitofrontal cortex, primary motor cortex, anterior cingulate gyrus, mediodorsal nucleus of the thalamus, and hippocampus. These areas are concerned with motivation, reward, sensory gating, movement, and attention, and also showed abnormalities in PET studies investigating glucose metabolism and rCBF (Gilbert et al. 2006).

Results from SPECT studies investigating the dopamine system in tics and TS varied. Most studies found increased DAT binding in the striatum of patients with TS compared to controls (Cheon et al. 2004; Heinz et al. 1998; Liu et al. 2010; Muller-Vahl et al. 2000; Serra-Mestres et al. 2004), although in some studies no difference in DAT binding was found (Hwang et al. 2008; Stamenkovic et al. 2001; Yeh et al. 2006). It is unclear what caused these varying results. One study found an association between DAT binding and self-injurious behavior and impulse control problems (Muller-Vahl et al. 2000). However, it appears that behavioral and psychiatric symptoms in TS are not directly related to measurable abnormalities in striatal DAT activity. Another study found a negative correlation between DAT binding and disease duration (Liu et al. 2010). DAT could be hyperfunctional during the first years of disease, after which some form of adaptation takes place (Liu et al. 2010; Yeh et al. 2006). This could explain the reduction of tics that is usually seen during puberty (Muller-Vahl et al. 2000). One SPECT study compared striatal DAT binding before and after a methylphenidate challenge. This study showed less reduction in DAT binding (reflecting occupancy of the DAT by methylphenidate) in patients with TS compared to controls, after phasic administration of methylphenidate (Yeh et al. 2007). If this theory of a hyperfunctional DAT system followed by adaptation is true, this could have contributed to the different results in the PET and SPECT studies investigating DAT binding in patients with Tourette syndrome. Other explanations for the discrepancies between studies could be sample size, age of patients (some studies investigated children, while others looked at adults), and use of dopamine blocking medication. In all SPECT studies, medication was stopped prior to scanning, but rest effect of medication cannot be completely ruled out. SPECT studies looking at the (postsynaptic) D2/3R did not find differences between patients with TS and controls (Muller-Vahl et al. 2000; Hwang et al. 2008; George et al. 1994), although one study found decreased tracer binding to these receptors in patients who had TS for more than 15 years compared to patients who had complaints less than 15 years and controls (Muller-Vahl et al. 2000). This could also be consistent with some form of adaptation of the dopamine system. One study in monozygotic twins with different levels of tic severity found a correlation between D2R binding in the caudate nucleus and severity of tics (Wolf et al. 1996).

Some PET and SPECT studies looked into the serotonin system. Tracer binding to the SERT in the midbrain and thalamus was decreased in patients with TS compared to controls (Wong et al. 2008; Muller-Vahl et al. 2005). There was a negative correlation between SERT binding and severity of tics (Heinz et al. 1998; Muller-Vahl et al. 2005), as well as a negative correlation between SERT binding and the severity of comorbid obsessive–compulsive symptoms (Muller-Vahl et al. 2005). Tracer binding to the serotonin receptor (5-HT_{2A}) was increased in the anterior cingulate cortex, orbitofrontal cortex, medial inferior frontal cortex, superior frontal cortex, and putamen in patients with TS compared to controls in one study (Haugbol et al. 2007), while another study only found weakly increased binding in patients with TS and comorbid OCD compared to controls in prefrontal, temporal, and cingulate cortices (Wong et al. 2008). Only one molecular imaging study compared SERT binding in TS patients with OCD (TS + OCD), TS patients without OCD (TS − OCD), and OCD patients without TS (OCD) to healthy controls using SPECT. SERT binding (measured with the selective SERT tracer ^{123}I-ADAM) was normal in patients with OCD and TS-OCD, but significantly increased in caudate nucleus, hypothalamus, and midbrain in TS + OCD. In TS patients with and without OCD, SERT binding in the pons was negatively correlated with tic severity (Muller-Vahl et al. 2019). One PET study used alfa-^{11}C-methyl-L-tryptophan (AMT) and PET to examine serotonin synthesis in children with TS compared to controls. AMT uptake was bilaterally reduced in the DLPFC and bilaterally increased in the thalamus (Behen et al. 2007). Altogether, these studies indicate that serotonin may play a role in the pathophysiology of Tourette syndrome (Heinz et al. 1998; Haugbol et al. 2007; Behen et al. 2007).

One PET study used ^{18}F-fluoroethoxybenzovesamicol in patients with TS to evaluate striatal cholinergic interneuron density and found no differences compared to healthy controls (Albin et al. 2017).

Concluding, both dopamine and serotonin are likely to play a role in the pathophysiology of TS. One of the current hypotheses is that TS is characterized by increased phasic dopamine release modulated by low serotonin levels. The low concentration of serotonin could explain the high percentages of comorbid psychiatric disorders, such as OCD (Wong et al. 2008). The role of acetylcholine has to be further investigated.

30.4 Myoclonus

30.4.1 Historical Background

Friedreich was the first to describe myoclonus in 1881 in a patient with possible myoclonic epilepsy (Faught 2003). Myoclonus is defined as brief muscle jerks and occurs in many neurologic and non-neurologic disorders. Over the years, most of the attention was on cortical myoclonus, in which Grinker in 1938 reported trains of electroencephalographic discharges coinciding with myoclonus in patients with familial myoclonus epilepsy. Since then different forms of myoclonus have been discovered as well as numerous underlying disorders (see below) (Shibasaki and Thompson 2011).

30.4.2 Classification, Clinical Features, and Etiology

There are three generally accepted classifications for myoclonus that are based on clinical characteristics, etiology, and anatomic localization. These three classifications are highly interrelated (Dijk and Tijssen 2010). When classifying myoclonus on clinical signs, it is important to note the distribution: focal, segmental, axial, or generalized. Myoclonus can sometimes be induced by action, especially in patients with posthypoxic encephalopathy, or by a tactile stimulus (stimulus-sensitive or reflex myoclonus). Furthermore, myoclonus can occur as muscle contractions (positive myoclonus) or as interruption of muscle tone (negative myoclonus) (Dijk and Tijssen 2010).

There are many disorders that can cause myoclonus, but they can roughly be divided into four etiological groups: physiological, symptomatic, epileptic, and essential. Physiological myoclonus is common in healthy individuals and consists of sleep jerks, hiccups, and other nonpathological forms of myoclonus. Symptomatic myoclonus accounts for approximately 70% of cases with a pathological origin. Underlying disorders that can cause myoclonus are for example, posthypoxic syndrome, Alzheimer's disease, drug-induced, and toxic–metabolic conditions. Epileptic myoclonus is the second most common pathological etiological category. Epileptic myoclonus can be the only symptom of epilepsy or can be a component of a seizure of any type. In essential myoclonus, myoclonus is the only or most important symptom. Most disorders in this category are hereditary and the most prevalent one is myoclonus-dystonia (see Chapter 29). One of the most prevalent causes of myoclonus is not included in this classification: psychogenic myoclonus. Approximately 8.5% of patients with myoclonus have psychogenic myoclonus and 17.2% of patients with a psychogenic movement disorder have myoclonus (Dijk and Tijssen 2010).

Anatomically myoclonus can be divided by electrophysiological tests in cortical (e.g., posthypoxic, epileptic, or in patients with neurodegenerative diseases), subcortical (e.g., myoclonus-dystonia), brainstem (e.g., hyperekplexia, opsoclonus-myoclonus syndrome), spinal (e.g., segmental or propriospinal myoclonus, the latter almost always has a psychogenic origin) or peripheral (e.g., hemifacial spasm) (Shibasaki and Thompson 2011).

The incidence and prevalence of myoclonus are mainly dependent on the incidence and prevalence of disorders causing myoclonus. The lifetime prevalence of pathological and persistent myoclonus was 8.6 cases per 100,000 population in a large study in the United States. In nursing homes, 0.5% of patients suffer from myoclonus. Transient (e.g., drug-induced) myoclonus is not included in this lifetime prevalence, but represents 27.6% of all patients with myoclonus who visit an emergency room for a movement disorder (Dijk and Tijssen 2010).

30.4.3 Pathophysiology

The pathophysiology of myoclonus is dependent on both the anatomical origin as well as the etiological cause of dystonia. It is beyond the scope of this chapter to deal with all the different pathophysiological processes that can eventually lead to myoclonus.

30.4.4 Treatment

Treatment of myoclonus mainly depends on the anatomical origin. Treatment of myoclonus is difficult and time-consuming. It often requires several drug trials before a drug with a beneficiary effect is found and most drugs only partly relieve symptoms, while at the same time causing side effects. In cortical myoclonus, first choice is the antiepileptic levetiracetam or piracetam, but the benzodiazepine clonazepam can also be used, especially in patients with posthypoxic cortical reflex myoclonus. Clonazepam is also the first choice in patients with myoclonus-dystonia, as well as most other forms of subcortical myoclonus and spinal myoclonus. Patients with peripheral myoclonus can be locally treated with botulinum toxin injections and patients with myoclonic epilepsy have to be treated with antiepileptics. This is only an indication for therapy and not an exhaustive overview. For this, we would like to refer to some of the excellent reviews on this topic (Dijk and Tijssen 2010).

30.4.5 Imaging

Imaging in some forms of myoclonus is dealt with in other chapters (e.g., myoclonus dystonia in the chapter on dystonia, and restless legs syndrome below). In this section, we will discuss findings in epileptic myoclonus, myoclonus in degenerative diseases (Alzheimer's disease and corticobasal degeneration), in prion disease (Creutzfeldt–Jakob disease and fatal familial insomnia), posthypoxic myoclonus, and opsoclonus-myoclonus syndrome.

30.4.5.1 Epileptic Myoclonus

In epilepsy two different forms of myoclonus can occur. Positive myoclonic jerks usually occur as focal seizures in patients with different forms of progressive myoclonus epilepsy. These patients often also suffer from generalized seizures. Another form is epileptic negative myoclonus, which is a short loss of muscle tone due to epilepsy. This causes, for example, the hands to drop when the arms and hands are extended. Both forms have been investigated with PET and SPECT.

In two patients with Lafora disease, a form of progressive myoclonus epilepsy, FDG PET imaging showed occipital hypometabolism. This is consistent with the visual hallucinations and visual agnosia these patients usually also have and is probably unrelated with the myoclonus or epilepsy (Jennesson et al. 2010). In four patients with Unverricht–Lundborg disease, another form of progressive myoclonus-epilepsy, tracer binding to D2/3R was evaluated with ^{11}C-raclopride and PET. Tracer binding was increased in the thalamus and striatum in patients compared to controls (Korja et al. 2007).

In patients with epileptic negative myoclonus on the right side of the body, hyperperfusion of the left premotor area, parietal cortex, and putamen were found using perfusion SPECT (Baumgartner et al. 1996; Yu et al. 2009). Surprisingly, FDG-PET in one of these patients showed hypometabolism of the left frontoparietal cortex (Yu et al. 2009). In one patient, ^{123}I-iomazenil (IMZ; a selective GABA-A receptor tracer) and SPECT showed reduced tracer binding in the premotor cortex (Usui et al. 2010).

In summary, imaging results in epileptic myoclonus are too limited to draw any definite conclusions.

30.4.5.2 Degenerative Diseases

Perfusion has been evaluated using SPECT in two important degenerative diseases that frequently cause myoclonus: Alzheimer's disease (AD) and corticobasal degeneration (CBD). We will only discuss results from studies that explicitly reported on patients with myoclonus. In patients with AD hypoperfusion was found in the frontal and parietal lobes (Hu et al. 2009; Kobayashi et al. 2000). In one study, this frontoparietal hypoperfusion was contralateral to the arm with the most severe myoclonus (Kobayashi et al. 2000).

In patients with CBD, more extensive hypoperfusion was found. The most consistent findings were frontoparietal and thalamus hypoperfusion (Hu et al. 2009; Huang et al. 2007; Storey et al. 1995). Areas that were implicated were the temporal lobe and cerebellum (Hu et al. 2009; Lu et al. 1998). Hypoperfusion was more prominent in the hemisphere contralateral to the most affected arm, with additional hypoperfusion in the interconnected ipsilateral cerebellum (Huang et al. 2007; Storey et al. 1995; Lu et al. 1998). Patients with CBD also have generalized cerebral atrophy, but hypoperfusion was found to be more extensive than would be expected based on atrophy (Storey et al. 1995). DAT binding was found to be reduced contralateral to the most affected arm or bilateral in the striatum (Huang et al. 2007).

Concluding, myoclonus in degenerative diseases like AD and CBD is correlated to frontoparietal hypoperfusion. Dopamine possibly plays a role in the pathophysiology of myoclonus in CBD. However, most of these findings have also been described in patients with AD or CBD, but without myoclonus.

30.4.5.3 Prion Disease

Creutzfeldt–Jakob disease (CJD) is a condition caused by misfolded prion proteins. CJD can be sporadic or hereditary. The misfolded prion proteins can cause varying symptoms of which the most prominent are memory and cognitive decline, and movement disorders including myoclonus, ataxia, and visual disturbances. The disease has a dramatic disease course and is uniformly fatal within months to years (Imran and Mahmood 2011). FDG PET imaging in a group of patients with CJD showed extensive hypometabolism that was most prominent in the temporal and parietal regions. Other affected areas included the occipital lobe, cerebellum, and basal ganglia. Myoclonus correlated to hypometabolism of the contralateral parietal lobe and basal ganglia (Henkel et al. 2002). In another patient, an FDG-PET scan showed hypermetabolism in the right frontoparietal cortex and left cerebellum early in the disease course. After the disease progressed, the patient developed seizures. A perfusion SPECT scan showed hypoperfusion of the right frontoparietal cortex, consistent with the study by Henkel and colleagues (Nagasaka et al. 2011). DAT binding was bilaterally reduced in the striatum of patients with CJD (Chen et al. 2010; Ragno et al. 2009) and tracer binding to the GABA-A receptor was reduced throughout the entire cerebral cortex, but not in the cerebellum (Itoh et al. 1998).

Fatal familial insomnia (FFI) is a genetic prion disease characterized by insomnia, oneiric stupor with autonomic and motor hyperactivity, pyramid tract symptoms, myoclonus, dysarthria, dysphagia, and ataxia. Like CJD, it has a fatal disease course within months to a few years (Imran and Mahmood 2011). With FDG-PET, a prominent hypometabolism of the thalamus with less extensive hypometabolism of the basal ganglia, frontotemporal cingulate cortex, and the cerebellum has been found in patients with FFI. The amount of hypometabolism correlates with the disease duration. SERT binding was reduced in the thalamus and hypothalamic regions in patients with FFI compared to controls, implicating the serotonin system in this rare disease (Montagna 2005; Montagna et al. 2003). As in degenerative diseases, these findings do not seem to be specific for myoclonus as the same results have been described in patients with prion diseases, but without myoclonus.

30.4.5.4 Posthypoxic Myoclonus

Posthypoxic myoclonus (Lance-Adams syndrome) is a form of cortical myoclonus that predominantly occurs during action. In patients with Lance-Adams syndrome increased metabolism of the pontine tegmentum spreading to the mesencephalon, ventrolateral thalamus, and medial temporal lobes, and decreased metabolism of the bilateral frontal lobes was found using FDG and PET (Frucht et al. 2004; Zhang et al. 2007). A perfusion SPECT scan in one patient showed hypoperfusion of the left temporal lobe (Zhang et al. 2007).

30.4.5.5 Opsoclonus-Myoclonus Syndrome

Opsoclonus-myoclonus syndrome (OMS) is a syndrome that usually occurs during or after a systemic infection or as a paraneoplastic phenomenon and is characterized by myoclonus of the limbs and myoclonic movements of the eyes (opsoclonus) (Dijk and Tijssen 2010). Perfusion SPECT scans in two patients with a recently developed OMS showed hyperperfusion of the cerebellum, mainly in the vermis (Oguro et al. 1997; van Toorn et al. 2005). Surprisingly, in a patient who already suffered more than 3 years from OMS a perfusion SPECT scan showed hypoperfusion of the cerebellum (Oguro et al. 1997). It could be that OMS is characterized by inflammation and hyperperfusion in the early stage, followed by hypoperfusion caused by cell death and gliosis (Oguro et al. 1997). Similar results were shown in one patient with an adnexal teratoma and paraneoplastic OMS using FDG-PET. In the acute stage, there was an increased glucose metabolism in the cerebellum that decreased after symptoms diminished with treatment of the teratoma. Twelve months after symptom onset, symptoms had completely resolved and there was a decrease in glucose metabolism of the visual cortex and still a slight increase of glucose metabolism in the deep cerebellar nuclei, albeit metabolism was lower than in the acute phase (Oh et al. 2017).

30.4.5.6 General Remarks on Imaging in Patients with Myoclonus

Imaging studies have been performed in patients with different underlying causes of myoclonus and it is interesting to see what the similarities are, as they could teach us more about the underlying brain abnormalities that lead to myoclonus. Hypoperfusion and/or hypometabolism of the frontoparietal cortex are found in different conditions with myoclonus. This has been found in patients with negative epileptic myoclonus, Alzheimer's disease, CBD, Creutzfeldt–Jakob disease, fatal familiar insomnia, and posthypoxic myoclonus. In several studies, the reduced perfusion or metabolism in the frontoparietal cortex was described to be contralateral to the most affected arm. Other areas that were often found to have abnormalities in perfusion or metabolism were the thalamus and the cerebellum. In most cases, there was reduced perfusion or metabolism in these regions. A third common factor was the involvement of the dopamine system in the striatum. D2/3R binding was increased in progressive myoclonus epilepsy and striatal DAT binding was reduced in corticobasal degeneration and Creutzfeldt–Jakob disease. However, thus far, results from different studies are too limited and too diverse to draw any hard conclusions on the origin of myoclonic jerks. Furthermore, most results merely seem to reflect abnormalities caused by the underlying condition and not by the myoclonus.

30.5 Restless Legs Syndrome and Periodic Limb Movements in Sleep

30.5.1 Historical Background

Restless legs syndrome (RLS) was first described in detail by Professor Ekbom, a Swedish neurologist, in his doctoral thesis in 1944. However, the first description of RLS dates back to 1685 in a publication by Sir Thomas Willis, who describes people who are so restless in bed that it looks as if they are being tortured (Teive et al. 2009). After this first description, several cases were published, most of which were thought to be psychogenic at that time, although the hereditary nature of the condition had also been noted. It was not until Ekbom published his first paper on RLS that it was recognized as a distinct neurological syndrome (Teive et al. 2009). Phillips et al. showed in 2000 that RLS occurs in up to 10% of the population and is heavenly underdiagnosed (Phillips et al. 2000; Shepard Jr. et al. 2005).

30.5.2 Clinical Features and Etiology

RLS is considered both a movement disorder as well as a sleep disorder. RLS is defined as an urge to move the legs accompanied with an unpleasant sensation in the legs or in another body part. Complaints are aggravated by rest, alleviated by movement and are worse in the evening or night (Avidan 2009). The incidence of RLS increases with age. Population prevalence of RLS varies between 1% and 15% in different studies and it is twice as common in females as males (Yeh et al. 2012).

RLS can be either primary or secondary. Primary RLS occurs early in life, with a peak at age 20, has a strong genetic component and family history is usually positive (Yeh et al. 2012). Secondary RLS develops later in life and is usually sporadic. Secondary RLS is often associated with another disorder, for example, peripheral neuropathy. There are some risk factors for developing RLS, for example, pregnancy, low serum iron, lower socioeconomic status, and poor medical as well as mental health and PD (Yeh et al. 2012).

Periodic limb movements in sleep (PLMS) are characteristic limb movements that occur at a typical rate of 0.5- to 5- or 10-s duration and recur periodically (5- to 90-s period) in a series (four or more) in any sleep state. The movements usually consist of extension of the big toe with partial flexion of the ankle, knee, and sometimes hip. These movements can be associated with a partial arousal or awakening; however, the patient is usually unaware of this. Patients can complain of excessive daytime sleepiness, headaches, and psychiatric symptoms, due to disturbed sleep. PLMS is estimated to occur in 4–11% of adults and is most common in patients with other sleep disorders, especially RLS (Avidan 2009).

30.5.3 Pathophysiology

The pathophysiology of RLS is largely unclear; however, there is some evidence for a role of the dopamine system in the pathophysiology of RLS. Higher concentrations of dopamine and homovanillic acid have been found in cerebrospinal fluid during daytime compared to nighttime in patients with RLS. This could indicate that a disturbed circadian rhythm of dopaminergic function is responsible for RLS symptoms. No genes have been identified yet, although some loci have been linked to RLS complaints in families with primary RLS (Avidan 2009).

30.5.4 Treatment

There are several different medical treatments for RLS, but they almost all share the risk of augmentation, which is the recurrence and worsening of symptoms after an initial period of improvement with treatment. Major classes of drugs that are being used in the treatment of RLS are dopamine agonists such as ropinirole and pramipexole, benzodiazepines such as clonazepam, anticonvulsants such as carbamazepine and gabapentin, opioids such as codeine, propoxyphene or oxycodone, bupropion and iron supplementation (Avidan 2009; Yeh et al. 2012). Treatment of PLMS is the same as for RLS, although one should be careful with prescribing benzodiazepines or opioids in patients with PLMS because of the high incidence of obstructive sleep apnea (Avidan 2009).

30.5.5 Imaging

Because of the proposed role of dopamine in the pathophysiology of RLS and PLMS, PET and SPECT imaging focused on the dopamine system. PET studies in patients with RLS showed decreased DAT binding in the caudate nucleus and putamen of patients compared to controls (Earley et al. 2011; Ruottinen et al. 2000; Turjanski et al. 1999). This was found in patients with and without comorbid PLMS and was found on scans both acquired at daytime and in the evening (Earley et al. 2011; Ruottinen et al. 2000). DAT binding in the striatum was not decreased, however, and there was no correlation between striatal DAT binding and severity of complaints (Earley et al. 2011). There were no differences in DAT binding between patients treated with levodopa at the time of scanning and patients without medical treatment (Turjanski et al. 1999). Results for PET tracer binding to D2/3R were somewhat conflicting. Two PET studies found decreased binding to D2/3R in the caudate nucleus, putamen, and nucleus accumbens of patients with RLS compared to controls (Turjanski et al. 1999; Oboshi et al. 2012). In these studies, there was no difference between patients with RLS treated with levodopa and patients without medical treatment (Turjanski et al. 1999). There was a negative correlation between D2/3R binding and severity of RLS symptoms and a positive correlation between D2/3R binding and the amount of improvement after treatment with the dopamine agonist pramipexole (Oboshi et al. 2012). In another PET study, D2/3R binding was however increased in the striatum, thalamus, and anterior cingulate cortex in patients with RLS compared to controls. This increased D2/3R binding was found both at daytime and in the evening (Cervenka et al. 2006). It is unclear what caused this difference in D2/3R binding; however, it might be partly explained by medication effects. In the studies, finding decreased D2/3R binding at least part of the patients had been exposed to dopaminergic medication, while in the study that found increased D2R binding all patients were medication-naïve (Cervenka et al. 2006).

SPECT studies also studied the dopamine system in patients with RLS and PLMS. Most SPECT studies found no difference in DAT binding between patients with RLS and PLMS compared to controls (Eisensehr et al. 2001; Linke et al. 2004; Michaud et al. 2002; Mrowka et al. 2005). One of these studies did find a lower putamen to caudate nucleus ratio in patients with RLS as compared to controls. In controls tracer binding in putamen was comparable to binding in caudate nucleus (Mrowka et al. 2005). One SPECT study found increased DAT binding in caudate nucleus, posterior putamen, and total striatum in elderly patients with moderately to severe RLS (Kim et al. 2012). Like the results from PET studies, results from SPECT studies looking at D2/3R binding were conflicting. Three SPECT studies found no difference in D2/3R binding in patients with RLS compared to controls (Eisensehr et al. 2001; Kim et al. 2012; Tribl et al. 2004), while two other studies found decreased D2/3R binding in the striatum of patients with RLS compared to controls (Michaud et al. 2002; Staedt et al. 1995). Both the studies with decreased D2R binding were performed in patients with RLS and PLMS (Michaud et al. 2002; Staedt et al. 1995), but so was one of the studies that did not find a difference in D2/3R binding (Tribl et al. 2004). Overall, most studies are consistent with the theory of central dopaminergic dysfunction as part of the pathophysiology in RLS and PLMS.

A few imaging studies did not focus on the dopamine system. One study used ^{123}I-beta-CIT and SPECT to evaluate the SERT in patients with RLS. There were no differences in SERT binding between patients with RLS and controls, but there was a negative correlation between scores on the International RLS Study Group Severity Scale and SERT binding in the pons and medulla. The authors hypothesized that an increase of serotonergic neurotransmission in the brainstem could cause deterioration of RLS symptoms through an effect on dopaminergic neurotransmission or through a direct effect on the activity of spinal and sensory neurons (Jhoo et al. 2010). Another study looked at the opioid system in patients with RLS using ^{11}C-diprenorphine (a nonselective opioid receptor ligand) and PET. There were no differences between tracer binding in patients with RLS and controls. There was, however, a negative correlation between severity of RLS symptoms and tracer binding in the medial pain system (medial thalamus, amygdala, caudate nucleus, anterior cingulate gyrus, insular cortex, and orbitofrontal cortex) in patients with RLS. Pain scores correlated negatively to tracer binding in the orbitofrontal cortex and anterior cingulate gyrus in patients with RLS (von Spiczak et al. 2005).

The only study using FDG and PET found no differences in regional glucose metabolism between patients with RLS and controls (Trenkwalder et al. 1999).

Concluding, imaging studies suggest that both the serotonin and the opioid system seem to play a role in the pathophysiology of RLS as does the dopamine system.

30.6 General Conclusion

PET and SPECT studies have been used extensively to unravel the pathophysiology of hyperkinetic movement disorders. As expected, results from these studies differ between different conditions, but it is interesting to see that there are also similarities between the different movement disorders. The most important difference lies in the areas of abnormal perfusion or metabolism in the different disorders. In tremor, the cerebellum is most implicated, while in myoclonus there is mainly abnormal perfusion or metabolism in the frontoparietal regions, and in TS a neuronal network including the basal ganglia, motor cortex, thalamus, and hippocampus may be implicated. The most outstanding similarity is that abnormalities of the dopaminergic system, and probably the serotonergic system as well, are likely to play a role in almost all hyperkinetic movement disorders. How changes in dopamine levels can lead to such diversity in symptomatology is yet to be discovered.

References

Abi-Jaoude E, Segura B, Obeso I et al (2015) Similar striatal D2/D3 dopamine receptor availability in adults with Tourette syndrome compared with healthy controls: a [(11) C]-(+)-PHNO and [(11) C]raclopride positron emission tomography imaging study. Hum Brain Mapp 36:2592–2601

Albin RL, Koeppe RA, Wernette K et al (2009) Striatal [11C]dihydrotetrabenazine and [11C]methylphenidate binding in Tourette syndrome. Neurology 72:1390–1396

Albin RL, Minderovic C, Koeppe RA (2017) Normal striatal vesicular acetylcholine transporter expression in Tourette syndrome. eNeuro 4(4):ENEURO.0178-17.2017

Asenbaum S, Pirker W, Angelberger P, Bencsits G, Pruckmayer M, Brucke T (1998) [123I]beta-CIT and SPECT in essential tremor and Parkinson's disease. J Neural Transm (Vienna) 105:1213–1228

Avidan AY (2009) Parasomnias and movement disorders of sleep. Semin Neurol 29:372–392

Baumgartner C, Podreka I, Olbrich A et al (1996) Epileptic negative myoclonus: an EEG-single-photon emission CT study indicating involvement of premotor cortex. Neurology 46:753–758
Behen M, Chugani HT, Juhasz C et al (2007) Abnormal brain tryptophan metabolism and clinical correlates in Tourette syndrome. Mov Disord 22:2256–2262
Benamer TS, Patterson J, Grosset DG et al (2000) Accurate differentiation of parkinsonism and essential tremor using visual assessment of [123I]-FP-CIT SPECT imaging: the [123I]-FP-CIT study group. Mov Disord 15:503–510
Boecker H, Wills AJ, Ceballos-Baumann A et al (1996) The effect of ethanol on alcohol-responsive essential tremor: a positron emission tomography study. Ann Neurol 39:650–658
Boecker H, Weindl A, Brooks DJ et al (2010) GABAergic dysfunction in essential tremor: an 11C-flumazenil PET study. J Nucl Med 51:1030–1035
Booij J, de Jong J, de Bruin K, Knol R, de Win MM, van Eck-Smit BL (2007) Quantification of striatal dopamine transporters with 123I-FP-CIT SPECT is influenced by the selective serotonin reuptake inhibitor paroxetine: a double-blind, placebo-controlled, crossover study in healthy control subjects. J Nucl Med 48:359–366
Brooks DJ, Playford ED, Ibanez V et al (1992) Isolated tremor and disruption of the nigrostriatal dopaminergic system: an 18F-dopa PET study. Neurology 42:1554–1560
Cervenka S, Palhagen SE, Comley RA et al (2006) Support for dopaminergic hypoactivity in restless legs syndrome: a PET study on D2-receptor binding. Brain 129:2017–2028
Chen JC, Hsu YT, Chiou TS et al (2010) Cortical and non-cortical myoclonus of Creutzfeldt-Jakob disease. Eur Neurol 64:265–267
Cheon KA, Ryu YH, Namkoong K, Kim CH, Kim JJ, Lee JD (2004) Dopamine transporter density of the basal ganglia assessed with [123I]IPT SPECT in drug-naive children with Tourette's disorder. Psychiatry Res 130:85–95
Colebatch JG, Findley LJ, Frackowiak RS, Marsden CD, Brooks DJ (1990) Preliminary report: activation of the cerebellum in essential tremor. Lancet 336:1028–1030
Crawford P, Zimmerman EE (2011) Differentiation and diagnosis of tremor. Am Fam Physician 83:697–702
Czarnecki K, Jones DT, Burnett MS, Mullan B, Matsumoto JY (2011) SPECT perfusion patterns distinguish psychogenic from essential tremor. Parkinsonism Relat Disord 17:328–332
Dale RC (2017) Tics and Tourette: a clinical, pathophysiological and etiological review. Curr Opin Pediatr 29:665–673
Deuschl G, Bain P, Brin M (1998) Consensus statement of the Movement Disorder Society on Tremor. Ad Hoc Scientific Committee. Mov Disord 13(Suppl 3):2–23
Deuschl G, Wenzelburger R, Loffler K, Raethjen J, Stolze H (2000) Essential tremor and cerebellar dysfunction clinical and kinematic analysis of intention tremor. Brain 123(Pt 8):1568–1580
Dijk JM, Tijssen MA (2010) Management of patients with myoclonus: available therapies and the need for an evidence-based approach. Lancet Neurol 9:1028–1036
Diler RS, Reyhanli M, Toros F, Kibar M, Avci A (2002) Tc-99m-ECD SPECT brain imaging in children with Tourette's syndrome. Yonsei Med J 43:403–410
Duncan R, Bone I, Melville ID (1988) Essential tremor cured by infarction adjacent to the thalamus. J Neurol Neurosurg Psychiatry 51:591–592
Dupuis MJ, Delwaide PJ, Boucquey D, Gonsette RE (1989) Homolateral disappearance of essential tremor after cerebellar stroke. Mov Disord 4:183–187
Dupuis MJ, Evrard FL, Jacquerye PG, Picard GR, Lermen OG (2010) Disappearance of essential tremor after stroke. Mov Disord 25:2884–2887
Earley CJ, Kuwabara H, Wong DF et al (2011) The dopamine transporter is decreased in the striatum of subjects with restless legs syndrome. Sleep 34:341–347
Eidelberg D, Moeller JR, Antonini A et al (1997) The metabolic anatomy of Tourette's syndrome. Neurology 48:927–934
Eisensehr I, Wetter TC, Linke R et al (2001) Normal IPT and IBZM SPECT in drug-naive and levodopa-treated idiopathic restless legs syndrome. Neurology 57:1307–1309
Elble R, Deuschl G (2011) Milestones in tremor research. Mov Disord 26:1096–1105

Fahn S (2011) Classification of movement disorders. Mov Disord 26:947–957
Faught E (2003) Clinical presentations and phenomenology of myoclonus. Epilepsia 44(Suppl 11):7–12
Frucht SJ, Trost M, Ma Y, Eidelberg D (2004) The metabolic topography of posthypoxic myoclonus. Neurology 62:1879–1881
George MS, Trimble MR, Costa DC, Robertson MM, Ring HA, Ell PJ (1992) Elevated frontal cerebral blood flow in Gilles de la Tourette syndrome: a 99Tcm-HMPAO SPECT study. Psychiatry Res 45:143–151
George MS, Robertson MM, Costa DC et al (1994) Dopamine receptor availability in Tourette's syndrome. Psychiatry Res 55:193–203
Gerasimou G, Costa DC, Papanastasiou E et al (2012) SPECT study with I-123-Ioflupane (DaTSCAN) in patients with essential tremor. Is there any correlation with Parkinson's disease? Ann Nucl Med 26:337–344
Gerschlager W, Munchau A, Katzenschlager R et al (2004) Natural history and syndromic associations of orthostatic tremor: a review of 41 patients. Mov Disord 19:788–795
Gilbert DL, Christian BT, Gelfand MJ, Shi B, Mantil J, Sallee FR (2006) Altered mesolimbocortical and thalamic dopamine in Tourette syndrome. Neurology 67:1695–1697
Gilles de la Tourette G (1885) Étude sur une affection nerveuse caracterisée par l'incoordination motrice accompagnée d'écholalie et de coprolalie. Arch Neurol 9:19–42. et 158–200
Group PS (2000) A multicenter assessment of dopamine transporter imaging with DOPASCAN/SPECT in parkinsonism. Neurology 55:1540–1547
Guridi J, Rodriguez-Oroz MC, Arbizu J et al (2008) Successful thalamic deep brain stimulation for orthostatic tremor. Mov Disord 23:1808–1811
Ha SW, Yang YS, Song IU, Chung YA, Oh JK, Chung SW (2015) Changes in regional brain glucose metabolism measured with F-18-FDG-PET in essential tremor. Acta Radiol 56:482–486
Haense C, Muller-Vahl KR, Wilke F et al (2016) Effect of deep brain stimulation on regional cerebral blood flow in patients with medically refractory Tourette syndrome. Front Psych 7:118
Hallett M, Dubinsky RM (1993) Glucose metabolism in the brain of patients with essential tremor. J Neurol Sci 114:45–48
Haugbol S, Pinborg LH, Regeur L et al (2007) Cerebral 5-HT2A receptor binding is increased in patients with Tourette's syndrome. Int J Neuropsychopharmacol 10:245–252
Heinz A, Knable MB, Wolf SS et al (1998) Tourette's syndrome: [I-123]beta-CIT SPECT correlates of vocal tic severity. Neurology 51:1069–1074
Henkel K, Zerr I, Hertel A et al (2002) Positron emission tomography with [(18)F]FDG in the diagnosis of Creutzfeldt-Jakob disease (CJD). J Neurol 249:699–705
Hienert M, Gryglewski G, Stamenkovic M, Kasper S, Lanzenberger R (2018) Striatal dopaminergic alterations in Tourette's syndrome: a meta-analysis based on 16 PET and SPECT neuroimaging studies. Transl Psychiatry 8:143
Hu WT, Rippon GW, Boeve BF et al (2009) Alzheimer's disease and corticobasal degeneration presenting as corticobasal syndrome. Mov Disord 24:1375–1379
Huang KJ, Lu MK, Kao A, Tsai CH (2007) Clinical, imaging and electrophysiological studies of corticobasal degeneration. Acta Neurol Taiwanica 16:13–21
Hwang WJ, Yao WJ, Fu YK, Yang AS (2008) [99mTc]TRODAT-1/[123I]IBZM SPECT studies of the dopaminergic system in Tourette syndrome. Psychiatry Res 162:159–166
Imran M, Mahmood S (2011) An overview of human prion diseases. Virol J 8:559
Isaias IU, Antonini A (2010) Single-photon emission computed tomography in diagnosis and differential diagnosis of Parkinson's disease. Neurodegener Dis 7:319–329
Isaias IU, Alterman RL, Tagliati M (2008a) Outcome predictors of pallidal stimulation in patients with primary dystonia: the role of disease duration. Brain 131:1895–1902
Isaias IU, Canesi M, Benti R et al (2008b) Striatal dopamine transporter abnormalities in patients with essential tremor. Nucl Med Commun 29:349–353
Itoh Y, Amano T, Shimizu T, Hashimoto J, Kubo A, Fukuuchi Y (1998) Single-photon emission computed tomography image of benzodiazepine receptors in a patient with Creutzfeldt-Jakob disease. Intern Med 37:896–900

Jeffries KJ, Schooler C, Schoenbach C, Herscovitch P, Chase TN, Braun AR (2002) The functional neuroanatomy of Tourette's syndrome: an FDG PET study III: functional coupling of regional cerebral metabolic rates. Neuropsychopharmacology 27:92–104

Jenkins IH, Frackowiak RS (1993) Functional studies of the human cerebellum with positron emission tomography. Rev Neurol (Paris) 149:647–653

Jennesson M, Milh M, Villeneuve N et al (2010) Posterior glucose hypometabolism in Lafora disease: early and late FDG-PET assessment. Epilepsia 51:708–711

Jhoo JH, Yoon IY, Kim YK et al (2010) Availability of brain serotonin transporters in patients with restless legs syndrome. Neurology 74:513–518

Katzenschlager R, Costa D, Gerschlager W et al (2003) [123I]-FP-CIT-SPECT demonstrates dopaminergic deficit in orthostatic tremor. Ann Neurol 53:489–496

Kim KW, Jhoo JH, Lee SB et al (2012) Increased striatal dopamine transporter density in moderately severe old restless legs syndrome patients. Eur J Neurol 19:1213–1218

Klieger PS, Fett KA, Dimitsopulos T, Kurlan R (1997) Asymmetry of basal ganglia perfusion in Tourette's syndrome shown by technetium-99m-HMPAO SPECT. J Nucl Med 38:188–191

Kobayashi K, Shimoda K, Higashima M et al (2000) Report of three cases of Alzheimer's disease with focal motor symptoms: clinical correlates of neuroimaging findings. World J Biol Psychiatry 1:164–169

Korja M, Kaasinen V, Lamusuo S, Parkkola R, Nagren K, Marttila RJ (2007) Substantial thalamostriatal dopaminergic defect in Unverricht-Lundborg disease. Epilepsia 48:1768–1773

Lampreave JL, Molina V, Mardomingo MJ et al (1998) Technetium-99m-HMPAO in Tourette's syndrome on neuroleptic therapy and after withdrawal. J Nucl Med 39:624–628

Lee MS, Kim YD, Im JH, Kim HJ, Rinne JO, Bhatia KP (1999) 123I-IPT brain SPECT study in essential tremor and Parkinson's disease. Neurology 52:1422–1426

Lerner A, Bagic A, Boudreau EA et al (2007) Neuroimaging of neuronal circuits involved in tic generation in patients with Tourette syndrome. Neurology 68:1979–1987

Linke R, Eisensehr I, Wetter TC et al (2004) Presynaptic dopaminergic function in patients with restless legs syndrome: are there common features with early Parkinson's disease? Mov Disord 19:1158–1162

Liu H, Dong F, Meng Z, Zhang B, Tan J, Wang Y (2010) Evaluation of Tourette's syndrome by (99m)Tc-TRODAT-1 SPECT/CT imaging. Ann Nucl Med 24:515–521

Louis ED (2018) Essential tremor then and now: how views of the most common tremor diathesis have changed over time. Parkinsonism Relat Disord 46(Suppl 1):S70–S74

Louis ED, Ferreira JJ (2010) How common is the most common adult movement disorder? Update on the worldwide prevalence of essential tremor. Mov Disord 25:534–541

Louis ED, Vonsattel JP (2008) The emerging neuropathology of essential tremor. Mov Disord 23:174–182

Louis ED, Vonsattel JP, Honig LS, Ross GW, Lyons KE, Pahwa R (2006) Neuropathologic findings in essential tremor. Neurology 66:1756–1759

Lu CS, Ikeda A, Terada K et al (1998) Electrophysiological studies of early stage corticobasal degeneration. Mov Disord 13:140–146

Mavroudis I, Petridis F, Kazis D (2019) Neuroimaging and neuropathological findings in essential tremor. Acta Neurol Scand 139:491–496

McNaught KS, Mink JW (2011) Advances in understanding and treatment of Tourette syndrome. Nat Rev Neurol 7:667–676

Merner ND, Girard SL, Catoire H et al (2012) Exome sequencing identifies FUS mutations as a cause of essential tremor. Am J Hum Genet 91:313–319

Meyer P, Bohnen NI, Minoshima S et al (1999) Striatal presynaptic monoaminergic vesicles are not increased in Tourette's syndrome. Neurology 53:371–374

Michaud M, Soucy JP, Chabli A, Lavigne G, Montplaisir J (2002) SPECT imaging of striatal pre- and postsynaptic dopaminergic status in restless legs syndrome with periodic leg movements in sleep. J Neurol 249:164–170

Montagna P (2005) Fatal familial insomnia: a model disease in sleep physiopathology. Sleep Med Rev 9:339–353

Montagna P, Gambetti P, Cortelli P, Lugaresi E (2003) Familial and sporadic fatal insomnia. Lancet Neurol 2:167–176

Moriarty J, Costa DC, Schmitz B, Trimble MR, Ell PJ, Robertson MM (1995) Brain perfusion abnormalities in Gilles de la Tourette's syndrome. Br J Psychiatry 167:249–254

Mrowka M, Jobges M, Berding G, Schimke N, Shing M, Odin P (2005) Computerized movement analysis and beta-CIT-SPECT in patients with restless legs syndrome. J Neural Transm (Vienna) 112:693–701

Muller-Vahl KR, Berding G, Brucke T et al (2000) Dopamine transporter binding in Gilles de la Tourette syndrome. J Neurol 247:514–520

Muller-Vahl KR, Meyer GJ, Knapp WH et al (2005) Serotonin transporter binding in Tourette syndrome. Neurosci Lett 385:120–125

Muller-Vahl KR, Szejko N, Wilke F et al (2019) Serotonin transporter binding is increased in Tourette syndrome with obsessive compulsive disorder. Sci Rep 9:972

Nagaratnam N, Kalasabail G (1997) Contralateral abolition of essential tremor following a pontine stroke. J Neurol Sci 149:195–196

Nagasaka T, Nagasaka K, Ohta E et al (2011) Cerebral hypermetabolism demonstrated by FDG PET in familial Creutzfeldt-Jakob disease. Clin Nucl Med 36:725–727

Oboshi Y, Ouchi Y, Yagi S et al (2012) In vivo mesolimbic D2/3 receptor binding predicts post-therapeutic clinical responses in restless legs syndrome: a positron emission tomography study. J Cereb Blood Flow Metab 32:654–662

Oguro K, Kobayashi J, Aiba H, Hojo H (1997) Opsoclonus-myoclonus syndrome with abnormal single photon emission computed tomography imaging. Pediatr Neurol 16:334–336

Oh SY, Boegle R, Eulenburg PZ, Ertl M, Kim JS, Dieterich M (2017) Longitudinal multi-modal neuroimaging in opsoclonus-myoclonus syndrome. J Neurol 264:512–519

Phillips B, Young T, Finn L, Asher K, Hening WA, Purvis C (2000) Epidemiology of restless legs symptoms in adults. Arch Intern Med 160:2137–2141

Pourfar M, Feigin A, Tang CC et al (2011) Abnormal metabolic brain networks in Tourette syndrome. Neurology 76:944–952

Ragno M, Scarcella MG, Cacchio G et al (2009) Striatal [123I] FP-CIT SPECT demonstrates dopaminergic deficit in a sporadic case of Creutzfeldt-Jakob disease. Acta Neurol Scand 119:131–134

Raudino F, Muscia F, Osio M (2009) Orthostatic tremor and I-123-FP-CIT-SPECT: report of a case. Neurol Sci 30:365–366

Roselli F, Pisciotta NM, Pennelli M et al (2010) Midbrain SERT in degenerative parkinsonisms: a 123I-FP-CIT SPECT study. Mov Disord 25:1853–1859

Ruottinen HM, Partinen M, Hublin C et al (2000) An FDOPA PET study in patients with periodic limb movement disorder and restless legs syndrome. Neurology 54:502–504

Schoberl F, Feil K, Xiong G et al (2017) Pathological ponto-cerebello-thalamo-cortical activations in primary orthostatic tremor during lying and stance. Brain 140:83–97

Schwartz M, Groshar D, Inzelberg R, Hocherman S (2004) Dopamine-transporter imaging and visuo-motor testing in essential tremor, practical possibilities for detection of early stage Parkinson's disease. Parkinsonism Relat Disord 10:385–389

Serra-Mestres J, Ring HA, Costa DC et al (2004) Dopamine transporter binding in Gilles de la Tourette syndrome: a [123I]FP-CIT/SPECT study. Acta Psychiatr Scand 109:140–146

Shepard JW Jr, Buysse DJ, Chesson AL Jr et al (2005) History of the development of sleep medicine in the United States. J Clin Sleep Med 1:61–82

Shibasaki H, Thompson PD (2011) Milestones in myoclonus. Mov Disord 26:1142–1148

Song IU, Ha SW, Yang YS, Chung YA (2015) Differences in regional glucose metabolism of the brain measured with F-18-FDG-PET in patients with essential tremor according to their response to beta-blockers. Korean J Radiol 16:967–972

Staedt J, Stoppe G, Kogler A et al (1995) Nocturnal myoclonus syndrome (periodic movements in sleep) related to central dopamine D2-receptor alteration. Eur Arch Psychiatry Clin Neurosci 245:8–10

Stamenkovic M, Schindler SD, Asenbaum S et al (2001) No change in striatal dopamine re-uptake site density in psychotropic drug naive and in currently treated Tourette's disorder patients: a [(123)I]-beta-CIT SPECt-study. Eur Neuropsychopharmacol 11:69–74

Storey E, Lichtenstein M, Desmond P, Lloyd J (1995) Clinical features and SPECT scanning in presumed cortico-basal ganglionic degeneration. J Clin Neurosci 2:321–328

Teive HA, Munhoz RP, Barbosa ER (2009) Professor Karl-Axel Ekbom and restless legs syndrome. Parkinsonism Relat Disord 15:254–257

Trenkwalder C, Walters AS, Hening WA et al (1999) Positron emission tomographic studies in restless legs syndrome. Mov Disord 14:141–145

Tribl GG, Asenbaum S, Happe S, Bonelli RM, Zeitlhofer J, Auff E (2004) Normal striatal D2 receptor binding in idiopathic restless legs syndrome with periodic leg movements in sleep. Nucl Med Commun 25:55–60

Trocello JM, Zanotti-Fregonara P, Roze E et al (2008) Dopaminergic deficit is not the rule in orthostatic tremor. Mov Disord 23:1733–1738

Turjanski N, Sawle GV, Playford ED et al (1994) PET studies of the presynaptic and postsynaptic dopaminergic system in Tourette's syndrome. J Neurol Neurosurg Psychiatry 57:688–692

Turjanski N, Lees AJ, Brooks DJ (1999) Striatal dopaminergic function in restless legs syndrome: 18F-dopa and 11C-raclopride PET studies. Neurology 52:932–937

Usui K, Matsuda K, Terada K et al (2010) Epileptic negative myoclonus: a combined study of EEG and [123I]iomazenil (123I-IMZ) single photon emission computed tomography indicating involvement of medial frontal area. Epilepsy Res 89:220–226

van Toorn R, Rabie H, Warwick JM (2005) Opsoclonus-myoclonus in an HIV-infected child on antiretroviral therapy—possible immune reconstitution inflammatory syndrome. Eur J Paediatr Neurol 9:423–426

von Spiczak S, Whone AL, Hammers A et al (2005) The role of opioids in restless legs syndrome: an [11C]diprenorphine PET study. Brain 128:906–917

Waln O, Wu Y, Perlman R, Wendt J, Van AK, Jankovic J (2015) Dopamine transporter imaging in essential tremor with and without parkinsonian features. J Neural Transm (Vienna) 122:1515–1521

Wegner F, Strecker K, Boeckler D et al (2008) Intact serotonergic and dopaminergic systems in two cases of orthostatic tremor. J Neurol 255:1840–1842

Wills AJ, Jenkins IH, Thompson PD, Findley LJ, Brooks DJ (1994) Red nuclear and cerebellar but no olivary activation-associated with essential tremor – a positron emission tomographic study. Ann Neurol 36:636–642

Wills AJ, Thompson PD, Findley LJ, Brooks DJ (1996) A positron emission tomography study of primary orthostatic tremor. Neurology 46:747–752

Wolf SS, Jones DW, Knable MB et al (1996) Tourette syndrome: prediction of phenotypic variation in monozygotic twins by caudate nucleus D2 receptor binding. Science 273:1225–1227

Wong DF, Singer HS, Brandt J et al (1997) D2-like dopamine receptor density in Tourette syndrome measured by PET. J Nucl Med 38:1243–1247

Wong DF, Brasic JR, Singer HS et al (2008) Mechanisms of dopaminergic and serotonergic neurotransmission in Tourette syndrome: clues from an in vivo neurochemistry study with PET. Neuropsychopharmacology 33:1239–1251

Yeh CB, Lee CH, Chou YH, Chang CJ, Ma KH, Huang WS (2006) Evaluating dopamine transporter activity with 99mTc-TRODAT-1 SPECT in drug-naive Tourette's adults. Nucl Med Commun 27:779–784

Yeh CB, Lee CS, Ma KH, Lee MS, Chang CJ, Huang WS (2007) Phasic dysfunction of dopamine transmission in Tourette's syndrome evaluated with 99mTc TRODAT-1 imaging. Psychiatry Res 156:75–82

Yeh P, Walters AS, Tsuang JW (2012) Restless legs syndrome: a comprehensive overview on its epidemiology, risk factors, and treatment. Sleep Breath 16:987–1007

Yu HY, Kwan SY, Lirng JF, Liao KK, Chu YK, Liao SQ (2009) Epileptic negative myoclonus: SPECT, PET, and video/EEG studies and the dramatic effects of levetiracetam. Epilepsy Behav 14:687–690

Zesiewicz TA, Elble RJ, Louis ED et al (2011) Evidence-based guideline update: treatment of essential tremor: report of the Quality Standards Subcommittee of the American Academy of Neurology. Neurology 77:1752–1755

Zhang X, Santaniello S (2019) Role of cerebellar GABAergic dysfunctions in the origins of essential tremor. Proc Natl Acad Sci U S A 116:13592–13601

Zhang YX, Liu JR, Jiang B et al (2007) Lance-Adams syndrome: a report of two cases. J Zhejiang Univ Sci B 8:715–720

Clinical Applications of [^{123}I]FP-CIT SPECT Imaging

31

Jan Booij, Marina A. J. Tijssen, and Henk W. Berendse

Contents

J. Booij (✉)
Department of Radiology and Nuclear Medicine, Amsterdam University Medical Centers. Academic Medical Center, University of Amsterdam, Amsterdam, The Netherlands
e-mail: j.booij@amsterdamumc.nl

M. A. J. Tijssen
Department of Neurology, University Medical Center Groningen, University of Groningen, Groningen, The Netherlands
e-mail: m.a.j.de.koning-tijssen@umcg.nl

H. W. Berendse
Department of Neurology, Amsterdam University Medical Centers, VU University Medical Center, Amsterdam, The Netherlands
e-mail: h.berendse@amsterdamumc.nl

R. A. J. O. Dierckx et al. (eds.), *PET and SPECT in Neurology*,
https://doi.org/10.1007/978-3-030-53168-3_31

Abstract

Dopamine transporter (DAT) imaging with [^{123}I]*N*-ω-fluoropropyl-2β-carbomethoxy-3β-(4-iodophenyl)nortropane ([^{123}I]FP-CIT) single-photon emission computed tomography (SPECT) is commonly used in routine clinical studies to exclude or detect a loss of striatal DATs in individual patients with a movement disorder or dementia. In this chapter, we describe the clinical applications of [^{123}I]FP-CIT SPECT imaging. To facilitate the interpretation of [^{123}I]FP-CIT SPECT images, we first describe the results of [^{123}I]FP-CIT SPECT studies in healthy controls. Thereafter, we describe the typical findings when applying this technique in movement disorders and dementia characterised by a loss of striatal DATs (e.g. Parkinson's disease and dementia with Lewy bodies). We will also describe the possibilities to analyse [^{123}I]FP-CIT SPECT scans in the setting of routine clinical practice. Finally, we briefly discuss the characterisation of extrastriatal [^{123}I]FP-CIT binding and its potential role in future studies.

31.1 Introduction

As described extensively in another chapter of this book series (Booij et al. 2020), the dopamine transporter (DAT) is mainly located in the membrane of presynaptic dopaminergic neurons (see Fig. 1 of Booij et al. 2020). Several radioligands for the DAT have been developed successfully for both positron emission tomography (PET) and single-photon emission computed tomography (SPECT) imaging (for details see Booij et al. 2020). Yet, only a single radiotracer for the DAT has been licensed both by the Federal Drug Administration (FDA) and the European Medicines Agency (EMA). This radiotracer is [^{123}I]*N*-ω-fluoropropyl-2β-carbomethoxy-3β-(4-iodophenyl)nortropane ([^{123}I]FP-CIT), which is marketed as DaTSCAN and DaTscan in Europe and the United States, respectively. [^{123}I]FP-CIT is a cocaine derivative that was first synthesised by the chemist John L. Neumeyer in the early 1990s (Neumeyer et al. 1994).

Currently, [^{123}I]FP-CIT SPECT is often used in routine clinical practice to exclude or detect the loss of nigrostriatal neurons in individual patients (Booij et al. 2001; Løkkegaard et al. 2002; Kupsch et al. 2012; Catafau et al. 2004).

In this chapter, we will discuss the potential clinical applications of [^{123}I]FP-CIT SPECT. We will first describe the results of studies performed in healthy control subjects and then discuss the role of [^{123}I]FP-CIT SPECT in differentiating between degenerative and non-degenerative movement disorders in clinical practice as well as its potential role in dementia. We will also discuss how [^{123}I]FP-CIT SPECT images can be analysed optimally as part of a routine clinical procedure. Finally, we will touch upon the potential role of extrastriatal [^{123}I]FP-CIT binding in future imaging studies.

31.2 Dopamine Transporter Imaging in Healthy Controls with [123I]FP-CIT SPECT

In routine clinical studies, it is important to recognise abnormalities of striatal [123I]FP-CIT binding on SPECT scans. Therefore, it is essential to be aware of the range of normal binding levels against which abnormal binding needs to be recognised. This will increase the diagnostic accuracy of [123I]FP-CIT SPECT imaging in routine clinical practice. In this paragraph, we will discuss the results of [123I]FP-CIT SPECT studies in healthy control subjects.

Autopsy studies in humans have shown a reduction in the number of pigmented neurons in the pars compacta of the substantia nigra with advancing age (McGeer et al. 1977; Fearnley and Lees 1991). In addition, autopsy studies showed that the concentration of striatal DATs declines with natural ageing (Allard and Marcusson 1989; De Keyser et al. 1990). In line with these pathological observations, [123I]FP-CIT SPECT studies performed in healthy controls revealed decreases in striatal DAT binding with age, ranging from 3.3% up to 9.6% per decade (Ishikawa et al. 1996; Lavalaye et al. 2000; Tissingh et al. 1998; Eusebio et al. 2012; van de Giessen et al. 2013; Kaasinen et al. 2015; Yamamoto et al. 2017). The two largest [123I]FP-CIT SPECT studies on this topic so far included 139 healthy controls (age range 20–83 years) and 256 healthy controls (age range 20–83 years), respectively, and reported an average decline of striatal DAT availability of 5.5–6.3% per decade (Varrone et al. 2013; Matsuda et al. 2018). Interestingly, one study included mainly Caucasians (Varrone et al. 2013), while the other included Asian subjects (Matsuda et al. 2018). Since the age-related decline in striatal DATs was comparable in both cohorts, this suggests that ageing effects on striatal DAT expression may be unrelated to race. Importantly, ageing had no effect on the caudate-to-putamen ratio of DAT binding (Fig. 31.1). This is in line with another large study in healthy controls

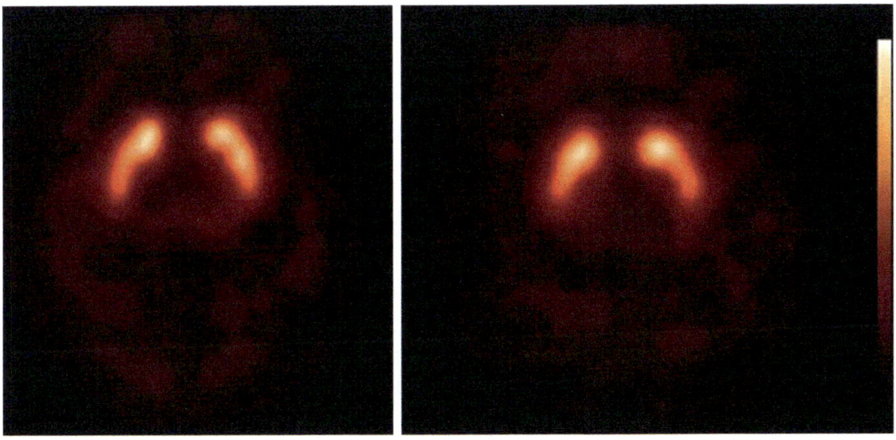

Fig. 31.1 [123I]FP-CIT SPECT scan obtained (3 h after injection) in a 21-year-old healthy female control (*left side*) and in a 78-year-old healthy female control (*right side*). Striatal binding of [123I]FP-CIT is symmetrical and clearly visible in both the caudate nucleus and putamen, in the young as well as the aged healthy control

using [^{123}I]β-CIT (a well-validated SPECT DAT tracer that is structurally closely related to [^{123}I]FP-CIT) and SPECT, which made clear that the rate of decline of DAT binding in the caudate nucleus and putamen with ageing was comparable (van Dyck et al. 2002). These findings suggest that it is important in routine clinical studies to take into account the effect of natural ageing on striatal DAT binding. A useful parameter, that is not influenced by natural ageing, is the caudate-to-putamen [^{123}I]FP-CIT binding ratio (Fig. 31.1).

Some [^{123}I]FP-CIT SPECT studies reported higher striatal binding ratios in women than in men (Lavalaye et al. 2000; Eusebio et al. 2012; Yamamoto et al. 2017; Matsuda et al. 2018), and this effect was more pronounced in younger than older controls (Lavalaye et al. 2000; Varrone et al. 2013; Matsuda et al. 2018), although this gender effect was not observed in all [^{123}I]FP-CIT studies (Pak et al. 2018). Also, an [^{123}I]β-CIT SPECT study performed in a large cohort of healthy controls (70 males and 52 females) did not find a significant effect of gender on striatal binding ratios (Best et al. 2005). Taken together, these data suggest that the diagnostic accuracy of [^{123}I]FP-CIT SPECT in routine clinical studies may be improved by taking gender effects into account, which may be particularly relevant in younger individuals.

[^{123}I]β-CIT SPECT studies in healthy controls demonstrated that the level of striatal DAT availability in the human brain may be associated with polymorphisms in the gene encoding for the DAT (van de Giessen et al. 2009; van Dyck et al. 2005; Jacobsen et al. 2000). However, a meta-analysis failed to establish a significant relationship between in vivo striatal DAT availability and polymorphisms in the gene encoding for the DAT in healthy controls (Costa et al. 2011). In a more recent meta-analysis, Faraone and co-workers concluded that the findings of SPECT studies on this topic were highly heterogeneous, and that the significant relationship between striatal DAT availability and polymorphisms in the gene encoding for the DAT may be limited to [^{123}I]β-CIT SPECT studies (Faraone et al. 2014). Also, to our knowledge no [^{123}I]FP-CIT SPECT study has been performed to look into this topic in a large group of healthy controls. Consequently, as it stands now, there is insufficient support to take gene effects into account in a setting in which [^{123}I]FP-CIT SPECT imaging is used for routine diagnostic purposes.

31.3 [^{123}I]FP-CIT SPECT Imaging in Parkinson's Disease and Atypical Parkinsonian Syndromes

31.3.1 [^{123}I]FP-CIT SPECT Imaging in Parkinson's Disease

An important neuropathological characteristic of Parkinson's disease (PD) is a severe loss of nigrostriatal dopamine neurons and consequently a decrease in striatal DATs (Kish et al. 1988; Kaufman and Madras 1991).

Several studies have established that [^{123}I]FP-CIT SPECT scanning can detect a loss of striatal DAT binding even in the early motor phase of PD (Eshuis et al. 2009; Isaias et al. 2007; Booij et al. 1997b; Tissingh et al. 1998; Pagano et al. 2018).

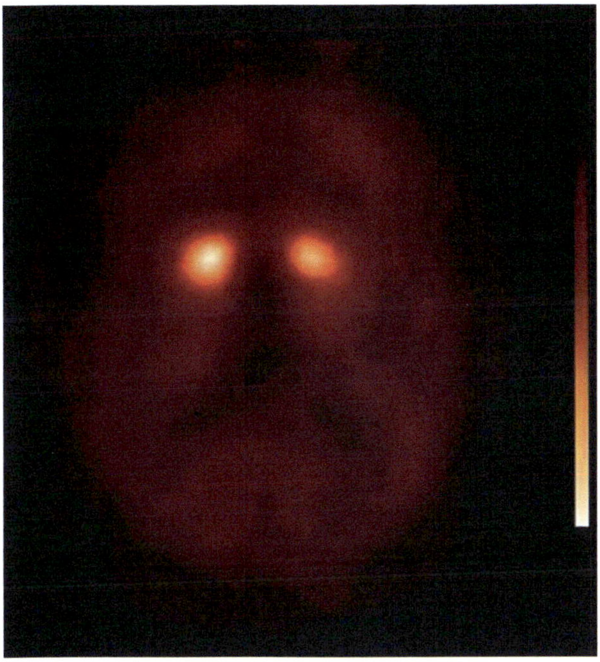

Fig. 31.2 [^{123}I]FP-CIT SPECT scan (3 h after injection) of a hemi-parkinsonian patient. Note the asymmetry of binding, as well as the severe loss of binding bilaterally in the putamen

Typically, the reduction in striatal DAT binding is stronger in the putamen than in the caudate nucleus and has an asymmetrical pattern (Fig. 31.2). Most often, DAT binding is lowest in the contralateral putamen (i.e. the side contralateral to the most affected side of the body). However, in individual PD patients, the decrease in DAT binding can be rather symmetrical or even lower on the ipsilateral than on the contralateral side. It has been suggested that this last phenomenon may be particularly true for PD patients with tremor-dominant features (Isaias et al. 2007). Interestingly, in many patients with clinically unilateral PD, there is a bilateral loss of putamen DAT binding (Tissingh et al. 1998; Filippi et al. 2005), which is consistent with studies in hemi-PD patients using [^{123}I]β-CIT as a ligand (Marek et al. 1996) (Fig. 31.2). However, for routine clinical studies, it is important to be aware of the fact that in some patients with unilateral PD, the loss of DAT binding may be restricted to one side of the brain (Fig. 31.3).

In early-stage PD patients, using age-corrected data, an approximately 60–65% loss of DAT availability can be found in the contralateral putamen (Booij et al. 2001; Tissingh et al. 1998). Additionally, recent studies have suggested that [^{123}I]FP-CIT SPECT scanning is sensitive enough to detect a loss of striatal DAT binding in the premotor phase of PD (Iranzo et al. 2010, 2017; Stiasny-Kolster et al. 2005; Doppler et al. 2017), consistent with findings from earlier [^{123}I]β-CIT SPECT studies (Berendse et al. 2001; Ponsen et al. 2004, 2010). Finally, the loss of striatal [^{123}I]FP-CIT binding in PD correlates with the degree of rigidity and hypokinesia, but not with the severity of resting or postural tremor (Spiegel et al. 2007; Isaias et al. 2007).

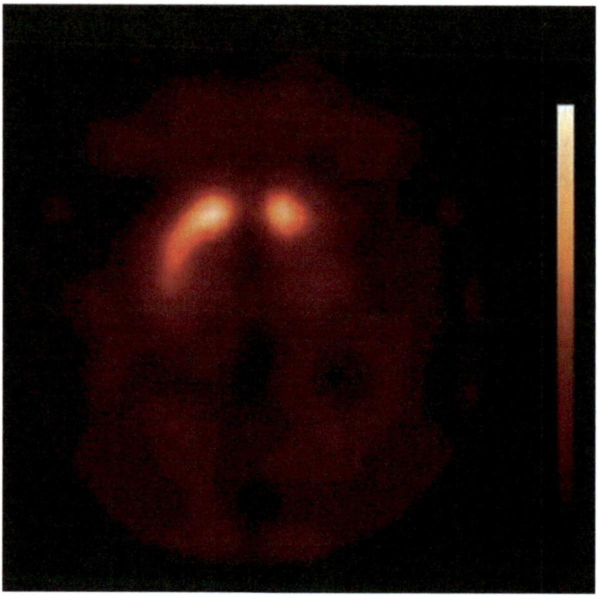

Fig. 31.3 [^{123}I]FP-CIT SPECT scan (3 h after injection) of an early-stage PD patient. Note that in this hemi-parkinsonian patient (motor signs only on the right side of the body), the loss of striatal binding is restricted to the contralateral (*left*) striatum

Although, in most studies in PD, loss of striatal DAT binding does not correlate with tremor scores (Spiegel et al. 2007; Isaias et al. 2007), it has, however, been suggested that a widespread degeneration of the nigrostriatal dopaminergic pathway might still play a role in the aetiology of rest tremor in PD (Isaias et al. 2007). Interestingly, tremor-dominant PD patients can have significantly lower DAT binding in the striatum *ipsilateral* to the rest tremor as compared to akinetic-rigid PD patients (Isaias et al. 2007). Moreover, in some patients with a strictly unilateral resting tremor (without bradykinesia and rigidity), reduced DAT binding may be restricted to the *ipsilateral* (instead of the contralateral) side of the striatum (Aguirregomozcorta et al. 2013; Lin and Chang 1997; Spiegel et al. 2007). These observations may be explained by degeneration/damage of 'crossed' dopaminergic fibres (Aguirregomozcorta et al. 2013).

In some large clinical trials into which patients were enrolled based on a clinical diagnosis of PD, 11–15% of patients showed no degeneration of the nigrostriatal pathway. In the ELLDOPA study, 15% of the included PD patients who were scanned with [^{123}I]β-CIT SPECT had normal baseline scans (Parkinson study group 2002). Importantly, the follow-up scans remained normal in the patients who were rescanned 4 year later. These patients have since been referred to as scans without evidence of dopaminergic deficit (SWEDD; Fahn 2005). Also, a more recent [^{123}I]FP-CIT SPECT study of 16 SWEDD cases showed that after a mean follow-up of 5.4 years, repeat DAT imaging was normal in 14 of these cases (87.5%) (Batla et al. 2014). Recent studies suggest that many of these patients do not suffer from PD but from other conditions including dystonic tremor, parkinsonism associated with fragile X mental retardation 1 gene expansions or even non-neurological diseases (Bajaj et al. 2010; Hall et al. 2010; Schneider et al. 2007; Sixel-Döring et al. 2011). These data emphasise the diagnostic power of DAT imaging.

In routine clinical studies, [^{123}I]FP-CIT SPECT is commonly used in inconclusive cases to differentiate PD from syndromes not characterised by nigrostriatal loss, for example, essential tremor or drug-induced parkinsonism (DIP) (Booij et al. 2001; Benamer et al. 2000; Marshall and Grosset 2003; Bajaj et al. 2013). In particular, the differentiation of PD from drug-induced parkinsonism (DIP) may present a diagnostic challenge to clinicians. Recent studies have shown that in this clinical situation, an abnormal [^{123}I]FP-CIT SPECT scan is indicative of an underlying neurodegenerative process as is common in PD (Bovi et al. 2010; Diaz-Corrales et al. 2010; Kägi et al. 2010; Tinazzi et al. 2009; Lim et al. 2013; Morley et al. 2016). DIP may persist beyond 6–9 months from the time of neuroleptic withdrawal, as was demonstrated in a recent report on two patients in whom DAT binding was normal (Lim et al. 2013). Importantly, for an accurate interpretation of [^{123}I]FP-CIT SPECT studies, it is not necessary to withdraw neuroleptics prior to the scanning procedure (Booij and Kemp 2008; Booij et al. 2010). Finally, a recent meta-analysis reported that [^{123}I]FP-CIT SPECT may be a useful imaging tool to differentiate PD from DIP (Brigo et al. 2014).

In summary, these findings suggest that [^{123}I]FP-CIT SPECT is a sensitive means to detect a loss of striatal DAT binding in PD. In routine clinical studies, [^{123}I]FP-CIT SPECT can be used to differentiate PD from other forms of parkinsonism that are not characterised by a loss of presynaptic dopaminergic neurons (e.g. essential tremor, psychogenic parkinsonism or DIP), in particular in clinically uncertain cases (Booij et al. 2001; Løkkegaard et al. 2002; Catafau et al. 2004; Cummings et al. 2011; Kägi et al. 2010; Marshall and Grosset 2003; Marshall et al. 2009; Kupsch et al. 2012; Bajaj et al. 2013).

31.3.2 [^{123}I]FP-CIT SPECT Imaging in Multiple System Atrophy and Progressive Supranuclear Palsy

Multiple system atrophy (MSA) and progressive supranuclear palsy (PSP) are neurodegenerative disorders associated with parkinsonism that are also characterised neuropathologically by a loss of nigrostriatal cells and consequently a loss of DATs (Kish et al. 1985; Ruberg et al. 1985; Warren et al. 2007; González et al. 2000).

[^{123}I]FP-CIT SPECT has been used in several studies to demonstrate a loss of striatal DATs in MSA-P (MSA with predominantly parkinsonian signs) and PSP versus healthy controls (Antonini et al. 2003; El Fakhri et al. 2006; Plotkin et al. 2005; van Laere et al. 2006; Bae et al. 2016; Kim et al. 2016). Generally speaking, the results obtained using [^{123}I]FP-CIT as a ligand in MSA-P are in line with findings in studies using [^{123}I]β-CIT (Scherfler et al. 2005; Knudsen et al. 2004; Varrone et al. 2001; Seppi et al. 2006; Joling et al. 2017). In a prospective study, [^{123}I]FP-CIT SPECT scanning was sensitive enough to detect MSA-P in the premotor phase (Iranzo et al. 2010). A subject with rapid eye movement sleep behaviour disorder but without parkinsonian signs had an abnormal [^{123}I]FP-CIT SPECT scan and developed MSA-P 2.5 years later.

Even in MSA-C (MSA-cerebellar subtype) patients without parkinsonian signs, a significant loss of striatal DAT binding compared to controls has been demonstrated using [^{123}I]FP-CIT SPECT (Muñoz et al. 2011). However, in comparison to patients with PD, MSA-P or PSP patients, the reported decrease in striatal DAT binding was relatively mild (an average loss of 20% of putamen DAT binding). Interestingly, the results of this SPECT study suggest that most but not all MSA-C patients without parkinsonism do have some degree of nigrostriatal dopaminergic denervation. The observation that a loss of DAT binding does not occur in all MSA-C cases (Bae et al. 2016; Joling et al. 2017; Vergnet et al. 2019) was confirmed by a post-mortem study in an autopsy-proven MSA-C case (Kolenc et al. 2012).

In most MSA-P and PSP patients, DAT binding in the putamen is lower than in the caudate nucleus. However, particularly in PSP, some studies suggested a more uniform loss of DATs in the putamen and caudate nucleus (Antonini et al. 2003), but this could not be reproduced by others (Seppi et al. 2006). Furthermore, some studies have shown that striatal DAT binding may differentiate MSA and/or PSP patients from PD patients at a group level (Goebel et al. 2011; Stoffers et al. 2005; Joling et al. 2017), although this is not a consistent finding in SPECT studies (Seppi et al. 2006). In any case, there is considerable overlap in striatal DAT binding values between groups, which suggests that in a routine clinical setting DAT imaging cannot be used to differentiate PD from MSA-P or PSP in individual cases (Stoffers et al. 2005). A recent post-mortem study of PD and MSA-P cases confirmed that the loss of striatal DAT was not significantly different between MSA and PD patients and also that the asymmetry of DAT binding was not significantly different between the two groups of patients (Perju-Dumbrava et al. 2012).

In summary, the results of the above-discussed studies suggest that [^{123}I]FP-CIT SPECT is a sensitive means to detect a loss of striatal DAT in MSA-P and PSP. However, it is important to emphasise that DAT imaging cannot be used to differentiate individual PD patients from MSA-P or PSP patients. Furthermore, striatal [^{123}I]FP-CIT binding can be normal in some MSA-C patients.

31.3.3 [^{123}I]FP-CIT SPECT Imaging in Corticobasal Degeneration

Corticobasal degeneration (CBD) is a rare syndrome, also characterised by nigrostriatal degeneration at autopsy (Oyanagi et al. 2001; Dickson et al. 2002). Indeed, an [^{123}I]FP-CT SPECT study that included the largest cohort of patients with a clinical diagnosis of probable CBD showed a loss of striatal DAT binding in 32 out of the 36 included patients (Cilia et al. 2011). In line with this observation, [^{123}I]β-CIT SPECT and other [^{123}I]FP-CIT SPECT studies in smaller groups of patients have also shown a loss of striatal DAT binding in CBD (Klaffke et al. 2006; Plotkin et al. 2005; Hammesfahr et al. 2016).

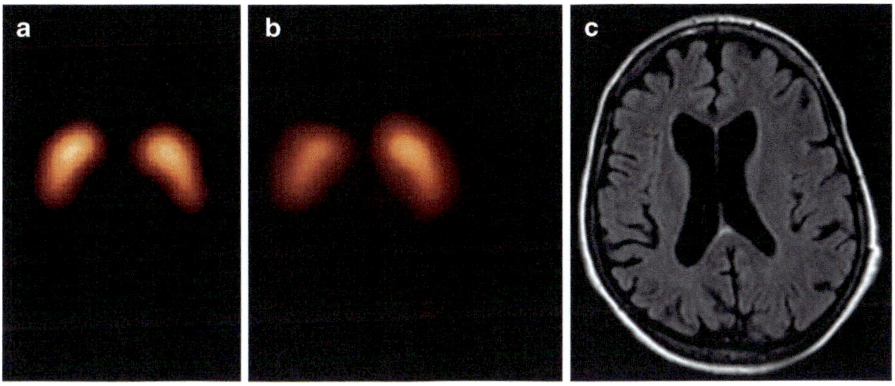

Fig. 31.4 [^{123}I]β-CIT SPECT scan of a healthy control (A) and a patient suffering from corticobasal degeneration (B), as well as an MR image of the same patient (C). The corticobasal degeneration has led to an asymmetrical degeneration of the nigrostriatal pathway (B) and a unilateral atrophy of the brain (C), both contralateral to the body side that showed clinical motor signs (Reprinted from 'Bewegingsstoornissen'; editors ECh Wolters and T van Laar, Amsterdam, 2002, The Netherlands)

Intriguingly, Cilia et al. (2011) demonstrated that the loss of striatal [^{123}I]FP-CIT binding in their sample of CBD patients was characterised by a larger variability, more uniform striatal reduction and a greater asymmetry of binding than in PD patients. Indeed, DAT SPECT images in some CBD patients may be quite characteristic for CBD (Fig. 31.4), whereas in many other CBD cases the [^{123}I]FP-CIT SPECT images may look similar to the images obtained in PD patients. Even of more interest, in some sporadic autopsy-proven CBD cases an ante-mortem [^{123}I]FP-CIT SPECT scan showed no evidence of a reduction in striatal DAT binding (O'Sullivan et al. 2008; Walker et al. 2002). In the study by Cilia et al. (2011), there were no remarkable differences in clinical or neuropsychological characteristics between CBD subjects with or without abnormal striatal [^{123}I]FP-CIT binding. Apparently, extrapyramidal motor symptoms in CBD may not always be associated with nigrostriatal degeneration and could involve supranigral factors (Cilia et al. 2011).

For routine clinical studies, it is important to underline that in many, but not all CBD cases, an [^{123}I]FP-CIT SPECT scan is abnormal (Hammesfahr et al. 2016). In some cases, the pattern of striatal DAT loss may even be characteristic for CBD (Fig. 31.4).

31.3.4 [^{123}I]FP-CIT SPECT Imaging in Vascular Parkinsonism and Traumatic Brain Injury

Significant vascular lesions in the striatum or in the substantia nigra pars compacta can be associated with a loss of striatal [^{123}I]FP-CIT binding (Marshall and Grosset 2003; Zijlmans et al. 2002; Booij et al. 2018; Fig. 31.5), although initial [^{123}I]β-CIT

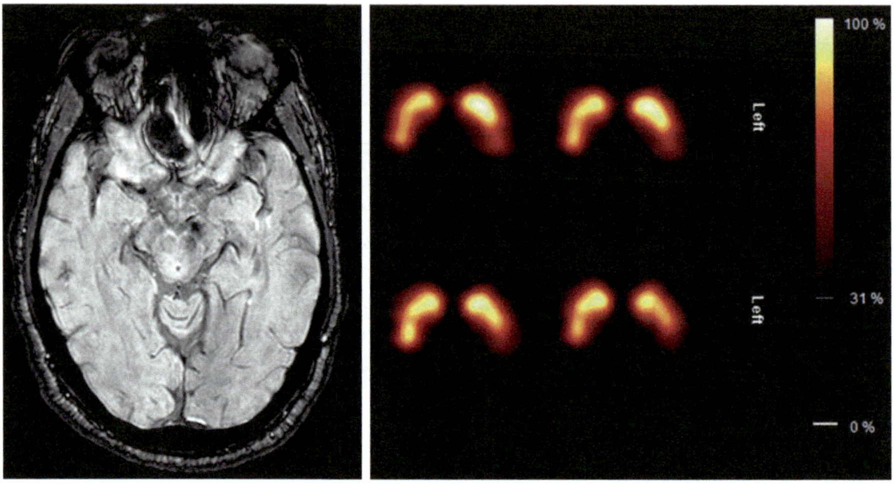

Fig. 31.5 MRI (susceptibility-weighted imaging) and [^{123}I]FP-CIT SPECT scan of the brain in a patient with vascular parkinsonism. The small lesion (hematoma) at the level of the substantia nigra (left panel) induced the abnormal SPECT scan. Please note that the [^{123}I]FP-CIT binding is normal in the right striatum, and abnormal in the posterior part of the left putamen. This pattern is atypical for Parkinson's disease since there is no gradual posterior-to-anterior loss of binding (reprinted from Booij et al. Imago 2018)

SPECT studies suggested that the vast majority of patients suffering from vascular parkinsonism had a normal [^{123}I]β-CIT SPECT scan (Gerschlager et al. 2002).

In a hallmark paper by Zijlmans and co-workers (Zijlmans et al. 2007), even patients fulfilling clinical criteria for vascular parkinsonism and without vascular lesions in the striatum could have an abnormal [^{123}I]FP-CIT SPECT scan, with bilateral loss of DAT binding, particularly in the putamen. A [^{123}I]FP-CIT SPECT study in a large cohort of PD patients and patients with vascular parkinsonism confirmed these findings and showed that around 60–70% of SPECT scans were abnormal in vascular parkinsonism (Benítez-Rivero et al. 2013). Importantly, scores based on visual pattern recognition discriminated better between PD and vascular parkinsonism cases than semi-quantitative scores based on the positioning of regions of interest. Lastly, in another [^{123}I]FP-CIT SPECT study in PD patients and patients with vascular parkinsonism, a significant number of patients with vascular lesions in the basal ganglia had a normal SPECT scan, which indicates that vascular lesions in the basal ganglia do not always cause abnormal striatal DAT binding (Antonini et al. 2012). In the same study, a normal [^{123}I]FP-CIT SPECT scan was associated with a lack of benefit from dopaminomimetic treatment in over 90% of these subjects (Antonini et al. 2012). Finally, a recent meta-analysis concluded that [^{123}I]FP-CIT SPECT may be a useful imaging tool to differentiate PD from vascular parkinsonism (Brigo et al. 2014).

All in all, a substantial number of patients with vascular parkinsonism have an abnormal [^{123}I]FP-CIT SPECT. Frequently, it is possible to differentiate vascular parkinsonism from PD using [^{123}I]FP-CIT SPECT. To do so, it may be of utmost importance to perform an careful visual inspection of the SPECT images (including structural images), and to recognise patterns of striatal DAT loss which are atypical for PD, but could support the diagnosis of vascular parkinsonism.

A recent study examined the effects of traumatic brain injury (TBI) on DAT binding (Jenkins et al. 2018). Forty-two moderate-severe TBI patients with cognitive impairments but without motor parkinsonism were examined. Around 20% of these patients had evidence of reduced DAT binding in the striatum as measured with [^{123}I]FP-CIT SPECT. Importantly, the caudate nucleus was affected more consistently than other striatal regions. Also, 11 patients had small, but visible, lesions in the striatum demonstrated by magnetic resonance imaging. Importantly, patients with lesions in these structures did not have different striatal DAT binding ratios compared to patients without lesions. These findings suggest that in the majority of patients with moderate/severe TBI, but without parkinsonism, the [^{123}I]FP-CIT SPECT scan is normal; in patients in whom such scans are rated as abnormal, the pattern of DAT loss may differ from what is typical for PD; and small lesions in the striatum may not influence significantly DAT loss as assessed by [^{123}I]FP-CIT SPECT.

In an older study, a severe reduction in striatal DAT binding, as measured by [^{123}I]β-CIT SPECT, was observed in a group of ten patients who were in a vegetative state or had persistent parkinsonism (Donnemiller et al. 2000).

31.3.5 [^{123}I]FP-CIT SPECT Imaging in DLB

Like other diseases characterised by Lewy body pathology (i.e. PD), also dementia with Lewy bodies (DLB) is associated with a loss of dopamine neurons and striatal DATs (Perry et al. 1998). By contrast, the loss of striatal DATs appears to be only subtle in patients suffering from Alzheimer's disease (Perry et al. 1998). In line with these autopsy findings, hallmark studies by Walker and colleagues demonstrated that ante-mortem DAT imaging with [^{123}I]FP-CIT SPECT substantially enhanced the accuracy of a diagnosis of DLB by comparison with clinical criteria alone (Walker et al. 2002, 2007). Many subsequent [^{123}I]FP-CIT SPECT studies confirmed the loss of striatal DATs in DLB (Auning et al. 2011; McKeith et al. 2007; Morgan et al. 2012; Roselli et al. 2009; van Laere et al. 2006; O'Brien et al. 2004; Siepel et al. 2013, 2016; Thomas et al. 2017; Jung et al. 2018). [^{123}I]FP-CIT SPECT may even detect a loss of striatal DAT binding in the preclinical phase of DLB (Iranzo et al. 2010; Thomas et al. 2019). Importantly, the results of [^{123}I]FP-CIT SPECT imaging may predict which patients with a clinical diagnosis of possible DLB will convert to probable DLB or to Alzheimer's disease (O'Brien et al. 2009). Finally, a meta-analysis indicated that the diagnostic accuracy of [^{123}I]FP-CIT SPECT in the diagnosis of DLB is high (Papathanasiou et al. 2012).

In most DLB patients, loss of striatal DAT binding is stronger in the putamen than in the caudate nucleus. Also, the loss of striatal DAT binding can be asymmetrical. However, in line with autopsy findings (Perry et al. 1998), the loss of striatal [^{123}I]FP-CIT binding can also be symmetrical with a relatively strong involvement

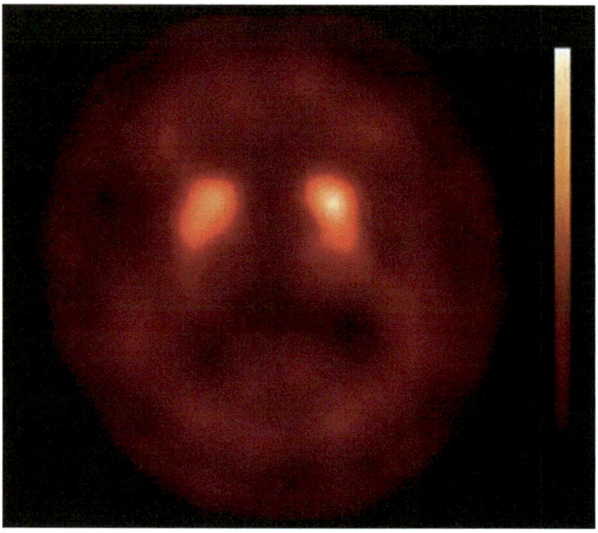

Fig. 31.6 [123I]FP-CIT SPECT scan obtained (3 h after injection) in a DLB patient. Note that due to the strong reduction in specific binding of [123I]FP-CIT in the striatum, the contrast between specific and non-specific binding is low. Also, the loss of binding is relatively symmetrical and involves both the caudate nucleus and putamen

of the caudate nucleus as compared to PD cases (Walker et al. 2004; Joling et al. 2018) (Fig. 31.6).

Although [123I]FP-CIT SPECT appears to be very sensitive in differentiating between DLB and Alzheimer's disease, the role in the differential diagnosis between PD with dementia (PDD), frontotemporal dementia and DLB is probably limited, since a recent study showed that a third of frontotemporal dementia cases had an abnormal [123I]FP-CIT SPECT scan (Morgan et al. 2012). Similarly, although at a group level loss of striatal DATs may be greater in PDD than DLB, the abnormalities on individual [123I]FP-CIT SPECT scans (i.e. lower DAT binding in the putamen than caudate nucleus) in PDD may be similar to the abnormalities observed in DLB (O'Brien et al. 2004; Colloby et al. 2012).

Importantly, an autopsy study in DLB, PDD and Alzheimer's cases showed that ante-mortem DAT imaging was associated with post-mortem nigral dopaminergic neuronal density (but not α-synuclein, tau or amyloid burden) in demented patients (Colloby et al. 2012). This observation may cast doubt on the potential of DAT imaging to differentiate DLB patients without parkinsonism from Alzheimer's disease cases. Nevertheless, most DLB patients without parkinsonism have abnormal DAT SPECT scans (O'Brien et al. 2004; McKeith et al. 2007). On the other hand, Alzheimer's disease patients with parkinsonism may have normal scans (McKeith et al. 2007; Ceravolo et al. 2004).

The results of recent studies suggest that in a subgroup of probable DLB patients the [123I]FP-CIT SPECT scan may be rated as normal initially, but becomes abnormal over time (Colloby et al. 2012; van der Zande et al. 2016; Thomas et al. 2017). This subgroup may consist of approximately 10% of DLB cases (van der Zande et al. 2016; Thomas et al. 2017), and the concept is that in these patients the Lewy bodies are expressed predominantly in the cortex, with initially only minimal involvement of the brainstem.

To summarise, there is evidence that [^{123}I]FP-CIT SPECT is helpful in differentiating DLB from Alzheimer's disease, but its role in differentiating DLB from frontotemporal dementia may be limited.

31.4 Methods to Analyse [^{123}I]FP-CIT SPECT Studies in Routine Clinical Practice

In routine clinical practice, many departments of nuclear medicine evaluate [^{123}I]FP-CIT SPECT scans by visual inspection only. Major reasons are a lack of age-matched control data and the fact that it is a simple way to analyse images. Although a visual qualitative analysis may seem inaccurate, this approach can in fact be very effective in excluding or confirming a loss of striatal DATs (Benamer et al. 2000; O'Brien et al. 2004; McKeith et al. 2007; Booij et al. 2017). An important advantage of visual analysis over a quantitative approach is that an abnormal pattern can be recognised rapidly. A recent study showed that a visual analysis approach was even more accurate in differentiating vascular parkinsonism from PD than a semi-quantitative approach (Benítez-Rivero et al. 2013). In addition, another large study on the diagnostic performance of [^{123}I]FP-CIT SPECT in patients with movement disorders or dementia showed that the results of combined reading (visual reading plus quantitative [^{123}I]FP-CIT SPECT data available to the reader) were not inferior to the results of the visual reading analysis, but the combined reading offered an increase in reader confidence (Booij et al. 2017). Moreover, the visual interpretation of [^{123}I]FP-CIT SPECT images can be further improved by visual rating of parametric distribution volume ratio images (Meyer et al. 2011). However, a visual analysis of [^{123}I]FP-CIT SPECT images may be less accurate in patients in which the degeneration is quite symmetrical and the involvement of the caudate nucleus and putamen more uniform. This type of pattern has been described in some DLB, PSP and MSA-C patients.

Even though visual assessment of [^{123}I]FP-CIT SPECT images remains an integral part of the study report, it is nowadays frequently supplemented by a quantification method (Tatsch and Poepperl 2012; Badiavas et al. 2011). Quantification does not only offer a more objective adjunct to an individual subjective judgement but also has the potential to detect subtle changes that can elude the human eye (Tatsch and Poepperl 2012) and may increase the reader confidence (Booij et al. 2017) and consistency between reporters (Taylor et al. 2018). In routine clinical DAT SPECT studies, semi-quantitative techniques using ROIs are commonly used due to their simplicity. Striatal ROIs were initially defined by manually drawing an irregular contour around the caudate nucleus and putamen and around a region devoid of DATs (occipital cortex or cerebellum). However, this method is strongly influenced by the intensity of striatal DAT binding. In other words, if there is decreased striatal [^{123}I]FP-CIT binding (e.g. in a PD case), the reader tends to draw smaller ROIs over striatal regions than in cases with more intense striatal [^{123}I]FP-CIT binding. Therefore, fixed (or predefined) ROIs are now used more frequently. These ROIs are derived from anatomical atlases or MR images and have led to a better standardisation. However, this technique is still investigator dependent and does not take into account interindividual differences in striatal volumes. From this perspective, it is of interest that several (semi)automated quantification tools have been developed and several methods have been proposed to quantify DAT studies by (semi)automated positioning of ROIs or volumes of interest (VOIs) (Badiavas et al. 2011; Habraken et al. 1999). Examples are BasGan (Calvini et al. 2007), BRASS (Radau et al. 2000) and DaTQUANT (Brogley 2019) (for a comprehensive review, see Tatsch and Poepperl 2012). Voxel-based analysis, for example, using statistical parametric mapping (SPM), has also been used to analyse [^{123}I]FP-CIT SPECT studies (Kas et al. 2007; van de Giessen et al. 2013). Automated voxel-based image analyses may increase the diagnostic accuracy of DAT imaging in differentiating between PD and other parkinsonian syndromes (Goebel et al. 2011). Finally, in recent years, machine learning paradigms have been developed and evaluated successfully to classify [^{123}I]FP-CIT SPECT studies (Taylor and Fenner 2017; Taylor et al. 2018; Iwabuchi et al. 2019). However, future studies are needed to evaluate the feasibility of voxel-based techniques as well as machine learning paradigms in routine clinical practice.

As mentioned before, for an optimal interpretation of [^{123}I]FP-CIT SPECT images, ageing effects should be taken into account, and gender effects may be relevant in younger subjects. However, it may be difficult for departments of nuclear medicine to acquire [^{123}I]FP-CIT SPECT data in healthy controls and to build their own control database. The Neuroimaging Committee of the EANM understood this problem and decided to initiate a programme to overcome it by setting up an investigator-initiated multicentre trial using EARL (EANM Research Ltd) as a platform (Tatsch 2012). This initiative resulted in a highly standardised European database which is available to allow correction of quantitative DAT binding for age and gender, mostly independent of the equipment used and the centre performing the scan (Dickson et al. 2012; Tatsch 2012; Varrone et al. 2013).

For an optimal interpretation of [^{123}I]FP-CIT SPECT images, it is important to take into account the potential effects of the medication used on [^{123}I]FP-CIT binding to the DAT (for a review see Booij and Kemp 2008). Luckily, most dopaminergic drugs that are commonly used by patients suffering from parkinsonian or dementia syndromes (e.g. levodopa, dopamine agonists or acetylcholinesterase inhibitors) will not significantly influence [^{123}I]FP-CIT binding to the DAT and therefore do not have to be discontinued prior to routine [^{123}I]FP-CIT SPECT studies (Booij and Kemp 2008). On the other hand, selective serotonin reuptake inhibitors may increase striatal [^{123}I]FP-CIT binding ratios.

31.5 Extrastriatal [^{123}I]FP-CIT Binding

In vitro experiments have shown that [^{123}I]FP-CIT has a high affinity for the DAT (low nanomolar range), a moderate affinity for the serotonin transporter (SERT) and a negligible affinity for the norepinephrine transporter (Abi-Dargham et al. 1996;

Scheffel et al. 1997). It is well accepted that striatal [^{123}I]FP-CIT binding predominantly reflects binding to the DAT (Booij et al. 1997a; Andringa et al. 2005).

In recent years, extrastriatal [^{123}I]FP-CIT binding has gained attention (Booij et al. 2007; Eusebio et al. 2012; Hesse et al. 2009; Koopman et al. 2012; Roselli et al. 2010; Kaasinen et al. 2015; Joling et al. 2017, 2018; Joutsa et al. 2015). For example, [^{123}I]FP-CIT binding in the SERT-rich midbrain and diencephalon can be blocked with a selective serotonin reuptake inhibitor (SSRI) in healthy volunteers (Booij et al. 2007). In addition to the severe loss of striatal [^{123}I]FP-CIT binding, there is significantly lower midbrain [^{123}I]FP-CIT binding in DLB and PSP compared to PD patients (Roselli et al. 2010), and lower hypothalamic binding in PSP and MSA-p than in PD (Joling et al. 2017). Future studies will have to determine whether analysis of extrastriatal [^{123}I]FP-CIT binding is helpful in routine clinical studies.

31.6 Concluding Remarks

[^{123}I]FP-CIT SPECT is a very sensitive means to detect a loss of striatal DAT binding. This tool is particularly helpful in uncertain clinical cases with slight parkinsonian features, as well as in the differential diagnosis between syndromes characterised by nigrostriatal neuronal loss (e.g. PD or DLB) and syndromes in which the nigrostriatal system is spared (e.g. essential tremor or Alzheimer's disease).

References

Abi-Dargham A, Gandelman MS, DeErausquin GA et al (1996) SPECT imaging of dopamine transporters in human brain with iodine-123-fluoroalkyl analogs of β-CIT. J Nucl Med 37:1129–1133

Aguirregomozcorta M, Stamelou M, Antonini A et al (2013) Patients with rest-tremor and scans with ipsilateral dopaminergic deficit. J Neurol 260:1132–1135

Allard P, Marcusson JO (1989) Age-correlated loss of dopamine uptake sites with [3H]GBR-12935 in human putamen. Neurobiol Aging 10:661–664

Andringa G, Drukarch B, Bol JG et al (2005) Pinhole SPECT imaging of dopamine transporters correlates with dopamine transporter immunohistochemical analysis in the MPTP mouse model of Parkinson's disease. NeuroImage 26:1150–1158

Antonini A, Benti R, De Notaris R et al (2003) 123I-Ioflupane/SPECT binding to striatal dopamine transporter (DAT) uptake in patients with Parkinson's disease, multiple system atrophy, and progressive supranuclear palsy. Neurol Sci 24:149–150

Antonini A, Vitale C, Barone P et al (2012) The relationship between cerebral vascular disease and parkinsonism: the VADO study. Parkinsonism Relat Disord 18:775–780

Auning E, Rongve A, Fladby T et al (2011) Early and presenting symptoms of dementia with Lewy bodies. Dement Geriatr Cogn Disord 32:202–208

Badiavas K, Molyvda E, Iakovou I, Tsolaki M, Psarrakos K, Karatzas N (2011) SPECT imaging evaluation in movement disorders: far beyond visual assessment. Eur J Nucl Med Mol Imaging 38:764–773

Bae YJ, Kim JM, Kim E et al (2016) Loss of nigral hyperintensity on 3 Tesla MRI of parkinsonism: comparison with 123I-FP-CIT SPECT. Mov Disord 31:684–692

Bajaj NP, Gontu V, Birchall J, Patterson J, Grosset DG, Lees AJ (2010) Accuracy of clinical diagnosis in tremulous parkinsonian patients: a blinded video study. J Neurol Neurosurg Psychiatry 81:1223–1228

Bajaj N, Hauser RA, Grachev ID (2013) Clinical utility of dopamine transporter single photon emission CT (DaT-SPECT) with (123I) ioflupane in diagnosis of parkinsonian syndromes. J Neurol Neurosurg Psychiatry 84:1288–1295

Batla A, Erro R, Stamelou M, Schneider SA, Schwingenschuh P, Ganos C, Bhatia KP (2014) Patients with scans without evidence of dopaminergic deficit: a long-term follow-up study. Mov Disord 29:1820–1825

Benamer TS, Patterson J, Grosset DG et al (2000) Accurate differentiation of parkinsonism and essential tremor using visual assessment of [123I]-FP-CIT SPECT imaging: the [123I]-FP-CIT study group. Mov Disord 15:503–510

Benítez-Rivero S, Marín-Oyaga VA et al (2013) Clinical features and 123I-FP-CIT SPECT imaging in vascular parkinsonism and Parkinson's disease. J Neurol Neurosurg Psychiatry 84:122–129

Berendse HW, Booij J, Francot CM, Bergmans PL, Hijman R, Stoof JC, Wolters EC (2001) Subclinical dopaminergic dysfunction in asymptomatic Parkinson's disease patients' relatives with a decreased sense of smell. Ann Neurol 50:34–41

Best SE, Sarrel PM, Malison RT et al (2005) Striatal dopamine transporter availability with [123I]β-CIT SPECT is unrelated to gender or menstrual cycle. Psychopharmacology 183:181–189

Booij J, Kemp P (2008) Dopamine transporter imaging with [123I]FP-CIT SPECT: potential effects of drugs. Eur J Nucl Med Mol Imaging 35:424–438

Booij J, Andringa G, Rijks LJ et al (1997a) [^{123}I]FP-CIT binds to the dopamine transporter as assessed by biodistribution studies in rats and SPECT studies in MPTP-lesioned monkeys. Synapse 27:183–190

Booij J, Tissingh G, Boer GJ et al (1997b) [123I]FP-CIT SPECT shows a pronounced decline of striatal dopamine transporter labelling in early and advanced Parkinson's disease. J Neurol Neurosurg Psychiatry 62:133–140

Booij J, Speelman JD, Horstink MW, Wolters EC (2001) The clinical benefit of imaging striatal dopamine transporters with [123I]FP-CIT SPET in differentiating patients with presynaptic parkinsonism from those with other forms of parkinsonism. Eur J Nucl Med 28:266–272

Booij J, de Jong J, de Bruin K, Knol R, de Win MM, van Eck-Smit BL (2007) Quantification of striatal dopamine transporters with 123I-FP-CIT SPECT is influenced by the selective serotonin reuptake inhibitor paroxetine: a double-blind, placebo-controlled, crossover study in healthy control subjects. J Nucl Med 48:359–366

Booij J, van Amelsvoort T, Boot E (2010) Co-occurrence of early-onset Parkinson disease and 22q11.2 deletion syndrome: potential role for dopamine transporter imaging. Am J Med Genet A 152A:2937–2938

Booij J, Dubroff J, Pryma D, Yu J, Agarwal R, Lakhani P, Kuo PH (2017) Diagnostic performance of the visual reading of $_{123}$I-ioflupane SPECT images with or without quantification in patients with movement disorders or dementia. J Nucl Med 58:1821–1826

Booij J, Reneman L, Adriaanse S, de Bie R (2018) Dopaminetransporterscintigrafie bij patiënten met parkinsonisme. Image 2:37–42

Booij J, van Wieringen JP, van de Giessen EM, Knol RJJ, Finnema SJ (2020) PET and SPECT imaging of the central dopamine system in humans. In: Dierckx RAJO, Otte A, de Vries EFJ, van Waarde A, Lammertsma AA (eds) PET and SPECT of neurobiological systems. Springer, New York, NY

Bovi T, Antonini A, Ottaviani S et al (2010) The status of olfactory function and the striatal dopaminergic system in drug-induced parkinsonism. J Neurol 257:1882–1889

Brigo F, Matinella A, Erro R, Tinazzi M (2014) [^{123}I]FP-CIT SPECT (DaTSCAN) may be a useful tool to differentiate between Parkinson's disease and vascular or drug-induced parkinsonisms: a meta-analysis. Eur J Neurol 21:1369–1376

Brogley JE (2019) DaTQUANT: the future of diagnosing Parkinson's disease. J Nucl Med Technol 47:21–26

Calvini P, Rodriguez G, Inguglia F, Mignone A, Guerra UP, Nobili F (2007) The basal ganglia matching tools package for striatal uptake semi-quantification: description and validation. Eur J Nucl Med Mol Imaging 34:1240–1253

Catafau AM, Tolosa E, DaTSCAN Clinically Uncertain Parkinsonian Syndromes Study Group (2004) Impact of dopamine transporter SPECT using 123I-Ioflupane on diagnosis and management of patients with clinically uncertain Parkinsonian syndromes. Mov Disord 19:1175–1182

Ceravolo R, Volterrani D, Gambaccini G et al (2004) Presynaptic nigro-striatal function in a group of Alzheimer's disease patients with parkinsonism: evidence from a dopamine transporter imaging study. J Neural Transm 111:1065–1073

Cilia R, Rossi C, Frosini D, Volterrani D et al (2011) Dopamine transporter SPECT imaging in corticobasal syndrome. PLoS One 6:e18301

Colloby SJ, McParland S, O'Brien JT, Attems J (2012) Neuropathological correlates of dopaminergic imaging in Alzheimer's disease and Lewy body dementias. Brain 135:2798–2808

Costa A, Riedel M, Müller U, Möller HJ, Ettinger U (2011) Relationship between SLC6A3 genotype and striatal dopamine transporter availability: a meta-analysis of human single photon emission computed tomography studies. Synapse 65:998–1005

Cummings JL, Henchcliffe C, Schaier S, Simuni T, Waxman A, Kemp P (2011) The role of dopaminergic imaging in patients with symptoms of dopaminergic system neurodegeneration. Brain 134:3146–3166

De Keyser JD, Ebinger G, Vauquelin G (1990) Age-related changes in the human nigrostriatal dopaminergic system. Ann Neurol 27:157–161

Diaz-Corrales FJ, Sanz-Viedma S, Garcia-Solis D, Escobar-Delgado T, Mir P (2010) Clinical features and 123I-FP-CIT SPECT imaging in drug-induced parkinsonism and Parkinson's disease. Eur J Nucl Med Mol Imaging 37:556–564

Dickson DW, Bergeron C, Chin SS et al (2002) Neuropathologic criteria for corticobasal degeneration. J Neuropathol Exp Neurol 61:935–946

Dickson JC, Tossici-Bolt L, Sera T et al (2012) Proposal for the standardisation of multi-centre trials in nuclear medicine imaging: prerequisites for a European 123I-FP-CIT SPECT database. Eur J Nucl Med Mol Imaging 39:188–197

Donnemiller E, Brenneis C, Wissel J, Scherfler C, Poewe W, Riccabona G, Wenning GK (2000) Impaired dopaminergic neurotransmission in patients with traumatic brain injury: a SPECT study using 123I-beta-CIT and 123I-IBZM. Eur J Nucl Med 27:1410–1414

Doppler K, Jentschke HM, Schulmeyer L et al (2017) Dermal phospho-alpha-synuclein deposits confirm REM sleep behaviour disorder as prodromal Parkinson's disease. Acta Neuropathol 133:535–545

El Fakhri G, Habert MO, Maksud P, Kas A, Malek Z, Kijewski MF, Lacomblez L (2006) Quantitative simultaneous 99mTc-ECD/123I-FP-CIT SPECT in Parkinson's disease and multiple system atrophy. Eur J Nucl Med Mol Imaging 33:87–92

Eshuis SA, Jager PL, Maguire RP, Jonkman S, Dierckx RA, Leenders KL (2009) Direct comparison of FP-CIT SPECT and F-DOPA PET in patients with Parkinson's disease and healthy controls. Eur J Nucl Med Mol Imaging 36:454–462

Eusebio A, Azulay JP, Ceccaldi M, Girard N, Mundler O, Guedj E (2012) Voxel-based analysis of whole-brain effects of age and gender on dopamine transporter SPECT imaging in healthy subjects. Eur J Nucl Med Mol Imaging 39:1778–1783

Fahn S (2005) Does levodopa slow or hasten the rate of progression of Parkinson's disease? J Neurol 252(Suppl 4):IV37–IV42

Faraone SV, Spencer TJ, Madras BK, Zhang-James Y, Biederman J (2014) Functional effects of dopamine transporter gene genotypes on in vivo dopamine transporter functioning: a meta-analysis. Mol Psychiatry 19:880–889

Fearnley JM, Lees AJ (1991) Ageing and Parkinson's disease: substantia nigra regional selectivity. Brain 114:2283–2301

Filippi L, Manni C, Pierantozzi M et al (2005) 123I-FP-CIT semi-quantitative SPECT detects preclinical bilateral dopaminergic deficit in early Parkinson's disease with unilateral symptoms. Nucl Med Commun 26:421–426

Gerschlager W, Bencsits G, Pirker W et al (2002) [123I]beta-CIT SPECT distinguishes vascular parkinsonism from Parkinson's disease. Mov Disord 17:518–523
Goebel G, Seppi K, Donnemiller E et al (2011) A novel computer-assisted image analysis of [123I]β-CIT SPECT images improves the diagnostic accuracy of parkinsonian disorders. Eur J Nucl Med Mol Imaging 38:702–710
González AM, Berciano J, Figols J, Pazos A, Pascual J (2000) Loss of dopamine uptake sites and dopamine D2 receptors in striatonigral degeneration. Brain Res 852:228–232
Habraken JB, Booij J, Slomka P, Sokole EB, van Royen EA (1999) Quantification and visualization of defects of the functional dopaminergic system using an automatic algorithm. J Nucl Med 40:1091–1097
Hall DA, Jennings D, Seibyl J, Tassone F, Marek K (2010) FMR1 gene expansion and scans without evidence of dopaminergic deficits in parkinsonism patients. Parkinsonism Relat Disord 16:608–611
Hammesfahr S, Antke C, Mamlins E et al (2016) FP-CIT- and IBZM-SPECT in corticobasal syndrome: results from a clinical follow-up study. Neurodegener Dis 16:342–347
Hesse S, Meyer PM, Strecker K et al (2009) Monoamine transporter availability in Parkinson's disease patients with or without depression. Eur J Nucl Med Mol Imaging 36:428–435
Iranzo A, Lomeña F, Stockner H et al (2010) Decreased striatal dopamine transporter uptake and substantia nigra hyperechogenicity as risk markers of synucleinopathy in patients with idiopathic rapid-eye-movement sleep behaviour disorder: a prospective study. Lancet Neurol 9:1070–1077
Iranzo A, Santamaría J, Valldeoriola F et al (2017) Dopamine transporter imaging deficit predicts early transition to synucleinopathy in idiopathic rapid eye movement sleep behavior disorder. Ann Neurol 82:419–428
Isaias IU, Benti R, Cilia R et al (2007) [123I]FP-CIT striatal binding in early Parkinson's disease patients with tremor vs. akinetic-rigid onset. Neuroreport 18:1499–1502
Ishikawa T, Dhawan V, Kazumata K et al (1996) Comparative nigrostriatal dopaminergic imaging with iodine-123-bCIT-FP/SPECT and fluorine-18-FDOPA/PET. J Nucl Med 37:1760–1765
Iwabuchi Y, Nakahara T, Kameyama M et al (2019) Impact of a combination of quantitative indices representing uptake intensity, shape, and asymmetry in DAT SPECT using machine learning: comparison of different volume of interest settings. EJNMMI Res 9:7
Jacobsen LK, Staley JK, Zoghbi SS et al (2000) Prediction of dopamine transporter binding availability by genotype: a preliminary report. Am J Psychiatry 157:1700–1703
Jenkins PO, De Simoni S, Bourke NJ (2018) Dopaminergic abnormalities following traumatic brain injury. Brain 141:797–810
Joling M, Vriend C, van den Heuvel OA et al (2017) Analysis of extrastriatal 123I-FP-CIT binding contributes to the differential diagnosis of parkinsonian diseases. J Nucl Med 58:1117–1123
Joling M, Vriend C, van der Zande JJ et al (2018) Lower 123I-FP-CIT binding to the striatal dopamine transporter, but not to the extrastriatal serotonin transporter, in Parkinson's disease compared with dementia with Lewy bodies. Neuroimage Clin 19:130–136
Joutsa J, Johansson J, Seppänen M, Noponen T, Kaasinen V (2015) Dorsal-to-ventral shift in midbrain dopaminergic projections and increased thalamic/raphe serotonergic function in early Parkinson disease. J Nucl Med 56:1036–1041
Jung Y, Jordan LG 3rd, Lowe VJ et al (2018) Clinicopathological and ^{123}I-FP-CIT SPECT correlations in patients with dementia. Ann Clin Transl Neurol 5:376–381
Kaasinen V, Joutsa J, Noponen T, Johansson J, Seppänen M (2015) Effects of aging and gender on striatal and extrastriatal [123I]FP-CIT binding in Parkinson's disease. Neurobiol Aging 36:1757–1763
Kägi G, Bhatia KP, Tolosa E (2010) The role of DAT-SPECT in movement disorders. J Neurol Neurosurg Psychiatry 81:5–12
Kas A, Payoux P, Habert MO et al (2007) Validation of a standardized normalization template for statistical parametric mapping analysis of 123I-FP-CIT images. J Nucl Med 48:1459–1467
Kaufman MJ, Madras BK (1991) Severe depletion of cocaine recognition sites associated with the dopamine transporter in Parkinson's-diseased striatum. Synapse 9:43–49

Kim JM, Jeong HJ, Bae YJ et al (2016) Loss of substantia nigra hyperintensity on 7 Tesla MRI of Parkinson's disease, multiple system atrophy, and progressive supranuclear palsy. Parkinsonism Relat Disord 26:47–54
Kish SJ, Chang LJ, Mirchandani L (1985) Progressive supranuclear palsy: relationship between extrapyramidal disturbances, dementia, and brain neurotransmitter markers. Ann Neurol 18:530–536
Kish SJ, Shannak K, Hornykiewicz O (1988) Uneven pattern of dopamine loss in the striatum of patients with idiopathic Parkinson's disease. Pathophysiologic and clinical implications. N Engl J Med 318:876–880
Klaffke S, Kuhn AA, Plotkin M, Amthauer H, Harnack D, Felix R, Kupsch A (2006) Dopamine transporters, D2 receptors, and glucose metabolism in corticobasal degeneration. Mov Disord 21:1724–1727
Knudsen GM, Karlsborg M, Thomsen G et al (2004) Imaging of dopamine transporters and D2 receptors in patients with Parkinson's disease and multiple system atrophy. Eur J Nucl Med Mol Imaging 31:1631–1638
Kolenc M, Popović M, Grmek M, Pirtošek Z, Trošt M (2012) A case of multiple system atrophy with normal dopamine transporter imaging. J Neurol 259:2719–2731
Koopman KE, la Fleur SE, Fliers E, Serlie MJ, Booij J (2012) Assessing the optimal time point for the measurement of extrastriatal serotonin transporter binding with 123I-FP-CIT SPECT in healthy, male subjects. J Nucl Med 53:1087–1090
Kupsch AR, Bajaj N, Weiland F et al (2012) Impact of DaTscan SPECT imaging on clinical management, diagnosis, confidence of diagnosis, quality of life, health resource use and safety in patients with clinically uncertain parkinsonian syndromes: a prospective 1-year follow-up of an open-label controlled study. J Neurol Neurosurg Psychiatry 83:620–628
Lavalaye J, Booij J, Reneman L, Habraken JB, van Royen EA (2000) Effect of age and gender on dopamine transporter imaging with [123I]FP-CIT SPET in healthy volunteers. Eur J Nucl Med 27:867–869
Lim TT, Ahmed A, Itin I, Gostkowski M, Rudolph J, Cooper S, Fernandez HH (2013) Is 6 months of neuroleptic withdrawal sufficient to distinguish drug-induced parkinsonism from Parkinson's disease? Int J Neurosci 123:170–174
Lin JJ, Chang DC (1997) Tremor caused by ipsilateral chronic subdural hematoma. Case illustration. J Neurosurg 87:474
Løkkegaard A, Werdelin LM, Friberg L (2002) Clinical impact of diagnostic SPET investigations with a dopamine re-uptake ligand. Eur J Nucl Med Mol Imaging 29:1623–1629
Marek KL, Seibyl JP, Zoghbi SS et al (1996) [123I]beta-CIT/SPECT imaging demonstrates bilateral loss of dopamine transporters in hemi-Parkinson's disease. Neurology 46:231–237
Marshall V, Grosset D (2003) Role of dopamine transporter imaging in routine clinical practice. Mov Disord 18:1415–1423
Marshall VL, Reininger CB, Marquardt M et al (2009) Parkinson's disease is overdiagnosed clinically at baseline in diagnostically uncertain cases: a 3-year European multicenter study with repeat [123I]FP-CIT SPECT. Mov Disord 24:500–508
Matsuda H, Murata M, Mukai Y et al (2018) Japanese multicenter database of healthy controls for [123I]FP-CIT SPECT. Eur J Nucl Med Mol Imaging 45:1405–1416
McGeer PL, McGeer EG, Suzuki J (1977) Aging and extrapyramidal function. Arch Neurol 34:33–35
McKeith I, O'Brien J, Walker Z et al (2007) Sensitivity and specificity of dopamine transporter imaging with 123I-FP-CIT SPECT in dementia with Lewy bodies: a phase III, multicentre study. Lancet Neurol 6:305–313
Meyer PT, Winz OH, Dafotakis M, Werner CJ, Krohn T, Schäfer WM (2011) Improved visual [^{123}I]FP-CIT SPECT interpretation for evaluation of parkinsonism by visual rating of parametric distribution volume ratio images. Q J Nucl Med Mol Imaging 55:301–309
Morgan S, Kemp P, Booij J et al (2012) Differentiation of frontotemporal dementia from dementia with Lewy bodies using FP-CIT SPECT. J Neurol Neurosurg Psychiatry 83:1063–1070

Morley JF, Cheng G, Dubroff JG, Wood S, Wilkinson JR, Duda JE (2016) Olfactory impairment predicts underlying dopaminergic deficit in presumed drug-induced parkinsonism. Mov Disord Clin Pract 28:603–606
Muñoz E, Iranzo A, Rauek S et al (2011) Subclinical nigrostriatal dopaminergic denervation in the cerebellar subtype of multiple system atrophy (MSA-C). J Neurol 258:2248–2253
Neumeyer JL, Wang S, Gao Y et al (1994) N-ω-fluoroalkyl analogs of (1R)-2β-carbomethoxy-3β-(4-iodophenyl)-tropane (β-CIT): radiotracers for positron emission tomography and single photon emission computed tomography imaging of dopamine transporters. J Med Chem 37:1558–1561
O'Brien JT, Colloby S, Fenwick J et al (2004) Dopamine transporter loss visualized with FP-CIT SPECT in the differential diagnosis of dementia with Lewy bodies. Arch Neurol 61:919–925
O'Brien JT, McKeith IG, Walker Z et al (2009) Diagnostic accuracy of 123I-FP-CIT SPECT in possible dementia with Lewy bodies. Br J Psychiatry 194:34–39
O'Sullivan SS, Burn DJ, Holton JL, Lees AJ (2008) Normal dopamine transporter single photon-emission CT scan in corticobasal degeneration. Mov Disord 23:2424–2426
Oyanagi K, Tsuchiya K, Yamazaki M, Keda K (2001) Substantia nigra in progressive supranuclear palsy, corticobasal degeneration, and parkinsonism-dementia complex of Guam: specific pathological features. J Neuropathol Exp Neurol 60:393–402
Pagano G, De Micco R, Yousaf T, Wilson H, Chandra A, Politis M (2018) REM behavior disorder predicts motor progression and cognitive decline in Parkinson disease. Neurology 91:894–905
Pak K, Nam HY, Shin S et al (2018) Effects of rs591323 on serotonin transporter availability in healthy male subjects. Ann Nucl Med 32:431–436
Papathanasiou ND, Boutsiadis A, Dickson J, Bomanji JB (2012) Diagnostic accuracy of 123I-FP-CIT (DaTSCAN) in dementia with Lewy bodies: a meta-analysis of published studies. Parkinsonism Relat Disord 18:225–229
Parkinson Study Group (2002) Dopamine transporter brain imaging to assess the effects of Pramipexole vs levodopa Parkinson disease progression. JAMA 287:1653–1661
Perju-Dumbrava LD, Kovacs GG, Pirker S, Jellinger K, Hoffmann M, Asenbaum S, Pirker W (2012) Dopamine transporter imaging in autopsy-confirmed Parkinson's disease and multiple system atrophy. Mov Disord 27:65–71
Perry E, Court J, Goodchild R et al (1998) Clinical neurochemistry: developments in dementia research based on brain bank material. J Neural Transm 105:915–933
Plotkin M, Amthauer H, Klaffke S et al (2005) Combined 123I-FP-CIT and 123I-IBZM SPECT for the diagnosis of parkinsonian syndromes: study on 72 patients. J Neural Transm 112:677–692
Ponsen MM, Stoffers D, Booij J, van Eck-Smit BL, Wolters EC, Berendse HW (2004) Idiopathic hyposmia as a preclinical sign of Parkinson's disease. Ann Neurol 56:173–181
Ponsen MM, Stoffers D, Wolters EC, Booij J, Berendse HW (2010) Olfactory testing combined with dopamine transporter imaging as a method to detect prodromal Parkinson's disease. J Neurol Neurosurg Psychiatry 81:396–399
Radau PE, Linke R, Slomka PJ, Tatsch K (2000) Optimization of automated quantification of 123I-IBZM uptake in the striatum applied to parkinsonism. J Nucl Med 41:220–227
Roselli F, Pisciotta NM, Perneczky R et al (2009) Severity of neuropsychiatric symptoms and dopamine transporter levels in dementia with Lewy bodies: a 123I-FP-CIT SPECT study. Mov Disord 24:2097–2103
Roselli F, Pisciotta NM, Pennelli M et al (2010) Midbrain SERT in degenerative parkinsonisms: a 123I-FP-CIT SPECT study. Mov Disord 25:1853–1859
Ruberg M, Javoy-Agid F, Hirsch E et al (1985) Dopaminergic and cholinergic lesions in progressive supranuclear palsy. Ann Neurol 18:523–529
Scheffel U, Lever JR, Abraham P et al (1997) N-substituted phenyltropanes as in vivo binding ligands for rapid imaging studies of the dopamine transporter. Synapse 25:345–349
Scherfler C, Seppi K, Donnemiller E et al (2005) Voxel-wise analysis of [123I]beta-CIT SPECT differentiates the Parkinson variant of multiple system atrophy from idiopathic Parkinson's disease. Brain 128:1605–1612

Schneider SA, Edwards MJ, Mir P, Cordivari C, Hooker J, Dickson J, Quinn N, Bhatia KP (2007) Patients with adult-onset dystonic tremor resembling parkinsonian tremor have scans without evidence of dopaminergic deficit (SWEDDs). Mov Disord 22:2210–2215

Seppi K, Scherfler C, Donnemiller E et al (2006) Topography of dopamine transporter availability in progressive supranuclear palsy: a voxelwise [123I]beta-CIT SPECT analysis. Arch Neurol 63:1154–1160

Siepel FJ, Rongve A, Buter TC, Beyer MK, Ballard CG, Booij J, Aarsland D (2013) (123I) FP-CIT SPECT in suspected dementia with Lewy bodies: a longitudinal case study. BMJ Open 3(4):pii: e002642

Siepel FJ, Dalen I, Grüner R, Booij J, Brønnick KS, Buter TC, Aarsland D (2016) Loss of dopamine transporter binding and clinical symptoms in dementia with Lewy bodies. Mov Disord 31:118–125

Sixel-Döring F, Liepe K, Mollenhauer B, Trautmann E, Trenkwalder C (2011) The role of 123I-FP-CIT-SPECT in the differential diagnosis of Parkinson and tremor syndromes: a critical assessment of 125 cases. J Neurol 258:2147–2154

Spiegel J, Hellwig D, Samnick S et al (2007) Striatal FP-CIT uptake differs in the subtypes of early Parkinson's disease. J Neural Transm 114:331–335

Stiasny-Kolster K, Doerr Y, Möller JC et al (2005) Combination of 'idiopathic' REM sleep behaviour disorder and olfactory dysfunction as possible indicator for alpha-synucleinopathy demonstrated by dopamine transporter FP-CIT-SPECT. Brain 128:126–137

Stoffers D, Booij J, Bosscher L, Winogrodzka A, Wolters EC, Berendse HW (2005) Early-stage [123I]beta-CIT SPECT and long-term clinical follow-up in patients with an initial diagnosis of Parkinson's disease. Eur J Nucl Med Mol Imaging 32:689–695

Tatsch K (2012) Standardisation and harmonisation boost the credibility of nuclear medicine procedures. Eur J Nucl Med Mol Imaging 39:186–187

Tatsch K, Poepperl G (2012) Quantitative approaches to dopaminergic brain imaging. Q J Nucl Med Mol Imaging 56:27–38

Taylor JC, Fenner JW (2017) Comparison of machine learning and semi-quantification algorithms for (I123)FP-CIT classification: the beginning of the end for semi-quantification? EJNMMI Phys 4:29

Taylor JC, Romanowski C, Lorenz E, Lo C, Bandmann O, Fenner J (2018) Computer-aided diagnosis for (123I)FP-CIT imaging: impact on clinical reporting. EJNMMI Res 8:36

Thomas AJ, Attems J, Colloby SJ et al (2017) Autopsy validation of 123I-FP-CIT dopaminergic neuroimaging for the diagnosis of DLB. Neurology 88:276–283

Thomas AJ, Donaghy P, Roberts G et al (2019) Diagnostic accuracy of dopaminergic imaging in prodromal dementia with Lewy bodies. Psychol Med 49:396–402

Tinazzi M, Antonini A, Bovi T et al (2009) Clinical and [123I]FP-CIT SPET imaging follow-up in patients with drug-induced parkinsonism. J Neurol 256:910–915

Tissingh G, Booij J, Bergmans P et al (1998) Iodine-123-N-omega-fluoropropyl-2beta-carbomethoxy-3beta-(4-iodophenyl)tropane SPECT in healthy controls and early-stage, drug-naive Parkinson's disease. J Nucl Med 39:1143–1148

van de Giessen E, de Win MM, Tanck MW, van den Brink W, Baas F, Booij J (2009) Striatal dopamine transporter availability associated with polymorphisms in the dopamine transporter gene SLC6A3. J Nucl Med 50:45–52

van de Giessen EV, Hesse S, Caan MW et al (2013) No association between striatal dopamine transporter binding and body mass index: a multi-center European study in healthy volunteers. NeuroImage 64:61–67

van der Zande JJ, Booij J, Scheltens P, Raijmakers PG, Lemstra AW (2016) [123]FP-CIT SPECT scans initially rated as normal became abnormal over time in patients with probable dementia with Lewy bodies. Eur J Nucl Med Mol Imaging 43:1060–1066

van Dyck CH, Seibyl JP, Malison RT et al (2002) Age-related decline in dopamine transporters: analysis of striatal subregions, nonlinear effects, and hemispheric asymmetries. Am J Geriatr Psychiatry 10:36–43 van Dyck CH, Malison RT, Jacobsen LK et al (2005) Increased dopamine transporter availability associated with the 9-repeat allele of the SLC6A3 gene. J Nucl Med 46:745–751

Van Laere K, Casteels C, De Ceuninck L et al (2006) Dual-tracer dopamine transporter and perfusion SPECT in differential diagnosis of parkinsonism using template-based discriminant analysis. J Nucl Med 47:384–392

Varrone A, Marek KL, Jennings D, Innis RB, Seibyl JP (2001) [(123)I]beta-CIT SPECT imaging demonstrates reduced density of striatal dopamine transporters in Parkinson's disease and multiple system atrophy. Mov Disord 16:1023–1032

Varrone A, Dickson JC, Tossici-Bolt L et al (2013) European multicentre database of healthy controls for [123I]FP-CIT SPECT (ENC-DAT): age-related effects, gender differences and evaluation of different methods of analysis. Eur J Nucl Med Mol Imaging 40:213–227

Vergnet S, Hives F, Foubert-Samier A (2019) Dopamine transporter imaging for the diagnosis of multiple system atrophy cerebellar type. Parkinsonism Relat Disord 63:199–203

Walker Z, Costa DC, Walker RW et al (2002) Differentiation of dementia with Lewy bodies from Alzheimer's disease using a dopaminergic presynaptic ligand. J Neurol Neurosurg Psychiatry 73:134–140

Walker Z, Costa DC, Walker RW et al (2004) Striatal dopamine transporter in dementia with Lewy bodies and Parkinson disease: a comparison. Neurology 62:1568–1572

Walker Z, Jaros E, Walker RW et al (2007) Dementia with Lewy bodies: a comparison of clinical diagnosis, FP-CIT single photon emission computed tomography imaging and autopsy. J Neurol Neurosurg Psychiatry 78:1176–1181

Warren NM, Piggott MA, Greally E, Lake M, Lees AJ, Burn DJ (2007) Basal ganglia cholinergic and dopaminergic function in progressive supranuclear palsy. Mov Disord 22:1594–1600

Yamamoto H, Arimura S, Nakanishi A et al (2017) Age-related effects and gender differences in Japanese healthy controls for [^{123}I] FP-CIT SPECT. Ann Nucl Med 31:407–412

Zijlmans J, Booij J, Valk J, Lees A, Horstink M (2002) Posttraumatic tremor without parkinsonism in a patient with complete contralateral loss of the nigrostriatal pathway. Mov Disord 17:1086–1088

Zijlmans J, Evans A, Fontes F, Katzenschlager R, Gacinovic S, Lees AJ, Costa D (2007) [123I]FP-CIT spect study in vascular parkinsonism and Parkinson's disease. Mov Disord 22:1278–1285

Part V

Inflammatory Disorders

PET Imaging of Microglia Activation and Infection in Neuropsychiatric Disorders with Potential Infectious Origin

32

Hans Christiaan Klein, Lot de Witte, Robert Bransfield, and Peter Paul De Deyn

Contents

H. C. Klein (✉)
Medical Imaging Centre, University Medical Hospital Groningen, University of Groningen, Groningen, The Netherlands

Lentis Mental Health and VNN Addiction Care, Groningen, The Netherlands

L. de Witte
Department of Psychiatry, University Medical Center Utrecht, University of Utrecht, Utrecht, The Netherlands

Department of Psychiatry, Icahn School of Medicine, New York, NY, USA

Mental Illness Research, Education and Clinical Center (MIRECC), James J Peters VA Medical Center, Bronx, NY, USA
e-mail: lotje.dewitte@mssm.edu

R. Bransfield
Department of Psychiatry, Rutgers-Robert Wood Johnson Medical School, Piscataway, NJ, USA

P. P. De Deyn
Department of Neurology, Alzheimer Center Groningen, University Medical Center Groningen, University of Groningen, Groningen, The Netherlands

Laboratory of Neurochemistry and Behavior, Department of Biomedical Sciences, Institute Born-Bunge, University of Antwerp, Born Bunge Foundation, Antwerp (Wilrijk), Belgium
e-mail: p.p.de.deyn@umcg.nl

R. A. J. O. Dierckx et al. (eds.), *PET and SPECT in Neurology*,
https://doi.org/10.1007/978-3-030-53168-3_32

Abstract

The central nervous system (CNS) is an immunoprivileged location for the possible sequestration of latent infections. The presence of pathogens may be involved in the etiology of neuropsychiatric diseases by inducing classical inflammatory responses, hypersensitivity, cellular toxicity, or direct alteration of cellular processes. Infection, persistence, and activation of microbes in the brain are not easy to assess in vivo, and the relation with clinical disease is very difficult to prove. An elegant way to determine an inflammatory response in the brain in vivo is by molecular imaging of microglia activation with [^{11}C]PK11195 and other radiopharmaceuticals that target the translocator protein (TSPO). In this chapter, we summarize the neuroimaging studies that target the TSPO in patients with neuropsychiatric diseases, and we propose positron emission tomography (PET) imaging with radiopharmaceuticals that target the metabolism of infectious agents directly.

32.1 General Introduction

During World War I, an epidemic of psychiatric disorders with a probable infectious origin occurred. This epidemic of "encephalitis lethargica" was meticulously described by Constantin von Economo, regarding the psychiatric, neurological, epidemiological, and postmortem microscopical phenomena of the disease (Dickman 2001; Triarhou 2006). In those days, 50% or more of the patients referred to mental hospitals appeared to have suffered from the epidemic (Economo 1929). Many patients subsequently acquired neurological symptoms such as parkinsonism, oculogyric crises, and lethargy. The inflammatory changes in the brain parenchyma (particularly in the midbrain) were also meticulously described. Von Economo showed that transmission of brain specimens of patients to small animals caused similar neuropathological and behavioral changes. The agent of transmission was nonfilterable; it passed filters that blocked the transmission of the bacterial diseases known at that time.

The dementia paralytica of the insane (DPI) is another example of an infectious neuropsychiatric disease. DPI is caused by the sexually transmitted spirochete *Treponema pallidum*. *T. pallidum* is a genus in the family of Spirochaetaceae. CNS infection (neurospirochetosis) was designated "the great imitator" of psychiatric disorders, and sequelae of obsessive–compulsive behavior, classical manic episodes, and paranoid delusional psychoses were frequent. Paralytic death ensued in nearly all patients suffering from DPI. A treatment was discovered by the 1927 Nobel laureate (Physiology and Medicine) Wagner Jauregg, which involved transmission of the *Plasmodium falciparum* parasite to the patient, inducing recurring malaria fevers. The working mechanism of fever therapy is probably immune modulation to eradicate the spirochete (Whitrow 1990). The therapy was lifesaving, and quite some patients regained full functioning after the therapy, although not all recovered, and in some, recovery was observed only during a certain period of time.

Borrelia genera are structurally similar to *Treponema* genera and both are part of the family of Spirochaetaceae. In contrast to sexual transmission of *Treponema* species, the *Borrelia* species is predominantly transmitted by ticks. *Borrelia burgdorferi* infections present as an erythema migrans skin lesion, and incidence of this primary lesions is increasing in many endemic areas, for example, in the Netherlands. There is some evidence that transmission of the spirochete by ticks is increasing and transmission of the spirochete to the brain of the human host is becoming more prevalent (Hildenbrand et al. 2009; Steere et al. 2004). Similar to DPI and encephalitis lethargica, a variety of symptoms can occur associated with neuroborreliosis (Markeljević et al. 2011; Almodovar et al. 2012; Miklossy 2008).

The degree of involvement of infections in neuropsychiatric diseases is currently a subject of debate. The difficulty in clarifying this issue is mainly due to the scarcity of methods to directly detect pathogens in the CNS in vivo. In comparison to peripheral tissue, biopsies of the brain are contraindicated presently and performed only in extremely rare case such as brain tumors. Infection of the brain parenchyma is not necessarily associated with detection of the pathogen in the cerebrospinal fluid (CSF). PET imaging may offer a solution to pursue infectious inflammatory changes in the living brain parenchyma. Uptake of the radiopharmaceutical [^{11}C]PK11195 is indicative of brain inflammation, and the number of studies with this imaging agent and second-generation radiopharmaceuticals targeting neuroinflammation is growing. Radiopharmaceuticals derived from antibiotics are available for imaging purposes, but not yet applied broadly for infection imaging. We propose a role for radiopharmaceuticals derived from—among others—nitroimidazole antibiotics as promising tools for imaging of infection of the CNS.

32.2 Establishment of CNS Infection

This first paragraph discusses the mechanisms involved in the dissemination of the pathogens to the brain and the mechanisms involved in the establishment of latent infection.

32.2.1 Neuroinvasive Species

The brain is often viewed as a sterile organ unless incidentally infected leading to diseases such as encephalitis. However, it is now known that the brain parenchyma is not pathogen free.

Using sensitive molecular techniques, it has been shown that respiratory viruses, herpes simplex viruses (HSV), *Borrelia* spirochetes, and many other pathogens can be present in brain tissue postmortem (Lakeman and Whitley 1995; Schmutzhard 2001).

Neuroinvasive microbes are microbes that can enter the CNS easily. Some microbes primarily reside within the CNS; others only incidentally invade the CNS. *Neurovirulent* microbes are pathogens that can cause diseases of the CNS. These include diseases established by direct infection of the CNS, such as viral and bacterial encephalitis, neuroborreliosis, and neurosyphilis, but also subacute sclerosing panencephalitis after measles infection. Furthermore, it is thought that the interaction between neurovirulent pathogens and the host may be involved in the pathophysiology of various neuropsychiatric diseases, such as Alzheimer's disease, depression, and schizophrenia.

Several classes of neurovirulent microbes have been described and include:

1. Viruses: human herpes viruses (herpes simplex virus, cytomegalovirus, etc.), polyomaviruses (JC/BK virus), flaviviruses (West Nile virus, Japanese encephalitis virus, etc.), human retroviruses (HIV, etc.), measles virus, influenza virus, rabies virus, and poliovirus.
2. Bacteria: *Treponema pallidum*, *B. burgdorferi*.
3. Parasites: *P. falciparum*, *Toxoplasma gondii*.
4. Fungi: *Cryptococcus neoformans*.
5. Human endogenous retroviruses: These viruses are not "real" neuroinvasive microbes, but are retroviruses that have infected the germline in the recent or ancient past and integrated their viral sequences in the human genome. In this way, the viral sequences also reach the CNS. These sequences have been implicated in various neuropsychiatric diseases, such as schizophrenia (Yolken et al. 2000) and multiple sclerosis (Anderton et al. 2011).

32.2.2 Neuroinvasion Mechanisms

Due to the blood–brain barrier (BBB), the brain is relatively protected from invading pathogens. However, microbes have evolved various strategies to invade the brain:

1. Although the BBB provides a barrier to most pathogens, some pathogens can invade the brain by this hematogenous route. The pathogen may penetrate the endothelium directly (transcytosis) or may first produce a productive infection in the endothelial cells. High levels of viremia/bacteremia are thought to be required

for direct spread via the hematogenous route; however, as a result of systemic infection, the permeability of the BBB can be increased (Moriarty et al. 2008).
2. In addition, certain pathogens can spread from the circulation into the brain via infiltration of leukocytes. HIV is thought to hide in leukocytes to spread throughout the body, including the CNS by passing the BBB to cause neuro-HIV ("Trojan horse") (Lindl et al. 2010).
3. The olfactory route is used by several pathogens to invade the brain. After a local infection in the skin or nasal mucosa, these pathogens spread by the olfactory nerve or by the perineuronal (cerebrospinal fluid) route to the CNS (Mori et al. 2005; Sips et al. 2011). Viruses also use other peripheral and cranial nerves for retrograde axonal transport to invade the CNS. For example, HSV uses the axons to the trigeminal nucleus to spread to the CNS (Theil et al. 2004).

32.2.3 Pathogen Reservoirs

Some microbes that have gained access to the brain transform into a state of relative inactivity. Only proteins are expressed that keep the microbe viable, but present in a latent state. Microbes may reside intracellularly (with, e.g., DNA as epigenome in the nucleus of the cell) or extracellularly (e.g., cysts of fungi), creating a reservoir, from which reactivations may occur. Various reservoirs in the brain are available for neuroinvasive pathogens:

1. HIV dementia is a disease, in which brain macrophages are loaded with viral RNA (Alexaki et al. 2008), but the virus often replicates at low speed.
2. HSV is "resting" in a latent form in many individuals without overt clinical symptoms in neurons of the sensory ganglia (especially trigeminal) (Theil et al. 2003). A continuous immune surveillance with cytotoxic-type T cells is necessary to keep the virus in latency and prevent it from replicating and disseminating (Posavad et al. 2003; Derfuss et al. 2007). Interestingly, HSV DNA can not only be detected in the trigeminal ganglion but can also be detected by PCR in the brain (Gordon et al. 1996). Intraparenchymal replication in HSV encephalitis predominantly affects the temporal lobes, cortex, and hippocampus, inducing bizarre behavior, language impairment, headache, paralysis, and memory deficits that can partly remain after resolution of the infection (Kapur et al. 1994).
3. It is clear that spirochetes of the *Borrelia* species can be present but latent in the brain. However, the reservoir is still unknown. A variety of possibilities exist: intracellular or extracellular and in defective cyst form or in replication competent spirochetal form (Miklossy et al. 2008).

32.2.4 Response to Pathogens

Although we now know that neurons can be partly regenerated after CNS injury, the CNS environment is in an anti-inflammatory state compared to other organs to protect against immune-mediated brain damage. The severity of infection, virulence factors of the microbe, but also host factors are thought to play an important role in directing the level and nature of how the immune system responds. Microbial invasion may be followed by an absence of a response, mild to severe classical inflammatory responses, but also hypersensitivity reactions and direct cellular toxicity. Since most neuropsychiatric diseases are at least partly dependent on genetic factors, it is likely that the infectious disease phenotype is modified by genetic factors, both of the host and the pathogens. Examples of responses to various neurotropic pathogens are as follows:

1. Infection of the CNS by HIV may lead to an inflammatory response, including production of cytokines, excitotoxic neurotransmitters, and oxygen radicals (Lindl et al. 2010). Combined administration of various therapeutic drugs may be necessary to acquire a good response of patients with neuro-HIV.
2. Despite the fact that HSV is present in a latent state in the majority of people, HSV encephalitis is very rare. It is thought that the virus is kept under control and trapped in the neuron by local T cells and macrophage-like cells. This cellular response occurs in the ganglion to prevent the virus from replicating and disseminating. Interesting is the fact that psychotropic drugs, such as lithium, may also improve resistance against HSV infections (Amsterdam 1990). Probably the immune-modulating properties of psychotropic drugs explain these favorable actions on viral diseases (Lieb 2002).
3. The immune response to spirochetal diseases is noteworthy. Seronegativity in serum and cerebrospinal fluid (CSF) does not rule out neurospirochetosis and can lead to a fatal outcome (Oksi et al. 1996). Immune responses in the periphery may also be absent in *Treponema pallidum* infection while the spirochete is actively moving within the ocular tissue (Smith and Israel 1967). Thus, immune responses toward spirochetes in the CNS are either restricted to the CNS or actively suppressed in the periphery.

32.3 Inflammatory Response to CNS Infection

This paragraph discusses the specialized cells in the brain that respond to the dissemination and establishment of infection of pathogens. Functions of cells in the blood–brain barrier, in the circumventricular organs, and in the brain, parenchyma shall be addressed. Immune response is orchestrated by microglia and the activation of microglia can be imaged with [^{11}C]PK11195.

32.3.1 Functions of the Blood–Brain Barrier

The brain parenchyma is protected from direct influx of compounds from the blood by the blood–brain barrier (BBB). The BBB is impermeable for diffusion of polar molecules such as cytokines and immune globulins due to the presence of tight junctions between the endothelial cells of the capillaries (Pardridge 1999). However, specific carriers can transport some molecules across the BBB. Carrier-mediated transport of polar molecules is heavily dependent on the expression of specific carriers for solutes in the blood (Kusuhara and Sugiyama 2005). Transcytosis (penetration through the cell, by phagocytosis and intracellular transport and exocytosis) is an "emergent" specialized property of the BBB (Hervé et al. 2008), modified by mostly unknown factors. The BBB creates a unique immune milieu in the brain parenchyma, dependent on the immune molecules and cells that are allowed to traverse the BBB.

An exception to the tightly controlled transport from the circulation to the CNS is the circumventricular organ. In the circumventricular organs of the brain, the capillary endothelium is fenestrated, giving direct access of cytokines and immune globulins into the parenchyma (although then barred by the next barrier, the basement membrane), and only in these regions can peripheral proteins and microbes enter the parenchyma directly (Sisó et al. 2010). Specialized "leaky barriers" in the hypothalamus provide the possibility to specifically sense blood milieu and CSF milieu (Rodríguez et al. 2010).

32.3.2 Functions of Microglia

Early during embryogenesis, myeloid cells of the macrophage/monocyte lineage seed the CNS, where they find residency (Monier et al. 2007). In the brain, these cells differentiate into microglia. The roles of microglia have only partly been unraveled. Microglia have important functions in neurodevelopment, neuroinflammation, and CNS repair. During embryogenesis, microglia are essential for neuronal synaptogenesis and neurogenesis (Tremblay and Majewska 2011). In adulthood, these trophic functions probably continue, and microglia are activated in regions of the brain that are experiencing remodeling, for example, after peripheral nerve lesions (Moneta et al. 1993). Recent murine studies demonstrated the importance of functional microglia in synaptic pruning (Paolicelli et al. 2011).

Microglia can reside in both resting and more activated state. Activated microglia may take part in the following:

1. Rescuing response
2. Response to remove debris
3. Toxic response (release of nitric oxide (NO) by microglia is detrimental)

A local response by microglia is not necessarily mirrored by changes in serum or cerebrospinal fluid, because of the BBB and brain–CSF barrier. It may be safely assumed that in the early prodromal phase of a subtle infectious process in the brain, no detectable immune changes occur in the periphery. The BBB restricts the diffusion into plasma, and the brain–CSF barrier restricts diffusion into the CSF of cytokines as potential markers of inflammation of the brain parenchyma.

Therefore, in vivo imaging techniques for inflammation are needed that combine the property of effective penetration through the BBB and of sufficient binding to microglia in the brain parenchyma. In this chapter, we will focus on the most applied radiopharmaceutical for detecting microglia activation, [^{11}C]PK11195.

32.3.3 Microglia Activation: Imaging with [^{11}C]PK11195

Radiopharmaceuticals—when sufficiently lipophilic and not a substrate for efflux pumps—easily penetrate the lipid biomembranes of the BBB. To image inflammation, the intermediately lipophilic isoquinolone PK11195 is available (log $P = 3.4$) among others (Doorduin et al. 2009b). This compound binds to the translocator protein (TSPO) of mitochondria in activated microglia cells and other immune cells and increases during inflammation (Cosenza-Nashat et al. 2009). In noninflammatory conditions, expression in brain is low, thereby offering "contrast" between inflamed and noninflamed tissues. Microglia activation as imaged with TSPO ligand is usually designated as "neuroinflammation." However, neuroinflammation reflects the sum of activation of glia, microglia, and perivascular macrophages in the brain, increasing numbers of glia, microglia, and perivascular macrophages (by influx from the periphery or cell division). All of these activations are reflected by increased expression of TSPO and subsequently increased trapping of [^{11}C]PK11195 in tissue, and the microglia provide the major uptake of [^{11}C]PK11195 (Cosenza-Nashat et al. 2009). In the last years, many radiopharmaceuticals alternative to [^{11}C]PK11195 were developed and applied in human research. Drawbacks of the alternatives are that binding is dependent on frequent gene polymorphisms in man that prevent reliable binding of the radiopharmaceutical in all carriers of the polymorphism (Song 2019). Clinical relevance of the carrier is not known and selecting only noncarrier for imaging hampers conclusions from the studies. The most classic way of neuroinflammation imaging with [^{11}C]PK11195 and arterial input normalization—by coregistration of arterial [^{11}C]PK11195 concentration during the scanning procedure—is still the most robust (Plavén-Sigray et al. 2018). Despite the promises of new radiopharmaceuticals, major caveats appeared and [^{11}C]PK11195 remains the most reliable (Best et al. 2019). Therefore, we limited the description of studies on neuroinflammation in brain diseases to [^{11}C]PK11195 imaging.

Activated microglia are either involved in proinflammatory responses, such as production of cytokines and cytotoxic compounds and NO, or involved in anti-inflammatory responses and excretion of growth factors such as brain-derived neurotropic factor (BDNF). Activated microglia can be divided in M1 and M2 phenotypes with inflammatory switch functions in the brain (Durafourt et al. 2012). Microglia with the M1 phenotype have in vitro destructive capacities as opposed to M2 phenotype microglia, which are protective/anti-inflammatory. To our knowledge, no radiopharmaceuticals have as yet been developed to target these receptors specifically.

32.4 Microglia Activation in Neuropsychiatric Disorders

Microglia activation imaging with [^{11}C]PK11195 has been helpful in gaining knowledge of the mechanisms of many neuropsychiatric disorders. The association between loss of function of brain regions and elevation of [^{11}C]PK11195 uptake supports the role of inflammation in the disease. The inflammation may be related to tissue loss and debris removal, neuroplasticity/remodeling, autoimmunity, presence of toxic metabolites, hypovitaminosis, or antimicrobial response. This paragraph summarizes the results of [^{11}C]PK11195 imaging studies in neuropsychiatric disorders in general, without direct proof of a specific infectious origin. In the next paragraph, the studies with [^{11}C]PK11195 in patients suffering from infectious disorders are summarized.

32.4.1 Neurodegenerative Disorders

It is well known that in many neurodegenerative diseases, inflammation is part of the pathophysiological process. Microglial activation has, for example, been found in gray matter of postmortem brain from patients with multiple sclerosis (MS). A study shows that MS in patients with active disease is reflected by increased [^{11}C]PK11195 uptake in gray matter of regions that correspond to disease symptomatology of individual patients (Politis et al. 2012). More recently, two studies show enhanced uptake in MS lesions that reduce 12.3% upon treatment with fingolimod (Sucksdorff et al. 2017) and 26.8% on natalizumab (Kaunzner et al. 2017). Also, in Parkinson's disease, with destruction of neurons in the substantia nigra and projecting areas such as striatum, increased uptake was found in basal ganglia, pons, and cortical regions. Elevated [^{11}C]PK11195 uptake was present chronically and not associated with loss of dopaminergic neurons nor with clinical symptoms (Gerhard et al. 2006). In Huntington's disease, caused by accumulation of huntingtin in neurons, the striatum is affected in the inflammatory process. The accumulation of [^{11}C]PK11195 is significantly associated with the number of CAG repeats and symptom severity (Pavese et al. 2006). Asymptomatic carriers of the CAG repeat already show profound microglial activation (and loss of dopaminergic terminals) which is correlated to the number of CAG repeats of the huntingtin gene (Tai et al. 2007). In corticobasal degeneration (CBD), the inflammatory changes also involve striatum, one of the major structures involved in the neurodegenerative process (Gerhard et al. 2004). The diagnosis of upper motor neuron disease is difficult to confirm by clinical investigation. [^{11}C]PK11195 PET imaging may help confirm the diagnosis by showing inflammatory lesions in specific areas of the cerebral cortex that correspond to the clinical signs (Turner et al. 2005). Also, in amyotrophic lateral sclerosis, the uptake of [^{11}C]PK11195 is increased in the regions of the brain that are responsible for clinical symptoms in patients and predictive of function loss (Turner et al. 2004). In the first microglia PET study in Alzheimer's disease patients, increases of [^{11}C]PK11195 were found in the parietotemporal and cingulate cortex, and also the entorhinal cortex was affected (Cagnin et al. 2001a, b). Cortical involvement of neuroinflammation was confirmed in a later study showing the frontal, temporoparietal, and cingulated regions affected. A positive correlation between cognitive impairment (MMSE) and microglia activation was elegantly shown (Edison et al. 2008). In other studies, subtle microglia activation was found in occipital cortex (Schuitemaker et al. 2013). In this and another study (Wiley et al. 2009), the patients with mild cognitive impairment showed no significant elevation of [^{11}C]PK11195 binding. A study involving consecutive imaging with the amyloid radiopharmaceutical [^{11}C]PiB (Pittsburg compound) for amyloid foci and [^{11}C]PK11195 for neuroinflammation showed that specifically the amyloid lesions in early MCI were subject to inflammation. An increase of the average binding potential by 0.18 was noted in the amyloid foci (Parbo et al. 2017). Later, in the transition toward full-blown Alzheimer Disease, the association between amyloid accumulation and neuroinflammation is less clear (Chaney et al. 2019). Therefore, the neuroinflammation within PiB positive amyloid plaques provides an early denominator of the MCI phase, and may reflect the early or triggering pathophysiology of Alzheimer disease progression.

In neurodegenerative diseases, microglia activation specifically in the afflicted brain regions is a more common finding. The localization of inflammatory lesions corresponds to the localization of the disease process: motor cortex in ALS, dispersed focal inflammatory sites in MS, parietotemporal lesions in Alzheimer's disease, alterations in the basal ganglia in Parkinson's disease, Huntington's disease, and corticobasal degeneration. The timing of neuroinflammation in these diseases appears to be dependent on the stage of the disease. In Parkinson's disease, the microglia activation occurs early in the disease, but does not correspond further to clinical stage. In Huntington's disease, neuroinflammatory changes occur very early, already in the symptom-free phase of aberrant gene carriers. In Alzheimer's disease, microglia activation appears as a more subtle and late general phenomenon, but focal in the MCI stage.

These examples illustrate that the imaging studies did not resolve the exact role of the microglia response, which is probably very dependent on the underlying pathophysiology, which may be autoimmune/infectious/toxic/genetic, or combinations of these factors. For example, the late response in Alzheimer's disease might correspond to tissue remodeling and clearing of cellular debris, while in the early MCI stage microglia activation, that is only detectable in the PiB positive amyloid foci, might represent a protective, even anti-inflammatory response. This focal tracer accumulation might, for example, represent a protective response in the early phase, which precedes conversion to full-blown dementia and could predict which patients will and will not convert to full-blown Alzheimer dementia. The results of neuroinflammation scanning in Huntington's carriers is also illustrative. In these patients, microglia activation is found very early, already in the symptom-free phase. In Huntington's disease, microglia activation might also represent a protective/adaptive response opposing toxic accumulation of huntingtin in neurons. The major limitation of [^{11}C]PK11195 imaging is that it does not differentiate between protective and detrimental activities of microglia. Development of specific radiopharmaceuticals that target only M1 (destructive) or M2 (protective) microglia may resolve this issue.

32.4.2 Vitamin Deficiency

Thiamine (vitamin B1) deficiency causes increased uptake of [^{3}H]PK11195 in autoradiography slices of specific nuclei (Leong et al. 1994) associated with the human syndrome of Korsakoff's dementia. Microglia activation is a core feature of thiamine-deficiency induced brain damage (Wang and Hazell 2010). Immediate supply of high-dose thiamine partially restores the histological changes of microglia and neurons in vulnerable nuclei (Ke et al. 2003). To our knowledge, no human studies have been performed studying in vivo microglia activation with positron emission tomography (PET) in thiamine deficiency and Korsakoff syndrome in man.

32.4.3 Encephalopathy

Liver infections of hepatitis C virus (HCV) may induce encephalopathy with emotional disorders and cognitive decline. The mechanism of this encephalopathic syndrome is unknown. Peripheral accumulation of ammonia (in cirrhosis), effect of peripheral cytokines released by the infection in the liver, and direct infection of the brain parenchyma with HCV are potential mechanisms. In vivo imaging with [^{11}C]PK11195 showed an increased binding in the caudate nucleus (Grover et al. 2012). This binding was associated with impaired metabolism (magnetic resonance spectroscopy, choline–creatine ratio increase) and impaired cognition, as was also shown in a more recent study (Pflugrad et al. 2016). HCV infection of the brain might be causing these metabolic and inflammatory changes.

Traumatic brain injury may also induce a prolonged encephalopathy associated with neuroinflammation. Prolonged activation of microglia in the thalamus was shown to persist for years after brain injury in some patients. Microglia activation is associated with ongoing suffering from encephalopathy in these subjects (Ramlackhansingh et al. 2011).

32.4.4 Psychiatric Disorders

In major psychiatric disorders, such as schizophrenia and depression, many studies showed reduction of hippocampal volume. In schizophrenia, hippocampal volume reduction occurs quite early in the disease, already before the occurrence of psychosis (Hurlemann et al. 2008). In major depression, hippocampal volume reductions are associated with recurrence of depressions (MacQueen et al. 2003). Interestingly, the hippocampus shows elevated uptake of [^{11}C]PK11195 in patients during psychotic episodes (Doorduin et al. 2009a), and uptake is insignificantly elevated in patients with resolved psychosis (Van Berckel et al. 2008). These studies were most reliable, because they employed an arterial input function for determination of specific binding of [^{11}C]PK11195 to the brain regions of interest. Reduction of hippocampal volume in patients with schizophrenia probably occurs during or soon after a psychosis and is detectable in prospective magnetic resonance imaging (MRI) studies. This may imply that the hippocampus is especially prone to volume reductions during the psychotic phase of schizophrenia, and this vulnerability is reflected by neuroinflammation. Regrettably, more recent studies (Holmes et al. 2016; Di Biase et al. 2017) used the reference tissue model, which compares the specific binding of [^{11}C]PK11195 to the region of interest with binding to cerebellar tissue, which is not neutral, not by definition free from inflammation and therefore prone to more variation than arterial input. The question in which stage—in our opinion during psychotic symptom phase with active inflammation—hippocampal volume reduction takes place in the disease process, is therefore not completely resolved yet. In patients with major depression, microglia activation appears to be globally occurring in brain, and is not limited to the hippocampus as we found in psychotic patients (Doorduin et al. 2009a), and in bipolar disorder patients (Haarman et al. 2014). Interesting results from [^{11}C]PK11195 study in depression is that microglia activation was limited to the patients with suicidal thought, implicating a neuroinflammatory component to suicidality (Holmes et al. 2018).

32.5 Microglia Activation in Neuroinfectious Disorders

Very little research is performed on imaging of infectious diseases directly and also studies with neuroinflammation imaging in patients during infection are scarce. This is peculiar, because PET imaging of neuroinflammation is relatively noninvasive and may support the diagnostic process of encephalitis before CSF alterations are found. Robust PK11195 imaging has some disadvantages, for example, arterial input necessity, and elaborate data analysis (cluster analysis) when the input function is not used. In this chapter, we will show some pioneering studies on neuroinflammation in the herpes encephalitis model and some research in HIV patients and suggest to apply [^{11}C]PK11195 imaging in the diagnosis of neuroborreliosis. Despite the disadvantages of PK11195, we did not yet succeed in finding a better tracer for neuroinflammation imaging of infection (Doorduin et al. 2009b, 2010).

32.5.1 Herpes Simplex Virus Infection

Herpes simplex virus encephalitis (HSE) is a classic example of an infection of the brain with a major impact on human behavior, emotion, and cognition. HSV is a common pathogen in man, is known to produce bizarre behavioral disturbances after brain infection, and can be diagnosed reliably with the detection of HSV antibodies or DNA in CSF. We used an HSE model in rats and studied changes in

[^{11}C]PK11195 trapping. We showed a signal of neuroinflammation in the affected areas, with highest signal at the entrance site of infection (olfactory bulbs, in olfactory route infection). Interestingly, also in the midbrain nuclei, a signal was found: Possibly the infection of this locus explains part of the behavioral changes, such as manic-like behavior in the open field in these rats. Interestingly, after administration of antipsychotics, the manic-like behavior and the neuroinflammatory changes in the brain were attenuated (Doorduin 2010).

HSE in humans is rare, and to our knowledge only one study with [^{11}C]PK11195 imaging has been performed. In this study, predominantly the temporal lobe and the hippocampus were affected. A follow-up MRI after 1 year clearly showed disappearance of hippocampus tissue in the inflamed area (Cagnin et al. 2001a). Microglia activation might reflect an adaptive response of the host after infection that results in the removal of dysfunctional neurons and circuitry.

32.5.2 HIV

In primate models of neuroAIDS, the retention of [^{11}C]PK11195 was proportional to the number of activated macrophages/microglia in the brain (Venneti et al. 2008). Two early studies in patients with HIV in comparison with healthy controls were performed with [^{11}C]PK11195 and yielded different results. In one study (Wiley et al. 2006), no difference in brain uptake was found between HIV patients and healthy controls. In the other study, a significantly elevated uptake of [^{11}C]PK11195 was found in five regions in the brain of HIV dementia patients as compared to healthy controls (Hammoud et al. 2005). Further research of microglia activation in HIV patients with [^{11}C]DPA-713 as TSPO tracer showed that microglia activation is related to dementia signs of the disease (Rubin et al. 2018).

32.5.3 Neuroborreliosis

It is quite surprising that no [^{11}C]PK11195 studies have been performed in neuroborreliosis patients. A case study with brain stem involvement of the *Borrelia* infection shows a [^{18}F]FDG PET hot spot in the brain stem (Plotkin et al. 2005). This spot resolved after successful antibiotic treatment. After treatment of neuroborreliosis and residual cognitive symptoms, on perfusion single-photon emission computed tomography (SPECT) images, a left frontal hypometabolism was shown. The hypometabolism was normalized in patients that gained relief from the cognitive symptoms. In the patients that remained symptomatic, the hypometabolism did not resolve (Logigian et al. 1997). A study with [^{11}C]DPA-713 as TSPO tracer showed increased TSPO binding in eight brain regions in post-Lyme treatment symptomatic patients, excluding the patients with the low affinity T/T polymorphism of TSPO (Coughlin et al. 2018).

32.6 Neuroinfection Imaging

This section addresses an emerging technique for neuropsychiatric research: imaging of infectious pathogens in the CNS with PET in the living brain. Two examples of infection imaging in the CNS are briefly discussed. It is beyond the scope of this section to allude to all further efforts for development of tracers for infection. The examples in this chapter show how specific radiopharmaceuticals were chosen, derived from antiviral or antibiotic drugs.

Nucleoside analogs are used for treatment of viral infections. Examples are the thymidine analogs that are used in clinical practice to inhibit replication of herpes viruses. These compounds bind irreversibly to the herpes virus thymidine kinase (TK) enzyme and thereby inhibit the enzyme to phosphorylate thymidine, which is essential for DNA replication of virus in nondividing neuronal cells. Acyclovir and penciclovir are examples of these thymidine analogs. Fluorinated penciclovir ([^{18}F]FHBG) is available as a radiotracer to image presence of HSV-TK. Fluorinated ganciclovir ([^{18}F]FHPG) is an alternative for the detection of TK in tissues using PET imaging (De Vries et al. 2006). These compounds have been successfully applied to determine efficacious gene therapy (insertion of TK gene in solid tumors for subsequent killing with acyclovir). We also showed that HSV-TK imaging was feasible in a rat model of HSE (Buursma et al. 2005). We showed that in patients with schizophrenia, uptake of [^{18}F]FHBG was significantly higher in the temporal lobe of patients with severe symptoms of psychosis (Doorduin 2010). Nucleoside radiopharmaceuticals are polar compounds and penetrate the intact BBB rather slowly, and the absolute uptake of [^{18}F]FHBG was very low.

Antibiotics could be used as base material for synthesis of radiopharmaceuticals aimed at detecting bacterial infections. The advantages of some antibiotics are their lipophilic character and easy penetration of the BBB. Interesting compounds to image bacterial infections might be [^{18}F]FMISO or [^{18}F]FAZA. These radiopharmaceuticals are derived from the antibiotic misonidazole and azomycin, respectively, and belong to the group of nitroimidazoles. Nitroimidazoles are active against a broad spectrum of gram-negative bacteria. Therefore, nitroimidazole accumulation may be an indicator of infection of all sensitive microbes. Because[^{18}F]FMISO is trapped in the mitochondrial electron transport chain in the host during conditions of hypoxia, [^{18}F]FMISO is in use as a hypoxia imaging radiopharmaceutical (Lee and Scott 2007).] [^{18}F]FMISO infection imaging has been described in a study with patients experiencing periodontal spirochetal infections (Liu et al. 1996) and [^{18}F]FAZA imaging in Echinococcus infections (Rolle et al. 2015). The extent of accumulation of [^{18}F]FMISO and [^{18}F]FAZA in infected pockets may reflect infectious burden. Nitroimidazole imaging has also been suggested to be promising in assessing the number of bacilli in tuberculosis granuloma (Ankrah et al. 2016).

It is a challenge with profound opportunities to study presence of viruses or bacteria in the CNS with specific radiopharmaceuticals. The nucleosides [^{18}F]FHPG and [^{18}F]FHBG and the nitroimidazoles [^{18}F]FMISO and [^{18}F]FAZA are promising probes to elucidate if specific neuropsychiatric diseases might have an infectious cause.

32.7 Clinical Note

If a clinician is confronted with a patient experiencing a neuropsychiatric syndrome of potential infectious origin, and a lesion on brain MRI does not discriminate between infection/malignancy and neurodegenerative disorders, PET imaging may already be useful. [^{11}C]PK11195 imaging has been performed in herpes encephalitis patients (Cagnin et al. 2001a). Although it is not feasible to apply PET imaging in the acute phase of the disease, it could be used to demonstrate ongoing inflammation and necessitate extended prescription of antiviral medication.

Infection imaging is used in clinical practice by infusing labeled leucocytes or by using an inflammation analysis algorithm for [^{18}F]FDG. PET imaging is of limited use in parenchymal brain infections because resting glucose metabolism in brain is high, which limits the contrast between inflamed tissue and surrounding healthy tissue. The clinician could regard a whole-body inflammation [^{18}F]FDG scan, as this may reveal any peripheral infectious site which disseminates, for example, to a brain abscess (Haroon et al. 2012). The pattern of distribution of peripheral foci of [^{18}F]FDG may give a cue to the type of infection. For example, if neuropsychiatric symptoms are associated with joint pains and occur in patients with an infection history of tick bite and the patient is seropositive for Borrelia species, then one might expect that [^{18}F]FDG whole body scans reveal hot spots in the affected joints.

32.8 Conclusion

Microglia activation occurs in the brains of patients suffering from schizophrenia, Parkinson's disease, Alzheimer's disease, and Korsakoff's dementia. It is very important to clarify the causes of this inflammatory process, and this requires intelligent use of available molecular imaging techniques. The brain is quite accessible for pathogens that acquire latency in the brain. Examples are HSV and *B. burgdorferi*. Pathogens in the brain are a neglected element in the etiopathogenesis of neuropsychiatric disorders, since access to the brain for biopsy is normally not possible. The application of PET imaging with nucleoside and nitroimidazole radiopharmaceuticals to determine virus and spirochete infection of the brain is a logical and promising avenue for further research.

Acknowledgments The intellectual and financial support from the Stanley Medical Research Institute and the Virgo consortium, funded by the Dutch Government project number FES0908 and the Netherlands Genomics Initiative (NGI) project number 050-060-452, is kindly acknowledged.

References

Alexaki A, Liu Y, Wigdahl B (2008) Cellular reservoirs of HIV-1 and their role in viral persistence. Curr HIV Res 6(5):388–400

Almodovar JL, Hehir MK, Nicholson KA, Stommel EW (2012) Acute bilateral painless radiculitis with abnormal Borrelia burgdorferi immunoblot. J Clin Neuromuscul Dis 14(2):75–77. https://doi.org/10.1097/CND.0b013e318279d634

Amsterdam J (1990) A possible antiviral action of lithium carbonate in herpes simplex virus infections. Biol Psychiatry 27(4):447–453. https://doi.org/10.1016/0006-3223(90)90555-G

Anderton JA, Bose S, Vockerodt M, Vrzalikova K, Wei W, Kuo M, Helin K et al (2011) The H3K27me3 demethylase, KDM6B, is induced by Epstein-Barr virus and over-expressed in Hodgkin's lymphoma. Oncogene 30(17):2037–2043. https://doi.org/10.1038/onc.2010.579

Ankrah AO, Glaudemans AWJM, Sathekge MM, Klein HC (2016) Imaging latent tuberculosis infection with radiolabeled nitroimidazoles. Clin Transl Imaging 4:157–159

Best L, Ghadery C, Pavese N, Tai YF, Strafella AP (2019) New and Old TSPO PET radioligands for imaging brain microglial activation in neurodegenerative disease. Curr Neurol Neurosci Rep 19(5):24. https://doi.org/10.1007/s11910-019-0934-y

Buursma AR, De Vries EFJ, Garssen J, Kegler D, Van Waarde A, Schirm J, Hospers GAP et al (2005) [18F]FHPG positron emission tomography for detection of herpes simplex virus (HSV) in experimental HSV encephalitis. J Virol 79(12):7721–7727. https://doi.org/10.1128/JVI.79.12.7721-7727.2005

Cagnin A, Myers R, Gunn RN, Lawrence AD, Stevens T, Kreutzberg GW, Jones T et al (2001a) In vivo visualization of activated glia by [11C] (R)-PK11195-PET following herpes encephalitis reveals projected neuronal damage beyond the primary focal lesion. Brain 124(Pt 10):2014–2027. http://www.ncbi.nlm.nih.gov/pubmed/11571219

Cagnin A, Brooks DJ, Kennedy AM, Gunn RN, Myers R, Turkheimer FE, Jones T et al (2001b) In-vivo measurement of activated microglia in dementia. Lancet 358(9280):461–467. https://doi.org/10.1016/S0140-6736(01)05625-2

Chaney A, Williams SR, Boutin H (2019) In vivo molecular imaging of neuroinflammation in Alzheimer's disease. J Neurochem 149(4):438–451. https://doi.org/10.1111/jnc.14615

Cosenza-Nashat M, Zhao M-L, Suh H-S, Morgan J, Natividad R, Morgello S, Lee SC (2009) Expression of the translocator protein of 18 kDa by microglia, macrophages and astrocytes based on immunohistochemical localization in abnormal human brain. Neuropathol Appl Neurobiol 35(3):306–328. https://doi.org/10.1111/j.1365-2990.2008.01006.x

Coughlin JM, Yang T, Rebman AW, Bechtold KT, Du Y, Mathews WB et al (2018) Imaging glial activation in patients with post-treatment Lyme disease symptoms: a pilot study using [11C]DPA-713 PET. J Neuroinflammation 15(1):346. https://doi.org/10.1186/s12974-018-1381-4

De Vries EFJ, Dierckx RA, Klein HC (2006) Nuclear imaging of inflammation in neurologic and psychiatric disorders. Curr Clin Pharmacol 1(3):229–242. http://www.ncbi.nlm.nih.gov/pubmed/18666748

Derfuss T, Segerer S, Herberger S, Sinicina I, Hüfner K, Ebelt K, Knaus H-G et al (2007) Presence of HSV-1 immediate early genes and clonally expanded T-cells with a memory effector phenotype in human trigeminal ganglia. Brain Pathol 17(4):389–398. https://doi.org/10.1111/j.1750-3639.2007.00088.x

Di Biase MA, Zalesky A, O'keefe G, Laskaris L, Baune BT, Weickert CS et al (2017) PET imaging of putative microglial activation in individuals at ultra-high risk for psychosis, recently diagnosed and chronically ill with schizophrenia. Transl Psychiatry 7(8):e1225. https://doi.org/10.1038/tp.2017.193

Dickman MS (2001) von Economo encephalitis. Arch Neurol 58(10):1696–1698. http://www.ncbi.nlm.nih.gov/pubmed/11594935

Doorduin J (2010) Herpes viruses and neuroinflammation: PET imaging and implication in schizophrenia. Dissertations, University of Groningen

Doorduin J, De Vries EFJ, Willemsen ATM, De Groot JC, Dierckx RA, Klein HC (2009a) Neuroinflammation in schizophrenia-related psychosis: a PET study. J Nucl Med 50(11):1801–1807. https://doi.org/10.2967/jnumed.109.066647

Doorduin J, Klein HC, Dierckx RA, James M, Kassiou M, De Vries EFJ (2009b) [11C]-DPA-713 and [18F]-DPA-714 as new PET tracers for TSPO: a comparison with [11C]-(R)-PK11195 in a rat model of herpes encephalitis. Mol Imaging Biol 11(6):386–398. https://doi.org/10.1007/s11307-009-0211-6

Doorduin J, Klein HC, De Jong JR, Dierckx RA, De Vries EFJ (2010) Evaluation of [11C]-DAA1106 for imaging and quantification of neuroinflammation in a rat model of herpes encephalitis. Nucl Med Biol 37(1):9–15. https://doi.org/10.1016/j.nucmedbio.2009.09.002
Durafourt BA, Moore CS, Zammit DA, Johnson TA, Zaguia F, Guiot M-C, Bar-Or A et al (2012) Comparison of polarization properties of human adult microglia and blood-derived macrophages. Glia 60(5):717–727. https://doi.org/10.1002/glia.22298
Economo C (1929) Die Encephalitis Lethargica, ihre Nachkrankheiten und ihre Behandlung. Engl J Med 201:708
Edison P, Archer HA, Gerhard A, Hinz R, Pavese N, Turkheimer FE, Hammers A et al (2008) Microglia, amyloid, and cognition in Alzheimer's disease: an [11C](R)PK11195-PET and [11C]PIB-PET study. Neurobiol Dis 32(3):412–419. https://doi.org/10.1016/j.nbd.2008.08.001
Gerhard A, Watts J, Trender-Gerhard I, Turkheimer F, Banati RB, Bhatia K, Brooks DJ (2004) In vivo imaging of microglial activation with [11C](R)-PK11195 PET in corticobasal degeneration. Mov Disord 19(10):1221–1226. https://doi.org/10.1002/mds.20162
Gerhard A, Trender-Gerhard I, Turkheimer F, Quinn NP, Bhatia KP, Brooks DJ (2006) In vivo imaging of microglial activation with [11C](R)-PK11195 PET in progressive supranuclear palsy. Mov Disord 21(1):89–93. https://doi.org/10.1002/mds.20668
Gordon L, McQuaid S, Cosby SL (1996) Detection of herpes simplex virus (types 1 and 2) and human herpesvirus 6 DNA in human brain tissue by polymerase chain reaction. Clin Diagn Virol 6(1):33–40. http://www.ncbi.nlm.nih.gov/pubmed/15566888
Grover VPB, Pavese N, Koh S-B, Wylezinska M, Saxby BK, Gerhard A, Forton DM et al (2012) Cerebral microglial activation in patients with hepatitis C: in vivo evidence of neuroinflammation. J Viral Hepat 19(2):e89–e96. https://doi.org/10.1111/j.1365-2893.2011.01510.x
Haarman BCMB, Riemersma-Van der Lek RF, de Groot JC, Ruhé HGE, Klein HC, Zandstra TE et al (2014) Neuroinflammation in bipolar disorder – a [(11)C]-(R)-PK11195 positron emission tomography study. Brain Behav Immun 40:219–225. https://doi.org/10.1016/j.bbi.2014.03.016
Hammoud DA, Endres CJ, Chander AR, Guilarte TR, Wong DF, Sacktor NC, McArthur JC et al (2005) Imaging glial cell activation with [11C]-R-PK11195 in patients with AIDS. J Neurovirol 11(4):346–355. https://doi.org/10.1080/13550280500187351
Haroon A, Zumla A, Bomanji J (2012) Role of fluorine 18 fluorodeoxyglucose positron emission tomography-computed tomography in focal and generalized infectious and inflammatory disorders. Clin Infect Dis 54(9):1333–1341. https://doi.org/10.1093/cid/cis193
Hervé F, Ghinea N, Scherrmann J-M (2008) CNS delivery via adsorptive transcytosis. AAPS J 10(3):455–472. https://doi.org/10.1208/s12248-008-9055-2
Hildenbrand P, Craven DE, Jones R, Nemeskal P (2009) Lyme neuroborreliosis: manifestations of a rapidly emerging zoonosis. AJNR Am J Neuroradiol 30(6):1079–1087. https://doi.org/10.3174/ajnr.A1579
Holmes SE, Hinz R, Drake RJ, Gregory CJ, Conen S, Matthews JC et al (2016) In vivo imaging of brain microglial activity in antipsychotic-free and medicated schizophrenia: a [11C](R)-PK11195 positron emission tomography study. Mol Psychiatry 21(12):1672–1679
Holmes SE, Hinz R, Conen S, Gregory CJ, Matthews JC, Anton-Rodriguez JM et al (2018) Elevated translocator protein in anterior cingulate in major depression and a role for inflammation in suicidal thinking: a positron emission tomography study. Biol Psychiatry 83(1):61–69. https://doi.org/10.1016/j.biopsych.2017.08.005
Hurlemann R, Jessen F, Wagner M, Frommann I, Ruhrmann S, Brockhaus A, Picker H et al (2008) Interrelated neuropsychological and anatomical evidence of hippocampal pathology in the at-risk mental state. Psychol Med 38(6):843–851. https://doi.org/10.1017/S0033291708003279
Kapur N, Barker S, Burrows EH, Ellison D, Brice J, Illis LS, Scholey K et al (1994) Herpes simplex encephalitis: long term magnetic resonance imaging and neuropsychological profile. J Neurol Neurosurg Psychiatry 57(11):1334–1342
Kaunzner UW, Kang Y, Monohan E, Kothari PJ, Nealon N, Perumal J et al (2017) Reduction of PK11195 uptake observed in multiple sclerosis lesions after natalizumab initiation. Mult Scler Relat Disord 15(6):27–33. https://doi.org/10.1016/j.msard.2017.04.008

Ke Z-J, DeGiorgio LA, Volpe BT, Gibson GE (2003) Reversal of thiamine deficiency-induced neurodegeneration. J Neuropathol Exp Neurol 62(2):195–207

Kusuhara H, Sugiyama Y (2005) Active efflux across the blood-brain barrier: role of the solute carrier family. NeuroRx 2(1):73–85. https://doi.org/10.1602/neurorx.2.1.73

Lakeman FD, Whitley RJ (1995) Diagnosis of herpes simplex encephalitis: application of polymerase chain reaction to cerebrospinal fluid from brain-biopsied patients and correlation with disease. J Infect Dis 171(4):857–863

Lee ST, Scott AM (2007) Hypoxia positron emission tomography imaging with 18f-fluoromisonidazole. Semin Nucl Med 37(6):451–461. https://doi.org/10.1053/j.semnuclmed.2007.07.001

Leong DK, Le O, Oliva L, Butterworth RF (1994) Increased densities of binding sites for the "peripheral-type" benzodiazepine receptor ligand [3H]PK11195 in vulnerable regions of the rat brain in thiamine deficiency encephalopathy. J Cereb Blood Flow Metab 14(1):100–105. https://doi.org/10.1038/jcbfm.1994.14

Lieb J (2002) Lithium and antidepressants: inhibiting eicosanoids, stimulating immunity, and defeating microorganisms. Med Hypotheses 59(4):429–432. https://doi.org/10.1016/S0306-9877(02)00148-2

Lindl KA, Marks DR, Kolson DL, Jordan-Sciutto KL (2010) HIV-associated neurocognitive disorder: pathogenesis and therapeutic opportunities. J Neuroimmune Pharmacol 5(3):294–309. https://doi.org/10.1007/s11481-010-9205-z

Liu RS, Chu LS, Yen SH, Chang CP, Chou KL, Wu LC, Chang CW et al (1996) Detection of anaerobic odontogenic infections by fluorine-18 fluoromisonidazole. Eur J Nucl Med 23(10):1384–1387. http://www.ncbi.nlm.nih.gov/pubmed/8781145

Logigian EL, Johnson KA, Kijewski MF, Kaplan RF, Becker JA, Jones KJ, Garada BM et al (1997) Reversible cerebral hypoperfusion in Lyme encephalopathy. Neurology 49(6):1661–1670. http://www.ncbi.nlm.nih.gov/pubmed/9409364

MacQueen GM, Campbell S, McEwen BS, Macdonald K, Amano S, Joffe RT, Nahmias C et al (2003) Course of illness, hippocampal function, and hippocampal volume in major depression. Proc Natl Acad Sci U S A 100(3):1387–1392. https://doi.org/10.1073/pnas.0337481100

Markeljević J, Sarac H, Rados M (2011) Tremor, seizures and psychosis as presenting symptoms in a patient with chronic lyme neuroborreliosis (LNB). Coll Antropol 35(Suppl 1):313–318. http://www.ncbi.nlm.nih.gov/pubmed/21648354

Miklossy J (2008) Biology and neuropathology of dementia in syphilis and Lyme disease. In: Duyckaerts C, Litvan I (eds) Handbook of clinical neurology (3rd series). Dementias, vol 89. Elsevier, Amsterdam, pp 825–844

Miklossy J, Kasas S, Zurn AD, McCall S, Yu S, McGeer PL (2008) Persisting atypical and cystic forms of Borrelia burgdorferi and local inflammation in Lyme neuroborreliosis. J Neuroinflammation 5:40. https://doi.org/10.1186/1742-2094-5-40

Moneta ME, Gehrmann J, Töpper R, Banati RB, Kreutzberg GW (1993) Cell adhesion molecule expression in the regenerating rat facial nucleus. J Neuroimmunol 45(1–2):203–206. http://www.ncbi.nlm.nih.gov/pubmed/8101190

Monier A, Adle-Biassette H, Delezoide A-L, Evrard P, Gressens P, Verney C (2007) Entry and distribution of microglial cells in human embryonic and fetal cerebral cortex. J Neuropathol Exp Neurol 66(5):372–382. https://doi.org/10.1097/nen.0b013e3180517b46

Mori I, Nishiyama Y, Yokochi T, Kimura Y (2005) Olfactory transmission of neurotropic viruses. J Neurovirol 11(2):129–137. https://doi.org/10.1080/13550280590922793

Moriarty TJ, Norman MU, Colarusso P, Bankhead T, Kubes P, Chaconas G (2008) Real-time high resolution 3D imaging of the Lyme disease spirochete adhering to and escaping from the vasculature of a living host. PLoS Pathog 4(6):e1000090. https://doi.org/10.1371/journal.ppat.1000090

Oksi J, Kalimo H, Marttila RJ, Marjamäki M, Sonninen P, Nikoskelainen J, Viljanen MK (1996) Inflammatory brain changes in Lyme borreliosis. A report on three patients and review of literature. Brain 119(Pt 6):2143–2154. http://www.ncbi.nlm.nih.gov/pubmed/9010017

Paolicelli RC, Bolasco G, Pagani F, Maggi L, Scianni M, Panzanelli P, Giustetto M et al (2011) Synaptic pruning by microglia is necessary for normal brain development. Science 333(6048):1456–1458. https://doi.org/10.1126/science.1202529
Parbo P, Ismail R, Hansen KV, Amidi A, Mårup FH, Gottrup H et al (2017) Brain inflammation accompanies amyloid in the majority of mild cognitive impairment cases due to Alzheimer's disease. Brain 140(7):2002–2011
Pardridge WM (1999) Blood-brain barrier biology and methodology. J Neurovirol 5(6):556–569. https://doi.org/10.3109/13550289909021285
Pavese N, Gerhard A, Tai YF, Ho AK, Turkheimer F, Barker RA, Brooks DJ et al (2006) Microglial activation correlates with severity in Huntington disease: a clinical and PET study. Neurology 66(11):1638–1643. https://doi.org/10.1212/01.wnl.0000222734.56412.17
Pflugrad H, Meyer G-J, Dirks M, Raab P, Tryc AB, Goldbecker A et al (2016) Cerebral microglia activation in hepatitis C virus infection correlates to cognitive dysfunction. J Viral Hepat 23(5):348–357. https://doi.org/10.1111/jvh.12496
Plavén-Sigray P, Matheson GJ, Cselényi Z, Jucaite A, Farde L, Cervenka S (2018) Test-retest reliability and convergent validity of (R)-[11C]PK11195 outcome measures without arterial input function. EJNMMI Res 8. https://doi.org/10.1186/s13550-018-0455-8
Plotkin M, Hautzel H, Krause BJ, Mohr S, Langen KJ, Müller H-W (2005) Fluorine-18-labeled fluorodeoxyglucose-positron emission tomography studies of acute brainstem Lyme neuroborreliosis [corrected] case report. J Neurosurg 102(5):927–929. https://doi.org/10.3171/jns.2005.102.5.0927
Politis M, Giannetti P, Su P, Turkheimer F, Keihaninejad S, Wu K, Waldman A et al (2012) Increased PK11195 PET binding in the cortex of patients with MS correlates with disability. Neurology 79(6):523–530. https://doi.org/10.1212/WNL.0b013e3182635645
Posavad CM, Wald A, Hosken N, Huang ML, Koelle DM, Ashley RL, Corey L (2003) T cell immunity to herpes simplex viruses in seronegative subjects: silent infection or acquired immunity? J Immunol 170(8):4380–4388. http://www.ncbi.nlm.nih.gov/pubmed/12682275
Ramlackhansingh AF, Brooks DJ, Greenwood RJ, Bose SK, Turkheimer FE, Kinnunen KM, Gentleman S et al (2011) Inflammation after trauma: microglial activation and traumatic brain injury. Ann Neurol 70(3):374–383. https://doi.org/10.1002/ana.22455
Rodríguez EM, Blázquez JL, Guerra M (2010) The design of barriers in the hypothalamus allows the median eminence and the arcuate nucleus to enjoy private milieus: the former opens to the portal blood and the latter to the cerebrospinal fluid. Peptides 31(4):757–776. https://doi.org/10.1016/j.peptides.2010.01.003
Rolle A-M, Soboslay PT, Reischl G, Hoffmann WH, Pichler BJ, Wiehr S (2015) Evaluation of the metabolic activity of Echinococcus multilocularis in rodents using positron emission tomography tracers. Mol Imaging Biol 17(4):512–520
Rubin LH, Sacktor N, Creighton J, Du Y, Endres CJ, Pomper MG, Coughlin JM (2018) Microglial activation is inversely associated with cognition in individuals living with HIV on effective antiretroviral therapy. AIDS (London, England) 32(12):1661–1667
Schmutzhard E (2001) Viral infections of the CNS with special emphasis on herpes simplex infections. J Neurol 248(6):469–477. http://www.ncbi.nlm.nih.gov/pubmed/11499636
Schuitemaker A, Kropholler MA, Boellaard R, Van der Flier WM, Kloet RW, Van der Doef TF, Knol DL et al (2013) Microglial activation in Alzheimer's disease: an (R)-[^{11}C]PK11195 positron emission tomography study. Neurobiol Aging 34(1):128–136. https://doi.org/10.1016/j.neurobiolaging.2012.04.021
Sips GJ, Wilschut J, Smit JM (2011) Neuroinvasive flavivirus infections. Rev Med Virol. https://doi.org/10.1002/rmv.712
Sisó S, Jeffrey M, González L (2010) Sensory circumventricular organs in health and disease. Acta Neuropathol 120:689–705. https://doi.org/10.1007/s00401-010-0743-5
Smith JL, Israel CW (1967) Spirochetes in the aqueous humor in seronegative ocular syphilis. Persistence after penicillin therapy. Arch Ophthalmol 77(4):474–477
Song YS (2019) Perspectives in TSPO PET imaging for neurologic diseases. Nucl Med Mol Imaging 53(6):382–385. https://doi.org/10.1007/s13139-019-00620-y

Steere AC, Coburn J, Glickstein L (2004) The emergence of Lyme disease. J Clin Invest 113(8):1093–1101. https://doi.org/10.1172/JCI21681

Sucksdorff M, Rissanen E, Tuisku J, Nuutinen S, Paavilainen T, Rokka J et al (2017) Evaluation of the effect of fingolimod treatment on microglial activation using serial PET imaging in multiple sclerosis. J Nucl Med 58(10):1646–1651. https://doi.org/10.2967/jnumed.116.183020

Tai YF, Pavese N, Gerhard A, Tabrizi SJ, Barker RA, Brooks DJ, Piccini P (2007) Microglial activation in presymptomatic Huntington's disease gene carriers. Brain 130(Pt 7):1759–1766. https://doi.org/10.1093/brain/awm044

Theil D, Derfuss T, Paripovic I, Herberger S, Meinl E, Schueler O, Strupp M et al (2003) Latent herpesvirus infection in human trigeminal ganglia causes chronic immune response. Am J Pathol 163(6):2179–2184. http://www.pubmedcentral.nih.gov/articlerender.fcgi?artid=1892378&tool=pmcentrez&rendertype=abstract

Theil D, Horn AKE, Derfuss T, Strupp M, Arbusow V, Brandt T (2004) Prevalence and distribution of HSV-1, VZV, and HHV-6 in human cranial nerve nuclei III, IV, VI, VII, and XII. J Med Virol 74(1):102–106. https://doi.org/10.1002/jmv.20152

Tremblay M-È, Majewska AK (2011) A role for microglia in synaptic plasticity? Commun Integr Biol 4(2):220–222. https://doi.org/10.4161/cib.4.2.14506

Triarhou LC (2006) The signalling contributions of Constantin von Economo to basic, clinical and evolutionary neuroscience. Brain Res Bull 69(3):223–243. https://doi.org/10.1016/j.brainresbull.2006.02.001

Turner MR, Cagnin A, Turkheimer FE, Miller CCJ, Shaw CE, Brooks DJ, Leigh PN et al (2004) Evidence of widespread cerebral microglial activation in amyotrophic lateral sclerosis: an [11C](R)-PK11195 positron emission tomography study. Neurobiol Dis 15(3):601–609. https://doi.org/10.1016/j.nbd.2003.12.012

Turner MR, Gerhard A, Al-Chalabi A, Shaw CE, Hughes RAC, Banati RB, Brooks DJ et al (2005) Mills' and other isolated upper motor neurone syndromes: in vivo study with 11C-(R)-PK11195 PET. J Neurol Neurosurg Psychiatry 76(6):871–874. https://doi.org/10.1136/jnnp.2004.047902

Van Berckel BN, Bossong MG, Boellaard R, Kloet R, Schuitemaker A, Caspers E, Luurtsema G et al (2008) Microglia activation in recent-onset schizophrenia: a quantitative (R)-[11C]PK11195 positron emission tomography study. Biol Psychiatry 64(9):820–822. https://doi.org/10.1016/j.biopsych.2008.04.025

Venneti S, Bonneh-Barkay D, Lopresti BJ, Bissel SJ, Wang G, Mathis CA, Piatak M et al (2008) Longitudinal in vivo positron emission tomography imaging of infected and activated brain macrophages in a macaque model of human immunodeficiency virus encephalitis correlates with central and peripheral markers of encephalitis and areas of synaptic degeneration. Am J Pathol 172(6):1603–1616. https://doi.org/10.2353/ajpath.2008.070967

Wang D, Hazell AS (2010) Microglial activation is a major contributor to neurologic dysfunction in thiamine deficiency. Biochem Biophys Res Commun 402(1):123–128. https://doi.org/10.1016/j.bbrc.2010.09.128

Whitrow M (1990) Wagner-Jauregg and fever therapy. Med Hist 34(3):294–310. http://www.pubmedcentral.nih.gov/articlerender.fcgi?artid=1036142&tool=pmcentrez&rendertype=abstract

Wiley CA, Lopresti BJ, Becker JT, Boada F, Lopez OL, Mellors J, Meltzer CC et al (2006) Positron emission tomography imaging of peripheral benzodiazepine receptor binding in human immunodeficiency virus-infected subjects with and without cognitive impairment. J Neurovirol 12(4):262–271. https://doi.org/10.1080/13550280600873868

Wiley CA, Lopresti BJ, Venneti S, Price J, Klunk WE, DeKosky ST, Mathis CA (2009) Carbon 11-labeled Pittsburgh compound B and carbon 11-labeled (R)-PK11195 positron emission tomographic imaging in Alzheimer disease. Arch Neurol 66(1):60–67. https://doi.org/10.1001/archneurol.2008.511

Yolken RH, Karlsson H, Yee F, Johnston-Wilson NL, Torrey EF (2000) Endogenous retroviruses and schizophrenia. Brain Res Brain Res Rev 31(2–3):193–199. http://www.ncbi.nlm.nih.gov/pubmed/10719148

PET Imaging in Multiple Sclerosis

33

Chris W. J. van der Weijden, Jan F. Meilof, and Erik F. J. de Vries

Contents

Abstract

Multiple sclerosis (MS) pathology is associated with inflammation and demyelination in the central nervous system (CNS), which leads to neurodegeneration. Various positron emission tomography (PET) tracers have been employed to image these processes. PET tracers for 18-kD translocator protein (TSPO) receptors, which are overexpressed on activated microglia, macrophages, and astrocytes, have been used to assess neuro-inflammation. PET imaging of TSPO expression depicted an increased activation of inflammatory cells in normal

C. W. J. van der Weijden (✉) · E. F. J. de Vries
Department of Nuclear Medicine and Molecular Imaging, University Medical Center Groningen, University of Groningen, Groningen, The Netherlands
e-mail: c.w.j.van.der.weijden@umcg.nl; e.f.j.de.vries@umcg.nl

J. F. Meilof
Department of Biomedical Sciences of Cells and Systems, University Medical Center Groningen, University of Groningen, Groningen, The Netherlands

Department of Neurology, Martini Ziekenhuis, Groningen, The Netherlands
e-mail: j.f.meilof@umcg.nl

R. A. J. O. Dierckx et al. (eds.), *PET and SPECT in Neurology*,
https://doi.org/10.1007/978-3-030-53168-3_33

appearing white matter (NAWM), grey matter (GM), and MS lesions. A reduction in inflammation in MS lesions was found to be a main determinant of treatment efficacy. Recently, advances have been made in myelin visualisation with PET. The first clinical studies to visualise myelin with PET show promising results. As for other neurodegenerative diseases, [^{18}F]FDG is still the main PET tracer used to assess neuronal damage. Current clinical use of PET in MS is mainly restricted to aiding in differential diagnosis or for determining the efficacy of immune suppressive treatments. Once myelin imaging has been validated as a reliable method for characterisation of myelin integrity, it would enable the evaluation of the efficacy of a new line of therapies that aim to repair myelin.

33.1 Introduction

Multiple sclerosis (MS) is the most common neurodegenerative disease in young adults (Ramagopalan et al. 2010). MS pathology is characterised by immune attacks on the myelin sheath covering the axon (Traugott et al. 1983). The initiation of the immune response seems to be driven by peripheral activation of the adaptive immune system (Dendrou et al. 2015). After migration to the central nervous system (CNS), activated T cells cause activation of antigen presenting cells, like microglia and macrophages, which then initiate recruitment of additional inflammatory cells (Fig. 33.1). During this process, myelin-specific antibodies are produced and together with cytotoxic cytokines, excitotoxins, reactive oxygen, and nitric oxide, which are released by activated microglia and macrophages, they cause the damage to myelin (Dendrou et al. 2015; Lassmann et al. 2012). Oligodendrocytes are able to repair the myelin sheaths of axons (remyelination) and thereby restore the protective and signal enhancement function of myelin (Prineas and Connell 1979). However, when myelin damage is too severe, it will be beyond the restoration capacity of oligodendrocytes. Damaged myelin makes axons vulnerable for any exposure to environmental effects and ultimately leads to neurodegeneration (Ferguson et al. 1997; Franklin and Ffrench-Constant 2008). All these processes (i.e. inflammation, myelin degradation, and neurodegeneration) are part of the MS pathology and are involved in relapses (episodes with a temporary increase in severity of symptoms) and disease progression.

When a patient presents with a history of only one relapse, this is called a clinically isolated syndrome (CIS). Subjects with CIS have an increased risk to develop MS, and therefore CIS is considered to be a prodromal stage of MS (Baecher-Allan et al. 2018). Almost all patients with CIS develop relapsing remitting MS (RRMS), although this may take many years. RRMS is with an 85% occurrence, the most prevalent form of MS. The remaining 15% of patients have a slowly progressive disease course from disease onset without relapses, which is called primary progressive MS (PPMS). In RRMS, clinical symptoms emerge during relapses, but subsequently diminish over time during remission due to reduction of inflammation and recovery of the myelin sheaths. Incomplete repair of myelin damage leads to

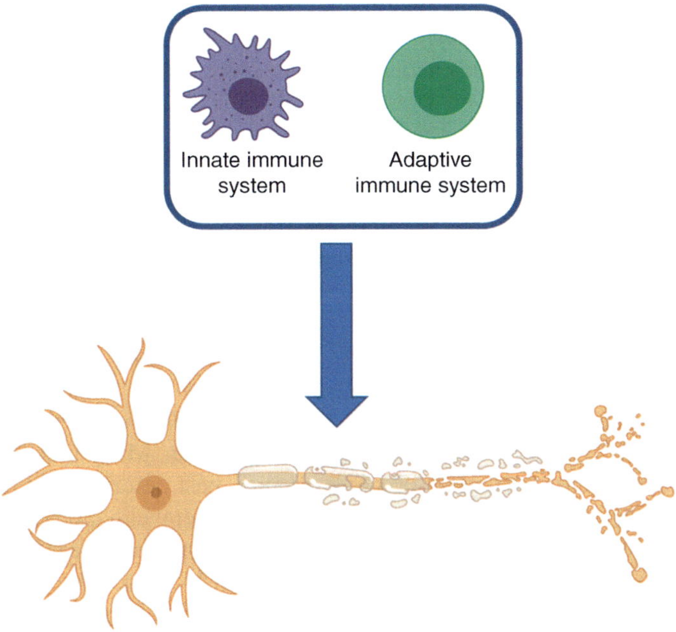

Fig. 33.1 Current view of the MS pathogenesis pathway. Inflammatory cells cause demyelination, which ultimately results in neurodegeneration

increased axonal damage and disease progression. When remissions no longer occur and axonal damage increases more gradually, MS patients are considered to have entered the secondary progressive (SP) stage of MS.

Due to the random location of inflammatory lesions occurring in the CNS, clinical symptoms in MS are highly diverse. The most typical symptoms are the ones involving the optic nerve, the urinary tract, and those resulting in sensory and motor symptoms (Huang et al. 2017; Miljković and Spasojević 2013). Disease severity is often expressed using the Expanded Disability Status Scale (EDSS) (Kurtzke 1983). The EDSS is scored from 0 (no disability or other impairments) to 10 (death due to MS). With a score of 5, the patient is hampered in his daily activities and walking distance due to symptoms of MS, and is not capable of completing full work days without special precautions.

A diagnosis of MS is based on the combination of clinical symptoms, the presence of typical lesions on MRI, and, if necessary, analysis of cerebrospinal fluid (Thompson et al. 2018). The mainstay in diagnosing MS is the demonstration of dissemination of lesions in place and in time clinically or with MRI. Current MRI protocols are very effective in supporting a diagnosis of MS and excluding other diseases. On MRI scans, the damage caused by inflammation is visualised as white matter lesions, which are hyper-intense on T2 fluid-attenuated inversion recovery (T2-FLAIR) images (Biediger et al. 2014). The visually non-affected white matter is typically called normal appearing white matter (NAWM), which does not mean biological changes are absent. Gadolinium (Gd) contrast enhancement is a marker for blood–brain barrier breakdown. This makes it possible to distinguish with MRI between active (Gd-enhanced) and non-active (non-enhanced) lesions (Kaunzner and Gauthier 2017). However, irrespective of their activity status, these lesions depict a combination of processes including inflammation, gliosis, demyelination, and axonal loss. MRI is therefore currently not able to visualise alterations in individual biological processes. The availability of highly specific ligands would enable distinguishing between individual biological alterations in MS pathology with molecular imaging techniques, in particular positron emission tomography (PET).

33.2 PET Tracers Used to Assess MS Pathology

PET imaging can enable imaging of individual biological processes. However, it is only possible to visualise one biological process per scan. Many tracers have been developed for specific biological processes. MS is best described using the three major biological processes involving inflammation, demyelination, and neurodegeneration. Within these processes, there are multiple aspects that can be visualised, and hence a wide variety of tracers have been used in MS. An overview of the tracers used in MS is displayed in Table 33.1. A more thorough discussion of the relevance of these tracers within MS pathology is provided in the following sections.

Table 33.1 PET tracers currently being employed for the visualisation of biological processes in MS pathology

Tracer	Imaging target	Relevant structures/cells
[^{11}C]PK11195	TSPO	Activated microglia, macrophages, astrocytes
[^{11}C]PBR28	TSPO	Activated microglia, macrophages, astrocytes
[^{18}F]PBR06	TSPO	Activated microglia, macrophages, astrocytes
[^{18}F]PBR111	TSPO	Activated microglia, macrophages, astrocytes
[^{18}F]GE-180	TSPO	Activated microglia, macrophages, astrocytes
[^{11}C]DPA713	TSPO	Activated microglia, macrophages, astrocytes
[^{18}F]DPA714	TSPO	Activated microglia, macrophages, astrocytes
[^{11}C]acetate	MCT	Activated astrocytes
[^{11}C]TMSX	Adenosine A_{2A} receptor	Cerebral stress coping mechanisms
[^{11}C]PiB	Amyloid beta and MBP	In MS pathology, assessment of myelin integrity
[^{18}F] Florbetaben	Amyloid beta and MBP	In MS pathology, assessment of myelin integrity
[^{18}F] Florbetapir	Amyloid beta and MBP	In MS pathology, assessment of myelin integrity
[^{11}C] flumazenil	Benzodiazepine receptor	Synaptic integrity
[^{11}C]DASB	Serotonin transporters	Neuronal presynaptic membrane
[^{18}F]FDG	Glucose consumption	Neurodegeneration
[^{11}C] methionine	Protein synthesis	Differential diagnosis between MS and brain tumours

MBP myelin basic protein, *MCT* monocarboxylate transporter, *MS* multiple sclerosis, *TSPO* 18-kDa translocator protein

33.3 PET Imaging to Assess Neuro-Inflammation

MS is characterised by neuro-inflammation aimed at the myelin layers around the axons. The 18-kD translocator protein (TSPO) is upregulated in activated inflammatory cells in the brain (Fig. 33.2), especially in microglia, but also in macrophages and to a lesser extent in astrocytes (Chechneva and Deng 2016). TSPO is found on mitochondrial membranes and has many functions, including the mediation of cholesterol transport from the cytosol into the mitochondria (Papadopoulos et al. 2006) and regulation of mitochondrial energy metabolism (Gut 2015). The latter function could be the reason why TSPO is upregulated in activated inflammatory cells. Thus, determination of TSPO expression is used to assess the amount of activated inflammatory cells (Fig. 33.3). Traditionally, [^{11}C]PK11195 PET imaging was the primary method for the evaluation of TSPO expression (Vowinckel et al. 1997). [^{11}C]PK11195 is currently still regularly used (Table 33.2), although a new generation of TSPO tracers with higher affinity has been developed as well. A major disadvantage of the new so-called "second generation" tracers is the genotype-dependent binding affinity. The second-generation tracers require therefore classification of patients into low- (LAB), medium- (MAB), and high-affinity binding (HAB) individuals. A single-nucleotide polymorphism in the TSPO gene (rs6971), which replaces alanine with threonine (Ala147Thr), was shown to be responsible for the variation in binding affinity resulting in LAB for homozygotes of this single nucleotide permutation (SNP) (Owen et al. 2012). A study assessing the frequency of the different TSPO binding affinities showed that 66% were HAB, 29% MAB, and 5% LAB (Owen et al. 2012). This means that, aside from the PET scan, also genotyping has to be performed for a correct analysis of the acquired images. In contrast, [^{11}C]PK11195 binding is not affected by this SNP and is therefore still a regularly used PET tracer for inflammation.

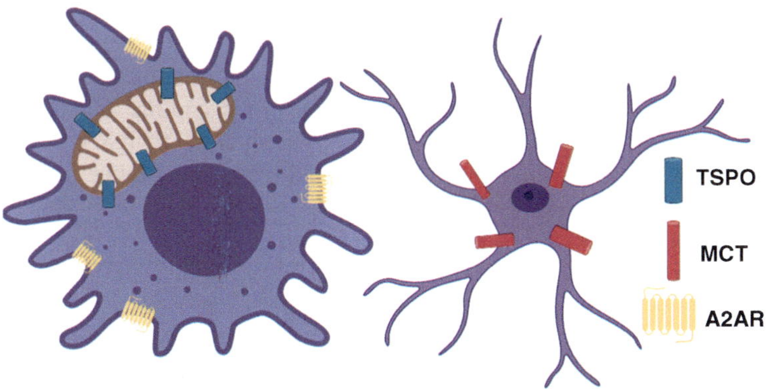

Fig. 33.2 PET imaging targets on inflammatory cells used in MS research. TSPO and monocarboxylate transporter (MCT) are markers for neuro-inflammation. Within activated inflammatory cells, TSPO is upregulated. Many PET tracers that bind TSPO have been developed to enable the visualisation of this upregulation and thus the activation status of inflammatory cells. A more specific method is imaging of MCT expression, which is upregulated in activated astrocytes. Microglial A2AR expression is supposed to modulate the inflammatory response

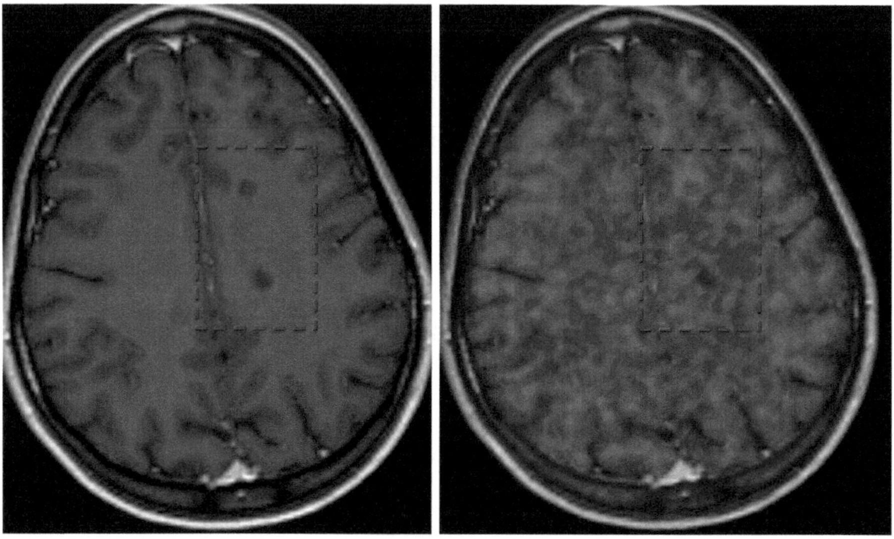

Fig. 33.3 Differentiation of two non-enhanced lesions on T1 MRI and [^{11}C]PK11195 PET. The upper lesion clearly depicts an increase in [^{11}C]PK11195 uptake, which means inflammatory activation, and thus depicts an active lesion. In contrast, the lower lesion does not show increased tracer uptake, and therefore is an inactive lesion (permission for the use of the images was obtained; source: DOI: https://doi.org/10.1007/s40336-015-0147-6) (Airas et al. 2015)

Studies assessing TSPO expression in MS with [^{11}C]PK11195 PET imaging displayed increased tracer uptake in NAWM, cortical grey matter (GM), and thalamus, which was associated with a longer disease duration and higher age (Giannetti et al. 2015; Politis et al. 2012; Rissanen et al. 2014). Other studies found only a significantly increased uptake in the whole brain, but not in individual regions (Sucksdorff et al. 2017). These findings illustrate that with advancing disease duration and age, more activated inflammatory cells are observed. More detailed analysis of the lesions themselves resulted in differential results for Gd-contrast-enhanced lesions vs. non-contrast-enhanced lesions. In general, lesions have a higher tracer uptake than NAWM, with contrast-enhanced lesions having an even higher [^{11}C]PK11195 uptake than non-enhanced lesions, supporting the concept that MRI contrast enhancement is a marker for inflammation (Vowinckel et al. 1997; Giannetti et al. 2015; Kaunzner et al. 2017). Increased [^{11}C]PK11195 uptake in cortical GM has also been observed in MS patients and was significantly correlated ($r = 0.84$, $p = 0.0089$) with EDSS scores (Politis et al. 2012). In RRMS patients, a higher [^{11}C]PK11195 uptake has been associated with smaller total black hole volumes, which are supposed to represent inactive non-remyelinated lesions with extensive axonal damage (Giannetti et al. 2014). In short, these studies show a global cerebral increase of activated inflammatory cells with disease progression, duration, and age, which corresponds to increased clinical disability. Furthermore, an increase of [^{11}C]PK11195 uptake in MS lesions corresponds with disease activity. As depicted in Table 33.2, there are also studies that do not show an increased uptake in GM

Table 33.2 Overview of the main results per study using [^{11}C]PK11195 PET to image inflammatory response in MS patients

Study	Tracer	Subjects	GM	NAWM	Non-enhanced lesions	Enhanced lesions
Giannetti et al. (2015)	[^{11}C] PK11195	8 HC 18 CIS	No differences observed	Increased [^{11}C] PK11195 uptake	n.a.	n.a.
Politis et al. (2012)	[^{11}C] PK11195	8 HC 10 RRMS	Increased [^{11}C] PK11195 uptake	Increased [^{11}C] PK11195 uptake	n.a.	n.a.
		8 SPMS	More increased [^{11}C] PK11195 uptake than in RRMS	More increased [^{11}C] PK11195 uptake than in RRMS		
E. Rissanen et al. (2014)	[^{11}C] PK11195	8 HC 10 SPMS	No differences observed	Increased [^{11}C] PK11195 uptake		Increased [^{11}C] PK11195 uptake
Sucksdorff et al. (2017)	[^{11}C] PK11195	8 HC 10 RRMS	No differences observed	No differences observed	n.a.	n.a.
Kaunzner et al. (2017)	[^{11}C] PK11195	5 HC 18 MS	n.a.	n.a.	Increased [^{11}C] PK11195 uptake	More increased [^{11}C] PK11195 uptake than non-enhanced lesions
Vowinckel et al. (1997)	[^{11}C] PK11195	2 MS	n.a.	n.a.	[^{11}C] PK11195 uptake not increased	Increased [^{11}C] PK11195 uptake

CIS clinically isolated syndrome, *HC* healthy control, *MS* multiple sclerosis, *n.a.* not applicable, *SPMS* secondary progressive MS, *RRMS* relapse remitting MS

(Giannetti et al. 2015; Rissanen et al. 2014; Sucksdorff et al. 2017), Sucksdorff et al. (2017) did not observe differences in NAWM, and Vowinckel et al. (1997) found only an increased uptake in contrast-enhanced lesions, but not in non-enhanced lesions. Giannetti et al. (2015) investigated CIS, which is a group early in the spectrum of the MS disease course, so it is logical that they found less differences in inflammation. This is in line with the findings of Politis et al. (2012) that observed increased tracer uptake in RRMS, which was further increased in secondary progressive MS (SPMS). Aside from that, the inconsistencies most likely arise from the extreme heterogeneous aspect of MS pathology and the small sample sizes in the studies. The amount and severity of inflammation vary per person and the low affinity of [^{11}C]PK11195 for TSPO makes it difficult to find uniform group-based differences.

The most frequently studied second-generation TSPO tracer is [^{11}C]PBR28 (Table 33.3). Increased [^{11}C]PBR28 uptake has been generally observed in MS patients, including in the whole cortex, thalamus, hippocampus, basal ganglia, NAWM, lesions, and more specifically in contrast-enhanced lesions (Oh et al. 2011;

Table 33.3 Overview of the main results of studies using second-generation TSPO tracers

Study	Tracer	Subjects	GM	NAWM	Non-enhanced lesions	Enhanced lesions
Herranz et al. (2016)	[^{11}C] PBR28	11 HC 12 RRMS	Increased tracer uptake	Increased tracer uptake	n.a.	n.a.
		15 SPMS	More increased tracer uptake than for RRMS	More increased tracer uptake than for RRMS		
Oh et al. (2011)	[^{11}C] PBR28	7 HC 11 MS	No differences observed	No differences observed	Tracer uptake not increased	Increased tracer uptake
Singhal et al. (2018)	[^{11}C] PBR28	6 RRMS	n.a.	Increased tracer uptake	n.a.	n.a.
	[^{18}F] PBR06			Increased tracer uptake		
Datta et al. (2017b)	[^{11}C] PBR28	20 HC 24 MS	n.a.	Increased tracer uptake	Increased tracer uptake	Increased tracer uptake
	[^{18}F] PBR111	10 HC 10 MS	n.a.	Increased tracer uptake	Increased tracer uptake	Increased tracer uptake
Colasanti et al. (2014)	[^{18}F] PBR111	11 HC 11 RRMS	n.a.	Increased	Lesional uptake increased (enhancement not specified)	
Unterrainer et al. (2018)	[^{18}F] GE-180	19 RRMS	n.a.	n.a.	Increased tracer uptake	Tracer uptake increased more than non-enhanced
Bunai et al. (2018)	[^{11}C] DPA713	6 HC 6 RRMS	Increased	n.a.	n.a.	n.a.
Hagens et al. (2018)	[^{18}F] DPA714	7 HC 3 SPMS 5 PPMS	n.a.	n.a.	Tracer uptake increased (enhancement not specified)	

GM grey matter, *HC* healthy control, *MS* multiple sclerosis, *n.a.* not applicable, *NAWM* normal appearing white matter, *RRMS* relapse remitting MS, *SPMS* secondary progressive MS

Herranz et al. 2016). This increased [^{11}C]PBR28 uptake also appeared to increase with disability and disease duration (Oh et al. 2011; Herranz et al. 2016). In addition, a higher uptake of [^{11}C]PBR28 in NAWM and GM has been observed in SPMS compared to RRMS, which might be explained by the relation between increased tracer uptake and disease duration and/or elevated immune cell activation in SPMS as compared to RRMS patients in a remission phase (Herranz et al. 2016). Furthermore, [^{11}C]PBR28 uptake in both NAWM and lesions were positively correlated with T2 lesion volumes in RRMS, indicating that a higher tracer uptake corresponds with a larger total T2 lesion volume in RRMS (Datta et al. 2017a). In SPMS, a higher activation of inflammatory cells (tracer uptake) was positively correlated with brain atrophy, illustrating that neurodegenerative effects are accompanying the increased activation of inflammatory cells and further explaining the relation between disease duration and EDSS score (Datta et al. 2017a). Thus, like [^{11}C]PK11195, increased [^{11}C]PBR28 uptake, corresponding with increased activated inflammatory cells, is related to disease progression, duration, and clinical disability and an increase of [^{11}C]PBR28 uptake in MS lesions corresponds with disease activity. As stated in the previous section about [^{11}C]PK11195, inconsistencies in the literature are also found for the higher affinity second-generation TSPO tracers (Table 33.3). Oh et al. (2011) did not find any differences in tracer uptake for GM and NAWM non-enhanced lesions, but did for contrast-enhanced lesions. This is, however, the only study showing discrepancies with other studies, and illustrates the relative uniformity in the data with higher affinity TSPO tracers compared with the first-generation tracers. Heterogeneity in MS pathology may explain the remaining inconsistencies between studies.

Direct comparisons of [^{11}C]PBR28 with [^{18}F]PBR06, [^{18}F]PBR111, and [^{18}F]GE-180 have been performed, but not with [^{11}C]PK11195 (Table 33.3). Both [^{11}C]PBR28 and [^{18}F]PBR06 have a high tracer uptake in NAWM; however, only [^{18}F]PBR06 uptake was correlated to EDSS score, meaning that [^{18}F]PBR06 could be more sensitive to slight changes in immune activation in the specific population studied (Singhal et al. 2018). A comparison of [^{11}C]PBR28 with [^{18}F]PBR111 showed that [^{11}C]PBR28 has a higher binding in thalamus compared to [^{18}F]PBR111, aside from that, both tracers showed an increased uptake in NAWM, and both showed a higher tracer uptake in both contrast and non-contrast-enhanced lesions (Datta et al. 2017b). The other study analysing solely [^{18}F]PBR111 TSPO binding confirmed the higher tracer uptake in both NAWM and lesions (Colasanti et al. 2014). [^{11}C]PBR28 and [^{18}F]GE-180 TSPO binding are highly comparable (Sridharan et al. 2019). Like [^{11}C]PBR28, [^{18}F]GE-180 tracer uptake is also increased in lesions, especially in contrast-enhanced lesions (Unterrainer et al. 2018). According to these findings, all tracers seem to perform comparable, although [^{18}F]PBR06 might be slightly more and [^{18}F]PBR111 slightly less sensitive than [^{11}C]PB28.

Other second-generation TSPO tracers are [^{11}C]DPA713 and [^{18}F]DPA714 (Table 33.3). [^{11}C]DPA713 showed a global cortical increase of tracer uptake in MS patients (Bunai et al. 2018). For [^{18}F]DPA714, an increased uptake was observed in lesions compared to NAWM, and specifically for HAB patients. [^{18}F]DPA714

Table 33.4 Studies assessing MCT to image neuro-inflammation

Study	Tracer	Subjects	GM	NAWM	Non-enhanced lesions	Enhanced lesions
Takata et al. (2014)	[^{11}C] acetate	6 HC 6 RRMS	Increased tracer uptake	Increased tracer uptake	n.a.	n.a.

GM grey matter, *HC* healthy control, n.a. not applicable, *NAWM* normal appearing white matter, *RRMS* relapse remitting MS

showed also an increased tracer binding in NAWM when compared to NAWM of HAB healthy subjects (Hagens et al. 2018). These findings indicate that with [^{11}C]DPA713 PET, a global increase of activated inflammatory cells is observed in MS, and with [^{18}F]DPA714 the increase in activated immune cells was only visible in NAWM of HAB patients. This suggests that [^{11}C]DPA713 might be more suitable for visualising inflammatory changes in MS than [^{18}F]DPA714. The fact that [^{18}F]DPA714 is a TSPO agonist, whereas the other TSPO tracers are antagonists may also play a role in explaining this difference in binding.

Despite the upregulation of TSPO in microglia, macrophages, and astrocytes, TSPO imaging is primarily used to assess microglial activation (Fig. 33.2). However, astrocytes also play a role in MS pathology. In MS, there is an increased cerebral expression of the monocarboxylate transporter (MCT) (Nijland et al. 2014). MCT functions as a transporter for monocarboxylates, such as acetate. Acetate is preferentially absorbed into astrocytes by MCT (Waniewski and Martin 1998). Therefore, [^{11}C]acetate could be used to assess astrocyte activation, due to the upregulation of MCT by activated astrocytes (Table 33.4). Using [^{11}C]acetate, increased tracer uptake was observed in both WM and GM in MS patients compared to healthy subjects, and the amount of [^{11}C]acetate uptake was positively correlated to the number of lesions (Takata et al. 2014). This suggests that aside from microglia, also astrocytes are activated in MS pathology, and the amount of activation increases with disease severity. Whether the increased activation of astrocytes in MS pathology is supporting repair of neuronal damage still remains to be investigated.

Following degradation of the myelin sheaths, axons are susceptible to adverse environmental impact, such as exposure to oxidative stress, ultimately leading to neurodegeneration. The inflammation in MS pathology is a major source of oxidative stress. Upon neuronal damage, adenosine is released leading to the attraction of microglia. One intrinsic manner to cope with inflammation and corresponding tissue damage is the microglial upregulation of adenosine signalling via the adenosine A_{2A} receptor (A2AR) (Garcia et al. 2007). Upregulation of A2AR results in attenuation of inflammation (Fig. 33.2) and thereby limits the damage caused by inflammation (Blackburn et al. 2009). In MS, A2AR upregulation has been demonstrated by PET imaging with the A2AR tracer [^{11}C]TMSX (Rissanen et al. 2013). This indicates that in MS, microglial upregulation of A2AR expression might attenuate the inflammation, thereby reducing tissue damage and enhancing axonal survival.

33.4 PET Imaging to Assess Myelin Integrity

One of the main characteristics of MS pathology is the degradation of myelin. However, a validated and specific imaging method to directly visualise myelin in vivo and therefore to assess its integrity is still lacking. Because of high binding of amyloid tracers to white matter in healthy subjects, amyloid tracers have been recently applied for assessment of myelin integrity (Matías-Guiu et al. 2015). Amyloid tracers are designed to bind amyloid-beta deposits in the brain, which is one of the hallmarks of Alzheimer's disease pathology. More specifically, amyloid tracers bind to the beta sheets in amyloid-beta depositions (Wu et al. 2011). Myelin basic protein (MBP), one of the most prominent protein in the myelin lipid layers, also contains beta sheet structures (Ridsdale et al. 2002). Therefore, the high uptake of amyloid tracers in white matter of healthy subjects is hypothesised to correspond with binding to MBP, and thus might be used as a measurement for assessing myelin integrity (Fig. 33.4).

Amyloid tracers for assessing myelin integrity generally display a decreased uptake in the white matter lesions compared to NAWM (Table 33.5). However, none of the studies also assessed the perfusion rate of lesions. Diminished perfusion in lesions could also lead to a lower tracer uptake in the lesions, even without demyelination. Current research with amyloid tracers leads to conflicting results regarding differentiation between NAWM in MS patients and WM of healthy subjects. [^{18}F]Florbetaben, for instance, showed differences between tracer uptake in NAWM

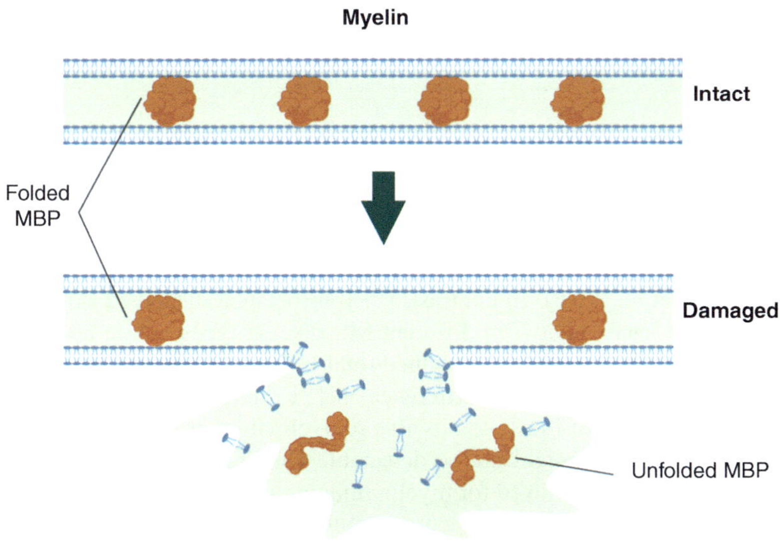

Fig. 33.4 Mechanism of action for myelin visualisation. The main target for myelin visualisation is supposedly myelin basic protein (MBP). The tracers bind to the beta sheets of intact MBP. When myelin is damaged, MBP loses its structure and thereby the tracer binding site (the figure is inspired by Stapulionis et al. (2008); Source: DOI: https://doi.org/10.4049/jimmunol.180.6.3946)

Table 33.5 Overview of studies with amyloid tracers employed for myelin imaging

Study	Tracer	Subjects	GM	NAWM	Non-enhanced lesions	Enhanced lesions
Bodini et al. (2016)	[^{11}C]PiB	8 HC 20 RRMS	No differences in tracer uptake	No differences in tracer uptake	Decreased tracer uptake	Decreased tracer uptake
Grecchi et al. (2017)	[^{11}C]PiB	20 RRMS	n.a.	n.a.	Decreased tracer uptake	Decreased tracer uptake
Zeydan et al. (2018)	[^{11}C]PiB	80 HC 12 MS	No differences in tracer uptake	No differences in tracer uptake	n.a.	n.a.
Matías-Guiu et al. (2015)	[^{18}F] Florbetaben	3 HC 5 RRMS 5 SPMS 2 PPMS	n.a.	Decreased tracer uptake	Decreased tracer uptake (enhancement not specified)	
Matías-Guiu et al. (2017)	[^{18}F] Florbetaben	1 MS	n.a.	n.a.	Decreased tracer uptake (enhancement not specified)	
Pietroboni et al. (2019)	[^{18}F] Florbetapir	7 RRMS 3 SPMS 2 PPMS	n.a.	n.a.	Decreased tracer uptake (enhancement not specified)	

GM grey matter, *HC* healthy control, *MS* multiple sclerosis, *n.a.* not applicable, *NAWM* normal appearing white matter, *PPMS* primary progressive MS, *RRMS* relapse remitting MS, *SPMS* secondary progressive MS

and WM, whereas [^{11}C]PiB did not (Matías-Guiu et al. 2015; Bodini et al. 2016). [^{18}F]Florbetaben, [^{18}F]Florbetapir, as well as [^{11}C]PiB, all showed a decreased tracer uptake in lesions relative to NAWM (Matías-Guiu et al. 2015, 2017; Bodini et al. 2016; Pietroboni et al. 2019; Zeydan et al. 2018; Grecchi et al. 2017). Furthermore, [^{11}C]PiB has shown to be able to capture remyelination and demyelination processes (Bodini et al. 2016). In contrast, [^{18}F]Florbetaben displayed differences in tracer uptake in lesions between different MS disease types, while no significant differences were observed in T2-weighted total lesion volumes between MS types (Matías-Guiu et al. 2015). This difference in [^{18}F]Florbetaben uptake in lesions between MS types might illustrate possible remyelination processes of lesions that occur in RRMS, which might not be detectable with T2 imaging. An example of [^{18}F]Florbetaben PET employed for myelin imaging is displayed in Fig. 33.5. Aside from the repurposing of amyloid tracers, recently the tracer [^{11}C]MeDAS has been specifically developed for the visualisation of myelin (Wu et al. 2010). PET studies with [^{11}C]MeDAS in preclinical models show that the tracer binds more specifically to MBP than other tracers (De Paula et al. 2014a, 2014b). Currently, the first clinical study with [^{11}C]MeDAS is still in progress (Trial register no. NL7262).

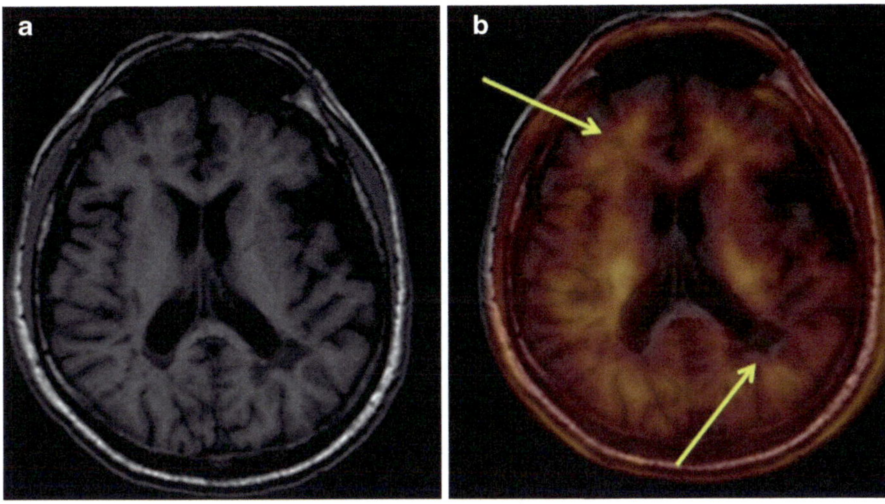

Fig. 33.5 A [^{18}F]Florbetaben PET image illustrating its ability to depict demyelination. On the left, a T1 MRI scan is displayed, with on the right a PET-MRI fusion image, illustrating both normal tracer uptake (left top corner) and a decreased tracer uptake (right bottom corner) at the lesion location as detected by T1 MRI (permission for the use of the images was obtained; Source: DOI: https://doi.org/10.1186/s12883-015-0502-2) (Matías-Guiu et al. 2015)

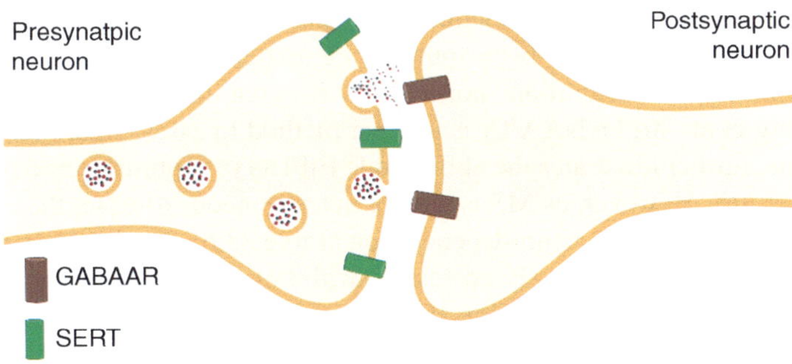

Fig. 33.6 Neuronal targets used for PET imaging in MS. $GABA_A$ receptor is essential for the propagation of action potentials, a reduced expression indicates a reduced synaptic density. SERT upregulation increases serotonin re-uptake and thereby enhances depressive symptoms

33.5 PET Imaging to Assess Neuronal Integrity

As a result of neurodegeneration, the amount of synapses decreases. One of the most important synaptic receptors is the γ-aminobutyric $acid_A$ ($GABA_A$) receptor. $GABA_A$ receptors (Fig. 33.6) are essential for propagating action potentials, and thus responsible for signal transduction (Mohler 2009). One of the sub-components of the $GABA_A$ receptor is the benzodiazepine receptor. Benzodiazepines enhance the effect of GABA binding to the $GABA_A$ receptor (Sigel and Ernst 2018). In MS, imaging with [^{11}C]flumazenil, an antagonist for the benzodiazepine receptor, resulted in a lower cortical tracer uptake compared to healthy subjects, indicating a reduction of synapses in MS (Freeman et al. 2015).

Depression and mood disorders can occur in MS, possibly as a direct result of the disease. Depression is associated with a decreased availability of serotonin. Serotonin is a major contributor to feelings of well-being and happiness (Mitchell and Phillips 2007). One cause for the decreased availability of serotonin is an increase of serotonin transporters (Fakhoury 2016). Serotonin transporters transport serotonin from the synaptic cleft to the presynaptic neuron, and thereby counteract the effects of serotonin (Fig. 33.6). Therefore, a decrease or inhibition of serotonin transporters increases serotonin concentrations in the synapses and thus stimulates serotonin functions. [^{11}C]DASB is a tracer binding to serotonin transporters. In MS, a study with [^{11}C]DASB showed a reduced tracer uptake in the cingulate cortex, the thalamus, and the insula and an increased uptake in the orbitofrontal cortex (Hesse et al. 2014). This indicates a reduction of serotonin transporters in limbic and paralimbic regions and an increase in frontal regions. This study also assessed the correlation between [^{11}C]DASB uptake and depression. In line with expectations, there was a positive correlation between insular tracer uptake and depression, which means the higher the amount of serotonin transporters in the insula, the more prominent the depressive symptoms.

Like in all other neurodegenerative diseases, [^{18}F]FDG, a tracer for imaging glucose consumption is also used in MS to study neuronal integrity (Roelcke et al. 1997). As neurons are the major consumers of glucose in the brain, a decreased uptake of [^{18}F]FDG depicts dysfunction or degeneration of neurons. Reduced cortical [^{18}F]FDG uptake has also been found to be associated with a reduced cortical *N*-acetylaspartate concentration normalised to creatine (NAA/Cr) in RRMS (Blinkenberg et al. 2011). NAA/Cr is another method to assess neuronal deterioration and thus further illustrates the ability of [^{18}F]FDG to capture neurodegenerative processes in MS. However, as MS is a quite heterogeneous disease, there is a wide variety of regions showing neurodegeneration (Table 33.6). The hypometabolism in those regions was also positively correlated with both the duration and severity of MS (Bakshi et al. 1998). The clinical effects of neurodegeneration studied with [^{18}F]FDG in MS are mostly related to mobility or fatigue, but also to some extent to cognition.

Several brain regions are involved in the initiation of movement, and therefore neurodegeneration in any of those regions can affect mobility. The combination of regions responsible for movement is called the motor network. For the initiation of movement, first the parietal and temporal lobes receive sensory information and then initiate the motor network by stimulation of the prefrontal cortex (Gray and Bjorklund 2014). The prefrontal cortex then creates a general plan of action, which is then converted by the premotor area into neural programmes for movement. The primary motor cortex propagates this to the cerebellum and basal ganglia for fine tuning. The optimised plan of action is then sent down the spinal cord for execution of the movement.

Table 33.6 Overview of studies assessing CNS glucose metabolism in MS using [^{18}F]FDG PET

Study	Subjects	Metabolism quantification method	Hypermetabolism
Bakshi et al. (1998)	6 HC 25 MS	Absolute	Whole brain, cortex, WM, subcortical
Derache et al. (2013)	17 RRMS	CMRglu	Negative correlations with fatigue
Roelcke et al. (1997)	16 HC 47 MS	Normalised to mean uptake (CMRglu)	Whole brain, prefrontal cortex, premotor cortex, putamen, supplementary motor area, basal ganglia
Kindred et al. (2014)	8 HC 8 RRMS	SUVmean	Spinal cord
Blinkenberg et al. (2001)	9 HC 23 MS	CMRglu	Cortex, prefrontal cortex, orbitofrontal cortex, caudatus, putamen, thalamus, hippocampus

CMRglu cerebral metabolic rate of glucose, *HC* healthy control, *MS* multiple sclerosis, *RRMS* relapse remitting MS, *SUVmean* mean standardised uptake value, *WM* white matter

Several studies found changes in metabolism in regions of the motor network (Table 33.6). For instance, a reduction in cortical glucose uptake was found to be associated with disease severity expressed as fatigue (Roelcke et al. 1997; Derache et al. 2013). This might be explained by the increased muscular demands caused by a decreased CNS efficacy, and therefore leads to earlier muscular exhaustion, hence fatigue (Rudroff et al. 2014). Also negative correlations have been observed between physical score and metabolism in left parietal regions, right frontal regions, and right temporal regions (Derache et al. 2013). This means the higher physical score, the lower the [^{18}F]FDG uptake in those regions, which might illustrate network disruptions in patients with fatigue. In addition, a decreased [^{18}F]FDG uptake was observed in the spinal cord of MS patients (Kindred et al. 2014). This might indicate that the autonomic nervous system and walking/motor dysfunctions that are often seen in patients with MS could originate from spinal cord neurodegeneration.

While assessing cognitive effects of MS pathology, a negative correlation was observed between cognition and metabolism in thalamus (Derache et al. 2013). This means lower cognitive performance, relates to higher [^{18}F]FDG uptake in the thalamus, and thus may illustrate cerebral compensation for maintaining cognitive function. A more thorough assessment of the effects of MS pathology on cognition revealed a relation between lesion-affected regions, adjacent cortical hypometabolism, and corresponding diminished cognitive performance (Blinkenberg et al. 2001). This study found no other clinical deterioration aside from cognition and therefore illustrates that cognitive deterioration may occur without any other signs of disease progression, most likely resulting from white matter lesion-induced neurodegeneration.

33.6 PET Imaging as a Tool to Aid in Differential Diagnosis

MRI lesions can show a pattern specific for MS. In some cases, lesions seem to resemble tumours, both radiologically and clinically (Di Patre et al. 2003). This type of MS is therefore called tumefactive MS. For the differentiation of the lesions of tumefactive MS from brain tumours, [^{11}C]methionine PET imaging might be employed. Tumours are associated with a high proliferation and protein synthesis (Waarde and Elsinga 2008). For PET imaging of protein synthesis, radiolabelled amino acids, like [^{11}C]methionine, are used. Methionine was shown to have a low uptake in the healthy brain, but in tumours methionine uptake is increased (Jager et al. 2001; Coope et al. 2007). Therefore, [^{11}C]Methionine PET is widely used to aid in the diagnosis of brain tumours, and thus might be used to differentiate between tumefactive MS and cerebral tumours. However, at the moment there is only evidence from case studies to support this concept.

For instance, in a case for which it was not possible to differentiate between a tumefactive MS lesion and a tumour with MRI, [^{11}C]methionine PET displayed no significant uptake in the lesion (Ninomiya et al. 2015). The diagnosis of this specific patient was therefore tumefactive MS, which significantly influenced the selection of treatment strategies. In another case, [^{11}C]methionine PET was used to differentiate a low-grade glioma from a suspected diagnosis of tumefactive MS (Tarkkonen et al. 2016). In this patient there was actually significant [^{11}C]methionine uptake in the lesion, which suggested a possible tumour (Fig. 33.7). In addition, a [^{11}C]PK11195 PET scan was performed, which showed no increased uptake, arguing against MS and leading ultimately to a glioma diagnosis. These cases clearly illustrate that the important contribution PET could potentially have in differential diagnosis in cases where other techniques are inconclusive.

33.7 PET Imaging to Assess Treatment Effects in MS

To study therapy effects on MS pathology, PET imaging can play an important role due to visualisation of alterations in individual biological processes (Table 33.7). Currently, the primary treatment strategy of MS is inhibition of the immune attacks on the myelin sheaths. Current disease modifying therapies are all anti-inflammatory. For example, treatment with fingolimod inhibits the migration of lymphocytes from the lymph nodes (Matloubian et al. 2004; Mandala et al. 2002). Due to the reduction of lymphocytes, the severity of inflammatory responses in MS is reduced. In a [^{11}C]PK11195 PET imaging study, increased tracer uptake in NAWM and GM areas was observed in MS patients prior to fingolimod treatment, as compared to healthy subjects (Sucksdorff et al. 2017). After 6 months of fingolimod treatment patients displayed a decrease in tracer uptake in lesions, but not in other brain areas. Therefore, the inhibition of lymphocyte migration by fingolimod has globally limited effects on the activation of microglia and macrophages outside of the lesions. The observed clinical improvements are therefore probably primarily caused by the reduction of activation of inflammatory cells within the lesions. This illustrates the

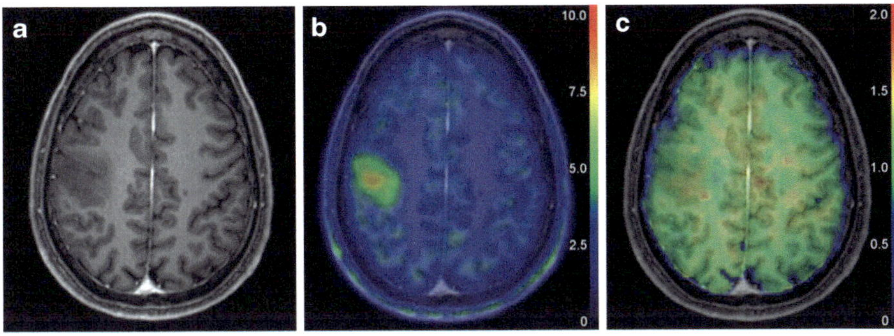

Fig. 33.7 MS differential diagnosis with PET imaging. (**a**) depicts a T1 MRI image with a hypointense lesion. (**b**) is a [^{11}C]methionine PET image, which clearly illustrates an increased uptake at the lesion. (**c**) [^{11}C]PK11195 PET image, illustrating no significant differences in uptake, and thus supported glioma diagnosis, which was confirmed by brain biopsy (permission for the use of the images was obtained; Source: DOI: https://doi.org/10.1016/j.msard.2016.07.016) (Tarkkonen et al. 2016)

Table 33.7 Overview of studies using PET to analyse therapy effects in MS

Study	Tracer	Subjects	Treatment	Treatment response
Sucksdorff et al. (2017)	[^{11}C] PK11195	10 RRMS	Fingolimod	Reduced lesional tracer uptake after 6 months of treatment, but not in other brain areas
Baumgartner et al. (2018)	[^{18}F]FDG	10 HC 9 RRMS	Interferon beta therapy	6 months IFN-beta. After treatment, decreased metabolism in cerebellum, increased metabolism in left inferior parietal cortex, right insula, left temporo-occipital cortex, left frontal cortex, and left striatum
Bunai et al. (2018)	[^{11}C] DPA713	6 HC 4 RRMS	Fingolimod	After 1 year treatment, a broad increased tracer uptake, especially in temporal and parietal cortex
		2 RRMS	Interferon beta therapy	
Ratchford et al. (2012)	[^{11}C] PK11195	9 RRMS	Glatiramer acetate	After 1 year of treatment, whole brain tracer uptake decreased, cerebral white matter, cortical grey matter. No change in binding in lesions
Kaunzner et al. (2017)	[^{11}C] PK11195	5 HC 18 MS	Natalizumab	After 6 months of treatment, decreased tracer uptake in both non- and enhanced lesions. No changes observed in NAWM, thalamus, and cortex

HC healthy control, *IFN-beta* interferon beta, *MS* multiple sclerosis, *NAWM* normal appearing white matter, *RRMS* relapse remitting MS importance of reducing the inflammatory status within lesions. In another study on the effect of interferon (IFN)-beta therapy, [^{18}F]FDG PET showed no differences between patients and healthy subjects at baseline (Baumgartner et al. 2018). However, after 6 months of treatment, using relative regional glucose metabolism (rCMRglu) as outcome measure, a decreased [^{18}F]FDG uptake was observed in the cerebellum and an increased [^{18}F]FDG uptake in various brain regions in MS patients compared to healthy subjects. Although this might suggest that IFN-beta would lead to a decrease in cerebellar neuronal integrity, due to the use of relative measurements instead of absolute, this effect could also represent a global increase in cerebral metabolic rate of glucose (CMRglu), combined with no increase in cerebellum and, thus, a relative decrease in cerebellum. Nevertheless, these results do not depict any effects of the efficacy of IFN-beta therapy on modulation of the inflammatory response. Another study, which analysed the effects of both fingolimod and IFN-beta, showed an increased [^{11}C]DPA713 uptake at baseline in patients, which was even further increased at follow-up (Bunai et al. 2018). Traditionally, TSPO tracers are used to visualise activated inflammatory cells, however, aside from the pro-inflammatory status (e.g. M1 microglia), activated inflammatory cells can also have a protective function (e.g. M2 microglia) and thus depict protective mechanisms. Nevertheless, the results of these studies show the complexity of disentangling the mechanisms of action of disease modifying therapies in MS.

[^{11}C]PK11195 PET has also been used for the analysis of the effects of glatiramer acetate, which is commonly used in MS treatment. Glatiramer acetate putatively binds to the major histocompatibility complex receptors and thereby inhibits the T-cell response to myelin antigens (Schrempf and Ziemssen 2007). The reduction of adaptive immune system activation should also reduce the activation of the innate immune system. A study analysing the effects of glatiramer acetate with [^{11}C]PK11195 displayed a decreased tracer uptake after 1 year of treatment compared to baseline (Ratchford et al. 2012). Therefore, these results support the concept of a decreased activation of the innate immune system over time due to glatiramer acetate treatment and thus illustrate its mechanism of action.

Antibodies are also commonly used in the treatment of MS. One of these antibodies is natalizumab, which very specifically binds to integrins expressed on the cerebral vasculature, and strongly decreases the influx of lymphocytes into the CNS (Peterson et al. 2002; Yednock et al. 1992). The influx reduction limits the effects of the adaptive immune system in the CNS and subsequently the activation of innate immune cells (Del Pilar Martin et al. 2008). [^{11}C]PK11195 PET imaging showed a decrease of tracer uptake in lesions after 6 months of treatment with natalizumab, but no changes were detected in NAWM, the thalamus, and GM (Kaunzner et al. 2017). These results illustrate that natalizumab treatment also has its main effect on inflammation in lesions compared to non-lesional tissue. While both fingolimod and natalizumab have proven clinical efficacy, this seems to be mainly caused by the reduction of the inflammation within lesions. Therefore, a more thorough assessment of the lesions with PET imaging instead of whole brain analysis would be more indicative for the efficacy of therapies.

33.8 Clinical Notes

The clinical application of PET scanning in MS at this moment is restricted to aiding diagnosis in difficult cases. PET imaging in MS has been mainly used in a research setting so far. If myelin binding ligands can deliver on their promise and quantifying myelin loss in lesions becomes feasible, such scan techniques can probably be used in phase II and III trials to aid in identifying drugs promoting myelin repair. Further down the road, myelin imaging using PET may be used to inform clinicians and patients about the individual treatment effect of myelin restoring treatment protocols. The place of inflammation imaging using PET in MS is more difficult to predict. MRI protocols are already capable of imaging inflammation in MS and do not have the disadvantage of using ionising radiation.

33.9 Conclusion

The use of PET imaging in MS is increasing, in particular, in a research setting. Currently, its primary role in clinical practice is in aiding with differential diagnosis between MS and brain tumours. PET imaging of activation of the innate immune system could be of particular interest in drug development, as the technique would enable objective efficacy evaluation of immune suppressive therapies. Due to the increasing interests in myelin imaging, a method to assess myelin integrity may soon become available. As myelin repair is likely the next target of interest in the treatment of MS, myelin PET could initially be used to determine the efficacy of various remyelination therapies, and in the end to monitor individual remyelination treatment responses.

References

Airas L, Rissanen E, Rinne JO (2015) Imaging neuroinflammation in multiple sclerosis using TSPO-PET. Clin Transl Imaging 3(6):461–473. https://doi.org/10.1007/s40336-015-0147-6

Baecher-Allan C, Kaskow BJ, Weiner HL (2018) Multiple sclerosis: mechanisms and immunotherapy. Neuron 97(4):742–768. https://doi.org/10.1016/j.neuron.2018.01.021

Bakshi R, Miletrch RS, Kinkel PR, Emmet ML, Kinkel WR (1998) High-resolution fluorodeoxyglucose positron emission tomography shows both global and regional cerebral hypometabolism in multiple sclerosis. J Neuroimaging 8(4):228–234. https://doi.org/10.1111/jon199884228

Baumgartner A, Frings L, Schiller F, Stich O, Mix M, Egger K, Schluh G, Rauer S, Meyer PT (2018) Regional neuronal activity in patients with relapsing remitting multiple sclerosis. Acta Neurol Scand 138(6):466–474. https://doi.org/10.1111/ane.13012

Biediger D, Collet C, Armspach J (2014) Multiple sclerosis lesion detection with local multimodal Markovian analysis and cellular automata 'GrowCut.' J Comput Surg. https://doi.org/10.1186/2194-3990-1-3

Blackburn MR, Vance CO, Morschl E, Wilson CN (2009) Adenosine receptors and inflammation. Handb Exp Pharmacol (193):215–269. https://doi.org/10.1007/978-3-540-89615-9_8

Blinkenberg M, Rune K, Jensen CV, Ravnborg MH, Kyllingsbaek S, Holm S, Paulson OB, Sørensen PS (2001) [Reduced metabolism in cerebral cortex correlates with MRI changes and cognitive dysfunction in patients with disseminated sclerosis]. Ugeskr Laeger 63(27):3788–3792

Blinkenberg M, Mathiesen HK, Tscherning T, Jønsson A, Svarer C, Holm S, Sellebjerg F, Paulson OB, Hanson LG, Sorensen PS (2011) Cerebral metabolism, magnetic resonance spectroscopy and cognitive dysfunction in early multiple sclerosis: an exploratory study. Neurol Res 34(1):52–58. https://doi.org/10.1179/1743132811y.0000000059

Bodini B, Veronese M, García-Lorenzo D, Battaglini M, Poirion E, Chardain A, Freeman L, Louapre C, Tchikviladze M, Papeix C, Dollé F, Zalc B, Lubetzki C, Bottlaender M, Turkheimer F, Stankoff B (2016) Dynamic imaging of individual remyelination profiles in multiple sclerosis. Ann Neurol 79:726–738. https://doi.org/10.1002/ana.24620

Bunai T, Terada T, Kono S, Yokokura M, Yoshikawa E, Futatsubashi M, Miyajima H, Ouchi Y (2018) Neuroinflammation following disease modifying therapy in multiple sclerosis: a pilot positron emission tomography study. J Neurol Sci 385:30–33. https://doi.org/10.1016/j.jns.2017.12.004

Chechneva O, Deng W (2016) Mitochondrial translocator protein (TSPO), astrocytes and neuroinflammation. Neural Regen Res 11(7):1056–1057. https://doi.org/10.4103/1673-5374.187027

Colasanti A, Guo Q, Muhlert N, Giannetti P, Onega M, Newbould RD, Ciccarelli O, Rison S, Thomas C, Nicholas R, Muraro PA, Malik O, Owen DR, Piccini P, Gunn RN, Rabiner EA, Matthews PM (2014) In vivo assessment of brain white matter inflammation in multiple sclerosis with 18F-PBR111 PET. J Nucl Med 55(7):1112–1118. https://doi.org/10.2967/jnumed.113.135129

Coope DJ, Cizek J, Eggers C, Vollmar S, Heiss W-D, Herholz K (2007) Evaluation of primary brain tumors using 11C-methionine PET with reference to a normal methionine uptake map. J Nucl Med 48(12):1971–1980. https://doi.org/10.2967/jnumed.107.043240

Datta G, Colasanti A, Kalk N, Owen D, Scott G, Rabiner EA, Gunn RN, Lingford-Hughes A, Malik O, Ciccarelli O, Nicholas R, Nei L, Battaglini M, Stefano ND, Matthews PM (2017a) 11 C-PBR28 and 18 F-PBR111 detect white matter inflammatory heterogeneity in multiple sclerosis. J Nucl Med 58(9):1477–1482. https://doi.org/10.2967/jnumed.116.187161

Datta G, Colasanti A, Rabiner EA, Gunn RN, Malik O, Ciccarelli O, Nicholas R, Van Vlierberghe E, Van Hecke W, Searle G, Santos-Ribeiro A, Matthews PM (2017b) Neuroinflammation and its relationship to changes in brain volume and white matter lesions in multiple sclerosis. Brain 140(11):2927–2938. https://doi.org/10.1093/brain/awx228

De Paula Faria D, Copray S, Sijbesma JWA, Willemsen ATM, Buchpiguel CA, Dierckx RAJO, De Vries EFJ (2014a) PET imaging of focal demyelination and remyelination in a rat model of multiple sclerosis: comparison of [11C]MeDAS, [11C]CIC and [11C]PIB. Eur J Nucl Med Mol Imaging 41(5):995–1003. https://doi.org/10.1007/s00259-013-2682-6

De Paula Faria D, De Vries EFJ, Sijbesma JWA, Dierckx RAJO, Buchpiguel CA, Copray S (2014b) PET imaging of demyelination and remyelination in the cuprizone mouse model for multiple sclerosis: a comparison between [11C]CIC and [11C]MeDAS. NeuroImage 87:395–402. https://doi.org/10.1016/j.neuroimage.2013.10.057

Del Pilar Martin M, Cravens PD, Winger R, Frohman EM, Racke MK, Eagar TN, Zamvil SS, Weber MS, Hemmer B, Karandikar NJ, Kleinschmidt-DeMasters BK, Stüve O (2008) Decrease in the numbers of dendritic cells and CD4 + T cells in cerebral perivascular spaces due to natalizumab. Arch Neurol 65(12):1596–1603. https://doi.org/10.1001/archneur.65.12.noc80051

Dendrou CA, Fugger L, Friese MA (2015) Immunopathology of multiple sclerosis. Nat Rev Immunol 5(9):545–558. https://doi.org/10.1038/nri3871

Derache N, Grassiot B, Mézenge F, Emmanuelle Dugué A, Desgranges B, Constans JM, Defer GL (2013) Fatigue is associated with metabolic and density alterations of cortical and deep gray matter in relapsing-remitting-multiple sclerosis patients at the earlier stage of the disease: a PET/MR study. Mult Scler Relat Disord 2(4):362–369. https://doi.org/10.1016/j.msard.2013.03.005

Di Patre PL, Castillo V, Delavelle J, Vuillemoz S, Picard F, Landis T (2003) "Tumor-mimicking" multiple sclerosis. Clin Neuropathol 22(5):235–239

Fakhoury M (2016) Revisiting the serotonin hypothesis: implications for major depressive disorders. Mol Neurobiol 53:2778–2786. https://doi.org/10.1007/s12035-015-9152-z

Ferguson B, Matyszak MK, Esiri MM, Perry VH (1997) Axonal damage in acute multiple sclerosis lesions. Brain 120(Pt 3):393–399. https://doi.org/10.1093/brain/120.3.393

Franklin RJM, Ffrench-Constant C (2008) Remyelination in the CNS: from biology to therapy. Nat Rev Neurosci 9(11):839–855. https://doi.org/10.1038/nrn2480

Freeman L, Garcia-Lorenzo D, Bottin L, Leroy C, Louapre C, Bodini B, Papeix C, Assouad R, Granger B, Tourbah A, Dollé F, Lubetzki C, Bottlaender M, Stankoff B (2015) The neuronal component of gray matter damage in multiple sclerosis: a [11C]flumazenil positron emission tomography study. Ann Neurol 78(4):554–567. https://doi.org/10.1002/ana.24468

Garcia GE, Truong LD, Li P, Zhang P, Du J, Chen J-F, Feng L (2007) Adenosine A 2A receptor activation and macrophage-mediated experimental glomerulonephritis. FASEB J 22(2):445–454. https://doi.org/10.1096/fj.07-8430com

Giannetti P, Politis M, Su P, Turkheimer F, Malik O, Keihaninejad S, Wu K, Reynolds R, Nicholas R, Piccini P (2014) Microglia activation in multiple sclerosis black holes predicts outcome in progressive patients: an in vivo [(11)C](R)-PK11195-PET pilot study. Neurobiol Dis 65:203–210. https://doi.org/10.1016/j.nbd.2014.01.018

Giannetti P, Politis M, Su P, Turkheimer FE, Malik O, Keihaninejad S, Wu K, Waldman A, Reynolds R, Nicholas R, Piccini P (2015) Increased PK11195-PET binding in normal-appearing white matter in clinically isolated syndrome. Brain 138(1):110–119. https://doi.org/10.1093/brain/awu331

Gray P, Bjorklund DF (2014) Psychology. Worth, New York

Grecchi E, Veronese M, Bodini B, García-Lorenzo D, Battaglini M, Stankoff B, Turkheimer FE (2017) Multimodal partial volume correction: application to [11C]PIB PET/MRI myelin imaging in multiple sclerosis. J Cereb Blood Flow Metab 37(12):3803–3817. https://doi.org/10.1177/0271678X17712183

Gut P (2015) Targeting mitochondrial energy metabolism with TSPO ligands. Biochem Soc Trans 43(4):537–542. https://doi.org/10.1042/bst20150019

Hagens MHJ, Golla SV, Wijburg MT, Yaqub M, Heijtel D, Steenwijk MD, Schober P, Brevé JJP, Schuit RC, Reekie TA, Kassiou M, van Dam AM, Windhorst AD, Killestein J, Barkhof F, van Berckel BNM, Lammertsma AA (2018) In vivo assessment of neuroinflammation in progressive multiple sclerosis: a proof of concept study with [18F]DPA714 PET. J Neuroinflammation 15(1):314. https://doi.org/10.1186/s12974-018-1352-9

Herranz E, Giannì C, Louapre C, Treaba CA, Govindarajan ST, Ouellette R, Loggia ML, Sloane JA, Madigan N, Izquierdo-Garcia D, Ward N, Mangeat G, Granberg T, Klawiter EC, Catana C, Hooker JM, Taylor N, Ionete C, Kinkel RP, Mainero C (2016) Neuroinflammatory component of gray matter pathology in multiple sclerosis. Ann Neurol 80(5):776–790. https://doi.org/10.1002/ana.24791

Hesse S, Moeller F, Petroff D, Lobsien D, Luthardt J, Regenthal R, Becker GA, Patt M, Thomae E, Seese A, Meyer PM, Bergh FT, Sabri O (2014) Altered serotonin transporter availability in patients with multiple sclerosis. Eur J Nucl Med Mol Imaging 41(5):827–835. https://doi.org/10.1007/s00259-013-2636-z

Huang WJ, Chen WW, Zhang X (2017) Multiple sclerosis: pathology, diagnosis and treatments (review). Exp Ther Med 13(6):3163–3166. https://doi.org/10.3892/etm.2017.4410

Jager PL, Vaalburg W, Pruim J, de Vries EG, Langen KJ, Piers DA (2001) Radiolabeled amino acids: basic aspects and clinical applications in oncology. J Nucl Med 42(3):432–445

Kaunzner UW, Gauthier SA (2017) MRI in the assessment and monitoring of multiple sclerosis: an update on best practice. Ther Adv Neurol Disord 10(6):247–261. https://doi.org/10.1177/1756285617708911

Kaunzner UW, Kang Y, Monohan E, Kothari PJ, Nealon N, Perumal J, Vartanian T, Kuceyeski A, Vallabhajosula S, Mozley PD, Riley CS, Newman SM, Gauthier SA (2017) Reduction of PK11195 uptake observed in multiple sclerosis lesions after natalizumab initiation. Mult Scler Relat Disord 15:27–33. https://doi.org/10.1016/j.msard.2017.04.008

Kindred JH, Koo PJ, Rudroff T (2014) Glucose uptake of the spinal cord in patients with multiple sclerosis detected by 18f-fluorodeoxyglucose PET/CT after walking. Spinal Cord 52(Suppl 3):S11–S13. https://doi.org/10.1038/sc.2014.130

Kurtzke JF (1983) Rating neurologic impairment in multiple sclerosis: an expanded disability status scale (EDSS). Neurology 33(11):1444–1452

Lassmann H, Van Horssen J, Mahad D (2012) Progressive multiple sclerosis: pathology and pathogenesis. Nat Rev Neurol 8:647–656. https://doi.org/10.1038/nrneurol.2012.168

Mandala S, Hajdu R, Bergstrom J, Quackenbush E, Xie J, Milligan J, Thornton R, Shei GJ, Card D, Keohane CA, Rosenbach M, Hale J, Lynch CL, Rupprecht K, Parsons W, Rosen H (2002) Alteration of lymphocyte trafficking by sphingosine-1-phosphate receptor agonists. Science 296(5566):346–349. https://doi.org/10.1126/science.1070238

Matías-Guiu JA, Cabrera-Martín MN, Matías-Guiu J, Oreja-Guevara C, Riola-Parada C, Moreno-Ramos T, Arrazola J, Carreras JL (2015) Amyloid PET imaging in multiple sclerosis: an 18F-florbetaben study. BMC Neurol 15:243. https://doi.org/10.1186/s12883-015-0502-2

Matías-Guiu JA, Cabrera-Martín MN, Cortés-Martínez A, Pytel V, Moreno-Ramos T, Oreja-Guevara C, Carreras JL, Matías-Guiu J (2017) Amyloid PET in pseudotumoral multiple sclerosis. Mult Scler Relat Disord 15:15–17. https://doi.org/10.1016/j.msard.2017.05.002

Matloubian M, Lo CG, Cinamon G, Lesneski MJ, Xu Y, Brinkmann V, Allende ML, Proia RL, Cyster JG (2004) Lymphocyte egress from thymus and peripheral lymphoid organs is dependent on S1P receptor 1. Nature 427(6972):355–360. https://doi.org/10.1038/nature02284

Miljković D, Spasojević I (2013) Multiple sclerosis: molecular mechanisms and therapeutic opportunities. Antioxid Redox Signal 19(18):2286–2334. https://doi.org/10.1089/ars.2012.5068

Mitchell RLC, Phillips LH (2007) The psychological, neurochemical and functional neuroanatomical mediators of the effects of positive and negative mood on executive functions. Neuropsychologia 45(4):617–629. https://doi.org/10.1016/j.neuropsychologia.2006.06.030

Mohler H (2009) Role of GABAA receptors in cognition. Biochem Soc Trans 37(Pt 6):1328–1333. https://doi.org/10.1042/BST0371328

Nijland PG, Michailidou I, Witte ME, Mizee MR, Van Der Pol SMA, Van Het Hof B, Reijerkerk A, Pellerin L, van der Valk P, de Vries HE, van Horssen J (2014) Cellular distribution of glucose and monocarboxylate transporters in human brain white matter and multiple sclerosis lesions. Glia 62(7):1125–1141. https://doi.org/10.1002/glia.22667

Ninomiya S, Hara M, Morita A, Teramoto H, Momose M, Takahashi T, Kamei S (2015) Tumefactive demyelinating lesion differentiated from a brain tumor using a combination of magnetic resonance imaging and ^{11}C-methionine positron emission tomography. Intern Med 54(11):1411–1414. https://doi.org/10.2169/internalmedicine.54.3712

Oh U, Fujita M, Ikonomidou VN, Evangelou IE, Matsuura E, Harberts E, Ohayon J, Pike VW, Zhang Y, Zoghbi SS, Innis RB, Jacobson S (2011) Translocator protein PET imaging for glial activation in multiple sclerosis. J Neuroimmune Pharmacol 6(3):354–361. https://doi.org/10.1007/s11481-010-9243-6

Owen DR, Yeo AJ, Gunn RN, Song K, Wadsworth G, Lewis A, Rhodes C, Pulford DJ, Bennacef I, Parker CA, Stjean PL, Cardon LR, Mooser VE, Matthews PM, Rabiner EA, Rubio JP (2012) An 18-kDa translocator protein (TSPO) polymorphism explains differences in binding affinity of the PET radioligand PBR28. J Cereb Blood Flow Metab 32(1):1–5. https://doi.org/10.1038/jcbfm.2011.147

Papadopoulos V, Baraldi M, Guilarte TR, Knudsen TB, Lacapère JJ, Lindemann P, Norenberg MD, Nutt D, Weizman A, Zhang MR, Gavish M (2006) Translocator protein (18 kDa): new nomenclature for the peripheral-type benzodiazepine receptor based on its structure and molecular function. Trends Pharmacol Sci 27(8):402–409. https://doi.org/10.1016/j.tips.2006.06.005

Peterson JW, Bö L, Mörk S, Chang A, Ransohoff RM, Trapp BD (2002) VCAM-1-positive microglia target oligodendrocytes at the border of multiple sclerosis lesions. J Neuropathol Exp Neurol 61(6):539–546. https://doi.org/10.1093/jnen/61.6.539

Pietroboni AM, Carandini T, Colombi A, Mercurio M, Ghezzi L, Giulietti G, Scarioni M, Arighi A, Fenoglio C, De Riz MA, Fumagalli GG, Basilico P, Serpente M, Bozzali M, Scarpini E, Galimberti D, Marotta G (2019) Amyloid PET as a marker of normal-appearing white matter early damage in multiple sclerosis: correlation with CSF β-amyloid levels and brain volumes. Eur J Nucl Med Mol Imaging 46(2):280–287. https://doi.org/10.1007/s00259-018-4182-1

Politis M, Giannetti P, Su P, Turkheimer F, Keihaninejad S, Wu K, Waldman A, Malik O, Matthews PM, Reynolds R, Nicholas R, Piccini P (2012) Increased PK11195 PET binding in the cortex of patients with MS correlates with disability. Neurology 79(6):523–530. https://doi.org/10.1212/WNL.0b013e3182635645

Prineas JW, Connell F (1979) Remyelination in multiple sclerosis. Ann Neurol 5(1):22–31. https://doi.org/10.1002/ana.410050105

Ramagopalan SV, Dobson R, Meier UC, Giovannoni G (2010) Multiple sclerosis: risk factors, prodromes, and potential causal pathways. Lancet Neurol 9(7):727–739. https://doi.org/10.1016/S1474-4422(10)70094-6

Ratchford JN, Endres CJ, Hammoud DA, Pomper MG, Shiee N, McGready J, Pham DL, Calabresi PA (2012) Decreased microglial activation in MS patients treated with glatiramer acetate. J Neurol 259(6):1199–1205. https://doi.org/10.1007/s00415-011-6337-x

Ridsdale RA, Beniac DR, Tompkins TA, Moscarello MA, Harauz G (2002) Three-dimensional structure of myelin basic protein. J Biol Chem 272:4269–4275. https://doi.org/10.1074/jbc.272.7.4269

Rissanen E, Virta JR, Paavilainen T, Tuisku J, Helin S, Luoto P, Parkkola R, Rinne JO, Airas L (2013) Adenosine A2A receptors in secondary progressive multiple sclerosis: a [11C]TMSX brain PET study. J Cereb Blood Flow Metab 33(9):1394–1401. https://doi.org/10.1038/jcbfm.2013.85

Rissanen E, Tuisku J, Rokka J, Paavilainen T, Parkkola R, Rinne JO, Airas L (2014) In vivo detection of diffuse inflammation in secondary progressive multiple sclerosis using PET imaging and the radioligand 11C-PK11195. J Nuclar Med 55(6):939–944. https://doi.org/10.2967/jnumed.113.131698

Roelcke U, Kappos L, Lechner-Scott J, Brunnschweiler H, Huber S, Ammann W, Plohmann A, Dellas S, Maguire RP, Missimer J, Radü EW, Steck A, Leenders KL (1997) Reduced glucose metabolism in the frontal cortex and basal ganglia of multiple sclerosis patients with fatigue: a 18 F-fluorodeoxyglucose positron emission tomography study. Neurology 48(6):1566–1571. https://doi.org/10.1212/WNL.48.6.1566

Rudroff T, Kindred JH, Koo PJ, Karki R, Hebert JR (2014) Asymmetric glucose uptake in leg muscles of patients with multiple sclerosis during walking detected by [18F]-FDG PET/CT. NeuroRehabilitation 35(4):813–823. https://doi.org/10.3233/NRE-141179

Schrempf W, Ziemssen T (2007) Glatiramer acetate: mechanisms of action in multiple sclerosis. Autoimmun Rev 6(7):469–475. https://doi.org/10.1016/j.autrev.2007.02.003

Sigel E, Ernst M (2018) The benzodiazepine binding sites of GABAA receptors. Trends Pharmacol Sci 39(7):659–671. https://doi.org/10.1016/j.tips.2018.03.006

Singhal T, O'Connor K, Dubey S, Belanger AP, Hurwitz S, Chu R, Tauhid S, Kijewski MF, Dicarli MF, Weiner HL, Bakshi R (2018) 18F-PBR06 versus 11C-PBR28 PET for assessing white matter translocator protein binding in multiple sclerosis. Clin Nucl Med 43(9):e289–e295. https://doi.org/10.1097/RLU.0000000000002179

Sridharan S, Raffel J, Nandoskar A, Record C, Brooks DJ, Owen D, Sharp D, Muraro PA, Gunn R, Nicholas R (2019) Confirmation of specific binding of the 18-kDa translocator protein (TSPO) radioligand [18F]GE-180: a blocking study using XBD173 in multiple sclerosis normal appearing white and grey matter. Mol Imaging Biol 21(5):935–944. https://doi.org/10.1007/s11307-019-01323-8

Stapulionis R, Oliveira CLP, Gjelstrup MC, Pedersen JS, Hokland ME, Hoffmann SV, Poulsen K, Jacobsen C, Vorup-Jensen T (2008) Structural insight into the function of myelin basic protein as a ligand for integrin alpha M beta 2. J Immunol 180(6):3946–3956

Sucksdorff M, Rissanen E, Tuisku J, Nuutinen S, Paavilainen T, Rokka J, Rinne J, Airas L (2017) Evaluation of the effect of fingolimod treatment on microglial activation using serial PET imaging in multiple sclerosis. J Nucl Med 58(10):1646–1651. https://doi.org/10.2967/jnumed.116.183020

Takata K, Kato H, Shimosegawa E, Okuno T, Koda T, Sugimoto T, Mochizuki H, Hatazawa J, Nakatsuji Y (2014) 11C-Acetate PET imaging in patients with multiple sclerosis. PLoS One 9(11):e111598. https://doi.org/10.1371/journal.pone.0111598

Tarkkonen A, Rissanen E, Tuokkola T, Airas L (2016) Utilization of PET imaging in differential diagnostics between a tumefactive multiple sclerosis lesion and low-grade glioma. Mult Scler Relat Disord 9:147–149. https://doi.org/10.1016/j.msard.2016.07.016

Thompson AJ, Banwell BL, Barkhof F, Carroll WM, Coetzee T (2018) Diagnosis of multiple sclerosis: 2017 revisions of the McDonald criteria. Lancet Neurol 17(2):162–173. https://doi.org/10.1016/s1474-4422(17)30470-2

Traugott U, Reinherz EL, Raine CS (1983) Multiple sclerosis. Distribution of T cells, T cell subsets and Ia-positive macrophages in lesions of different ages. J Neuroimmunol 4(3):201–221. https://doi.org/10.1016/0165-5728(83)90036-X

Unterrainer M, Mahler C, Vomacka L, Lindner S, Havla J, Brendel M, Böning G, Ertl-Wagner B, Kümpfel T, Milenkovic VM, Rupprecht R, Kerschensteiner M, Bartenstein P, Albert NL (2018) TSPO PET with [18F]GE-180 sensitively detects focal neuroinflammation in patients with relapsing–remitting multiple sclerosis. Eur J Nucl Med Mol Imaging 45(8):1423–1431. https://doi.org/10.1007/s00259-018-3974-7

Vowinckel E, Reutens D, Becher B, Verge G, Evans A, Owens T, Antel JP (1997) PK11195 binding to the peripheral benzodiazepine receptor as a marker of microgila activation in multiple sclerosis and experimental autoimmune encephalomyelitis. J Neurosci Res 50(2):345–353. https://doi.org/10.1002/(SICI)1097-4547(19971015)50:2<345::AID-JNR22>3.0.CO;2-5

Waarde A, Elsinga P (2008) Proliferation markers for the differential diagnosis of tumor and inflammation. Curr Pharm Des 14(31):3326–3339. https://doi.org/10.2174/138161208786549399

Waniewski RA, Martin DL (1998) Preferential utilization of acetate by astrocytes is attributable to transport. J Neurosci 18(14):5225–5233. https://doi.org/10.1523/jneurosci.18-14-05225.1998

Wu C, Wang C, Popescu DC, Zhu W, Somoza EA, Zhu J, Condie AG, Flask CA, Miller RH, MacKlin W, Wang Y (2010) A novel PET marker for in vivo quantification of myelination. Bioorg Med Chem 18(24):8592–8599. https://doi.org/10.1016/j.bmc.2010.10.018

Wu C, Bowers MT, Shea JE (2011) On the origin of the stronger binding of PIB over thioflavin T to protofibrils of the Alzheimer Amyloid-β peptide: a molecular dynamics study. Biophys J 100(5):1316–1324. https://doi.org/10.1016/j.bpj.2011.01.058

Yednock TA, Cannon C, Fritz LC, Sanchez-Madrid F, Steinman L, Karin N (1992) Prevention of experimental autoimmune encephalomyelitis by antibodies against α4β1 integrin. Nature 356(6364):63–66. https://doi.org/10.1038/356063a0

Zeydan B, Lowe VJ, Schwarz CG, Przybelski SA, Tosakulwong N, Zuk SM, Senjem ML, Gunter JL, Roberts RO, Mielke MM, Benarroch EE, Rodriguez M, Machulda MM, Lesnick TG, Knopman DS, Petersen RC, Jack CR, Kantarci K, Kantarci OH (2018) Pittsburgh compound-B PET white matter imaging and cognitive function in late multiple sclerosis. Mult Scler J 24(6):739–749. https://doi.org/10.1177/1352458517707346

PET and SPECT Imaging of Neurotoxicity

34

Erik F. J. de Vries, Rudi A. J. O. Dierckx, and Didima M. G. de Groot

Contents

E. F. J. de Vries (✉)
Nuclear Medicine and Molecular Imaging, University Medical Center Groningen, University of Groningen, Groningen, The Netherlands
e-mail: e.f.j.de.vries@umcg.nl

R. A. J. O. Dierckx
Nuclear Medicine and Molecular Imaging, University Medical Center Groningen, Groningen, The Netherlands

Department of Radiology and Nuclear Medicine, Ghent University, Ghent, Belgium
e-mail: r.a.dierckx@umcg.nl

D. M. G. de Groot
Netherlands Organization for Applied Scientific Research (TNO), Zeist, The Netherlands

Neurotoxicology|Safety Pharmacology, Stevensbeek, The Netherlands

R. A. J. O. Dierckx et al. (eds.), *PET and SPECT in Neurology*,
https://doi.org/10.1007/978-3-030-53168-3_34

Abstract

From conception until death, we are exposed to neurotoxins that can potentially induce toxic encephalopathy. Neurotoxins can cause acute adverse effects or show delayed symptoms. They can even induce impaired brain development in the offspring of exposed pregnant females. Both in patients and in animals, it can be difficult to establish the effects of toxins on the (developing) brain. Functional imaging with positron emission tomography (PET) or single-photon emission computed tomography (SPECT) could provide useful tools for preclinical testing of (developmental) neurotoxicity of potential toxic substances. These techniques could also aid clinicians in determining the damage that was done to brain functioning by exposure to a neurotoxin, and they may provide insight in the mechanisms that are involved in the intoxication. This book chapter reviews the potential applications of PET and SPECT imaging in (developmental) neurotoxicity testing and in the evaluation of functional deficits in the brain after exposure to neurotoxins.

Abbreviations

$[^{11}C]$DOPA	L-$[^{11}C]$-3,4-dihydroxyphenylalanine
$[^{18}F]$FDG	2′-$[^{18}F]$fluoro-2′-deoxyglucose
$[^{18}F]$FDOPA	L-6-$[^{18}F]$fluoro-3,4-dihydroxyphenylalanine
BBB	Blood–brain barrier
LPS	Lipopolysaccharide
MAM	Methylazoxymethanol
MPTP	1-Methyl-4-phenyl-1,2,3,6-tetrahydropyridine
MRI	Magnetic resonance imaging
PCBs	Polychlorinated biphenyls
PET	Positron emission tomography
SPECT	Single-photon emission computed tomography
TCDD	2,3,7,8-tetrachlorodibenzo-*p*-dioxin

34.1 Introduction

In our daily lives, we are continuously exposed to chemicals and toxins from the environment, medication, drinking water, and food (Prüss-Ustün et al. 2011). In most cases, exposure does not have any detrimental effect, because the human body has several defense mechanisms against potentially harmful substances. Examples of such effective protection mechanisms are the immune system and the liver that support detoxification and excretion of harmful substances. In addition to the central defense mechanisms, some critical organs have their own firewall. The brain, for example, is well protected behind the blood–brain barrier (BBB), which prevents brain entry by pathogens, particles, and large hydrophilic molecules. In addition, the BBB contains several efflux pumps that actively extrude xenobiotics from the brain (Leslie et al. 2005). These defense mechanisms, however, are not perfect. Occasionally, a toxic substance can penetrate the BBB and interfere with neurotransmission or cause damage to the brain. This can culminate in the destruction of neurons and eventually in loss of function. This process is called neurotoxicity and can be defined as the ability of substances to exert a destructive or poisonous effect upon nervous tissue. The common perception is that neurotoxicity is induced by exposure to harmful substances that originate outside the body. However, several compounds produced by our own body are also capable of inflicting brain injury. These endogenous toxic substances include glutamate, reactive oxygen species, and beta-amyloid. The production of these harmful endogenous substances and the neurotoxicity induced by them play an important role particularly in neurodegenerative diseases but also in psychiatric disorders that are associated with inflammation and/or brain atrophy. Imaging of these diseases has already been discussed in other chapters of this book series. This chapter will therefore focus only on neurotoxicity induced by exposure to exogenous substances.

34.1.1 Exposure to Neurotoxins

Whether a potentially harmful substance will actually induce neurotoxicity depends on numerous factors. The nature and importance of these factors can strongly differ between individual substances. In general, however, the dose, duration, and time window of exposure determine the severity of adverse effects (Tennekes and Sánchez-Bayo 2013). Neurotoxins can have an immediate effect after acute exposure to high levels of a hazardous compound. The cause of an acute toxic exposure can be either accidental in case of calamities or intentional, for example, as a result of a suicide attempt by a drug overdose. In case of acute exposure, the cause of neurotoxicity can easily be ascribed to a particular neurotoxin and as a result it may sometimes be possible to take specific countermeasures to reverse or reduce the (long-term) damage. In contrast to acute neurotoxicity, chronic exposure to low doses of a xenobiotic may remain asymptomatic for an extended period of time. During this latency period, brain injury accumulates until a threshold is reached and delayed symptoms of neurotoxicity become overt. At this stage, damage to the brain is often already irreversible. Some evidence indicates that neurotoxicity can even develop into neurodegenerative diseases like Alzheimer's disease and Parkinson's disease (Bartels 2011). In many cases, chronic exposure to a potential neurotoxin is unintentional, and therefore it can be difficult to correlate delayed neurotoxicity to a specific cause. Retrospective studies may give an indication of the potential culprit(s), but these studies may be prone to bias and therefore the results should be interpreted with care (Lees-Haley and Williams 1997). In some situations, the cause–effect relationship between a specific xenobiotic and neurological symptoms has been indisputably proven. A notorious example is the neurological syndrome, called Minamata disease, which is caused by methyl mercury poisoning (Ekino et al. 2007). This syndrome was first discovered in 1953 in the Minamata Bay region (Japan), where polluted industrial wastewater caused bioaccumulation of high levels of methyl mercury in fish and shellfish. The seafood was subsequently consumed by the local population, resulting in high uptake of methyl mercury. More recently, Spencer and coworkers reported evidence for a causal relationship between environmental chemicals and Western Pacific amyotrophic lateral sclerosis–Parkinson dementia (ALS–PD) complex in three genetically isolated areas (Guam, Kii, W. Papua). What these regions had in common was that the locals used cycad seed kernels for food consumption and medical care. Metabolites in the cycad seed kernels with genotoxic and neurotoxic properties like cycasin and methylazoxymethanol (MAM) appeared to cause ALS–PD (Kisby and Spencer 2011). Not only environmental pollution but also chronic occupational exposure to potentially harmful substances presents a serious risk of neurotoxicity. Workers in particular occupations (e.g., painters, industrial workers, and farmers) are frequently exposed to hazardous compounds, such as organic solvents, chemicals, pesticides, and herbicides, that potentially can be causatives of neurotoxicity (Meyer-Baron et al. 2012). Chronic exposure to harmful substances, however, can also be voluntary. Especially abuse of recreational drugs can be a potential risk factor for neurotoxicity, because of either the drug itself or contaminations in the drug. For example, long-term use of XTC was found to seriously impair brain functioning (Sarkar and Schmued 2010). Because of the addictive nature of recreational drugs, it is often difficult to convince users of the potential risk. Brain imaging in addiction will be covered by another chapter in this book series, and therefore neurotoxicity as a result of the chronic use of drugs of abuse will not be addressed in detail in this chapter.

34.1.2 Developmental Neurotoxicity

Not only the level and duration of exposure to harmful substances are important for the development of neurotoxicity, but also the specific phase in life at which the exposure occurs is a crucial factor. The brain is particularly vulnerable during development. Different brain regions have different functions and develop at different moments of time by specific processes of proliferation, migration, and differentiation. Moreover, the capacity of the blood–brain barrier to protect the brain from xenobiotics is low in the immature brain (Ek et al. 2012). Neurotoxins can not only induce direct damage to the immature brain but also interfere with normal development of the brain (Bondy and Campbell 2005). Exposure of pregnant and lactating women to chemicals, pharmaceuticals, or toxins can therefore be potentially harmful to their own brain, as well as to the development of the brain of their children. Moreover, brain development is still incomplete when a child is born. The brain continues to develop until early adulthood; brain development ends approximately at the age of 20–25 years. As a consequence, exposure to hazardous compounds presents a higher risk for (developmental) neurotoxicity to the fetus and infants than to adults. Despite the differences in vulnerability between infants and adults, existing international guidelines for toxicity testing mainly focus on exposure of adult animals and on physical malformations of the newborn after in utero exposure. However, the safety information from adults does not always adequately predict the safety profiles for pediatric groups, especially for immature systems such as the developing brain (Coecke et al. 2006).

34.1.3 Assessment of Neurotoxicity

Currently, several in vitro and in vivo methods are used to assess the neurotoxicity of a specific compound (Bull 2006). In vitro tests are usually performed on primary brain cells isolated from rodents or on cell lines, which can be of various origin. Cytotoxicity can be used as a general endpoint, but also more specific parameters, like morphology and electrophysiology, are applied (De Groot et al. 2013). Although these in vitro tests may give a first indication of the neurotoxicity potential of a specific compound, the predictive value of these assays is often limited. In vivo evaluation of neurotoxicity is usually performed in rodents, especially when referring to regulatory testing of chemicals for (developmental) neurotoxicity, although more recently the use of zebra fish embryos and larvae is explored (De Esch et al. 2012). In vivo tests in general comprise assessment of structural hallmarks by neuropathology and a series of functional tests addressing different domains of the nervous system to assess behavioral, physiological, and neurological endpoints, including impaired motor, sensory, and cognitive function. An important limitation of the behavioral tests is that they can only show symptoms of toxicity, rather than directly reveal neurotoxicity in the brain itself. As a consequence, the observed behavioral effects could as well originate from other factors than impaired brain functioning. Moreover, most behavioral tests were only validated for adult animals and may therefore not be suitable to assess *developmental* neurotoxicity. Both the behavioral tests and the proposed morphological tests are not very sensitive (De Groot et al. 2005). Besides these shortcomings, the existing neurotoxicity tests are also extremely laborious and require the sacrifice of hundreds of animals. As a result, the potential to cause detrimental effects on the (developing) brain has been investigated for only a limited number of chemicals, for example for organic solvents (De Groot 2017). For hazard identification and risk assessment of potentially harmful substances, more sensitive tests that could detect abnormalities directly in the brain would be highly advantageous (Radonjic et al. 2013).

Information about neurotoxicity in humans is scarce. Well-designed prospective studies in humans are not possible for ethical reasons. Most data originate from retrospective evaluation of accidents or incidents. Large epidemiological studies have provided relevant information on the detrimental effects of chemicals on the *developing* brain (i.e., effects in fetuses, children, and adolescents), but only for a limited number of compounds: heavy metals (lead, methylmercury, cadmium), dioxins, and dioxin-like polychlorinated biphenyls (PCBs), organochlorines (DDT/DDE/HCB), organophosphates, carbamates, and some others (bisphenol A, OH-PCBs, phthalates, flame retardants, perfluoro compounds). Epidemiological studies in humans concerning the neurotoxic potency of compounds on the developing brain are by definition long-lasting and very costly, as they involve the study of more than one generation. Supportive evidence is obtained from animal studies, which increasingly employ a combination of modern technologies like in vivo imaging, microdosing, sensor technologies, modern statistics, and various -omics.

In case of suspected neurotoxicity, a patient will first be assessed by clinical evaluation, including standard neurological examination (Bull 2006). When necessary, the examination can be extended with neuropsychological, electrophysiological, and behavioral tests. Imaging can also be added, as it enables investigation of neurotoxicity-related effects on brain structure and function in a noninvasive manner. The results of structural or functional neuroimaging investigations can be integrated with the data from the neurobehavioral evaluation to get better insight into the extent of the neurotoxicity and the affected brain structures, which can provide a better understanding of the observed symptoms.

34.1.4 Imaging of Neurotoxicity

Magnetic resonance imaging (MRI) is the most frequently applied neuroimaging technique to assess neurotoxicity. Structural MRI can provide high-resolution anatomical information about (changes in) individual brain structures. Special MRI techniques, such as BOLD, diffusion tensor imaging, and magnetic resonance spectroscopy, can also provide some insight in functional brain parameters. PET and SPECT are highly sensitive functional brain imaging techniques that are largely complementary to MRI. PET and SPECT are based on measurement of the kinetics and distribution of radiolabeled diagnostic probes (tracers) that participate in a specific biochemical or physiological process. Processes that can be monitored by PET and SPECT include receptor expression and occupancy, transporter and enzyme activity, blood flow, glucose metabolism. To measure a specific target or process of interest with PET or SPECT, a suitable tracer is required. When suitable tracers are available, PET and SPECT can not only give insight in the extent of neurodegeneration but also detect impairment of neurotransmission. Despite the potential advantages, the use of PET and SPECT in neurotoxicity assessment is still limited. In preclinical studies, toxicologists still largely rely on behavioral tests and histopathology of postmortem tissues. If neuroimaging is performed in humans, MRI is often selected as the method of choice. This chapter aims to give the reader insight in some opportunities that PET and SPECT may offer for assessment of neurotoxicity after exposure to exogenous neurotoxins. Exposure during different episodes of our lifetime, from fetus to adult, will be addressed.

34.2 Intrauterine Imaging of Exposure to Xenobiotics

34.2.1 Imaging of the Blood–Placenta Barrier

The developing fetus is connected to the outside world via the placenta, which is responsible for oxygen supply, nutrient uptake, and waste excretion. Since there is no direct intermingling between maternal and fetal blood, the placenta also serves as an efficient barrier protecting the fetus from microbes and many (but not all) xenobiotic substances. Still, maternal exposure to harmful chemicals and drugs may affect brain development of the fetus, if neurotoxins can cross the placenta and accumulate in the fetal brain. Part of the defense system of the placenta is formed by a series of efflux pumps that actively remove many harmful substances from the placenta back into the maternal blood pool (Leslie et al. 2005). One of these efflux pumps is the P-glycoprotein pump. Chung and coworkers investigated the activity of the P-glycoprotein pump in the blood–placenta barrier in pregnant macaques using PET imaging with the P-glycoprotein substrate [^{11}C]verapamil (Chung et al. 2010). The macaques were imaged twice: at day 75 (mid-gestation) and day 150 (late gestation) after conception. If P-glycoprotein in the placenta functions properly, the efflux pump prevents accumulation of the PET tracer in the fetus. Cyclosporine A is a competitive inhibitor of the P-glycoprotein pump and thus hampers the efflux of the PET tracer, resulting in an increase in tracer uptake in the fetus. In their study, Chung et al. used the cyclosporine A-induced increase in [^{11}C]verapamil uptake in the fetal liver (relative to maternal blood) as a measure for P-glycoprotein activity. At late gestation, cyclosporine induced a significantly larger increase in [^{11}C]verapamil uptake in the fetal liver than at mid-gestation, suggesting that P-glycoprotein activity was higher at late gestation. These results would implicate that at mid-gestation, the fetus is more vulnerable towards toxic compounds that are substrate of P-glycoprotein than at late gestation.

The P-glycoprotein pump in the placenta can also be affected by external factors, like infections. Wang and coworkers (Wang et al. 2005) showed that in the placenta of pregnant female rats, *mdr1a* and *mdr1b* RNA levels (encoding P-glycoprotein) were strongly downregulated 24 hours after intraperitoneal administration of the *E. coli* endotoxin lipopolysaccharide (LPS). Ex vivo biodistribution with ^{99m}Tc-sestamibi, a SPECT tracer for P-glycoprotein, confirmed the endotoxin-induced reduction in P-glycoprotein efflux activity. Four hours after tracer injection, the ratio of radioactivity concentration in the fetus to that in the placenta was 3.5-fold higher in LPS-treated rats than in saline-treated controls. LPS also caused an increased retention of the tracer in several maternal organs. The results of this study indicate that inflammation causes a suppression of P-glycoprotein activity, resulting in an increased permeability of the blood–placenta barrier for potentially harmful substances. As a consequence, maternal infection during pregnancy could lead to an increased risk of exposure of the fetus to potentially harmful neurotoxins.

34.2.2 Imaging Intrauterine Fetal Accumulation of Neurotoxins

Toxic substances may be able to penetrate the blood–placenta barrier, despite the presence of efflux pumps in the placenta. To assess the potential risk of maternal exposure to a particular substance, it would be helpful to estimate the exposure of the fetus. Therefore, it is essential to determine whether a particular compound can cross the placenta and to what extent it accumulates in the fetus. Accurate determination of fetal accumulation of a compound can be done by postmortem analysis after miscarriage or—in case of animal studies—after sacrifice of the animal. PET imaging can provide a means to measure the fetal exposure to a harmful substance in a noninvasive manner. For this purpose, it is required to radiolabel the particular compound with a PET isotope. Hartvig and coworkers provided proof of concept for this approach (Hartvig et al. 1989). To assess the transfer of drugs from the mother to the fetus, they radiolabeled [^{11}C]morphine and [^{11}C]heroin. The radiolabeled drugs were administered to pregnant rhesus monkeys, and radioactivity was measured over time in maternal blood, placenta, and fetal liver. Both drugs showed rapid accumulation in the fetus, followed by rapid washout. A noteworthy observation was that fetal plasma concentrations of [^{11}C]morphine could even exceed the maternal plasma concentration. This result would implicate that the risk for the fetus can be substantially higher than estimated based on the maternal blood levels.

Although the study by Hartvig et al. demonstrated that PET can be used to assess the intra-utero exposure of a fetus to a harmful substance, it did not specifically investigate the exposure of the fetal brain (Hartvig et al. 1989). Benveniste and coworkers injected pregnant bonnet macaques intravenously with [^{11}C]cocaine and investigated the accumulation of the tracer in the fetal brain with PET (Benveniste et al. 2005). In order to anatomically localize tracer accumulation, PET images were coregistered with the corresponding MRI images. Uptake of [^{11}C]cocaine in the fetal brain gradually increased over a period of 15–20 minutes after tracer injection. Tracer uptake in the fetal brain was slower and lower (11–22% lower distribution volume ratio) than uptake in the maternal brain. Uptake in fetal striatum was higher than that in cerebellum, reflecting the differential expression of binding sites (dopamine transporters) in these brain regions. Since PET only measures radioactivity, fetal brain uptake likely comprises a mixture of intact [^{11}C]cocaine and its metabolites. Still, this study nicely demonstrated the concomitant exposure of the fetal brain after maternal administration of the drug cocaine and thus provides supportive evidence for a causative relationship between cocaine use by pregnant women and the behavioral and cognitive deficits observed in their offspring (Buckingham-Howes et al. 2013).

Paraquat is a herbicide that has structural similarities with the neurotoxin 1-methyl-4-phenyl-1,2,3,6-tetrahydropyridine (MPTP). Paraquat has been shown to be toxic to dopaminergic cells in vitro (Gómez-Sánchez et al. 2010) and was therefore suspected to be a potential neurotoxin that could be implicated in the induction of Parkinson's disease. Bartlett and colleagues radiolabeled paraquat and used PET/CT (computed tomography) to investigate the exposure of the fetal brain to [^{11}C]paraquat in two rhesus monkeys (Bartlett et al. 2011). The CT images were used to delineate the fetal skull and subsequently to define the outline of the fetal brain. PET images at later time points showed that [^{11}C]paraquat did indeed accumulate in the fetus. However, uptake of [^{11}C]paraquat in the fetal brain was minimal (K_is 0.0016 min^{-1}) and not significantly different from uptake in the maternal brain (K_is 0.0009 min^{-1}). Thus, this imaging study suggests that prenatal exposure to the herbicide paraquat is unlikely to induce any neurotoxicity that could evolve in Parkinson's disease.

Metformin is an antidiabetic drug that has been widely used during pregnancy. Overgaard and coworkers used PET imaging with ^{11}C-labeled metformin in pregnant chinchilla to investigate the accumulation of this antidiabetic drug in the fetus (Overgaard et al. 2019). They demonstrated that [^{11}C]metformin did not accumulate in the chinchilla fetus. These results are in sharp contrast to the available evidence that indicates that the drug can readily pass the placenta in pregnant women (Charles et al. 2006). Analysis of placental mRNA, however, revealed that chinchilla and human expressed different subtypes of organic cation transporters. This family of transporters is involved in the transport of metformin across the blood–placenta barrier. These results clearly show that extrapolation of the findings from animal studies to humans should be done with extreme care.

34.2.3 Imaging Pharmacological Response to Intrauterine Fetal Exposure

The aforementioned studies demonstrated that PET can be a suitable tool to investigate the exposure of the fetal brain to a potential neurotoxin. However, a major disadvantage of the aforementioned approaches is that the toxic compound under investigation needs to be labeled with a PET isotope. This can be a time-consuming process and may not even be possible in some cases. As an alternative, a surrogate biomarker could be used to demonstrate the fetal brain exposure to a neurotoxin. Measurement of fetal brain glucose metabolism by PET with the glucose analogue 2′-[^{18}F]fluoro-2′-deoxyglucose ([^{18}F]FDG) could be an attractive approach, since this PET tracer is widely available. Benveniste and coworkers showed that [^{18}F]FDG PET could be used to assess fetal brain metabolism in pregnant bonnet macaques, if the PET images are properly coregistered with MRI images for anatomical localization (Benveniste et al. 2003). [^{18}F]FDG readily crosses the placenta and shows a distribution in the fetus that is comparable to that in adult animals. [^{18}F]FDG uptake in maternal brain was 23% higher than [^{18}F]FDG uptake in fetal brain (standardized uptake value 1.95 vs. 1.58). The [^{18}F]FDG PET approach seems feasible to investigate the in utero exposure of potential neurotoxins. In fact, the same group used [^{18}F]FDG PET to study the pharmacological effects of cocaine on brain metabolism of the fetus (Benveniste et al. 2010). Thus, pregnant bonnet macaques were intravenously (i.v.) injected with 1 mg/kg cocaine at the time of [^{18}F]FDG injection. In unchallenged control animals, brain glucose metabolism was twofold higher in the maternal brain than in the fetal brain (10.1 ± 7.6 vs. 5.1 ± 3.1 μg/100 g per minute). Exposure of the pregnant animals to cocaine increased the glucose metabolism in both maternal and fetal brains by approximately 100%. So, this study demonstrates that cocaine abuse during pregnancy can have a direct pharmacological effect on both maternal and fetal brain. This could affect the normal development of the fetal brain and result in detrimental effects in the offspring.

So far, all PET imaging studies on the accumulation of xenobiotics in the fetus have been carried out in animals, usually monkeys. An important reason for the lack of intrauterine PET imaging studies in humans is the radiation burden to the fetus that is intrinsically associated with PET imaging. A recent PET-MRI study showed that the absorbed dose to the fetus for [^{18}F]FDG PET is highly variable between subjects and is substantially higher in early pregnancies (Zanotti-Fregonara et al. 2015). Yet, the authors concluded that the absorbed dose is "below the threshold for noncancer health effects," although it remains a matter of debate whether the radiation exposure of the fetus is within acceptable limits. A potential way to overcome this hurdle is provided by the development of total-body PET (Cherry et al. 2018). The concept of this latest generation PET camera is to extend the number of detector rings in order to cover the entire body (or at least most of it). The extension of the field-of-view results in an increase in sensitivity of up to 40-fold compared to a conventional PET camera. Consequently, the injected tracer dose could be reduced 40 times, which would result in an absorbed radiation dose to the fetus that would be in the same range as other sources of radioactivity a pregnant woman is exposed to (e.g., an intercontinental flight). At such a low radiation burden, intrauterine PET imaging in humans may become feasible in the near future.

34.3 Developmental Neurotoxicity After Maternal Exposure to Xenobiotics

34.3.1 Methodology

PET can not only be used to assess the acute effect of a neurotoxin to the fetal brain, but it may also be used as a tool to evaluate the long-term effects of perinatal exposure on brain development. As PET is a noninvasive technique, it allows repetitive imaging of the same animals between birth and adulthood. Moreover, PET can measure neurotoxic effects directly in the brain and thus will likely have more statistical power than indirect methods like behavioral tests. As a consequence, implementation of PET in neurotoxicity testing paradigms may result in a strong reduction in the number of laboratory animals required. When a certain neurotoxic effect is expected, a specific process in the brain can be monitored by PET, provided that a dedicated PET tracer is available. However, in most cases the effect of a neurotoxin is not known in advance or the required PET tracer is not available. In these cases, PET imaging of a generic process that is likely affected by many neurotoxins should still be feasible. [^{18}F]FDG PET imaging can be used as a surrogate biomarker for brain glucose metabolism (and thus brain activity). As brain activity is likely to be affected by direct neurotoxicity and by inappropriate brain development, [^{18}F]FDG PET could be a valuable, generally applicable tool to assess developmental neurotoxicity. However, standardization of the imaging protocol is essential. For accurate determination of the glucose metabolism with [^{18}F]FDG PET, arterial blood sampling and pharmacokinetic modeling are required, but arterial blood sampling precludes any longitudinal studies. Moreover, conscious animals should preferably be used in these studies, because brain activity—and thus [^{18}F]FDG uptake—in awake animals is higher than in anesthetized animals. To overcome these potential hurdles, Schiffer and coworkers investigated different simplified procedures to estimate cerebral glucose metabolism in conscious animals (Schiffer et al. 2007). They developed a practical procedure that allowed good estimation of glucose metabolism in conscious animals. Thus, awake rats were intraperitoneally injected with [^{18}F]FDG. After 60 minutes of tracer distribution, animals were anesthetized and a 30-minute static scan was acquired. During the distribution time, a behavioral test can be performed. Best results are obtained if the tracer concentration in brain is corrected for radioactivity and glucose concentration in a blood sample that is taken 60 minutes after tracer injection.

34.3.2 Methylazoxymethanol

In a feasibility study, we have tested the potential of [^{18}F]FDG PET as a tool for developmental neurotoxicity testing, using the known proliferation inhibitor methylazoxymethanol (MAM) as the developmental neurotoxin (De Vries et al. 2008). Pregnant female rats were exposed to MAM (5 mg/kg body weight/day) on gestation days 13–15, which was known to cause reduced neuron numbers in brain areas under proliferation, the effects being larger at adolescent age (postnatal day [PND] 21) compared to young adult age (PND 61), suggesting a delay in structural brain development (De Groot et al. 2005). The offspring was subjected to serial [^{18}F]FDG PET imaging between postnatal days 18 and 61. On postnatal day 18, [^{18}F]FDG brain uptake was 24–32% reduced in the MAM-treated group as compared to saline-treated control animals (Fig. 34.1). Cerebral [^{18}F]FDG uptake remained lower in the MAM treatment group until day 61, although the difference between groups gradually diminished (10% reduction at day 61). Thus, in this study functional [^{18}F]FDG PET could clearly reveal a delay in structural brain development after in utero exposure of the pups to MAM. Interestingly, [^{18}F]FDG PET could already detect significant differences in brain glucose metabolism between the treatment group and the control group when only four animals per group were used, whereas a conventional open-field assay—also representing brain functioning—could not detect any significant effect in motor activity, even when ten animals per group were used. This indicates that PET could provide a more sensitive functional endpoint for developmental neurotoxicity than the behavioral test indicated by international guidelines for developmental neurotoxicity testing (OECD 2007; US EPA 1998).

34.3.3 Methylmercury

After this successful feasibility study, [^{18}F]FDG PET imaging—together with field potential analysis and microarray gene expression profiling—was

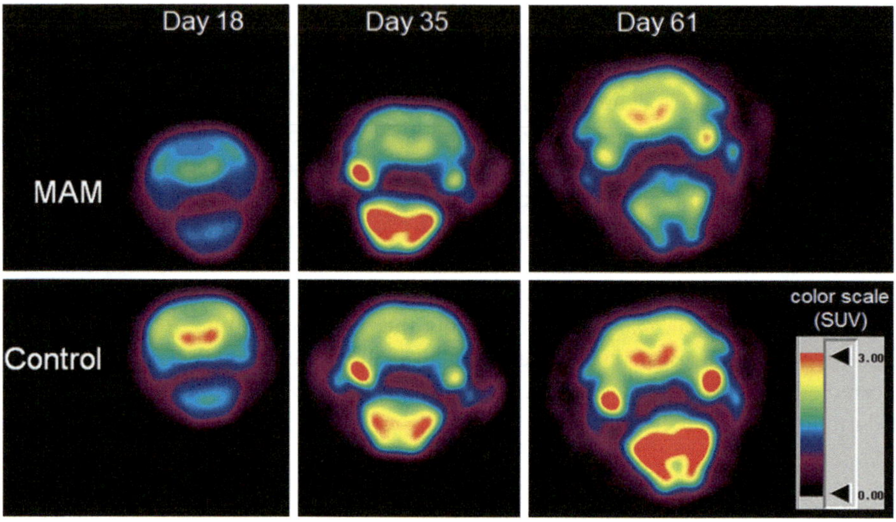

Fig. 34.1 [^{18}F]FDG PET imaging of the brain in the offspring of female rats that were exposed to methylazoxymethanol (MAM) during pregnancy. PET images were acquired between postnatal day 18 and 61. Images show a cross section of the brain that includes striatum

supplemented to a regulatory developmental toxicity study with methylmercury (according to US Environmental Protection Agency: Health Effects Test Guidelines OPPTS 870.6300 Developmental Neurotoxicity Study, EPA 712-C-98-239 1998). The aim was to investigate the added value of the imaging technique and to help unravel the mechanism of action of the neurotoxin (Radonjic et al. 2013). Four [^{18}F]FDG PET scans (postnatal days 18, 22, 37, and 61) were performed on control animals and on a group of animals that was exposed to 1.5 mg/kg methylmercury per day from gestation day 6 until lactation day 10. In the methylmercury-treated group, a trend towards a reduced glucose metabolism was observed in the hippocampus and cerebellum ($0.05 < p < 0.1$), whereas a trend towards increased tracer uptake in these brain regions was observed on day 22. On postnatal day 37, [^{18}F]FDG PET revealed significantly reduced tracer uptake in the hippocampus and cerebellum of methylmercury-treated animals as compared to healthy control animals. At day 61, the difference in tracer uptake between groups was largely diminished and—although still apparent—no longer statistically significant. Interestingly, the curves of [^{18}F]FDG uptake as a function of age (PND) had exactly the same shape, but the curve of the methylmercury-treated group was shifted by 15 days. This result suggests that maternal exposure to methylmercury induced a delay in brain development in the offspring. PET imaging data were in agreement with microarray gene expression profiling results, which also pointed towards a delayed brain development in the exposed animals. These effects were not detected by the classical tests in the developmental neurotoxicity testing guidelines, confirming the sensitivity of [^{18}F]FDG PET as a neurodevelopmental endpoint.

We have shown that this imaging methodology is widely applicable in neurotoxicity studies. Besides the aforementioned studies, we have also used the same study design to investigate developmental neurotoxicity effects of maternal and juvenile exposure to organotin compounds (De Groot et al. 2011, 2012b) and to ethanol (De Groot et al. 2012a). In both studies, [^{18}F]FDG PET could detect abnormalities in brain glucose metabolism, whereas conventional tests appeared far less sensitive or failed to show any effect of the neurotoxin. Thus, these studies strongly support the use of imaging endpoints in developmental toxicity testing.

34.4 Neurotoxicity After Adulthood Intoxication

PET and SPECT imaging have not been applied often to investigate neurotoxicity after adulthood exposure to neurotoxins; especially the number of animal studies is limited. Most studies describe the imaging findings of encephalopathy of workers after occupational intoxication, although some studies also investigated the effects of neurotoxicity after environmental exposure. The main neurotoxins involved are organic solvents and metals. The studies are in general retrospective in nature, as patients are usually studied only after the clinical diagnosis has already been established.

34.4.1 Organic Solvents

So far only a few case reports have been published on the use of [^{18}F]FDG PET for imaging the detrimental effects of chronic exposure to organic solvents, but these reports clearly show the strength of PET. Morrow and coworkers (Morrow et al. 1990) described a patient who was accidentally exposed to tetrabromoethane and experienced somatic, cognitive, and personality disorders. [^{18}F]FDG PET was performed, because neurological examination, CT, electroencephalogram (EEG), and electromyography (EMG) could not detect any abnormalities. PET showed decreased tracer uptake in the temporal and parietal cortices, basal ganglia, amygdala, and hippocampus, when compared to reference values of 24 healthy volunteers. This reduction in tracer uptake was consistent with neurobehavioral abnormalities (memory, motor function, and emotional reaction). A similar case report was published by Varney and coworkers, who performed [^{18}F]FDG PET on a worker who developed an encephalopathy after more than 750 occupational exposures to organic solvents over a period of 15 years (Varney et al. 1998). Despite multiple neurological abnormalities, findings from EEG and MRI appeared normal. Yet, the patient showed a marked reduction in brain glucose metabolism in the hippocampus and frontal and parietal cortices, even after 4 years of cessation of exposure. Both these case studies showed that [^{18}F]FDG PET can clearly identify an organic cause for neurological complaints, even when findings from EEG and MRI are normal. This could have important consequences for the workers involved, as it may help them obtain financial compensation for their work-related illness.

Solvent-induced encephalopathy has also been investigated by SPECT, which is more widely available and cheaper than PET. Hagstadius and colleagues used ^{133}Xe SPECT to measure resting state cerebral blood flow in 28 men who developed mild toxic encephalopathy after extensive exposure to organic solvents for 7–50 years and compared the results with 72 normal volunteers and with 50 male paint factory workers without complaints (Hagstadius et al. 1989). At diagnosis, the patients had significantly reduced cerebral blood flow in both hemispheres, as compared to controls. The largest reductions were observed in the prefrontal, frontotemporal, and inferior temporal regions. At follow-up after 24–84 months, the difference in cerebral blood flow was largely resolved, suggesting that some improvement in brain function occurred after cessation of exposure. Callender and coworkers investigated 33 workers who developed clinical toxic encephalopathy after exposure to a variety of neurotoxins, of which the majority was exposed to organic solvents (Callender et al. 1993). Cerebral blood flow measured with ^{99m}Tc-HMPAO SPECT showed abnormal findings in 94% (31/33) of the workers. Reduced flow was mainly observed in the frontal and temporal lobes, basal ganglia, and thalamus. The location of the abnormal cerebral blood flow was in agreement with the observed symptoms and behavioral effects. EEG and structural imaging were substantially less sensitive than SPECT, as abnormalities were observed in only 8, 7, and 29% of the patients with EEG, CT, and MRI, respectively. Neuropsychological evaluation showed abnormalities in only 79% of the patients and thus was less sensitive than SPECT as well. In two patients, both SPECT and [^{18}F]FDG PET were performed. In one patient, PET and SPECT showed the same abnormalities, whereas in the other patient, PET detected more abnormal brain regions than SPECT. These results were confirmed by Fincher et al., who used ^{99m}Tc-HMPAO SPECT to investigate cerebral blood flow in 25 subjects exposed to mixed organic solvents and 25 controls (Fincher et al. 1997). They observed reduced early phase tracer uptake in temporal, frontal, and thalamic brain regions of solvent-exposed subjects, suggestive of impaired cerebral blood flow. Taken together, these data indicate that ^{99m}Tc-HMPAO SPECT is a very sensitive tool to detect pathological effects of exposure to chemicals. [^{18}F]FDG PET might even be more sensitive, but an adequate head-to-head comparison between the two nuclear imaging techniques in a larger group of patients is still required.

Haut and colleagues used [^{15}O]water PET to measure the cerebral blood flow in six patients with toxic encephalopathy as a result of exposure to organic solvents and six age- and education-matched healthy controls (Haut et al. 2000). Since the symptoms of the patients were related to their verbal working memory, subjects were instructed to perform a verbal working memory task during the PET scan. The performance on the tasks was comparable for patients and controls. Patients showed a normal blood flow pattern in the posterior brain regions typical for the verbal working memory tasks but an abnormal blood flow pattern in the frontal lobe, which was ascribed to frontal dysfunction. Although this study nicely showed abnormal brain activation associated with a specific task, these types of studies are now largely being replaced by fMRI studies, which do not require the exposure of patients to radiation.

Measurement of metabolism and blood flow with PET or SPECT can provide general information about abnormalities that are induced by exposure to organic solvents. PET and SPECT can also give more specific information, for example, about the involvement of a specific circuitry or neurotransmitter system. Visser and coworkers investigated the frontal lobe–striatum–thalamus circuitry with SPECT, magnetic resonance spectroscopy, and diffusion tensor imaging (Visser et al. 2008). Three groups were investigated: 10 patients with chronic solvent-induced encephalopathy, 10 asymptomatic solvent-exposed house painters, and 11 nonexposed carpenters. SPECT with the tracer [^{123}I]iodobenzamide was used to measure the postsynaptic dopamine D_2 receptor binding (expressed as striatal-to-occipital uptake ratios). Remarkably, both solvent-induced encephalopathy patients and asymptomatic solvent-exposed painters showed a strong reduction in dopamine D_2 receptor binding in striatum, as compared to nonexposed controls. Dopamine D_2 receptor binding was negatively correlated with the solvent exposure index. In encephalopathy patients, but not in solvent-exposed workers, dopamine D_2 receptor binding was inversely correlated with attention and simple psychomotor speed performance. These results implicate that the striatal dopaminergic system is already affected by solvent exposure before symptoms become overt and that these effects in presymptomatic subjects can already be detected by [^{123}I]iodobenzamide SPECT. Edling and colleagues also investigated the dopaminergic system in the striatum of 17 male patients with neuropsychiatric symptoms after long-term (23 ± 8 years) occupational exposure to organic solvents (8 with and 9 without the final diagnosis toxic encephalopathy) and 11 healthy controls (Edling et al. 1997a). No presymptomatic exposed subjects were included. In this study, PET imaging with the tracers L-[^{11}C]-3,4-dihydroxyphenylalanine ([^{11}C]DOPA), [^{11}C]nomifensine, and [^{11}C]raclopride was used to evaluate dopamine synthesis, presynaptic dopaminergic terminals (more precisely presynaptic dopamine reuptake), and postsynaptic D_2 receptors, respectively. There were no differences in the striatal uptake of [^{11}C]DOPA, [^{11}C]nomifensine, or [^{11}C]raclopride between patients with or without the diagnosis toxic encephalopathy. After correction for age differences, the dopamine synthesis in patients was 25% higher than that in healthy controls. The number of presynaptic dopaminergic nerve terminals was not affected in patients. Unfortunately, the paper did not report any comparison of the postsynaptic D_2 receptors between patients and controls. However, when the results of these studies are combined, one could speculate that exposure to organic solvents results in a downregulation in postsynaptic D_2 receptor expression, or a reduction of D_2 receptor affinity, which causes an increase in dopamine production as a compensatory response.

Caseni and coworkers investigated dopamine transporter density in striatum of Parkinson patients with a history of exposure to hydrocarbon solvents, nonexposed Parkinson patients and controls using [^{123}I]Ioflupane SPECT (Canesi et al. 2007). Patients in the exposed group were subjected to exposure to solvents for more than 10 hours per week for at least 10 years. Both groups of Parkinson patients showed striatal tracer uptake well below that in healthy controls. In Parkinson patients chronically exposed to hydrocarbon solvents, the uptake of [^{123}I]Ioflupane in striatum was significantly more reduced than in nonexposed patients. The decrease in tracer binding was greater in putamen than in caudate. This study shows that occupational exposure to organic solvents results in an increased decrease in dopamine transporter density in striatum of Parkinson patients.

Edling et al. also investigated the acute effect of short-term exposure to toluene on dopamine synthesis and presynaptic dopaminergic nerve terminals (Edling et al. 1997b). Eleven male healthy volunteers were exposed to 100 ppm toluene while performing light exercise (pedaling on a bicycle ergometer at a workload of 50 W). [^{11}C]DOPA and [^{11}C]nomifensine PET were performed before and immediately after the acute exposure to toluene. None of the tracers showed any significant differences between baseline and postexposure PET scans. Thus, it was concluded that short exposure to toluene does not have an acute effect on dopamine synthesis or the number of presynaptic dopaminergic nerve terminals. Schiffer and coworkers used [^{18}F]FDG PET to study both the acute and long-term effects of toluene on brain metabolism in rats (Schiffer et al. 2006). Thus, adolescent rats were six times exposed to 5000 ppm toluene for 30 minutes on every other day. [^{18}F]FDG PET scans of the brain were made at baseline and 2 hours, 24 hours, 3 weeks, and 2 months after the last exposure. Tracer injection and distribution occurred in conscious animals. Toluene immediately induced a significant reduction in [^{18}F]FDG uptake (−21%) in all brain regions, although more pronounced in the subcortical regions. Abnormalities in tracer uptake were in agreement with the known distribution of toluene in the brain. The reduction in tracer uptake persisted throughout the experiment (−39%), although some recovery was observed after 2 months (−31%). The recovery was stronger in thalamus, hippocampus, and midbrain than in the cortical regions.

Airas and coworkers reported the use of L-6-[^{18}F]fluoro-3,4-dihydroxyphenylalanine ([^{18}F]FDOPA) PET in a case of methanol intoxication (Airas et al. 2008). The patient had consumed two cups of windshield washer containing methanol and developed blindness and severe extrapyramidal symptoms, such as hypokinesia and rigidity. [^{18}F]FDOPA PET was acquired 3.5 months after the intoxication and showed strongly reduced tracer uptake in striatum (putamen −60%; caudate −40%), indicating severely impaired dopamine synthesis. PET was in accordance with MRI findings that revealed substantial necrosis in the putamen. These results point towards severely injured dopaminergic neurostriatal neurons, causing the extrapyramidal symptoms in this patient. The patient responded well on treatment with L-DOPA.

Taken together, these studies indicate that PET and SPECT imaging can play an important role in identifying neurotoxic effects that are induced by exposure to organic solvents. In fact, PET and SPECT appear more sensitive than EEG and structural imaging with CT and MRI. Despite wide variability in exposure, most studies indicate that predominantly the frontal and temporal cortical regions and the dopaminergic system are affected by organic solvents. In general, imaging findings could well explain the neurobehavioral effects.

34.4.2 Metals

34.4.2.1 Manganese

Several studies have been published on the use of PET or SPECT for imaging of neurotoxicity after exposure to manganese dust. Manganese intoxication can lead to extrapyramidal symptoms that might mimic Parkinsonism.

Wooten and coworkers investigated the biodistribution and pharmacokinetics of manganese(II) in mice after intravenous injection or inhalation of a [^{52}Mn]manganese chloride solution (Wooten et al. 2017). Ex vivo analysis and PET imaging showed that substantial amounts of manganese accumulate inside the brain after both intravenous injection and inhalation of aerosols (0.9% ID/g and 0.3% ID/g after 24 hours, respectively). These results demonstrate that manganese salts can indeed cross the blood–brain barrier and may support findings of manganese-induced neurotoxicity.

Wolters et al. investigated dopamine synthesis and cerebral glucose metabolism in four workers exposed to manganese, using [^{18}F]FDOPA PET and [^{18}F]FDG PET, respectively (Wolters et al. 1989). [^{18}F]FDOPA PET did not show any abnormalities in striatal dopamine synthesis, whereas [^{18}F]FDG PET revealed a reduction in cortical glucose metabolism. In another study, four patients with Parkinsonian symptoms after chronic occupational exposure to manganese dust received both a [^{11}C]raclopride and a [^{18}F]FDOPA PET scan (Shinotoh et al. 1997). [^{18}F]FDOPA PET was normal in all patients, indicating normal presynaptic dopamine synthesis. In contrast, [^{11}C]raclopride PET showed reduced postsynaptic dopamine D_2 receptor binding in caudate (−12%) and putamen (−11%), although this effect was only statistically significant for caudate. The patients in this study did not respond to treatment with L-DOPA, which is in agreement with the observation that manganese causes postsynaptic damage. These results were partly confirmed by studies in monkeys (Shinotoh et al. 1995). [^{18}F]FDOPA, [^{11}C]raclopride, and [^{18}F]FDG PET were performed on three rhesus monkeys that were exposed to manganese by seven intravenous injections of 10–14 mg/kg $MnCl_2$. [^{18}F]FDOPA PET did not show any abnormalities, indicating that dopamine synthesis is not affected. [^{11}C]raclopride uptake in striatum was slightly reduced in one out of three animals 4 days after the last manganese administration, but returned to normal levels 4 days later. In contrast to the study by Wolters, [^{18}F]FDG PET did not reveal any effects on glucose metabolism in striatum or cerebral cortex in these monkeys, which could be ascribed to the shorter duration of the exposure to manganese. A subsequent study in these rhesus monkeys showed that animals that develop Parkinsonian symptoms after manganese intoxication do not respond to L-DOPA (Olanow et al. 1996), as was also observed in patients. Autopsy revealed gliosis in globus pallidus and substantia nigra pars reticularis, whereas the dopaminergic nigrostriatal system remains unaffected. Taken together, these studies show that the mild Parkinsonian symptoms induced by manganese intoxication in humans and monkeys are likely mainly due to downstream effects in the nigrostriatal pathway.

Despite similarities in clinical presentation of patients with chronic manganese intoxication and patients with idiopathic Parkinsonism, imaging can be used in the differential diagnosis between the two pathologies, as was nicely shown in two case reports by Kim and coworkers (Kim et al. 1998). The first case was a worker who was occupationally exposed to manganese in the production of welding rods and presented with Parkinsonian features. [^{18}F]FDOPA PET showed normal uptake in striatum and it was concluded that this patient suffered from manganese-induced Parkinsonism, rather than from idiopathic Parkinsonism (Kim et al. 1998). The second case consisted of a welder who also presented Parkinsonian features. Because of suspected chronic manganese intoxication, [^{18}F]FDOPA PET was performed. PET images showed reduced tracer uptake in left putamen, indicating presynaptic damage. It was therefore concluded that this patient had idiopathic Parkinsonism (Kim et al. 1999).

With the availability of newer generation PET-CT systems with better resolution, the effects of manganese intoxication on subregions of the presynaptic dopaminergic system have also been evaluated. Criswell et al. performed [^{18}F]FDOPA PET in 20 asymptomatic welders exposed to manganese fumes and compared them with 20 idiopathic Parkinson patients and 20 healthy controls (Criswell et al. 2011). They observed a small, but significant reduction in [^{18}F]FDOPA consumption in the caudate of welders when compared to controls. In asymptomatic welders, caudate was more affected than anterior putamen, which was in turn more affected than posterior putamen. Interestingly, this regional pattern of reduced [^{18}F]FDOPA uptake was distinct from Parkinson patients, in which the reversed order was observed. Thus, the authors suggested that reduced [^{18}F]FDOPA uptake in caudate may be an early marker of manganese neurotoxicity. In a subsequent publication, the same group investigated presynaptic striatal [^{18}F]FDOPA uptake in 27 manganese-exposed welders, 14 other manganese exposed workers, and 31 nonexposed controls (Criswell et al. 2018a). Both manganese-exposed groups showed lower [^{18}F]FDOPA uptake in caudate than controls. However, the reduced [^{18}F]FDOPA uptake in caudate was not associated with the manganese exposure dose or with clinical Parkinsonism symptoms, according to the Unified Parkinson Disease Rating Scale motor subscore 3 (UPDRS3).

Huang et al. used PET imaging with the type 2 vesicle monoamine transporter ligand [^{18}F]FP-(+)-DTBZ to investigate presynaptic dopaminergic dysfunction in four manganism patients, eight Parkinson patients, and eight healthy controls (Huang et al. 2015). PET Imaging indicated that nigrostriatal tracer uptake was reduced in Parkinson patients, but not in chronic manganism patients, indicating that presynaptic neurons in striatum are not degenerated in patients suffering from manganese exposure.

Huang and colleagues investigated the integrity of the presynaptic dopamine transporter function with ^{99m}Tc-TRODAT-1 SPECT in 4 patients with manganese-induced Parkinsonian features, 12 patients with Parkinson's disease, and 12 healthy controls (Huang et al. 2003). The ^{99m}Tc-TRODAT-1 uptake in putamen was only mildly reduced in manganese-exposed patients, as compared to healthy controls, whereas the uptake in caudate and total striatum was not significantly affected. In contrast, both caudate and putamen were strongly affected in patients with Parkinson's disease, who had much lower tracer uptake in total striatum and in caudate and putamen individually, as compared to manganese-exposed patients. This study demonstrated that presynaptic dopamine transporter activity is strongly reduced in Parkinson's disease but remains largely unaffected after chronic manganese exposure, thus confirming the results of [^{18}F]FDOPA PET studies. Therefore, the authors suggest that ^{99m}Tc-TRODAT-1 SPECT could be a relatively cheap and reliable tool to discriminate Parkinson's disease from manganese-induced neurotoxicity.

Criswell et al. also investigated the postsynaptic D2 receptor density in manganese-exposed welders and other workers using PET with the tracer *N*-[^{11}C]methylbenperidol (Criswell et al. 2018b). This tracer is insensitive to variation in dopamine level, as it cannot be displaced by the endogenous ligand. After correction for age, the binding potential of *N*-[^{11}C]methylbenperidol in substantia nigra was significantly greater in manganese-exposed workers than in nonexposed controls. Tracer binding in substantia nigra increased with increasing duration of manganese exposure and UPDRS3 score. These results suggest that D2 receptors in substantia nigra are involved in manganese-induced Parkinsonism.

34.4.2.2 Thallium

Acute thallium poisoning can cause polyneuropathy that is associated with myelin damage and axonal degeneration (Kuo et al. 2005). Recently, [^{18}F]FDG PET was applied to investigate cerebral glucose metabolism in two patients with acute thallium poisoning via the drinking water (Liu et al. 2013). Both patients showed severe cognitive impairment, which partially recovered during the 18-month follow-up. [^{18}F]FDG PET at month 5 (patient 1) and month 2 (patient 2) after intoxication showed a marked reduction in glucose metabolism in the cingulate gyrus and frontal and parietal lobes, as compared to healthy controls. Patient 2 received a follow-up scan 2 months after the first scan, showing partial recovery of the abnormalities in glucose metabolism. In contrast to PET, structural MRI did not reveal any abnormalities.

34.4.2.3 Arsenic

In the Japanese city of Kamisu, many inhabitants were intoxicated with diphenylarsinic acid by drinking water from a contaminated well. Diphenylarsinic intoxication mainly caused cerebellar and brainstem symptoms, such as ataxic gait, titubation, scanning speech, and tremors, but in some subjects also cerebral symptoms such as insomnia, visual and memory impairment (Ishii et al. 2004). To investigate diphenylarsinic acid-induced neurotoxicity, cerebral blood flow was assessed with *N*-isopropyl-*p*-[^{123}I]iodoamphetamine SPECT in 35 symptomatic and 43 asymptomatic subjects drinking contaminated well water for at least 1 year and 38 in healthy controls (Ishii et al. 2019). The asymptomatic group did not show any significant differences in cerebral blood flow, when compared to healthy controls. However, symptomatic exposed subjects revealed a significant reduction in cerebral blood flow in inferior occipital gyrus and cuneus as compared to healthy controls, and significantly lower cerebral blood flow in superior frontal gyrus as compared to the asymptomatic group. Moreover, cerebral blood flow in inferior occipital gyrus was negatively correlated with diphenylarsinic acid concentrations in hair and nails. This study was nicely able to link exposure to an environmental poison to adverse physiological effects in the brain, in particular reduced blood flow in the occipital lobe.

34.4.2.4 Mercury

Chronic exposure to metallic mercury can cause neurological symptoms like ataxia, tremor, coordination problems, and memory impairment (Bose-O'Reilly et al. 2017). Since these symptoms are also observed in Parkinson's disease, Lin and coworkers used ^{99m}Tc-TRODAT SPECT to investigate dopamine transporter concentrations in lamp factory workers who were exposed to mercury vapors and age- and gender-matched controls (Lin et al. 2011). ^{99m}Tc-TRODAT SPECT revealed a moderate but significant negative correlation between mercury levels in urine and the tracer uptake in striatum, caudate, and putamen. Cumulative mercury exposure was also negatively correlated with ^{99m}Tc-TRODAT uptake in striatum and caudate. Consequently, mercury-exposed workers exhibited significantly lower ^{99m}Tc-TRODAT uptake in striatum, caudate, and putamen than age-matched controls. Yet, the mercury-exposed workers did not show any clinical manifestation of Parkinsonism yet. These results suggest that ^{99m}Tc-TRODAT SPECT could provide an early indicator for mercury-induced neurotoxicity.

34.4.3 Pesticides

Pesticides, such as paraquat, rotenone, and maneb, have been associated with neurotoxicity and increased risk of Parkinson's disease. In fact, these pesticides were shown to cause degeneration of dopaminergic neurons in animals and were therefore used to generate animal models for Parkinson's disease (Uversky 2004). To investigate whether similar effects could be found in humans, Lewis et al. studied the integrity of striatal dopaminergic terminals in agricultural workers exposed to these pesticides by assessing dopamine transporter density with [^{123}I]ioflupane SPECT (Lewis et al. 2017). [^{123}I]ioflupane SPECT, however, did not reveal any significant difference in dopamine transporter binding in any striatal subregion between controls, low- and high-exposure agricultural workers. Dopamine transporter binding also did not correlate with the days of pesticide exposure. This study therefore could not demonstrate any degenerative effect of pesticide exposure on dopaminergic neurons in humans.

Another group of pesticides that are associated with neurotoxicity are organophosphates, such as glyphosate ("Roundup") and diisopropylfluorophosphate. Intoxication with these organophosphates can lead to inhibition of acetylcholinesterase and cause convulsions, recurrent seizures, affective disorders, and cognitive deficits (Glusczak et al. 2006; Chen 2012). Flannery and coworkers longitudinally investigated the neuroinflammatory response after acute intoxication of adult rats with [^{11}C]PK11195 PET (Flannery et al. 2016). The PET tracer [^{11}C]PK11195 binds to the 18-kDa mitochondrial membrane translocator protein, which is overexpressed on activated microglia, the resident macrophages of the brain. PET imaging showed an increased uptake of [^{11}C]PK11195 in animals that were exposed to diisopropylfluorophosphate. The increase in tracer uptake was highest on day 7, but some increased uptake was still present on day 21 after exposure. These results indicate that the pesticide induced persistent inflammatory response in the brain. Interestingly, the three animals with least severe seizures in this study did not show this temporal pattern of increased [^{11}C]PK11195 uptake in the PET images, indicating that neuroinflammation is positively correlated with seizure severity. However, PET imaging results did not correlate with cognitive impairment, suggesting that the observed cognitive impairment is not dependent on the diisopropylfluorophosphate-induced neuroinflammatory response.

34.4.4 Dioxins and PCBs

Dioxins and polychlorinated biphenyls (PCBs) are members of the family of polychlorinated aromatic hydrocarbons. Dioxins and PCBs are side products of the incomplete burning of waste containing chlorinated organic compounds. Dioxins are also formed in forest fires and volcanic eruptions, whereas PCBs have also been produced for industrial applications. Dioxins and PCBs are persistent in the environment and accumulate in the food chain. Human exposure occurs mainly via consumption of fatty food, especially meat, fish, dairy products, and eggs. Dioxins and PCB have been associated with a wide range of toxic effects, including immune toxicity, carcinogenicity, and developmental toxicity (Larsen 2006). Whether these compounds also induce neurotoxicity is a matter of discussion. To gain more insight in the effect of dioxins on the brain, Urban and coworkers performed ^{99m}Tc-ECD SPECT to assess abnormalities in cerebral blood flow in a cohort of 15 workers who were accidentally exposed to 2,3,7,8-tetrachlorodibenzo-*p*-dioxin (TCDD) in a chemical plant 35 years before (Urban et al. 2007). Nine of these patients showed signs of polyneuropathy and had more than 2× higher TCDD plasma concentrations than the other exposed subjects. Yet, SPECT showed abnormalities in cerebral blood flow in 14 of 15 patients, of which 4 had unilateral and 10 had bilateral foci of reduced cerebral blood flow. Patients had on average 2.5 perfusion defects, which were predominantly located in the region of the middle cerebral artery. In a follow-up study, the last eight survivors of this cohort were investigated again 50 years after the exposure to TCDD (Pelclova et al. 2018). All subjects showed impairment in neurological tests, and four subjects showed clinical signs of polyneuropathy and two subjects of mononeuropathy in the upper extremities. ^{99m}Tc-HMPAO SPECT revealed foci with decreased cerebral blood flow in both hemispheres in all patients. In six out of eight patients the cerebral blood flow defects had worsened since the previous follow-up 6 years before. These data suggest that the dioxin TCDD can induce chronic and progressive damage that is still measurable with SPECT 50 years after the fact.

On the basis of the results of preclinical studies, Seegal and coworkers hypothesized that PCBs could have a detrimental effect on the dopaminergic system in the brain. Therefore, they performed [^{123}I]β-CIT SPECT scans to assess the dopamine transporter density in a group of 89 workers who were occupationally exposed to PCBs in a capacitor factory (Seegal et al. 2010). SPECT showed that striatal dopamine transporter density was inversely correlated with serum PCB concentrations in women, whereas no such correlation was observed in men. Similar correlations were observed in caudate and putamen, independent of the subclass of PCBs subjects were exposed to. All women in this study were postmenopausal and the authors suggest that the gender difference observed in this study could be due to the fact the women have lost the neuroprotective effect of estrogens after menopause. These findings stress the need to take gender into consideration when exploring the effect of environmental factors on the brain.

34.5 Neurotoxicity in Suicide Survivors

34.5.1 Cyanide

A few case reports have been published that describe PET imaging of neurotoxicity in survivors of suicide attempts. A case report described the use of PET imaging of a survivor of a suicide attempt by ingestion of 1.5 g of potassium cyanide (Rosenberg et al. 1989). After treatment, the patient developed a severe Parkinsonian syndrome. MRI and PET imaging demonstrated that cyanide intoxication caused severe injury to dopaminergic neurons. [^{18}F]FDOPA PET showed reduced tracer uptake in striatum, indicating that dopamine synthesis is impaired, as is also observed in patients with Parkinson's disease. These results were in agreement with another case report, in which postmortem analysis of the brains of a survivor of a suicide attempt with cyanide showed major destruction of globus pallidus and putamen (Uitti et al. 1985). Zaknun et al. described the case of a 35-year-old woman who survived the ingestion of a lethal dose of potassium cyanide (Zaknun et al. 2005). ^{99m}Tc-HMPAO SPECT revealed reduced perfusion in frontal and striatal brain regions 9 days after intoxication and an additional perfusion defect in the precentral cortex after 7 weeks. [^{123}I]β-CIT SPECT showed reduced uptake in striatum on day 18 and a further reduction on day 54 after cyanide intoxication. [^{18}F]FDG PET showed reduced glucose metabolism, especially in striatum, frontal and anterior temporal lobes 19 days after cyanide ingestion. In line with these findings, another case report described a 20-year-old male surviving a suicide attempt with cyanide, who developed Parkinsonian syndrome (Sarikaya et al. 2006). [^{18}F]FDG PET of this patient revealed virtually no tracer uptake in putamen and reduced uptake in caudate and cerebellum. Taken together, the imaging findings in these case reports indicate that cyanide intoxication causes progressive degeneration of presynaptic nigrostriatal dopaminergic nerve terminals, which could be accompanied by frontal and cerebellar hypometabolism and/or hypoperfusion.

34.5.2 Carbon Monoxide

Carbon monoxide intoxication is a frequently applied suicide method. In Taiwan and Hong Kong, the number of suicides by inhalation of burning charcoal gasses, resulting in carbon monoxide poisoning, is strongly increasing since 1998 (Liu et al. 2007). A substantial fraction (10–30%) of the patients who were intoxicated with carbon monoxide develops delayed neuropsychiatric problems. Since the neuropsychiatric symptoms of carbon monoxide intoxication can resemble those of Parkinson's disease, Yang and coworkers hypothesized that the nigrostriatal dopaminergic neurons are more affected in patients with delayed neuropsychological abnormalities. Therefore, they used ^{99m}Tc-TRODAT SPECT to assess the striatal dopamine transporter density in 27 charcoal burning suicide patients (Yang et al. 2011). SPECT showed that dopamine transporter binding was lower in striatum of patients with neuropsychiatric symptoms than in patients without symptoms. Interestingly, when the initial loss of consciousness was included as a variable, the predictive value of dopamine transporter binding for neuropsychiatric effects was largely increased. In a subsequent study by the same group, ^{99m}Tc-TRODAT SPECT was performed in the first week after carbon monoxide intoxication and again 6 months later (Yang et al. 2015). Striatal dopamine transporter binding at baseline and after 6 months' follow-up was significantly lower in carbon monoxide poisoning patients than in healthy controls. There was no significant difference between baseline and follow-up SPECT, indicating that striatal degeneration did not progress any further after the acute intoxication phase. Changes in striatal dopamine transporter binding between baseline and follow-up were found to positively correlate with scores on the Wisconsin Card Sorting Test, a test for executive function.

Chen et al. analyzed networks of neurodegeneration with MRI and [^{18}F]FDG PET in 49 suicide survivors exposed to carbon monoxide by charcoal burning and 15 age-matched controls (Chen et al. 2015). [^{18}F]FDG PET demonstrated a pattern of hypometabolism in anterior brain regions, including prefrontal, cingulate, insular and temporal regions, caudate, and thalamus. These regions largely overlapped with gray matter atrophy as detected by MRI. The metabolic rate defects were more severe and extended for patients with higher clinical dementia rating scores. [^{18}F]FDG uptake in the orbital–frontal and dorsolateral prefrontal regions, anterior insular, temporal–parietal, and posterior cingulate cortex was significantly correlated with the Mini-Mental State Examination scores. Verbal memory learning, Stroop test, digit backward, and clinical dementia rating sum of box scores were also correlated with [^{18}F]FDG uptake in inferior and lateral frontal regions. These results indicate that carbon monoxide intoxication caused a specific degeneration pattern mainly in anterior brain regions that is associated with cognitive impairment in neuropsychological tests.

34.5.3 Pesticides

Wang et al. reported the imaging findings of two patients who were intoxicated with organophosphates, resulting in blindness of the patients (Wang et al. 1999). One patient tried to commit suicide by drinking a bottle of insecticide (Phosdrin R); the other patient was attacked by her boyfriend and injected with another insecticide (*O*-ethyl-*O*-nitrophenyl phenylphosphonate). In both patients, the finding from MRI of the visual areas was normal. In contrast, PET showed decreased glucose metabolism in the visual cortex areas in both patients and thus provided an organic cause for their blindness.

Mittal and coworkers investigated the cerebral blood flow in patients acutely exposed to organophosphate (chlorpyrifos, dichlorvos, phorate) poisoning, either by ingestion due to a suicide attempt ($n = 17$) or by accidental exposure due to a spraying accident ($n = 11$). ^{99m}Tc-ECD SPECT were acquired between days 5 and 13 after admission and revealed abnormal cerebral blood flow in 96% of the patients (Mittal et al. 2011). More perfusion defects were observed in men than in women and blood flow deficits were most common in the occipital lobes. However, abnormal cerebral blood flow observed by SPECT could not predict cognitive decline, as blood flow deficits did not correlate with neurocognitive dysfunction, either in the admission phase or at 3 months' follow-up.

34.5.4 Drug Overdose

Recently, a case report was published that described the use of [^{18}F]FDG PET in a survivor of a suicide attempt with an overdose of the antidepressant fluoxetine (Szólics et al. 2012). An overdose of the selective serotonin reuptake inhibitor fluoxetine (Prozac) causes serotonin toxicity, resulting in necrosis in the globus pallidus and white matter ischemia, was observed by MRI. [^{18}F]FDG PET was performed 37 years after the suicide attempt, but still showed reduced tracer uptake in the frontal, temporal, and parietal cortices and caudate.

Thus, these reports show that PET can provide sensitive functional information about the brain regions that are affected by the neurotoxin, even a long time after exposure. This information may help the clinician explain the neurobehavioral abnormalities of the patient.

34.6 Concluding Remarks

Neurotoxicity has long been a research area primarily for neurologists, pathologists, and toxicologists. Imaging of neurotoxicity has mainly been restricted to evaluation of structural abnormalities by MRI or CT. So far, the role of nuclear medicine in this field has been limited. Still, several studies have demonstrated the potential of PET and SPECT imaging. Since prospective clinical trials on the potential neurotoxicity of agents are ethically unacceptable, the neurotoxic effect of compounds is generally tested in animals, if at all. In preclinical studies, PET and SPECT seem to be especially attractive for evaluation of the developmental neurotoxicity effects of potential neurotoxins. Not only can PET be applied to assess the intrauterine exposure of a fetus to a neurotoxin, but PET also promises to be a very sensitive endpoint for developmental neurotoxicity testing. Several studies have already shown that [^{18}F]FDG PET can detect functional brain abnormalities after pre- or perinatal exposure to a toxin, when standard tests according to international guidelines for toxicity testing fail to show any effect. Because of its noninvasive nature, PET allows longitudinal testing, which, in addition to the high sensitivity of the technique, can result in a strong reduction of the number of animals required for the evaluation of the developmental neurotoxic potency of a substance. Because of the potential reduction in animals and workload, PET may even be cost-effective. The clinical application of PET and SPECT has mainly remained restricted to retrospective evaluation of patients who developed neurological symptoms after occupational, environmental, or accidental exposure to neurotoxins, mainly organic solvents and heavy metals, and to survivors of suicide attempts. Most studies show that PET and SPECT can detect functional abnormalities, even when EEG, CT, and MRI are normal. Thus, PET and SPECT are often able to detect an organic cause where other modalities fail. For patients, this can be of great importance when disputes on establishing the cause of the disorder and financial compensation are involved. Furthermore, functional PET and SPECT imaging can help to elucidate the extent of the encephalopathy and the mechanism responsible for intoxication-induced pathology. For mechanistic studies, back-translation to animal studies using functional imaging can provide additional information or confirmation of clinical results. So, functional imaging can help the clinician to better understand the cognitive, behavioral, and functional deficits of the patient. In some particular cases, PET and SPECT imaging can even provide a useful tool for the differential diagnosis between toxic encephalopathy and neurodegenerative diseases, as was nicely demonstrated for manganese intoxication and Parkinson's disease. Despite the potential of PET and SPECT imaging of neurotoxicity, the supporting evidence for the application of these imaging techniques in the clinic is still limited and mainly restricted to case reports and studies on small patient samples. Ideally, large clinical trials should be performed to establish the added value of PET and SPECT. However, this will be extremely difficult, since the number of patients who are acutely or chronically exposed to a particular neurotoxic substance and develop neurological deficits is fortunately very low, due to increasingly strict regulations.

Innovative technologies like microdosing in combination with PET or SPECT imaging may play an important role in the near future to explore the toxic potential of new medicines, as the effect of very low dosages of a compound in individual subjects can be measured in a very sensitive way. Combinations of imaging and -omics in such studies are very promising as they can help to unravel underlying neurotoxicity pathways which, in turn, will support the translation of results from animal to human and vice versa. A significant role for PET and SPECT in the science of (developmental) neurotoxicology seems warranted.

References

Airas L, Paavilainen T, Marttila RJ, Rinne J (2008) Methanol intoxication-induced nigrostriatal dysfunction detected using 6-[^{18}F]fluoro-L-dopa PET. Neurotoxicology 29:671–674

Bartels AL (2011) Blood-brain barrier P-glycoprotein function in neurodegenerative disease. Curr Pharm Des 17:2771–2777

Bartlett RM, Murali D, Nickles RJ, Barnhart TE, Holden JE, DeJesus OT (2011) Assessment of fetal brain uptake of paraquat in utero using in vivo PET/CT imaging. Toxicol Sci 122:551–556
Benveniste H, Fowler JS, Rooney WD, Moller DH, Backus WW, Warner DA, Carter P, King P, Scharf B, Alexoff DA, Ma Y, Vaska P, Schlyer D, Volkow ND (2003) Maternal-fetal in vivo imaging: a combined PET and MRI study. J Nucl Med 44:1522–1530
Benveniste H, Fowler JS, Rooney W, Ding YS, Baumann AL, Moller DH, Du C, Backus W, Logan J, Carter P, Coplan JD, Biegon A, Rosenblum L, Scharf B, Gatley JS, Volkow ND (2005) Maternal and fetal ^{11}C-cocaine uptake and kinetics measured in vivo by combined PET and MRI in pregnant nonhuman primates. J Nucl Med 46:312–320
Benveniste H, Fowler JS, Rooney WD, Scharf BA, Backus WW, Izrailtyan I, Knudsen GM, Hasselbalch SG, Volkow ND (2010) Cocaine is pharmacologically active in the nonhuman primate fetal brain. Proc Natl Acad Sci U S A 107:1582–1587
Bondy SC, Campbell A (2005) Developmental neurotoxicology. J Neurosci Res 81:605–612
Bose-O'Reilly S, Bernaudat L, Siebert U, Roider G, Nowak D, Drasch G (2017) Signs and symptoms of mercury-exposed gold miners. Int J Occup Med Environ Health 30:249–269
Buckingham-Howes S, Berger SS, Scaletti LA, Black MM (2013) Systematic review of prenatal cocaine exposure and adolescent development. Pediatrics 131:e1917–e1936
Bull S (2006) Review of environmental chemicals and toxicity. Focus on neurological diseases. Health Protection Agency publication HPA-ChaPD-001. http://www.hpa.org.uk/webc/HPAwebFile/HPAweb_C/1194947320712
Callender TJ, Morrow L, Subramanian K, Duhon D, Ristovv M (1993) Three-dimensional brain metabolic imaging in patients with toxic encephalopathy. Environ Res 60:295–319
Canesi M, Benti R, Marotta G, Cilia R, Isaias IU, Gerundini P, Pezzoli G, Antonini A (2007) Striatal dopamine transporter binding in patients with Parkinson's disease and severe occupational hydrocarbon exposure. Eur J Neurol 14:297–299
Charles B, Norris R, Xiao X, Hague W (2006) Population pharmacokinetics of metformin in late pregnancy. Ther Drug Monit 28:67–72
Chen Y (2012) Organophosphate-induced brain damage: mechanisms, neuropsychiatric and neurological consequences, and potential therapeutic strategies. Neurotoxicology 33:391–400
Chen NC, Huang CW, Huang SH, Chang WN, Chang YT, Lui CC, Lin PH, Lee CC, Chang YH, Chang CC (2015) Cognitive severity-specific neuronal degenerative network in charcoal burning suicide-related carbon monoxide intoxication: a multimodality neuroimaging study in Taiwan. Medicine (Baltimore) 94:e783
Cherry SR, Jones T, Karp JS, Qi J, Moses WW, Badawi RD (2018) Total-body PET: maximizing sensitivity to create new opportunities for clinical research and patient care. J Nucl Med 59:3–12
Chung FS, Eyal S, Muzi M, Link JM, Mankoff DA, Kaddoumi A, O'Sullivan F, Hsiao P, Unadkat JD (2010) Positron emission tomography imaging of tissue P-glycoprotein activity during pregnancy in the non-human primate. Br J Pharmacol 159:394–404
Coecke S, Eskes C, Gartlon J, Kinsner A, Price A, Van Vliet E, Prieto P, Boveri M, Bremer S, Adler S, Pellizzer C, Wendel A, Hartung T (2006) The value of alternative testing for neurotoxicity in the context of regulatory needs. Environ Toxicol Pharmacol 21:153–167
Criswell SR, Perlmutter JS, Videen TO, Moerlein SM, Flores HP, Birke AM, Racette BA (2011) Reduced uptake of [^{18}F]FDOPA PET in asymptomatic welders with occupational manganese exposure. Neurology 76:1296–1301
Criswell SR, Nielsen SS, Warden M, Perlmutter JS, Moerlein SM, Flores HP, Huang J, Sheppard L, Seixas N, Checkoway H, Racette BA (2018a) [^{18}F]FDOPA positron emission tomography in manganese-exposed workers. Neurotoxicology 64:43–49
Criswell SR, Warden MN, Searles Nielsen S, Perlmutter JS, Moerlein SM, Sheppard L, Lenox-Krug J, Checkoway H, Racette BA (2018b) Selective D2 receptor PET in manganese-exposed workers. Neurology 91:e1022–e1030
De Esch C, Slieker R, Wolterbeek A, Woutersen R, De Groot DM (2012) Zebrafish as potential model for developmental neurotoxicity testing: a mini review. Neurotoxicol Teratol 34:545–553
De Groot DMG (2017) Scientific review on the link between the narcotic effects of solvents and (developmental) neurotoxicity. Final report. Prepared for ECHA. Contract

Number: ECHA.6677-E3. March 2017; 241p. https://echa.europa.eu/de/publications/technical-scientific-reports

De Groot DM, Bos-Kuijpers MH, Kaufmann WS, Lammers JH, O'Callaghan JP, Pakkenberg B, Pelgrim MT, Waalkens-Berendsen ID, Waanders MM, Gundersen HJ (2005) Regulatory developmental neurotoxicity testing: a model study focussing on conventional neuropathology endpoints and other perspectives. Environ Toxicol Pharmacol 19:745–755

De Groot DM, Heerschap A, Krul C, Radonjic M, De Vries EF (2011) PET and MRI improve safety testing with far less animals (<50%). ALTEX 28:256

De Groot DM, Bogaart M, Nederlof R, Slieker RC, Wolterbeek AP, Dierckx RA, Van Waarde A, De Vries EF (2012a) In vivo [^{18}F]FDG microPET imaging in developmental neurotoxicity: a feasibility study in rat with ethanol. Reprod Toxicol 34:160–161

De Groot DM, Kuper CF, Radonjic M, Stierum R, Wolterbeek A, Heerschap A, Veltien A, Dierckx RA, De Vries EF (2012b) Imaging and omics in developing and juvenile rats after exposure to TBTO. Toxicol Lett 211:S155

De Groot MWGDM, Westerink RHS, Dingemans MML (2013) Don't judge a neuron only by its cover: neuronal function in *in vitro* developmental neurotoxicity testing. Toxicol Sci 132(1):1–7

De Vries EFJ, Van Waarde A, Willemsen ATM, Dierckx RA, Wolterbeek A, Wesselius A, De Groot DMG (2008) Protection of the unborn child from harmful drugs: a role for PET? Eur J Nucl Med Mol Imaging 35(suppl 2):S141

Edling C, Hellman B, Arvidson B, Andersson J, Hartvig P, Lilja A, Valind S, Långström B (1997a) Do organic solvents induce changes in the dopaminergic system? Positron emission tomography studies of occupationally exposed subjects. Int Arch Occup Environ Health 70:180–186

Edling C, Hellman B, Arvidson B, Johansson G, Andersson J, Hartvig P, Valind S, Långström B (1997b) Positron emission tomography studies of healthy volunteers—no effects on the dopamine terminals and synthesis after short-term exposure to toluene. Hum Exp Toxicol 16:171–176

Ek CJ, Dziegielewska KM, Habgood MD, Saunders NR (2012) Barriers in the developing brain and neurotoxicology. Neurotoxicology 33:586–604

Ekino S, Susa M, Ninomiya T, Imamura K, Kitamura T (2007) Minamata disease revisited: an update on the acute and chronic manifestations of methyl mercury poisoning. J Neurol Sci 262:131–144

Fincher CE, Chang TS, Harrell EH, Kettelhut MC, Rea WJ, Johnson A, Hickey DC, Simon TR (1997) Comparison of single photon emission computed tomography findings in cases of healthy adults and solvent-exposed adults. Am J Ind Med 31:4–14

Flannery BM, Bruun DA, Rowland DJ, Banks CN, Austin AT, Kukis DL, Li Y, Ford BD, Tancredi DJ, Silverman JL, Cherry SR, Lein PJ (2016) Persistent neuroinflammation and cognitive impairment in a rat model of acute diisopropylfluorophosphate intoxication. J Neuroinflammation 13:267

Glusczak L, dos Santos Miron D, Crestani M, Braga da Fonseca M, de Araújo Pedron F, Duarte MF, Vieira VL (2006) Effect of glyphosate herbicide on acetylcholinesterase activity and metabolic and hematological parameters in piava (Leporinus obtusidens). Ecotoxicol Environ Saf 65:237–241

Gómez-Sánchez R, Bravo-San Pedro JM, Niso-Santano M, Soler G, Fuentes JM, González-Polo RA (2010) The neuroprotective effect of talipexole from paraquat-induced cell death in dopaminergic neuronal cells. Neurotoxicology 31:701–708

Hagstadius S, Orbaek P, Risberg J, Lindgren M (1989) Regional cerebral blood flow at the time of diagnosis of chronic toxic encephalopathy induced by organic-solvent exposure and after the cessation of exposure. Scand J Work Environ Health 15:130–135

Hartvig P, Lindberg BS, Lilja A, Lundqvist H, Långström B, Rane A (1989) Positron emission tomography in studies on fetomaternal disposition of opioids. Dev Pharmacol Ther 12:74–80

Haut MW, Leach S, Kuwabara H, Whyte S, Callahan T, Ducatman A, Lombardo LJ, Gupta N (2000) Verbal working memory and solvent exposure: a positron emission tomography study. Neuropsychology 14:551–558

Huang CC, Weng YH, Lu CS, Chu NS, Yen TC (2003) Dopamine transporter binding in chronic manganese intoxication. J Neurol 250:1335–1339

Huang CY, Liu CH, Tsao E, Hsieh CJ, Weng YH, Hsiao IT, Yen TC, Lin KJ, Huang CC (2015) Chronic manganism: A long-term follow-up study with a new dopamine terminal biomarker of 18F-FP-(+)-DTBZ (18F-AV-133) brain PET scan. J Neurol Sci 353:102–106

Ishii K, Tamaoka A, Otsuka F, Iwasaki N, Shin K, Matsui A, Endo G, Kumagai Y, Ishii T, Shoji S, Ogata T, Ishizaki M, Doi M, Shimojo N (2004) Diphenylarsinic acid poisoning from chemical weapons in Kamisu, Japan. Ann Neurol 56:741–745

Ishii K, Nemoto K, Iwasaki N, Takeda T, Masuda T, Shibata Y, Tamaoka A (2019) Decreased regional cerebral blood flow in patients with diphenylarsinic acid intoxication. Eur J Neurol 26:136–141

Kim JW, Kim Y, Cheong HK, Ito K (1998) Manganese induced parkinsonism: a case report. J Korean Med Sci 13:437–439

Kim Y, Kim JW, Ito K, Lim HS, Cheong HK, Kim JY, Shin YC, Kim KS, Moon Y (1999) Idiopathic parkinsonism with superimposed manganese exposure: utility of positron emission tomography. Neurotoxicology 20:249–252

Kisby GE, Spencer PS (2011) Is neurodegenerative disease a long-latency response to early-life genotoxin exposure? Int J Environ Res Public Health 10:3889–3921

Kuo HC, Huang CC, Tsai YT, Chu CC, Hsieh ST, Chu NS (2005) Acute painful neuropathy in thallium poisoning. Neurology 65:302–304

Larsen JC (2006) Risk assessments of polychlorinated dibenzo- p-dioxins, polychlorinated dibenzofurans, and dioxin-like polychlorinated biphenyls in food. Mol Nutr Food Res 50:885–896

Lees-Haley PR, Williams CW (1997) Neurotoxicity of chronic low-dose exposure to organic solvents: a skeptical review. J Clin Psychol 53:699–712

Leslie EM, Deeley RG, Cole SP (2005) Multidrug resistance proteins: role of P-glycoprotein, MRP1, MRP2, and BCRP (ABCG2) in tissue defense. Toxicol Appl Pharmacol 204:216–237

Lewis MM, Sterling NW, Du G, Lee EY, Shyu G, Goldenberg M, Allen T, Stetter C, Kong L, Snipes SA, Jones BC, Chen H, Mailman RB, Huang X (2017) Lateralized basal ganglia vulnerability to pesticide exposure in asymptomatic agricultural workers. Toxicol Sci 159:170–178

Lin CY, Liou SH, Hsiech CM, Ku MC, Tsai SY (2011) Dose-response relationship between cumulative mercury exposure index and specific uptake ratio in the striatum on Tc-99m TRODAT SPECT. Clin Nucl Med 36:689–693

Liu KY, Beautrais A, Caine E, Chan K, Chao A, Conwell Y, Law C, Lee D, Li P, Yip P (2007) Charcoal burning suicides in Hong Kong and urban Taiwan: an illustration of the impact of a novel suicide method on overall regional rates. J Epidemiol Community Health 61:248–253

Liu CH, Lin KJ, Wang HM, Kuo HC, Chuang WL, Weng YH, Shih TS, Huang CC (2013) Brain fluorodeoxyglucose positron emission tomography (^{18}FDG-PET) in patients with acute thallium intoxication. Clin Toxicol 51:167–173

Meyer-Baron M, Kim EA, Nuwayhid I, Ichihara G, Kang SK (2012) Occupational exposure to neurotoxic substances in Asian countries - challenges and approaches. Neurotoxicology 33:853–861

Mittal T, Gupta N, Kohli A, Bhalla A, Singh B, Singh S (2011) Correlation of defects in regional cerebral blood flow determined by 99mTc SPECT with residual neurocognitive testing abnormalities during and 3 months post exposure in acutely poisoned patients with organophosphates. Clin Toxicol (Phila) 49:464–470

Morrow LA, Callender T, Lottenberg S, Buchsbaum MS, Hodgson MJ, Robin N (1990) PET and neurobehavioral evidence of tetrabromoethane encephalopathy. J Neuropsychiatry Clin Neurosci 2:431–435

Olanow CW, Good PF, Shinotoh H, Hewitt KA, Vingerhoets F, Snow BJ, Beal MF, Calne DB, Perl DP (1996) Manganese intoxication in the rhesus monkey: a clinical, imaging, pathologic, and biochemical study. Neurology 46:492–498

Organisation for Economic Co-operation and Development (OECD) (2007) OECD guidelines for the testing of chemicals, section 4: health effects test no.426: developmental neurotoxicity study. https://doi.org/10.1787/9789264067394

Overgaard MD, Duvald CS, Vendelbo MH, Pedersen SB, Jakobsen S, Alstrup AKO, Mikkelsen E, Ovesen PG, Pedersen M (2019) Biodistribution of [^{11}C]-Metformin and mRNA expression of placentae metformin transporters in the pregnant chinchilla. Contrast Media Mol Imaging 2019:9787340

Pelclova D, Urban P, Fenclova Z, Vlckova S, Ridzon P, Kupka K, Meckova Z, Bezdicek O, Navratil T, Rosmus J, Zakharov S (2018) Neurological and neurophysiological findings in workers with chronic 2,3,7,8-tetrachlorodibenzo-p-dioxin intoxication 50 years after exposure. Basic Clin Pharmacol Toxicol 122:271–277

Prüss-Ustün A, Vickers C, Haefliger P, Bertollini R (2011) Knowns and unknowns on burden of disease due to chemicals: a systematic review. Environ Health 10:9

Radonjic M, Cappaert NL, De Vries EF, De Esch CE, Kuper FC, Van Waarde A, Dierckx RA, Wadman WJ, Wolterbeek AP, Stierum RH, De Groot DM (2013) Delay and impairment in brain development and function in rat offspring after maternal exposure to methylmercury. Toxicol Sci 133:112–124

Rosenberg NL, Myers JA, Martin WR (1989) Cyanide-induced parkinsonism: clinical, MRI, and 6-fluorodopa PET studies. Neurology 39:142–144

Sarikaya I, Apaydin H, Topal U, Karaoglan O (2006) Cyanide-induced parkinsonism and F-18 FDG PET/CT findings. Clin Nucl Med 31:363–364

Sarkar S, Schmued L (2010) Neurotoxicity of ecstasy (MDMA): an overview. Curr Pharm Biotechnol 11:460–469

Schiffer WK, Lee DE, Alexoff DL, Ferrieri R, Brodie JD, Dewey SL (2006) Metabolic correlates of toluene abuse: decline and recovery of function in adolescent animals. Psychopharmacology (Berl) 186:159–167

Schiffer WK, Mirrione MM, Dewey SL (2007) Optimizing experimental protocols for quantitative behavioral imaging with ^{18}F-FDG in rodents. J Nucl Med 48:277–287

Seegal RF, Marek KL, Seibyl JP, Jennings DL, Molho ES, Higgins DS, Factor SA, Fitzgerald EF, Hills EA, Korrick SA, Wolff MS, Haase RF, Todd AC, Parsons P, McCaffrey RJ (2010) Occupational exposure to PCBs reduces striatal dopamine transporter densities only in women: a beta-CIT imaging study. Neurobiol Dis 38:219–225

Shinotoh H, Snow BJ, Hewitt KA, Pate BD, Doudet D, Nugent R, Perl DP, Olanow W, Calne DB (1995) MRI and PET studies of manganese-intoxicated monkeys. Neurology 45:1199–1204

Shinotoh H, Snow BJ, Chu NS, Huang CC, Lu CS, Lee C, Takahashi H, Calne DB (1997) Presynaptic and postsynaptic striatal dopaminergic function in patients with manganese intoxication: a positron emission tomography study. Neurology 48:1053–1056

Szólics M, Chaudhry M, Ljubisavljevic M, Corr P, Samir HA, Van Gorkom KN (2012) Neuroimaging findings in a case of fluoxetine overdose. J Neuroradiol 39:254–257

Tennekes HA, Sánchez-Bayo F (2013) The molecular basis of simple relationships between exposure concentration and toxic effects with time. Toxicology 309:39–51

Uitti RJ, Rajput AH, Ashenhurst EM, Rozdilsky B (1985) Cyanide-induced parkinsonism: a clinicopathologic report. Neurology 35:921–925

Urban P, Pelclová D, Lukás E, Kupka K, Preiss J, Fenclová Z, Smerhovský Z (2007) Neurological and neurophysiological examinations on workers with chronic poisoning by 2,3,7,8-TCDD: follow-up 35 years after exposure. Eur J Neurol 14:213–218

US Environmental Protection Agency (US EPA) (1998) Health effect test guidelines OPPTS 870.6300 developmental neurotoxicity study. Docket ID:EPA 712-C-98-239

Uversky VN (2004) Neurotoxicant-induced animal models of Parkinson's disease: understanding the role of rotenone, maneb and paraquat in neurodegeneration. Cell Tissue Res 318:225–241

Varney NR, Morrow LA, Pinkston JB, Wu JC (1998) PET scan findings in a patient with a remote history of exposure to organic solvents. Appl Neuropsychol 5:100–106

Visser I, Lavini C, Booij J, Reneman L, Majoie C, De Boer AG, Wekking EM, De Joode EA, Van der Laan G, Van Dijk FJ, Schene AH, Den Heeten GJ (2008) Cerebral impairment in chronic solvent-induced encephalopathy. Ann Neurol 63:572–580

Wang AG, Liu RS, Liu JH, Teng MM, Yen MY (1999) Positron emission tomography scan in cortical visual loss in patients with organophosphate intoxication. Ophthalmology 106:1287–1291

Wang JH, Scollard DA, Teng S, Reilly RM, Piquette-Miller M (2005) Detection of P-glycoprotein activity in endotoxemic rats by ^{99m}Tc-sestamibi imaging. J Nucl Med 46:1537–1545

Wolters EC, Huang CC, Clark C, Peppard RF, Okada J, Chu NS, Adam MJ, Ruth TJ, Li D, Calne DB (1989) Positron emission tomography in manganese intoxication. Ann Neurol 26:647–651

Wooten AL, Aweda TA, Lewis BC, Gross RB, Lapi SE (2017) Biodistribution and PET imaging of pharmacokinetics of manganese in mice using Manganese-52. PLoS One 12:e0174351

Yang KC, Ku HL, Wu CL, Wang SJ, Yang CC, Deng JF, Lee MB, Chou YH (2011) Striatal dopamine transporter binding for predicting the development of delayed neuropsychological sequelae in suicide attempters by carbon monoxide poisoning: A SPECT study. Psychiatry Res 194:219–223

Yang KC, Wang SJ, Hsieh WC, Lirng JF, Yang CC, Deng JF, Lin CL, Chou YH (2015) Longitudinal changes in the dopamine transporter and cognition in suicide attempters with charcoal burning. Psychiatry Res 231:160–167

Zaknun JJ, Stieglbauer K, Trenkler J, Aichner F (2005) Cyanide-induced akinetic rigid syndrome: clinical, MRI, FDG-PET, beta-CIT and HMPAO SPECT findings. Parkinsonism Relat Disord 11:125–129

Zanotti-Fregonara P, Laforest R, Wallis JW (2015) Fetal radiation dose from 18F-FDG in pregnant patients imaged with PET, PET/CT, and PET/MR. J Nucl Med 56:1218–1222

PET and SPECT in Hepatic and Uraemic Encephalopathy

35

Georg Berding, Frank Bengel, and Karin Weissenborn

Contents

Abstract

Liver or kidney failure can disturb brain function to a variable extent. If organ failure is treated successfully, brain function is normally, at least in part, restored. A broad spectrum of radiotracer imaging methods has been employed to measure correlates of brain function and thereby elucidate the pathophysiology of hepatic or uraemic encephalopathy. Measurements of regional cerebral perfusion as well

G. Berding (✉) · F. Bengel
Department of Nuclear Medicine, Hannover Medical School, Hannover, Germany
e-mail: berding.georg@mh-hannover.de; Bengel.Frank@mh-hannover.de

K. Weissenborn
Department of Neurology, Hannover Medical School, Hannover, Germany
e-mail: Weissenborn.Karin@mh-hannover.de

R. A. J. O. Dierckx et al. (eds.), *PET and SPECT in Neurology*,
https://doi.org/10.1007/978-3-030-53168-3_35

as energy metabolism in hepatic encephalopathy (HE) mostly revealed reductions in areas (particularly the frontal cortex and cingulum) relevant for the typically observed functional deficits (e.g. in attention or movement initiation). Positron emission tomography (PET) studies demonstrated that in HE, brain uptake of the neurotoxic ammonia increases with its plasma concentration. Some studies using the biomarker C-11-PK11195 indicate the presence of neuroinflammation in HE. Different neuroreceptor systems have been studied in HE throughout demonstrating reduced binding—particularly to central gamma-aminobutyric acid (GABA)-A receptors and dopamine as well as serotonin transporters. In patients with chronic renal failure and particularly those with depressive mood, reductions of cerebral blood flow and energy metabolism have been demonstrated, primarily located in the frontal cortex.

35.1 Introduction

Both the liver and kidneys are required to maintain human homeostasis in particular by preventing accumulation of toxic molecules with potentially detrimental effects on the central nervous system (CNS). Failure of these organs can therefore be the pathophysiologic basis of brain dysfunction ranging from mild subclinical impairments to devastating, potentially life-threatening complications. In contrast to degenerative brain diseases, there are quite effective treatment options available, for example, transplantation to tackle the underlying cause (organ failure) and thereby brain dysfunction. Nevertheless, these treatment options are demanding and sometimes accompanied by serious side effects themselves. As a consequence, it is of major importance to improve an understanding of the pathophysiology of brain disease caused by liver or renal failure for optimisation of therapy management with regard to minimal collateral brain damage. In this context, functional molecular imaging of the brain using radiotracer methods can give crucial information. Changes in regional brain perfusion, substrate and energy metabolism or in specific neurotransmission systems as well as neuroinflammatory response can be detected. Either single-photon emission computed tomography (SPECT) or positron emission tomography (PET) can be employed for this purpose. The aim of this review is to summarise the present knowledge on the use of these methods with regard to brain alterations in patients with failure or at least substantial dysfunction of the liver or kidneys.

35.2 Hepatic Encephalopathy

35.2.1 Pathophysiology

Major players in the pathogenesis of hepatic encephalopathy (HE) are (1) ammonia, (2) neuroinflammation, (3) GABAergic neurotransmission and (4) branched-chain amino acids (Gillmann et al. 2012; McPhail et al. 2010; Patel et al. 2012). It is assumed that in patients with liver failure, increased ammonia levels in the blood result into increased levels in the brain and specifically in astrocytes where ammonia is converted to glutamine. Moreover, it has been suggested that increased glutamine levels are associated with oxidative stress, astrocyte swelling and consequently brain oedema. A second important factor is a neuroinflammatory reaction in the brain, in the frame of a systemic inflammatory response syndrome, triggered by pro-inflammatory cytokines including tumour necrosis factor (α) and interleukins (1β and 6) originating from the liver. Changes in neurotransmission include particularly the GABA- and glutamatergic pathways (Llansola et al. 2015). Finally, the composition of amino acids in the blood has been related to the pathophysiology and prognosis of HE. In particular, reductions in valine concentrations and the ratio between branched-chain and aromatic amino acids (Fischer's ratio) have been demonstrated to be associated with HE. Low concentrations of branched chain amino acids were linked to sarcopenia and thus a reduction of muscular metabolism of ammonia (Kinny-Köster et al. 2016). Consequently, supplementation of branched-chain amino acids is used to suppress this route of HE pathogenesis. All of the four aforementioned factors in the pathophysiology of HE have been addressed in radiotracer imaging studies by some means or other. Table 35.1 gives an overview in the employed radiopharmaceuticals, addressed patient groups and main results.

35.2.2 Regional Cerebral Blood Flow: SPECT and PET

Studies of brain perfusion using SPECT tracers require limited resources and provide nevertheless a robust insight into cerebrovascular changes and regional functional activity. PET enables absolute measurements of regional cerebral blood flow (CBF), but it is technically more complex, for example, requiring an onsite cyclotron and invasive blood sampling, and higher priced. Both methods allow to assess treatment effects on the brain with an objective measure and correlate this to clinical symptoms and neuropsychological testing.

The comparability of SPECT studies on resting-state brain perfusion in patients with liver disease is sometimes limited by the fact that presence and extent of HE are not properly documented. Nevertheless, in the spectrum of patients with liver cirrhosis, if documented without HE, with minimal HE or overt HE, mostly relative regional hypoperfusion of cerebral cortex has been observed with SPECT (Catafau et al. 2000; Ohta et al. 1998; Iwasa et al. 2000, 2005; Nakagawa et al. 2004; Trzepacz et al. 1994; Yazgan et al. 2003). Some studies report (coexisting) hyperperfusion in areas of the limbic system, for example, the basal ganglia (Catafau et al. 2000; Ohta et al. 1998; Kohira et al. 1994; Yazgan et al. 2003). Hypoperfusion involves most frequently parts of the frontal cortex (Iwasa et al. 2000; Nakagawa et al. 2004), particularly prefrontal (Catafau et al. 2000; Nakagawa et al. 2004); parietal cortex (Ohta et al. 1998; Iwasa et al. 2000; Nakagawa et al. 2004); cingulum (Nakagawa et al. 2004), particularly the anterior cingulate (Iwasa et al. 2005), and sometimes the temporal cortex (Iwasa et al. 2000; Trzepacz et al. 1994). PET studies obtaining

Table 35.1 Overview of the results of brain imaging studies with SPECT or PET in hepatic encephalopathy reported in the literature

Imaging procedure	Author, year	Patients	Key finding
Tc-99m-HMPAO-, Tc-99m-ECD-, I-123-IMP- or I-133-xenon-SPECT	Catafau et al. (2000)	Subclinical HE	Regional hypo-/hyperperfusion
	Ikeda et al. (2001)	Before and after liver transplantation	No change in perfusion
	Iwasa et al. (2000, 2005)	Liver cirrhosis	Regional hypoperfusion
	Iwasa et al. (2003)	Liver cirrhosis	Hypoperfusion improved after BCAA therapy
	Jalan et al. (2003)	Liver cirrhosis	Regional hypoperfusion after amino acid load
	Kohira et al. (1994)	HE	Regional hyperperfusion
	Nakagawa et al. (2004)	Minimal HE	Regional hypoperfusion
	Ohta et al. (1998)	Portal–systemic encephalopathy	Regional hypo-/hyperperfusion improved after therapy
	Strauss et al. (1999)	Fulminant hepatic failure	Reduced anterior-to-posterior perfusion ratio
	Trzepacz et al. (1994)	Subclinical HE	Regional hypoperfusion
	Yazgan et al. (2003)	Subclinical HE	Regional hypo-/hyperperfusion
O-15-water with/without N-13-ammonia PET	Ahl et al. (2004)	Liver cirrhosis, minimal HE	Reduced regional CBF in lenticular nucleus and cerebellar vermis, no change in PS product
	Dam et al. (2013)	Liver cirrhosis, acute HE	Reduced global CBF, normalised after recovery from HE
	Goldbecker et al. (2010)	Liver fibrosis, no HE	No changes in global or regional CBF and PS product
	Iversen et al. (2009)	Liver cirrhosis, acute HE	Reduced global and regional CBF (frontal, parietal, temporal and occipital cortices, striatum and thalamus)
	Keiding et al. (2006)	Liver cirrhosis, acute HE	Correlation between ammonia in blood and trapping in brain, no change in PS product
	Lockwood et al. (1979)	Liver disease	Correlation between ammonia in blood and trapping in brain
	Lockwood et al. (1991)	Minimal HE	Increased PS product

Table 35.1 (continued)

Imaging procedure	Author, year	Patients	Key finding
F-18-fluorodeoxy-glucose (FDG) or O-15-oxygen PET	Kato et al. (2000)	Subclinical HE	Reduced regional glucose metabolism
	Giewekemeyer et al. (2007)	Early HE	Reduced regional glucose metabolism
	Iversen et al. (2009)	Overt HE	Reduced regional oxygen metabolism
	Senzolo et al. (2009)	Before and after liver transplantation	Improvement of glucose metabolism
	Vankadari et al. (2018)	Decompensated liver cirrhosis	Glucose metabolism reduced in cerebral cortex, increased in basal ganglia
	Zhang et al. (2019)	Cirrhosis without overt HE	Glucose metabolism reduced in cerebral cortex, increased in basal ganglia
C-11-PK11195 PET	Berding et al. (2010)	HCV-infected	Increased marker binding
	Berding et al. (2012)	Alcohol-toxic cirrhosis	No increased marker binding
	Cagnin et al. (2006)	HE	Increased marker binding
	Iversen et al. (2006)	HE	No increased marker binding
C-11-flumazenil PET	Jalan et al. (2000)	HE	Increased radioligand binding
	MacDonald et al. (1997)	HE	Increased radioligand binding
	Samson et al. (1987)	HE	Increased radioligand binding
I-123-β-CIT or I-123-IBZM SPECT	Weissenborn et al. (2000)	HE	Reduced dopamine transporter and receptor binding
I-123-β-CIT SPECT	Weissenborn et al. (2006)	HCV-infected	Reduced dopamine and serotonin transporter binding
	Heeren et al. (2011)	HCV-infected	
F-18-CPFPX PET	Boy et al. (2008)	Liver cirrhosis	Reduced adenosine receptor binding

HE hepatic encephalopathy, *BCAA* branched-chain amino acid, *CBF* cerebral blood flow, *PS product* blood–brain barrier permeability surface area product, *HCV* hepatitis C virus

absolute measures of cerebral blood flow in patients with liver disease substantiate the presence of flow impairments (Ahl et al. 2004; Dam et al. 2013; Goldbecker et al. 2010; Iversen et al. 2009; Keiding et al. 2006; Lockwood et al. 1991). Ahl et al. (2004) found in liver cirrhosis patients with HE compared with those without HE reduced CBF within lenticular nucleus and cerebellar vermis. Widespread reductions of regional CBF were observed in cirrhotic patients with an acute episode of HE compared with healthy subjects—encompassing areas within the frontal, parietal, temporal and occipital cortices as well as striatum and thalamus (Iversen et al. 2009). With respect to global changes of CBF in patients with liver disease, findings are consistently pointing to a decrease. Not significant decreases of 7% in patients with liver fibrosis without HE (Goldbecker et al. 2010) and around 20% in minimal or early HE (Ahl et al. 2004; Lockwood et al. 1991) were reported. A significant decrease of 35–40% in global CBF was found during acute episodes of HE, reversing to an insignificant decrease of 11% after recovery from HE (Dam et al. 2013; Iversen et al. 2009).

A positive correlation between regional cerebral perfusion assessed by SPECT imaging and scores obtained in neuropsychological testing has been reported by some authors (Catafau et al. 2000; Iwasa et al. 2005; Trzepacz et al. 1994). Results of brain perfusion measurements in general might suggest the possibility of a higher susceptibility of phylogenetically younger brain regions in particular the frontal cortex to pathophysiologic changes induced by late-stage liver disease which is in line with observed neuropsychological deficits in attention and visuopractic domains observed in neuropsychological testing (Trzepacz et al. 1994; Strauss et al. 1999).

Two interventional studies have focused on acute changes of brain (patho)physiology in patients with advanced liver disease. Jalan et al. (2003) simulated in patients with liver cirrhosis a gastrointestinal bleeding by oral administration of amino acids (mimicking haemoglobin). This resulted into a significant increase of blood ammonia levels and deterioration in neuropsychological test results. Sequential SPECT studies prior to administration of amino acids and 4 hours later revealed reduced perfusion in both temporal lobes, left superior frontal gyrus, right parietal and cingulate gyrus. The study stresses the relevance of ammonia and the time course of the pathophysiology. Strauss et al. (1999) studied in patients with fulminant hepatic failure whether the use of hyperventilation to prevent or postpone the development of cerebral oedema and intracranial hypertension has an influence on cerebral perfusion. They employed xenon-133 and Tc-99-HMPAO SPECT for that purpose. No significant difference between perfusion during normoventilation vs. hyperventilation was observed. Nevertheless, perfusion was impaired in the frontal cortex of patients compared with healthy controls and was restored to normal in patients after hepatic recovery and disappearance of HE.

Effects of treatment for liver failure on HE and brain perfusion have been investigated as well. In a study of patients with liver cirrhosis without overt HE, treatment with branched-chain amino acids resulted in a 13–20% increase of blood flow as demonstrated using sequential brain perfusion SPECT (Iwasa et al. 2003). PET has been used to study the impact of transjugular intrahepatic portosystemic shunting (TIPS) as a therapy option for end-stage liver disease, which is carrying a risk for the development of HE. No change of cerebral blood flow before and after TIPS was found—although flow values varied considerably preinterventionally (Iversen et al. 2011). Moreover, a study of patients with citrullinaemia type II brain perfusion SPECT before and 6–36 months after liver transplantation failed to show significant changes—however, no marked decreases of perfusion had been present preoperatively (Ikeda et al. 2001). Finally, a recent meta-analysis of studies on CBF in HE including non-emission tomographic methods as well (like magnetic resonance imaging [MRI] arterial spin labelling and nitrogen oxide (N_2O) based measurements) revealed a considerable degree of variation across studies (Bjerring et al. 2018). However, predominantly reductions of CBF in HE were reported, with the exemption of HE following portocaval shunting with a tendency towards increased CBF and the observation that MRI and N_2O-based methods resulted in higher CBF during HE.

35.2.3 Ammonia: PET

Due to the central role of ammonia in the pathophysiology of HE, N-13-labelled ammonia has been employed to further elucidate the pathogenesis. If N-13 ammonia is used in conjunction with measurements of blood flow using O-15-water, the permeability of the blood–brain barrier (BBB) for ammonia can be assessed by calculation of the so-called permeability surface (PS) product (Berding et al. 2009).

This concept has been applied in the context of HE first by Lockwood et al. (1991) in patients with minimal HE. They reported a globally increased permeability supporting a key role of ammonia in HE pathogenesis and even relevance in cases with moderately or a lack of increased ammonia blood levels. This paper had a major impact on the conception of pathophysiology in HE; however, the results have not been reproduced and criticised for methodological reasons. Two points of criticism have been addressed: (1) the lack of measuring metabolites in this study might disregard radioactive metabolites entering the brain and (2) the lack of dynamic acquisition eliminated the possibility to apply full bio-kinetic modelling including consideration of backflux of tracer to the blood (Sørensen and Ott 2012).

Ahl et al. (2004) found no significant difference in global PS product between liver cirrhosis patients with and without minimal HE. However, the PS product in the thalamus was even increased in patients without HE, possibly implicating that increased permeability of the blood–brain barrier might be an early phenomenon of disease. Nevertheless, a later study of the same group comparing the PS product in patients with liver fibrosis with that in healthy controls revealed no significant difference (Goldbecker et al. 2010). Likewise, studies of patients with liver cirrhosis carried out at the University Hospital Aarhus did not show significant changes of the PS product in patients without HE and those with acute overt HE during the episode as well as after recovery compared to healthy control subjects (Dam et al. 2013; Keiding et al. 2006).

Interestingly, with respect to ammonia trapping in the brain, studies comparing ammonia concentration in the blood and the metabolic rate of ammonia in the brain (derived by multiplication of net ammonia influx and arterial ammonia concentration) demonstrated a linear correlation (Keiding et al. 2006; Lockwood et al. 1979). Proceeding from the lack of specific change in blood–brain barrier permeability for ammonia shown by the aforementioned studies using a state-of-the-art approach for quantification, this implies that the pathophysiologically relevant concentration of ammonia in the brain is simply driven by the blood ammonia concentration.

35.2.4 Energy Metabolism: PET

Measurements of energy metabolism have been employed to improve an understanding of pathophysiology and therapy effects in HE. First, Kato et al. (2000) demonstrated hypometabolism in the frontal and temporal cortices as well as the basal ganglia of patients with subclinical HE compared to control subjects. Partly divergent, in more recent studies (as far as declared also in patients with subclinical HE), extended cortical hypometabolism (particularly parietal and occipital) but hypermetabolism in the basal ganglia was found (Vankadari et al. 2018, Zhang et al. 2019). A study of Giewekemeyer et al. (2007) aimed to identify brain regions relevant for bradykinesia, as an early sign of HE. They performed F-18-flurodeoxyglucose (FDG) PET studies at rest in patients with normal neurological status and either no or minimal HE according to portosystemic encephalopathy (PSE) syndrome test. Significant correlations between motor function (finger and hand tapping) and glucose metabolism could be demonstrated for brain areas relevant for movement initiation (cingulate gyrus, frontomedial, frontodorsal and parietal cortices). Iversen et al. (2009) studied oxygen consumption using oxygen-15 (O-15) PET in patients with cirrhosis without HE and with an acute episode of HE. They reported a clear reduction during the acute episode but not in patients without HE. Moreover, oxygen consumption was negatively correlated to plasma concentrations of ammonia. The authors conclude that the reduction is associated with the pathophysiology of HE and not the cirrhosis as such. Interestingly the authors published a few years later data of oxidative metabolisms that have been obtained in the same patients using C-11-acetate always after the O-15 PET studies reported earlier (Iversen et al. 2014). This elegant approach allows to disentangle the oxidative metabolism of neurons and astrocytes, since in the brain, acetate is metabolised in the astrocytes because the only monocarboxylate transporter (MCT) of neurons, MCT2, fails to recognise acetate to the same extent as MCT1 located in endothelial cells and astrocytes. The net rate constant of oxidation of C-11-acetate was not different between patients with cirrhosis and HE and control subjects, implicating that the observed reduction observed in patients based on O-15 is related to changes in neurons.

The impact of therapy for end-stage liver disease on brain energy metabolism was investigated by Senzolo et al. (2009). He studied in cirrhotic patients without overt HE but neuropsychological deficits cerebral glucose metabolism using F-18-FDG PET before and 1 year after liver transplantation. Significant beneficial effects of transplantation on initially impaired metabolism in most of the cortical (frontal, temporal, occipital) and subcortical regions corresponding with improvements in neuropsychological testing could be demonstrated.

35.2.5 Neuroinflammation: PET

In patients with hepatic disorders affecting the brain, a widely used first-generation marker of activated microglia (C-11-PK11195) has been applied. However, this marker has certain limitations, such as a relatively high non-specific uptake/low signal-to-noise ratio and complexity of quantification. Therefore, intense search for alternative markers is going on (Chauveau et al. 2008; Owen and Matthews 2011). The target for these radiotracers is the 18-kDa translocator protein (TSPO), which is present at very low levels in the normal healthy CNS but shows highly enhanced expression in the neuroinflammatory state. TSPO is located intracellularly at the mitochondrial membrane. Due to TSPO presence in peripheral tissues like the kidney and high affinity to benzodiazepines, it has originally been named as peripheral benzodiazepine receptor. Its functions are not fully understood, but they include the control of cholesterol transport, neurosteroid synthesis and maybe also the release of pro-inflammatory cytokines (Politis et al. 2012; Venneti et al. 2013).

Results of experimental studies imply an involvement of TSPO in the pathogenesis of encephalopathy in hepatic disease. Exposure of cultured astrocytes to ammonia results in increased TSPO expression. Exposure of mice to ammonia results in increased H-3-PK11195 binding/TSPO expression in the brain (Desjardins and Butterworth 2002). Consequently, C-11-PK11195 has been applied in patients with HE—nevertheless, results reported in the literature so far are ambiguous. Cagnin et al. (2006) observed in patients with minimal HE significantly increased C-11-PK11195 binding in the basal ganglia and the prefrontal cortex. In contrast, Iversen et al. (2006) found in patients with alcoholic liver cirrhosis during an acute episode of clinically overt HE no significant difference in C-11-PK11195 binding compared to healthy control subjects. Controversial findings might be related to different inclusion criteria, encompassing patients with hepatitis (3 out of 5) in the study of Cagnin et al. (2006), while this condition is not declared in the paper of Iversen et al. (2006). In a study employing C-11-PK11195 in a homogeneous group of hepatitis C-infected patients with fatigue, significantly increased binding was observed in the basal ganglia (thalamus) and frontal cortex (Berding et al. 2010). A study from the same group comparing liver cirrhosis patients according to the cause of liver disease, patients with cirrhosis due to hepatitis C showed increased C-11-PK11195 binding in frontal and occipital cortices, while no increase was found in those with alcoholic cirrhosis (Berding et al. 2012). Figure 35.1 displays results of C-11-PK11195 PET obtained in patients with hepatitis C, alcoholic cirrhosis and healthy control subjects. Patients with hepatitis C were also studied by Grover et al. (2012). They observed no change of C-11-PK11195 binding in the cerebral cortex but increased binding in the caudate and the thalamus. More recently, Pflugrad et al. (2016) described increased C-11-PK11195 binding in putamen, caudate, thalamus and (right) frontal cortex of hepatitis C-infected patients without deficits in a combined score of cognitive domains, including attention, concentration, learning ability and memory. Thus, in summary, the presently available data suggest that neuroinflammation in the brain depends on the cause of liver cirrhosis and is specifically driven by hepatitis C virus infection.

35.2.6 Neurotransmission: PET and SPECT

Specific detection of molecular processes in signal transduction between neurons is one of the exclusive goals for radiotracer studies. With respect to HE, there are hypotheses for preferential damage of specific neurotransmission systems.

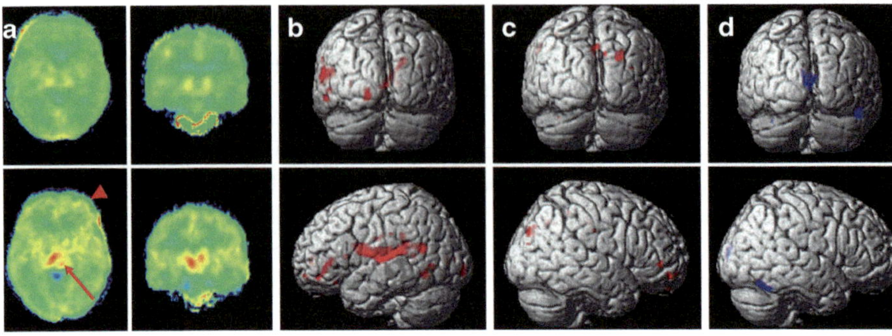

Fig. 35.1 C-11-PK11195 PET imaging of neuroinflammation in hepatic encephalopathy indicates the relevance of underlying liver disease. In panel (**a**), results of individual PET studies in a healthy control subject (upper row) and a patient with hepatitis C and fatigue symptomatology (lower row) are displayed. In the patient, increased binding in thalamus (red arrow) and frontal cortex (arrowhead) can be seen. Panels (**b–d**) show group comparisons with statistical parametric mapping. Regionally increased tracer binding ($p < 0.001$, uncorrected) is evident in hepatitis C-infected patients with cirrhosis vs. normal controls (**b**) and vs. patients with alcohol-toxic cirrhosis (**c**). The comparison between patients with alcohol-toxic cirrhosis and normal controls revealed reduced activity in the first group (**d**)

Particularly, the gamma-aminobutyric acid (GABA)/central benzodiazepine receptor system has been implicated to play a role in HE pathophysiology. The assumption of an increased GABAergic tone has primarily been based on the observation of beneficial effects of benzodiazepine antagonists such as flumazenil in patients with HE and animal models of HE (Albrecht and Jones 1999). Several partly controversial explanations for this increased tone have been given. A decrease in hepatic metabolism of benzodiazepines and an increase in benzodiazepine precursors provided by the intestinal flora (both resulting into increased natural benzodiazepines in the brain), an increased permeability of the blood–brain barrier for GABA and a modulation of the GABA-A receptors by ammonia or neurosteroids (Albrecht and Jones 1999; Ahboucha and Butterworth 2004; Patel et al. 2012).

In line with pathophysiological concepts, the first PET study employing C-11-flumazenil as tracer for benzodiazepine receptor binding in patients with HE showed a two- to threefold increase in uptake (Samson et al. 1987). In another study using the same radioligand along with blood sampling and bio-kinetic modelling in patients with recurrent HE, significant increases in benzodiazepine receptor binding in the thalamus, cerebellum and pons as well as minor and statistically insignificant increases in the cerebral cortex, putamen and whole brain could be demonstrated (MacDonald et al. 1997). This has been confirmed in a study by Jalan et al. (2000), observing significantly increased C-11-flumazenil binding in the cerebral cortex, basal ganglia and cerebellum of HE patients compared to control subjects.

With respect to other neurotransmission systems, the available imaging data are less sound. The monoaminergic systems (dopaminergic, serotonergic) have been thought to be afflicted in the pathophysiology of motor and cognitive deficits observed in HE patients. First evidence for an involvement of the dopaminergic system came from a post-mortem study (Mousseau et al. 1993). Corresponding results were obtained in an in vivo case study demonstrating impaired pre- and postsynaptic striatal dopaminergic transmission (Weissenborn et al. 2000). In patients with hepatitis C infection and fatigue, reduced dopamine and serotonin transporter binding was found (Weissenborn et al. 2006; Heeren et al. 2011). Patients with transporter binding below the normal reference range showed reduced performance in neuropsychological testing. However, with respect to serotonin, experimental findings indicate increased synthesis as well as metabolism of this transmitter (Lozeva-Thomas 2004). Nevertheless, the precise changes expected in HE at serotonin transporter/receptor level still have to be defined.

A major importance with respect to the pathophysiology of HE is assumed for the glutamatergic system. It has been shown experimentally that ammonia increases glutamate release resulting in overstimulation of glutamate receptors specifically *N*-methyl-D-aspartate (NMDA) receptors. This has been proposed as a potential background for seizures in HE. Beneficial effects of a NMDA receptor antagonists (MK-801) have been demonstrated by in vivo model of HE. The chronic state of HE is believed to result in a downregulation of glutamatergic NMDA receptors (Albrecht and Jones 1999). In vivo imaging studies of glutamatergic receptors in HE patients are lacking so far. In part difficulties in finding a suitable radioligand in the past decades are responsible for this; however, new options are foreseeable (Sobrio et al. 2010).

A solitary study has investigated adenosine receptors in the brains of patients with liver cirrhosis (Boy et al. 2008). The authors expected an alteration of this neuromodulatory receptor system contributing to neurotransmitter imbalance observed in these patients. As a matter of fact, they observed widely distributed significant reductions of adenosine receptor binding in the cortical and subcortical regions ranging between 20 and 50% compared to control subjects.

35.2.7 Open Questions: PET and SPECT in Hepatic Encephalopathy

As laid out earlier, the pathophysiology of HE has been widely reviewed using radiotracer methods. Nevertheless, basically new aspects remain to be addressed. Three main points might be taken into consideration. (1) The effects of liver transplantation on brain function are not well investigated. Only two studies have been performed so far. One study demonstrated no effect on brain perfusion in contrast to the clinically known beneficial effects and the other study demonstrated beneficial effects on brain metabolism (Ikeda et al. 2001; Senzolo et al. 2009). Of importance would be prognostic information. (2) There is a large body of experimental evidence for neuroinflammation to play a key role in HE. The in vivo data in patients generated with C-11-PK11195 so far produced partly conflicting results. New second-generation markers of neuroinflammation are available but have not been employed in HE so far. (3) Finally, data on in vivo changes in neurotransmission systems occurring in HE patients are fragmentary. Especially with respect to the glutamatergic systems, further insights might hold promise even for the development of new drug therapies.

35.3 Uraemic Encephalopathy

35.3.1 Pathophysiology and Symptomatology

Renal failure is associated with a broad spectrum of neurological complications, including encephalopathy, movement disorders, neuropathy, myelinolysis, myopathy, atherosclerosis and cerebrovascular accidents (Brouns and De Deyn 2004; Seifter and Samuels 2011). The pathophysiology of these complications is assumed to base on an accumulation of uraemic toxins, disturbances of intermediary metabolism and hormonal regulation. In conjunction with specific therapies of renal failure, additional pathogenetic factors have to be considered. For example, the disequilibrium syndrome in conjunction with haemodialysis, which is presumed to result from the fast reversion of urea plasma concentration and an intracellular acidosis in the cerebral cortex—or in the context of renal transplantation: toxicity of immunosuppressive drugs and opportunistic infections (Brouns and De Deyn 2004). More recently, the important role of organic anion transporters (OAT-3) came into focus. These transporters are located at the blood–brain and blood–cerebrospinal fluid barriers (BBB, BCSPFB) (Seifter and Samuels 2011; Hosoya and Tachikawa 2011). Dysfunction of these transporters by uraemic toxins is assumed to cause an accumulation of uraemic toxins itself, for example, guanidine compounds. Inhibitory effects of these compounds on GABA-A receptors and activating effects on NMDA receptors might explain enhanced cortical excitability and play in general an important role in the pathogenesis of uraemic encephalopathy (UE) (De Deyn et al. 2009; Hosoya and Tachikawa 2011; Seifter and Samuels 2011). Some of the aforementioned factors in the pathophysiology of UE have been addressed in radiotracer imaging studies. Table 35.2 gives an overview of the employed radiopharmaceuticals, addressed patient groups and main results.

35.3.2 Blood Flow: SPECT and PET

Since there is a strong indication for a pathophysiologic relevance of changes in the cerebrovascular system, blood flow has been one of the main targets in imaging studies of UE using either SPECT or PET. A number of SPECT studies focus on patients with end-stage renal failure before or on haemodialysis with depression. Particularly, frontal and/or temporal hypoperfusions have been identified in these patients (Fazekas et al. 1996; Kim et al. 2008; Nam et al. 2011; Song et al. 2009). However, one of these studies showed that hypoperfusion can be present even in non-depressed pre-dialytic patients, and another study showed that perfusion deficits are reversed in pre-dialytic patients after initiation of haemodialysis (Song et al. 2009; Nam et al. 2011). Furthermore, end-stage renal failure can be associated with movement disturbances. In this context, a case report of Lee et al. (2006) indicates a possible affection of the basal ganglia, specifically hyperperfusion. However, other researchers report, in contrast, hypoperfusion in the basal ganglia in patients

Table 35.2 Overview of the results of brain imaging studies with SPECT or PET in uraemic encephalopathy reported in the literature

Imaging procedure	Author, year	Patients	Key finding
Tc-99m-HMPAO- or Tc-99m-ECD-SPECT	Fazekas et al. (1996)	Haemodialysis	Regional hypoperfusion
	Kim et al. (2008)	Pre-dialytic and depressive	Regional hypoperfusion
	Lass et al. (1999)	End-stage renal failure	Multiple infarct pattern
	Lee et al. (2006)	Renal failure and movement disorder	Regional hyperperfusion in basal ganglia
	Nam et al. (2011)	Pre-dialytic and depressive	Increased perfusion after dialysis if depression reduced
	Nishikawa et al. (2000)	Haemolytic uraemic syndrome	No abnormalities
	Song et al. (2009)	Pre-dialytic and depressive	Regional hypoperfusion
	Choi et al. (2015)	Uraemic syndrome and parkinsonism	Hypoperfusion in basal ganglia
O-15-water PET	Kuwabara et al. (2002)	Chronic renal failure and anaemia	Reduced cerebrovascular perfusion reserve
	Moore et al. (2002)	Renal failure in Fabry disease	Increased cerebrovascular perfusion reserve
	Moore et al. (2001)	Renal failure in Fabry disease	Enzyme replacement reversed increased perfusion
Oxygen-15 PET	Kanai et al. (2001)	Chronic renal failure	Oxygen metabolism reduced, extraction increased
F-18-fluorodeoxy-glucose (FDG) PET	Minamimoto et al. (2007)	Suspected renal failure	Reduced regional glucose metabolism
	Song et al. (2008)	Pre-dialytic chronic kidney disease	Reduced regional glucose metabolism
	Wang et al. (2004)	Diabetic uraemia	Reduced regional glucose metabolism
C-11-CFT (2-carbomethoxy-3-(4-fluorophenyl) tropane), C-11-raclopride	Ishii et al. (2016)	Diabetic uraemic syndrome and parkinsonism	Reduced pre- and postsynaptic dopaminergic function

with renal failure (Song et al. 2009; Fazekas et al. 1996). In a case study of a patient with haemolytic uraemic syndrome (HUS), no abnormalities in brain perfusion were detected (Nishikawa et al. 2000). Lass et al. (1999) described a pattern of multiple discrete cortical perfusion defects as typical for patients in end-stage renal failure rather than involvement of more extended brain regions.

A PET study of cerebrovascular perfusion reserve revealed a general reduction of this parameter in patients with chronic renal failure (CRF) (Kuwabara et al. 2002). Reversely, in Fabry disease, an X-linked enzyme deficiency of alpha-galactosidase associated with renal failure, an increase of flow reserve was observed (Moore et al. 2002). Moreover, increased resting blood flow observed in the latter group was observed to be significantly lowered after enzyme replacement therapy (Moore et al. 2001).

35.3.3 Energy Metabolism: PET

Oxygen metabolism and glucose utilisation have been studied in patients with chronic renal failure (CRF) using PET. CRF patients showed in the hemisphere significantly reduced regional cortical metabolic rate of oxygen ($rCMRO_2$) and significantly increased regional oxygen extraction fraction (rOEF) (Kanai et al. 2001). There was a tendency of lowest values in the frontal cortex. Minamimoto et al. (2007) selected during a period of 2.5 years out of patients receiving F-18-FDG PET scans for cancer a subgroup of 20 patients with suspected renal failure (i.e. blood serum creatinine level in excess of 1.1 mg/dL). They found significantly reduced standardised uptake values (SUV) in the brain cortex and white matter of patients as compared to healthy volunteers. Song et al. (2008) studied patients with pre-dialytic chronic kidney disease using F-18-FDG brain scans. They observed significant decreases in glucose metabolism primarily in the prefrontal cortex and additionally in the anterior cingulate and the temporal and parietal cortices. Metabolism in the orbitofrontal cortex was inversely correlated with the Hamilton Depression Rating Scale. Finally, Wang et al. (2004) performed F-18-FDG PET brain scans in two patients with diabetic uraemia. Tracer uptake in patients was significantly reduced compared to a control group of healthy subjects in the striatum and in the cerebral cortex (with occipital predominance in one and frontal in the other case).

35.3.4 PET and SPECT in Uraemic Encephalopathy With Parkinsonism

The pathophysiology of parkinsonism in uraemic encephalopathy has been addressed in two case studies. Choi et al. (2015) demonstrated hypoperfusion in the basal ganglia—as known to be present in atypical Parkinson syndromes—by means of Tc-99m-HMPAO SPECT. Ishii et al. (2016) observed decreased binding to striatal dopamine transporters as well as dopamine D_2 receptors using specific PET radioligands in a patient with diabetic uraemic syndrome presenting with parkinsonism—again a constellation of findings characteristic for atypical Parkinson syndromes (Brooks 2012). The case studies illustrate the potential of SPECT and PET to objectivise regional specific neuronal damage according to clinical symptomatology in encephalopathy, for example, of uraemic origin.

35.3.5 Open Questions: PET and SPECT in Uraemic Encephalopathy

Brain effects of renal failure are studied to a much lesser extent using emission tomographic methods when compared to the effects of liver failure. Particularly, studies of neuroinflammatory changes in vivo are lacking. Nevertheless, the current knowledge on the pathophysiology of brain-related symptoms in patients with renal failure strongly implies a relevance of such processes, which can be targeted by radiotracers. This would be specifically of interest in patients receiving immunosuppression or with respect to GABAergic or glutamatergic neurotransmission.

References

Ahboucha S, Butterworth RF (2004) Pathophysiology of hepatic encephalopathy: a new look at GABA from the molecular standpoint. Metab Brain Dis 19:331–343

Ahl B, Weissenborn K, van den Hoff J, Fischer-Wasels D, Köstler H, Hecker H, Burchert W (2004) Regional differences in cerebral blood flow and cerebral ammonia metabolism in patients with cirrhosis. Hepatology 40:73–79

Albrecht J, Jones EA (1999) Hepatic encephalopathy: molecular mechanisms underlying the clinical syndrome. J Neurol Sci 170:138–146

Berding G, Banati RB, Buchert R, Chierichetti F, Grover VPBB, Kato A, Keiding S, Taylor-Robinson SD (2009) Radiotracer imaging studies in hepatic encephalopathy: ISHEN practice guidelines. Liver Int 29:621–628

Berding G, Boellaard R, Wilke F, Pflugrad H, Fitz E, Meyer GJ, Buchert R, Knapp WH, Geworski L, Weissenborn K (2010) Evidence for a relevance of neuroinflammation in the pathogenesis of fatigue in hepatitis C infected patients. Eur J Nucl Med Mol Imaging 37(suppl 2):S209

Berding G, Afshar K, Boellaard R, Wilke F, Pflugrad H, Meyer GJ, Geworski L, Bengel F, Weissenborn K, Tryc A (2012) Cerebral C-11-PK11195 binding is significantly increased in patients with hepatitis C-cirrhosis but not in alcohol toxic. J Nucl Med 53(Suppl 1):1946

Bjerring PN, Gluud LL, Larsen FS (2018) Cerebral blood flow and metabolism in hepatic encephalopathy - a meta-analysis. J Clin Exp Hepatol 8:286–293

Boy C, Meyer PT, Kircheis G, Holschbach MH, Herzog H, Elmenhorst D, Kaiser HJ, Coenen HH, Haussinger D, Zilles K, Bauer A (2008) Cerebral A1 adenosine receptors (A1AR) in liver cirrhosis. Eur J Nucl Med Mol Imaging 35:589–597

Brooks DJ (2012) Parkinson's disease: diagnosis. Parkinsonism Relat Disord 18:S31–S33

Brouns R, De Deyn PP (2004) Neurological complications in renal failure: a review. Clin Neurol Neurosurg 107:1–16

Cagnin A, Taylor-Robinson SD, Forton DM, Banati RB (2006) In vivo imaging of cerebral "peripheral benzodiazepine binding sites" in patients with hepatic encephalopathy. Gut 55:547–553

Catafau AM, Kulisevsky J, Berna L, Pujol J, Martin JC, Otermin P, Balanzo J, Carrio I (2000) Relationship between cerebral perfusion in frontal-limbic-basal ganglia circuits and neuropsychologic impairment in patients with subclinical hepatic encephalopathy. J Nucl Med 41:405–410

Chauveau F, Boutin H, Van Camp N, Dollé F, Tavitian B (2008) Nuclear imaging of neuroinflammation: a comprehensive review of [^{11}C]PK11195 challengers. Eur J Nucl Med Mol Imaging 35:2304–2319

Choi EK, Oh JK, Chung YA, Song IU (2015) Brain SPECT and MRI findings in a uremic patient with parkinsonism. Clin Nucl Med 40:e453–e454

Dam G, Keiding S, Munk OL, Ott P, Vilstrup H, Bak LK, Waagepetersen HS, Schousboe A, Sørensen M (2013) Hepatic encephalopathy is associated with decreased cerebral oxygen metabolism and blood flow, not increased ammonia uptake. Hepatology 57:258–265

De Deyn PP, Vanholder R, Eloot S, Glorieux G (2009) Guanidino compounds as uremic (neuro) toxins. Semin Dial 22:340–345

Desjardins P, Butterworth RF (2002) The "peripheral-type" benzodiazepine (omega 3) receptor in hyperammonemic disorders. Neurochem Int 41:109–114

Fazekas G, Fazekas F, Schmidt R, Flooh E, Valetitsch H, Kapeller P, Krejs GJ (1996) Pattern of cerebral blood flow and cognition in patients undergoing chronic haemodialysis treatment. Nucl Med Commun 17:603–608

Giewekemeyer K, Berding G, Ahl B, Ennen JC, Weissenborn K (2007) Bradykinesia in cirrhotic patients with early hepatic encephalopathy is related to a decreased glucose uptake of frontomesial cortical areas relevant for movement initiation. J Hepatol 46:1034–1039

Gillmann A, Gerharz CD, Müssig K (2012) Diagnostics and treatment of hepatic encephalopathy. Dtsch Med Wochenschr 137:29–33

Goldbecker A, Buchert R, Berding G, Bokemeyer M, Lichtinghagen R, Wilke F, Ahl B, Weissenborn K (2010) Blood-brain barrier permeability for ammonia in patients with different grades of liver fibrosis is not different from healthy controls. J Cereb Blood Flow Metab 30:1384–1393

Grover VP, Pavese N, Koh SB, Wylezinska M, Saxby BK, Gerhard A, Forton DM, Brooks DJ, Thomas HC, Taylor-Robinson SD (2012) Cerebral microglial activation in patients with hepatitis C: in vivo evidence of neuroinflammation. J Viral Hepat 19:e89–e96

Heeren M, Weissenborn K, Arvanitis D, Bokemeyer M, Goldbecker A, Tountopoulou A, Peschel T, Grosskreutz J, Hecker H, Buchert R, Berding G (2011) Cerebral glucose utilisation in hepatitis C virus infection-associated encephalopathy. J Cereb Blood Flow Metab 31:2199–2208

Hosoya K, Tachikawa M (2011) Roles of organic anion/cation transporters at the blood-brain and blood-cerebrospinal fluid barriers involving uremic toxins. Clin Exp Nephrol 15:478–485

Ikeda S, Yazaki M, Takei Y, Ikegami T, Hashikura Y, Kawasaki S, Iwai M, Kobayashi K, Saheki T (2001) Type II (adult onset) citrullinaemia: clinical pictures and the therapeutic effect of liver transplantation. J Neurol Neurosurg Psychiatry 71:663–670

Ishii K, Ishii K, Shioya A, Nemoto K, Tamaoka A (2016) Decreased dopamine transporter and receptor ligand binding in Parkinsonism with diabetic uremic syndrome. Ann Nucl Med 30:320–324

Iversen P, Hansen DA, Bender D, Rodell A, Munk OL, Cumming P, Keiding S (2006) Peripheral benzodiazepine receptors in the brain of cirrhosis patients with manifest hepatic encephalopathy. Eur J Nucl Med Mol Imaging 33:810–816

Iversen P, Sørensen M, Bak LK, Waagepetersen HS, Vafaee MS, Borghammer P, Mouridsen K, Jensen SB, Vilstrup H, Schousboe A, Ott P, Gjedde A, Keiding S (2009) Low cerebral oxygen consumption and blood flow in patients with cirrhosis and an acute episode of hepatic encephalopathy. Gastroenterology 136:863–871

Iversen P, Keiding S, Mouridsen K, Ott P, Vilstrup H (2011) Transjugular intrahepatic portosystemic shunt does not alter cerebral blood flow. Clin Gastroenterol Hepatol 9:1001–1003

Iversen P, Mouridsen K, Hansen MB, Jensen SB, Sorensen M, Bak LK, Waagepetersen HS, Schousboe A, Ott P, Vilstrup H, Keiding S, Gjedde A (2014) Oxidative metabolism of astrocytes is not reduced in hepatic encephalopathy: a PET study with [^{11}C]acetate in humans. Front Neurosci 8:353

Iwasa M, Matsumura K, Kaito M, Ikoma J, Kobayashi Y, Nakagawa N, Watanabe S, Takeda K, Adachi Y (2000) Decrease of regional cerebral blood flow in liver cirrhosis. Eur J Gastroenterol Hepatol 12:1001–1006

Iwasa M, Matsumura K, Watanabe Y, Yamamoto M, Kaito M, Ikoma J, Gabazza EC, Takeda K, Adachi Y (2003) Improvement of regional cerebral blood flow after treatment with branched-chain amino acid solutions in patients with cirrhosis. Eur J Gastroenterol Hepatol 15:733–737

Iwasa M, Matsumura K, Nakagawa Y, Yamamoto M, Tanaka H, Horiike S, Ikoma J, Kaito M, Takeda K, Adachi Y (2005) Evaluation of cingulate gyrus blood flow in patients with liver cirrhosis. Metab Brain Dis 20:7–17

Jalan R, Turjanski N, Taylor-Robinson SD, Koepp MJ, Richardson MP, Wilson JA, Bell JD, Brooks DJ (2000) Increased availability of central benzodiazepine receptors in patients with chronic hepatic encephalopathy and alcohol related cirrhosis. Gut 46:546–552

Jalan R, Olde Damink SW, Lui HF, Glabus M, Deutz NE, Hayes PC, Ebmeier K (2003) Oral amino acid load mimicking hemoglobin results in reduced regional cerebral perfusion and deterioration in memory tests in patients with cirrhosis of the liver. Metab Brain Dis 18:37–49

Kanai H, Hirakata H, Nakane H, Fujii K, Hirakata E, Ibayashi S, Kuwabara Y (2001) Depressed cerebral oxygen metabolism in patients with chronic renal failure: a positron emission tomography study. Am J Kidney Dis 38(4 suppl 1):S129–S133

Kato A, Suzuki K, Kaneta H, Obara H, Fujishima Y, Sato S (2000) Regional differences in cerebral glucose metabolism in cirrhotic patients with subclinical hepatic encephalopathy using positron emission tomography. Hepatol Res 17:237–245

Keiding S, Sørensen M, Bender D, Munk OL, Ott P, Vilstrup H (2006) Brain metabolism of ^{13}N-ammonia during acute hepatic encephalopathy in cirrhosis measured by positron emission tomography. Hepatology 43:42–50

Kim SJ, Song SH, Kim JH, Kwak IS (2008) Statistical parametric mapping analysis of the relationship between regional cerebral blood flow and symptom clusters of the depressive mood in patients with pre-dialytic chronic kidney disease. Ann Nucl Med 22:201–206

Kinny-Köster B, Bartels M, Becker S, Scholz M, Thiery J, Ceglarek U, Kaiser T (2016) Plasma amino acid concentrations predict mortality in patients with end-stage liver disease. PLoS One 11(7):e0159205

Kohira I, Matsuo E, Shiro Y, Uemura N, Matsumoto S, Kitamura Y, Matsumoto Y, Ishizu H, Sakai K, Kuroda S et al (1994) Hepatic encephalopathy with increased cerebral blood flow in SPECT and MRI abnormalities in the basal ganglia. Jpn J Psychiatry Neurol 48:33–36

Kuwabara Y, Sasaki M, Hirakata H, Koga H, Nakagawa M, Chen T, Kaneko K, Masuda K, Fujishima M (2002) Cerebral blood flow and vasodilatory capacity in anemia secondary to chronic renal failure. Kidney Int 61:564–569

Lass P, Buscombe JR, Harber M, Davenport A, Hilson AJ (1999) Cognitive impairment in patients with renal failure is associated with multiple-infarct dementia. Clin Nucl Med 24:561–565

Lee PH, Shin DH, Kim JW, Song YS, Kim HS (2006) Parkinsonism with basal ganglia lesions in a patient with uremia: evidence of vasogenic edema. Parkinsonism Relat Disord 12:93–96

Llansola M, Montoliu C, Agusti A, Hernandez-Rabaza V, Cabrera-Pastor A, Gomez-Gimenez B, Malaguarnera M, Dadsetan S, Belghiti M, Garcia-Garcia R, Balzano T, Taoro L, Felipo V (2015) Interplay between glutamatergic and GABAergic neurotransmission alterations in cognitive and motor impairment in minimal hepatic encephalopathy. Neurochem Int 88:15–19

Lockwood AH, McDonald JM, Reiman R, Gelbard AS, Laughlin JS, Duffy TE, Plum F (1979) The dynamics of ammonia metabolism in man. Effects of liver disease and hyperammonemia. J Clin Invest 63:449–460

Lockwood AH, Yap EW, Wong WH (1991) Cerebral ammonia metabolism in patients with severe liver disease and minimal hepatic encephalopathy. J Cereb Blood Flow Metab 11(2):337–341

Lozeva-Thomas V (2004) Serotonin brain circuits with a focus on hepatic encephalopathy. Metab Brain Dis 19:413–420

Macdonald GA, Frey KA, Agranoff BW, Minoshima S, Koeppe RA, Kuhl DE, Shulkin BL, Lucey MR (1997) Cerebral benzodiazepine receptor binding in vivo in patients with recurrent hepatic encephalopathy. Hepatology 26:277–282

McPhail MJ, Bajaj JS, Thomas HC, Taylor-Robinson SD (2010) Pathogenesis and diagnosis of hepatic encephalopathy. Expert Rev Gastroenterol Hepatol 4:365–378

Minamimoto R, Takahashi N, Inoue T (2007) FDG-PET of patients with suspected renal failure: standardized uptake values in normal tissues. Ann Nucl Med 21:217–222

Moore DF, Scott LT, Gladwin MT, Altarescu G, Kaneski C, Suzuki K, Pease-Fye M, Ferri R, Brady RO, Herscovitch P, Schiffmann R (2001) Regional cerebral hyperperfusion and nitric oxide pathway dysregulation in Fabry disease: reversal by enzyme replacement therapy. Circulation 104:1506–1512

Moore DF, Altarescu G, Herscovitch P, Schiffmann R (2002) Enzyme replacement reverses abnormal cerebrovascular responses in Fabry disease. BMC Neurol 2:4

Mousseau DD, Perney P, Layrargues GP, Butterworth RF (1993) Selective loss of pallidal dopamine D2 receptor density in hepatic encephalopathy. Neurosci Lett 162:192–196

Nakagawa Y, Matsumura K, Iwasa M, Kaito M, Adachi Y, Takeda K (2004) Single photon emission computed tomography and statistical parametric mapping analysis in cirrhotic patients with and without minimal hepatic encephalopathy. Ann Nucl Med 18:123–129

Nam HY, Song SH, Kim SJ, Kwak IS, Kim IJ, Lee SB, Lee DW, Kim BS, Pak K, Kim YK, Yun HS (2011) Effect of dialysis on cerebral blood flow in depressive end-stage renal disease patients. Ann Nucl Med 25:165–171

Nishikawa M, Hayashi T, Yoshitomi T, Inoue T, Ichiyama T, Furukawa S (2000) Perioperative evaluation of cerebral hemodynamics by transcranial Doppler ultrasonography in patient with hemolytic uremic syndrome. No To Hattatsu 32:520–523

Ohta H, Matsumoto R, Kato T, Tomono N, Shimizu T (1998) Tc-99m HMPAO brain perfusion SPECT images in a patient with portal-systemic encephalopathy. Clin Nucl Med 23:634–636

Owen DR, Matthews PM (2011) Imaging brain microglial activation using positron emission tomography and translocator protein-specific radioligands. Int Rev Neurobiol 101:19–39

Patel D, McPhail MJ, Cobbold JF, Taylor-Robinson SD (2012) Hepatic encephalopathy. Br J Hosp Med (Lond) 73:79–85

Pflugrad H, Meyer GJ, Dirks M, Raab P, Tryc AB, Goldbecker A, Worthmann H, Wilke F, Boellaard R, Yaqub M, Berding G, Weissenborn K (2016) Cerebral microglia activation in hepatitis C virus infection correlates to cognitive dysfunction. J Viral Hepat 23:348–357

Politis M, Su P, Piccini P (2012) Imaging of microglia in patients with neurodegenerative disorders. Front Pharmacol 3:96

Samson Y, Bernuau J, Pappata S, Chavoix C, Baron JC, Maziere MA (1987) Cerebral uptake of benzodiazepine measured by positron emission tomography in hepatic encephalopathy. N Engl J Med 316:414–415

Seifter JL, Samuels MA (2011) Uremic encephalopathy and other brain disorders associated with renal failure. Semin Neurol 31:139–143

Senzolo M, Pizzolato G, Ferronato C, Chierichetti F, Boccagni P, Dam M, Burra P (2009) Long-term evaluation of cognitive function and cerebral metabolism in liver transplanted patients. Transplant Proc 41:1295–1296

Sobrio F, Gilbert G, Perrio C, Barré L, Debruyne D (2010) PET and SPECT imaging of the NMDA receptor system: an overview of radiotracer development. Mini Rev Med Chem 10:870–886

Song SH, Kim IJ, Kim SJ, Kwak IS, Kim YK (2008) Cerebral glucose metabolism abnormalities in patients with major depressive symptoms in pre-dialytic chronic kidney disease: statistical parametric mapping analysis of F-18-FDG PET, a preliminary study. Psychiatry Clin Neurosci 62:554–561

Song SH, Kwak IS, Kim SJ, Kim YK, Kim IJ (2009) Depressive mood in pre-dialytic chronic kidney disease: statistical parametric mapping analysis of Tc-99m ECD brain SPECT. Psychiatry Res 173:243–247

Sørensen M, Ott P (2012) Cerebral ammonia metabolism in cirrhosis. In: Keiding S, Sørensen M (eds) Functional molecular imaging in hepatology. Bentham Science Publishers, Sharjah, pp 153–159. eISBN: 978-1-60805-290-5

Strauss GI, Høgh P, Møller K, Knudsen GM, Hansen BA, Larsen FS (1999) Regional cerebral blood flow during mechanical hyperventilation in patients with fulminant hepatic failure. Hepatology 30:1368–1373

Trzepacz PT, Tarter RE, Shah A, Tringali R, Faett DG, Van Thiel DH (1994) SPECT scan and cognitive findings in subclinical hepatic encephalopathy. J Neuropsychiatry Clin Neurosci 6:170–175

Vankadari K, Mittal BR, Kumar R, Singh H, Bhattacharya A, Dhiman RK (2018) Detection of hepatic encephalopathy on ^{18}F-FDG PET/CT brain images in a patient with decompensated liver cirrhosis. Clin Nucl Med 43:e486–e4e7

Venneti S, Lopresti BJ, Wiley CA (2013) Molecular imaging of microglia/macrophages in the brain. Glia 61:10–23

Wang HC, Hsu JL, Shen YY (2004) Acute bilateral basal ganglia lesions in patients with diabetic uremia: an FDG-PET study. Clin Nucl Med 29:475–478

Weissenborn K, Berding G, Köstler H (2000) Altered striatal dopamine D_2 receptor density and dopamine transport in a patient with hepatic encephalopathy. Metab Brain Dis 15:173–178

Weissenborn K, Ennen JC, Bokemeyer M, Ahl B, Wurster U, Tillmann HL, Trebst C, Hecker H, Berding G (2006) Monoaminergic neurotransmission is altered in hepatitis C virus infected patients with chronic fatigue and cognitive impairment. Gut 55:1624–1630

Yazgan Y, Narin Y, Demirturk L, Saracoglu M, Ercan M, Akyatan N, Dalkanat N, Ozel AM, Cetin M (2003) Value of regional cerebral blood flow in the evaluation of chronic liver disease and subclinical hepatic encephalopathy. J Gastroenterol Hepatol 18:1162–1167

Zhang W, Ning N, Li X, Li M, Duan X, Guo Y, Dang Y, Li Y, Gao J, Ye J, Yang J (2019) Impaired brain glucose metabolism in cirrhosis without overt hepatic encephalopathy: a retrospective ^{18}F-FDG PET/CT study. Neuroreport 30:776–782

Part VI

Epilepsy

PET in Epilepsy

36

Matthias Koepp, Marian Galovic,
and Maria Ilyas-Feldmann

Contents

M. Koepp (✉)
Department of Clinical and Experimental Epilepsy, Institute of Neurology, University College London, London, UK
e-mail: m.koepp@ucl.ac.uk

M. Galovic
Department of Clinical and Experimental Epilepsy, Institute of Neurology, University College London, London, UK

Department of Neurology, University Hospital Zurich, Zurich, Switzerland
e-mail: Marian.Galovic@usz.ch

M. Ilyas-Feldmann
Department of Clinical and Experimental Epilepsy, Institute of Neurology, University College London, London, UK

Epilepsy-Center Berlin-Brandenburg, Department of Neurology, Charité—Universitätsmedizin Berlin, Berlin, Germany
e-mail: m.feldmann@alumni.ucl.ac.uk

R. A. J. O. Dierckx et al. (eds.), *PET and SPECT in Neurology*,
https://doi.org/10.1007/978-3-030-53168-3_36

Abstract

The major drawback in clinical positron emission tomography (PET) imaging is that of specificity: in epilepsy, PET shows both the cause and consequence of seizure activity in the focus and projection area of the seizure onset. This can make treatment decisions for resective surgery difficult.

18F-Fluorodeoxyglucose ([^{18}F]FDG) PET has been long integrated in presurgical neuroimaging in many centres and proved to be clinically useful in identifying focal glucose metabolic abnormalities.

[^{11}C]Flumazenil, which delineates γ-aminobutyric acid receptor A (GABA-A) availability, may provide a biochemical marker of epileptogenicity and strengthens the hypothesis that inhibitory mechanisms are disturbed in the epileptic focus. Although [^{11}C]flumazenil, and other novel PET ligands for opioid and serotonin neurotransmission, showed great potential in selected patient subgroups, these tracers have not yet reached the stage of routine clinical application.

Ultimately, the challenge for PET imaging in epilepsy, like for most central nervous system (CNS) diseases, is overcoming drug-resistance due to poor delivery and/or retention of pharmaceuticals across the blood-brain barrier. There is the potential of PET to be relevant for the selection of certain novel treatment strategies, beyond the localisation of the focus for resective surgery.

36.1 Clinical Impact of PET in Epilepsy

Deoxyglucose radiolabelled with 18-fluorine ([^{18}F]FDG) administered to patients interictally is the sole application of PET in widespread routine clinical use in epilepsy. The technique provides a measure of cerebral glucose metabolism, which is reduced in the epileptogenic region interictally, in 60–90% of patients with temporal lobe epilepsy (TLE). Ictal [^{18}F]FDG PET is unhelpful as cerebral uptake of the radioligand takes place over many minutes post-injection.

Unfortunately, the area of hypometabolism demonstrated with [^{18}F]FDG PET is usually considerably larger than the pathological abnormality, site of neuronal loss and epileptogenic zone. In those patients with definitive magnetic resonance imaging (MRI) lesions, the technique adds little. However, its place remains in the presurgical evaluation of patients with non-definitive MRI abnormalities and/or discordant data, in particular patients with normal MRI—both in temporal and neocortical epilepsies and subtle focal cortical dysplasia. Imaging with [^{18}F]FDG PET has shown that patients with TLE who were seizure-free after temporal lobe resection had a greater proportion of hypometabolic area surgically removed than individuals who continued to have seizures (Willmann et al. 2007). This finding raises the possibility of tailoring the extent of resection according to the area of hypometabolism, especially in anatomically complex cases. Such a tailored approach would be challenging, however, as the volume of hypometabolism is often extensive and frequently extends into eloquent cerebral areas. The findings in patients with TLE might simply reflect the possibility that the greater the extent of resection, the greater the chance of seizure remission.

The available evidence for clinical effectiveness of PET is inadequate to reliably inform clinical practice. This is astonishing considering that since the 1980s, [^{18}F]FDG PET has been the imaging workhorse of presurgical evaluations in patients with epilepsy, although over the past 20 years, these imaging techniques have been largely superseded by high-quality MRI. Indeed, FDG PET is redundant if a lesion shown on MRI is concordant with clinical and electroencephalogram (EEG) data (Willmann et al. 2007). The value of FDG PET data is enhanced by voxel-based comparisons of individual patient scans with normative data and coregistration of PET images with MRI scans (Salamon et al. 2008). These advances have helped to decide on placement of intracranial EEG electrodes, but have not yet been shown to improve surgical outcomes. There is a lack of studies evaluating the impact of these tests on clinical decision-making and patient outcomes; only one such study meets this criterion, reporting the impact of imaging (FDG PET) on the decision-making process (O'Brien et al. 2008). Of the 110 patients who received FDG PET, the decision for or against surgery was considered to be influenced by the results of the FDG PET scan in 78 patients (71%): 48 influenced the decision in favour of surgery and 28 in favour of no surgery, and 2 patients had doubt cast on prior decisions and eligibility for surgery became uncertain. The positive decision predictive value for PET was 65% (95% CI 53–77%) and negative decision predictive value was 60% (95% CI 45–72%). It showed that if the FDG PET result does not lead to a positive or negative decision to undertake surgery, invasive EEG is offered. This strategy appeared the most cost-effective at conventional cost-effectiveness thresholds of £20,000–30,000. When the additional benefits conferred over the longer term for patients who received surgery compared to medical management alone (i.e. the benefits over and above those attributed to the additional success rate of surgery in increasing the probability of patients becoming seizure-free at 1 year) were excluded, medical management appeared to be the more appropriate management strategy for patients in whom the decision to proceed to surgery was still unclear following the results of FDG PET.

36.2 Impact of Novel PET Ligands

The development of specific PET ligands to identify focal abnormalities and, hence, to inform surgical treatment has been a long-term aspiration in epilepsy surgery. Several PET receptor ligands have been used to investigate the neurochemical basis of the epilepsies and have partially entered clinical routine. The aim is to assess neurotransmitter systems that are directly responsible for modulating synaptic activity, specific ligand–receptor relationships that seem to be important for epileptogenesis and spread of epileptic activity and generic mechanisms relevant for the development of pharmaco-resistance.

36.2.1 Imaging GABAergic Neurotransmission

[^{11}C]Flumazenil (FMZ) binds to the γ-aminobutyric acid receptor complex and can identify occult surgically relevant abnormalities. In the context of identifying epileptogenic tissue, binding of [^{11}C]FMZ was significantly lower in the epileptic focus than in the contralateral homotopic reference region and the remaining neocortex (Savic et al. 1988). It identified occult but surgically relevant abnormalities of benzodiazepine receptors (Ryvlin et al. 1998), and in malformations of cortical development, abnormalities were more extensive than subtle structural abnormality revealed with MRI (Hammers et al. 2001). Reduced binding can be seen at the epileptogenic focus and the seizure onset region, however, in a more restricted distribution than the corresponding area of [^{18}F]FDG hypometabolism, and sometimes also in projection areas (Savic et al. 1995). In addition, the degree of GABA receptor reduction showed a positive correlation with seizure frequency (Laufs et al. 2011). Furthermore, there was a close correlation between time since last seizure and magnitude of change in FMZ binding (Bouvard et al. 2005). Therefore, this method may not only be suitable for noninvasive localisation of the seizure focus but also provides a biochemical marker of epileptogenicity, strengthening the hypothesis that inhibitory mechanisms are disturbed in the epileptic focus. In unilateral hippocampal sclerosis, reduction of binding of [^{11}C]FMZ has been shown to be confined to the hippocampus (Koepp et al. 1996) and to be over and above that caused by neuron loss and hippocampal atrophy (Koepp et al. 1998a). In malformations of cortical development, abnormalities of benzodiazepine receptors, as demonstrated with [^{11}C]FMZ PET, were more extensive than the structural abnormality revealed with MRI (Hammers et al. 2001). Moreover, [^{11}C]FMZ PET was shown to be more accurate than [^{18}F]FDG PET for the detection of cortical regions of seizure onset and frequent spiking in patients with extra-TLE (Muzik et al. 2000), whereas both [^{18}F]FDG and [^{11}C]FMZ PET showed low sensitivity in the detection of cortical areas of rapid seizure spread (Koepp et al. 2000).

Currently, the clinical role of [^{11}C]FMZ for the detection of temporal and extratemporal foci is viewed controversially. Even though [^{11}C]FMZ binding has revealed focal abnormalities in 80% of patients with refractory TLE and normal high-quality MRI, this method has not been considered consistently helpful in localising epileptic foci (Koepp et al. 2000). In addition, the short half-time of ^{11}C (20 min) hampers the wide use of [^{11}C]FMZ for clinical routine. The possible implementation of [^{18}F]FMZ in clinical routine will most probably provide a more definite answer about the clinical benefit of benzodiazepine receptor imaging (Vivash et al. 2013).

The use of interictal [^{11}C]FMZ PET in patients with idiopathic generalised epilepsy, together with voxel-based morphometry MRI studies, has truly challenged the concept of generalised epilepsies revealing predominantly frontal increases in FMZ binding suggestive of focal microdysgenesis (Koepp et al. 1997; Savic et al. 1994). In a similar vein, the prevailing concept in focal epilepsies of epileptogenic zones, defined 'posthum' through seizure freedom following complete resection, has been challenged in a recent analysis of FMZ PET studies. Laufs and colleagues averaged both PET and functional MRI (fMRI) data across a group of patients with different sites of seizure onset and identified an area in the human piriform (primary olfactory) cortex that was active in association with interictal EEG spikes and showed reduced FMZ binding associated with increased seizure frequency (Laufs et al. 2011). This region was located in close proximity to the physiologically defined deep piriform cortex from which convulsants are known to initiate temporal lobe seizures, and blockade of glutamate receptors or application of a GABA receptor agonist reduces limbic motor seizures in rodents and nonhuman primates (Piredda and Gale 1985).

36.2.2 Imaging Serotonergic Neurotransmission

One major drawback in clinical imaging is that of specificity. MRI, FDG and FMZ PET all show both the cause and consequence of seizure activity, in the focus and projection area of the seizure onset. Furthermore, often multiple lesions are detected, and the significance of these changes is unclear.

Alpha[^{11}C]methyl-L-tryptophan (AMT) is an analogue of the essential amino acid tryptophan, the precursor of serotonin. AMT PET was originally developed to study abnormalities of brain serotonin synthesis. Preliminary studies in patients with neocortical epilepsy demonstrated that epileptogenic cortical areas show increased AMT uptake in some patients, even if MRI or FDG PET are non-localising (Fedi et al. 2001; Juhász et al. 2003). An increase in alpha [^{11}C]AMT uptake has been suggested to indicate the epileptic focus in situations where more than one possible focus is present, such as in patients with tuberous sclerosis. In one study, 25% of children with refractory focal epilepsy and normal MRI had a focal increase in AMT binding, and positive findings had a high specificity for the identification of the epileptic focus (Wakamoto et al. 2008). The sensitivity of AMT PET appears to be below 50% in non-lesional epilepsy, but its high specificity for detecting the lobe of seizure onset makes it an attractive imaging modality when other, more conventional imaging techniques fail to provide a clear localising information and also in presurgical evaluation of patients for reoperation after a failed surgery (Juhász et al. 2003). Recent studies suggested that increased AMT uptake may be relatively common in patients with epileptogenic cortical malformations (Chugani et al. 2013).

Experimental data in animals indicate that 5-HT$_{1A}$ receptors are located predominantly in limbic areas and that serotonin, via these receptors, mediates an antiepileptic and anticonvulsant effect. The literature on 5-HT$_{1A}$ receptor binding has recently been reviewed in detail (Hammers 2012). 5-HT$_{1A}$ receptors have been investigated with [^{18}F]FCWAY (Toczek et al. 2003). Twelve patients with TLE were correctly lateralised but not localised, including three patients with normal hippocampal volumes. Asymmetry indices for [^{18}F]fluorocyclohexanecarboxylic acid (FCWAY) were greater than those for FDG PET or hippocampal volumes.

Another study used the novel 5-HT$_{1A}$ radioligand [^{18}F]MPPF (20-methoxyphenyl-(*N*-20-pyridinyl)-*p*-[18F]fluorobenzamidoethylpiperazine), an antagonist of the 5-HT$_{1A}$ receptors, to assess the extent of 5-HT$_{1A}$ receptor binding changes in patients with TLE and hippocampal ictal onset. Patients had TLE of various aetiologies, and all underwent video-EEG evaluation with depth electrodes implanted. Binding was reduced in the epileptogenic areas, and magnitude of decrease was related to both electrophysiological data (greatest in areas of ictal onset and spread) and structural data (greatest in lesions with volume loss, followed by lesions). Binding potential (BP) reductions were found in all nine patients; they corresponded to or included the ictal onset zone in five and propagation areas in two and were maximal in the onset areas but failed to reach significance in two. In four patients, contralateral abnormalities were seen; in one of these patients who was explored with contralateral depth electrodes, one seizure did start contralaterally. [^{18}F]MPPF PET correctly indicated lateralisation in all three patients without lesions on MRI. In patients with normal hippocampal volume, the BP decrease was restricted to the temporal pole (Merlet et al. 2004a). The decrease was more pronounced in the seizure onset zone and in regions where the discharge propagated than in regions where only interictal paroxysms or no epileptic activity was recorded (Merlet et al. 2004b). Therefore, these results indicate that [^{18}F]MPPF binding not only reflects structural changes but also reflects neuronal loss.

The reduction in 5-HT_{1A} BP in patients with mesial TLE may be explained, on the one hand, by a decrease in receptor density due to downregulation due to hyperexcitability or, on the other hand, by an increase in endogenous serotonin as a reactional process to modulate hyperexcitability.

Comparison between [^{18}F]FDG and [^{18}F]MPPF PET data showed the clear-cut superiority of the latter for localising visually the epileptogenic area in patients with mesial TLE. The specificity of [^{18}F]FDG PET was lower than that of [^{18}F]MPPF PET, with only 23% of patients showing hypometabolism restricted to the hippocampus, amygdala and temporal pole, versus 38% demonstrating such abnormalities with [^{18}F]MPPF PET (Didelot et al. 2008). Taken together, these studies suggest that 5-HT_{1A} receptor PET could play a role in lateralising TLE when other imaging modalities are nonconclusive.

36.2.3 Imaging Opioid Neurotransmission

PET studies using opioid receptor ligands with different selectivity support findings from animal experiments suggesting a predominantly anticonvulsant effect of opioid peptides. The earliest human PET study indicating selective modulation of the opiate system in partial epilepsy was that of Frost et al. (1988), who demonstrated, with the μ-selective ligand [^{11}C]carfentanil, increased μ-opioid receptor availability in the areas of the epileptogenic temporal lobe exhibiting interictal hypometabolism. Increased receptor availability could point either to a decreased interictal tone of endogenous opioids, to an increased number of μ-opioid receptors, or both. In contrast to this finding, no comparable asymmetry was detectable with the nonspecific opioid receptor ligand [^{11}C] diprenoprhine (DPN) and the κ- and μ-selective ligand [^{18}F]carfentanil (CFX) (Mayberg et al. 1991; Theodore et al. 1992). A study with the δ-selective opioid receptor ligand [^{11}C]methylnaltrindole also showed increased receptor availability in the epileptogenic temporal lobe, but with a different regional pattern (Madar et al. 1997).

The in vivo demonstration in humans of selective regional alterations of κ- and μ-receptor binding in TLE supports the hypothesis derived from animal studies that endogenous ligand binding to these receptor subtypes plays a role in the tonic anticonvulsive mechanism that limits the spread of seizure activity from the epileptogenic focus. One important advantage of PET is that it allows for localising changes in neurotransmitter levels that accompany changes in neural activity. All the studies listed so far were performed in the interictal (between seizure) state. A limitation of the aforementioned studies is that they do not provide evidence for dynamic changes in opioid receptor availability, which would form a more compelling argument for the relevance of opioid receptor-mediated neurotransmission in epilepsy. Some studies used frequency of seizures and time since last seizure as indirect marker for epileptogenicity, as ictal (during seizure) investigations are difficult to perform due to the paroxysmal nature of the epilepsies. Seizure provocation is possible for some generalised epilepsies and reflex epilepsies, such as reading epilepsy, which is an ideal model to study functional changes that occur at or around the time of seizures.

Our group addressed the issue by demonstrating decreased [^{11}C]DPN binding in the left parietal–temporal–occipital cortex, a reading-associated area, during reading-induced seizures, in patients with reading epilepsy (Koepp et al. 1998b). Extrapolating this finding suggests the release of endogenous peptides during the ictal period in the epileptogenic (or at least, symptomatogenic) region, that is, the temporal lobe in TLE. Further evidence is provided by the finding of increased elimination of diprenorphine from the association cortex during hyperventilation-induced absence seizures and also by the finding of decreased [^{18}F]CFX binding in the presumed epileptogenic zone during a fortuitous ictal scan (Theodore et al. 1992; personal communication). More recently, our group demonstrated increased opioid peptide receptor binding postictally (i.e. within 24 h after a seizure) in the ipsilateral fusiform gyrus and temporal pole in patients with TLE (Hammers et al. 2007). Opioid receptor binding, which was also elevated relative to that of healthy controls, returned to baseline within the interictal period (6–56 days).

In summary, there is evidence for a dynamic relationship between opioid peptide receptor availability and seizures. Interictal studies suggest increased μ- and δ-opiate receptor availability in the ipsilateral temporal lobe during the interictal period in TLE. Ictal studies of reading-induced and absence epilepsies suggest decreased μ-, δ- and κ-opiate receptor availability during seizures. Postictal opioid peptide receptor binding is increased in the ipsilateral temporal lobe in TLE. The finding of changes in opioid receptor availability over a time course of hours following spontaneous seizures suggests an important role of the endogenous opioid receptor-mediated neurotransmission in temporal lobe seizures.

36.2.4 Imaging P-gp Function

The challenge in treating most CNS diseases is overcoming drug-resistance due to poor delivery and/or retention of pharmaceuticals. In epilepsy, about one third of patients are drug-resistance. The drug transporter hypothesis proposes that drug-resistance is related to increased expression of multidrug efflux transporter proteins such as P-glycoprotein (P-gp). These proteins are thought to prevent antiepileptic drug (AED) entry by actively extruding AEDs from their target site (Sisodiya et al. 2002). Multidrug efflux transporters are highly expressed in capillary endothelial cells and astrocytic foot processes that form the blood brain barrier (BBB). They limit intracellular concentration of substrates by pumping them out of the cell through an active energy-dependent mechanism. Epilepsy was the first CNS disorder for which drug-resistance was associated with enhanced expression of P-gp in the brain (Tishler et al. 1995). Pathologically elevated expression of P-gp has been found in resected brain tissue of patients with drug-resistant TLE undergoing surgery (Sisodiya et al. 2002) as well as in limbic brain regions of mouse and rat models of TLE (Loscher and Potschka 2005a). It is not clear whether the endothelial and parenchymal overexpression of P-gp is a consequence of epilepsy, of uncontrolled seizures or of chronic treatment with AEDs or whether it is constitutive, that is, present before the onset of epilepsy (Loscher and Potschka 2005b). Noninvasive brain imaging of multidrug efflux transporter function in drug-resistant and seizure-free epilepsy patients are a strategy to evaluate whether the overexpression of multidrug efflux transporters at the BBB as postulated in the transporter hypothesis have any functional consequences that underlie drug-resistance in epilepsy. Additionally, PET tracers for multidrug efflux transporters could be useful to identify epilepsy patients with increased multidrug efflux transporter activity who will benefit from treatment with multidrug efflux transporter modulation drugs and therefore hold great promises for individualised medicine (Sisodiya and Bates 2006).

P-gp function at the BBB of healthy humans has been imaged and quantified using the high-affinity P-gp substrates [(^{11})C]-verapamil and [^{11}C]-*N*-desmethyl-loperamide, which are very effectively transported by P-gp at the BBB. This results in low brain uptake of this radiotracer thus making it difficult to identify regional differences in cerebral P-gp function. A possible strategy to overcome the limitation of the low brain uptake of these P-gp substrate radiotracers is to perform PET scans after partial blockade by P-gp-modulating drugs, such as cyclosporine A (CsA) or tariquidar (Loscher and Langer 2010). The third-generation P-gp inhibitor tariquidar is safer than the non-selective CsA for use in human subjects and was shown to lack interaction with metabolism and plasma protein binding of (R)-[^{11}C]verapamil (Bankstahl et al. 2008; Wagner et al. 2009). Blocking P-gp with an inhibitor allows the radiotracer to enter the BBB and hence increase its uptake and signal in the brain. A proof of concept study was performed in rats 48 h after pilocarpine-induced status epilepticus (SE), supporting the hypothesis of regionally increased cerebral P-gp function in epilepsy. Both control and post-SE rats underwent (R)-[^{11}C]verapamil PET scans after administration of tariquidar at 3 mg/kg (Bankstahl et al. 2011). Regional PET data was analysed, and P-gp expression was independently quantified in the same brain regions using immunohistochemical staining (Bankstahl et al. 2011). In brain regions with increased P-gp expression (cerebellum, thalamus and hippocampus) in SE rats, the influx rate constants from blood to brain (K_1-values) of (R)-[^{11}C]verapamil were significantly decreased relative to control animals.

The caveat in the interpretation of (R)-[^{11}C]verapamil is that the peripheral metabolism of the radiotracer is significantly faster in epilepsy patients compared to healthy controls. This is most likely caused by hepatic cytochrome P450 enzyme induction of AEDs (Abrahim et al. 2008). The difficulty is that these radiometabolites which are generated from the (R)-[^{11}C]verapamil are also taken up into the brain tissue independent of P-gp function and compromise the quantitative measurement of P-gp function especially when comparing different study groups such as patient and healthy controls. To limit the effect of radio-labelled metabolites, a kinetic analysis with a single-tissue compartment model on the first 10 min of dynamic PET data should be used (Muzi et al. 2009).

A pilot study by Langer et al. (2007) used PET and the radiotracer (R)-[^{11}C]verapamil to test for differences in P-gp activity between epileptogenic and non-epileptogenic brain regions of patients with drug-resistant unilateral TLE. Although statistical significance was not reached, the findings were in-line with the hypothesis of P-gp overexpression. Influx rate constants from the blood to brain (K_1) and efflux rate constants from the brain to blood (K_2) were increased ipsilateral to the seizure focus in several temporal lobe regions known to be involved in seizure generation and propagation. Additionally, asymmetries were most prominent in the parahippocampal and ambient gyrus, amygdala, medial anterior temporal lobe and lateral anterior temporal lobe. In contrast to temporal lobe volumes of interest, asymmetries were minimal in regions located outside the temporal lobe.

Our recent voxel-based data revealed that at baseline K_1 was significantly reduced in drug-resistance compared to seizure-free TLE in temporal lobe regions and higher P-gp activity was associated with higher seizure frequency. After TQD, whole-brain K_1 increases were significantly reduced in drug-resistance TLE patients compared to controls (21.9% vs. 56.8% after 2 mg/kg TQD and 42.6% vs. 57.9% after 3 mg/kg TQD) which was most pronounced in the sclerotic hippocampus (24.5% vs. 65%, $p < 0.0001$). The reduced K_1 at baseline and reduced increases in K_1 after TQD in pharmacoresistant TLE compared to seizure-free TLE patients and controls support the hypothesis of P-gp overexpression in drug-resistant epilepsy (Feldmann et al. 2013). A follow-up (R)-[^{11}C]verapamil PET study analysed P-gp activity in seven patients undergoing epilepsy surgery (Bauer et al. 2014). They showed that optimal surgical outcome was associated with higher temporal lobe P-gp function before surgery, higher P-gp-positive staining in surgically resected hippocampal specimens, and reduction in global P-gp function postoperatively, compared with nonoptimal surgery outcome. Their result also indicated that P-gp expression is dynamic and changes with seizure frequency or AED treatment.

Our results were externally reproduced in a study using (R)-[^{11}C]verapamil PET and the non-selective P-gp inhibitor CsA in six patients with drug-resistant epilepsy and five patients with drug-sensitive epilepsy compared to eight healthy controls (Shin et al. 2016). All patients with drug-resistant epilepsy had significantly different asymmetry from the healthy controls, whereas all patients with drug-sensitive epilepsy had an asymmetry similar to that in healthy controls. In the temporal lobe, the asymmetry indices of patients with left temporal lobe drug-resistant epilepsy were more positive than those of healthy controls (healthy controls: 4.0413 ± 1.7452; patients: 7.2184 ± 1.8237; $p = 0.048$), and those of patients with right temporal drug-resistant epilepsy were more negative (patients: -1.6496 ± 3.4136; $p = 0.044$).

In addition, specific regions that had significant asymmetry were different between the lateral and medial temporal lobe epilepsy groups (Shin et al. 2016). By using this imaging technique with (R)-[^{11}C]verapamil PET we can identify individual patients where drug-resistance is caused by P-gp overactivity and potentially individualise treatment. Moreover, comparative studies between drug-resistant and seizure-free epilepsy patients can enable testing for a correlation between P-gp function and the pharmacoresponse. This imaging technique can also guide patient selection for future clinical studies. In particular, PET imaging of P-gp function may allow individualised application of approaches to overcome P-gp-associated drug-resistance.

36.2.5 Imaging NMDA Receptor Function

The *N*-methyl-D-aspartate (NMDA) receptor complex binds glutamate, the most important excitatory neurotransmitter in the brain. NMDA receptors have been showed to be involved in epileptogenesis and antagonists of the NMDA receptor have been used to treat seizures, particularly refractory status epilepticus. Developing a suitable ligand for in vivo imaging in humans has, however, proven difficult.

One study detected reduced binding of [^{11}C]-labelled ketamine in the ipsilateral temporal lobe of patients with TLE (Kumlien et al. 1999). This could reflect either reduced NMDA receptor density, reduced perfusion or focal atrophy.

More recently [^{18}F]GE-179, a novel ligand binding to activated (i.e. open) NMDA receptors, has been successfully employed in people with epilepsy (McGinnity et al. 2015). Its longer half-life makes it potentially more broadly available and might increase its clinical applicability. Increased activation of NMDA receptors was demonstrated in 8 people with epilepsy using this tracer. This could reflect ongoing epileptogenesis in these refractory cases. Conversely, tracer uptake was reduced in three epilepsy patients taking antidepressants. This could point to an interaction of antidepressants with the NMDA receptor. Further studies of this ligand are currently ongoing.

36.2.6 Imaging Dopaminergic Neurotransmission

The dopaminergic system is tough to play a role in seizure termination by modulating thalamo-cortical connections. Thus, alterations of the dopaminergic system in epilepsy could point to a disturbed mechanism of ictal termination.

Several PET studies demonstrated reduced dopaminergic neurotransmission in the basal ganglia of people with epilepsy. A variety of different radioligands were employed and a broad mix of clinical syndromes were examined, adding support to the robustness of the findings. These observations included presynaptic dopaminergic deficits using [^{18}F]fluoro-L-DOPA (Bouilleret et al. 2005, 2008), decreased D2/D3-receptor binding using [^{18}F]fallypride (Werhahn et al. 2006; Yakushev et al. 2010; Landvogt et al. 2010; Bernedo Paredes et al. 2015), decreased D1-receptor binding using [^{11}C]SCH23390 (Fedi et al. 2008), and reduced dopamine transporter activity with [^{11}C]PE2I (Ciumas et al. 2008, 2010; Odano et al. 2012). The syndromes studied included not only TLE, but also juvenile myoclonic epilepsy, idiopathic generalised epilepsy and autosomal dominant nocturnal frontal lobe epilepsy. Studying regions outside of the basal ganglia is difficult because of a low concentration of dopaminergic synapses in the neocortex. However, two studies also found reduced tracer uptake in the epileptogenic zone of TLE patients (Werhahn et al. 2006, Landvogt et al. 2010).

36.2.7 Imaging Inflammation

Measuring inflammation in epilepsy using PET focused on the translocator protein (TSPO), a marker that is overexpressed on activated microglia and reactive astrocytes. Three studies from the same research group demonstrated increased TSPO tracer binding ([^{11}C]PBR28 and [^{11}C]DPA-713) in the epileptogenic zone of people with mesial TLE and neocortical epilepsy (Hirvonen et al. 2012; Gershen et al. 2015; Dickstein et al. 2019). In one of these studies, the authors also found increased binding in the hemisphere contralateral to the epileptogenic zone, whereas it was less pronounced than on the ipsilateral side (Gershen et al. 2015). In one patient studied longitudinally, significantly increased tracer uptake was observed 36 h after a seizure compared to an interictally rescan (Butler et al. 2013). Overall, these findings point to increased inflammation and microglia activation in people with epilepsy, particularly within the epileptic focus and shortly after seizures. Another case series observed increased TSPO expression using [^{11}C]PK11195 PET in two patients with histologically confirmed Rasmussen's encephalitis (Banati et al. 1999), substantiating the role of neuroinflammation in this syndrome.

36.3 Outlook

Future research needs to be considered in relation to how the research informs the different levels of the diagnostic evaluation framework and ultimately how this links to the decision problem(s) faced by clinicians. It is integral to the evaluation of diagnostic technologies in the workup for epilepsy surgery that their impact on clinical decision-making, and on further treatment decisions, is considered; findings from these studies should be used alongside assessments of the long-term clinical effects and of costs of such treatments.

References

Abrahim A, Luurtsema G, Bauer M, Karch R, Lubberink M, Pataraia E, Joukhadar C, Kletter K, Lammertsma A, Baumgartner C, Muller M, Langer O (2008) Peripheral metabolism of (R)-[11C]verapamil in epilepsy patients. Eur J Nucl Med Mol Imaging 35:116–123

Banati RB, Goerres GW, Myers R et al (1999) [11C](R)-PK11195 positron emission tomography imaging of activated microglia in vivo in Rasmussen's encephalitis. Neurology 53(9):2199–2203

Bankstahl JP, Kuntner C, Abrahim A, Karch R, Stanek J, Wanek T, Wadsak W, Kletter K, Muller M, Loscher W, Langer O (2008) Tariquidar-induced P-glycoprotein inhibition at the rat blood-brain barrier studied with (R)-11C-verapamil and PET. J Nucl Med 49:1328–1335

Bankstahl JP, Bankstahl M, Kuntner C, Stanek J, Wanek T, Meier M, Ding XQ, Muller M, Langer O, Loscher W (2011) A novel positron emission tomography imaging protocol identifies seizure-induced regional overactivity of P-glycoprotein at the blood-brain barrier. J Neurosci 31:8803–8811

Bauer M, Karch R, Zeitlinger M, Liu J, Koepp MJ, Asselin M-C, Sisodiya SM et al (2014) In vivo P-glycoprotein function before and after epilepsy surgery. Neurology 83:1326–1331

Bernedo Paredes VE, Buchholz H-G, Gartenschläger M, Breimhorst M, Schreckenberger M, Werhahn KJ (2015) Reduced D2/D3 receptor binding of Extrastriatal and striatal regions in temporal lobe epilepsy. PLoS One 10(11):e0141098. https://doi.org/10.1371/journal.pone.0141098

Bouilleret V, Semah F, Biraben A et al (2005) Involvement of the basal ganglia in refractory epilepsy: an 18F-fluoro-L-DOPA PET study using 2 methods of analysis. J Nucl Med 46(3):540–547

Bouilleret V, Semah F, Chassoux F et al (2008) Basal ganglia involvement in temporal lobe epilepsy: a functional and morphologic study. Neurology 70(3):177–184. https://doi.org/10.1212/01.wnl.0000297514.47695.48

Bouvard et al (2005) Seizure-related short-term plasticity of benzodiazepine receptors in partial epilepsy: a [11C]flumazenil-PET study. Brain 128:1330–1343

Butler T, Ichise M, Teich AF et al (2013) Imaging inflammation in a patient with epilepsy due to focal cortical dysplasia. J Neuroimaging 23(1):129–131

Chugani HT, Luat AF, Kumar A, Govindan R, Pawlik K, Asano E (2013) α-[11C]-Methyl-L-tryptophan-PET in 191 patients with tuberous sclerosis complex. Neurology 81(7):674–680

Ciumas C, Wahlin T-BR, Jucaite A, Lindstrom P, Halldin C, Savic I (2008) Reduced dopamine transporter binding in patients with juvenile myoclonic epilepsy. Neurology 71(11):788–794

Ciumas C, Wahlin T-BR, Espino C, Savic I (2010) The dopamine system in idiopathic generalized epilepsies: identification of syndrome-related changes. NeuroImage 51(2):606–615

Dickstein LP, Liow J-S, Austermuehle A et al (2019) Neuroinflammation in neocortical epilepsy measured by PET imaging of translocator protein. Epilepsia 313(3):285–287

Didelot A, Ryvlin P, Lothe A, Merlet I, Hammers A, Mauguiere F (2008) PET imaging of brain 5-HT1A receptors in the preoperative evaluation of temporal lobe epilepsy. Brain 131:2751–2764

Fedi M, Reutens D, Okazawa H et al (2001) Localizing value of alpha-methyl-L-tryptophan PET in intractable epilepsy of neocortical origin. Neurology 57:1629–1636

Fedi M, Berkovic SF, Scheffer IE et al (2008) Reduced striatal D1 receptor binding in autosomal dominant nocturnal frontal lobe epilepsy. Neurology 71(11):795–798

Feldmann M, Asselin MC, Liu J, Wang S, McMahon A, Anton-Rodriguez J, Walker M, Symms M, Brown G, Hinz R, Matthews J, Bauer M, Langer O, Thom M, Jones T, Vollmar C, Duncan JS, Sisodiya SM, Koepp MJ (2013) P-glycoprotein expression and function in patients with temporal lobe epilepsy: a case-control study. Lancet Neurol 12(8):777–785

Frost JJ, Mayberg HS, Fisher RS et al (1988) Mu-opiate receptors measured by positron emission tomography are increased in temporal lobe epilepsy. Ann Neurol 23:231–237

Gershen LD, Zanotti-Fregonara P, Dustin IH et al (2015) Neuroinflammation in temporal lobe epilepsy measured using positron emission tomographic imaging of Translocator protein. JAMA Neurol 72(8):882–888

Hammers A (2012) Epilepsy. NeuroMethods. https://doi.org/10.1007/7657_2012_58

Hammers A, Koepp MJ, Richardson MP et al (2001) Central benzodiazepine receptors in malformations of cortical development: a quantitative study. Brain 124:1555–1565

Hammers A, Asselin MC, Hinz R et al (2007) Upregulation of opioid receptor binding following spontaneous epileptic seizures. Brain 130:1009–1016

Hirvonen J, Kreisl WC, Fujita M et al (2012) Increased in vivo expression of an inflammatory marker in temporal lobe epilepsy. J Nucl Med 53(2):234–240

Juhász C, Chugani DC, Muzik O et al (2003) Alpha-methyl-L-tryptophan PET detects epileptogenic cortex in children with intractable epilepsy. Neurology 60:960–968
Koepp MJ, Richardson MP, Brooks DJ, Poline JB, Van Paesschen W, Friston KJ et al (1996) Cerebral benzodiazepine receptors in hippocampal sclerosis. An objective in vivo analysis. Brain 119:1677–1687
Koepp MJ, Richardson MP, Brooks DJ, Cunningham VJ, Duncan JS (1997) Central benzodiazepine/gamma-aminobutyric acid A receptors in idiopathic generalized epilepsy: an [11C]flumazenil positron emission tomography study. Epilepsia 38:1089–1097
Koepp MJ, Hand KS, Labbé C, Richardson MP, Van Paesschen W, Baird VH et al (1998a) In vivo [11C]flumazenil-PET correlates with ex vivo [3H]flumazenil autoradiography in hippocampal sclerosis. Ann Neurol 43:618–626
Koepp MJ, Richardson MP, Brooks DJ, Duncan JS (1998b) Focal cortical release of endogenous opioids during reading-induced seizures. Lancet 352:952–955
Koepp MJ, Hammers A, Labbe C, Woermann FG, Brooks DJ, Duncan JS (2000) 11CFlumazenil PET in patients with refractory temporal lobe epilepsy and normal MRI. Neurology 54:332–339
Kumlien E, Hartvig P, Valind S, Oye I, Tedroff J, Långström B (1999) NMDA-receptor activity visualized with (S)-[N-methyl-11C]ketamine and positron emission tomography in patients with medial temporal lobe epilepsy. Epilepsia 40(1):30–37
Landvogt C, Buchholz H-G, Bernedo V, Schreckenberger M, Werhahn KJ (2010) Alteration of dopamine D2/D3 receptor binding in patients with juvenile myoclonic epilepsy. Epilepsia 51(9):1699–1706
Langer O, Bauer M, Hammers A, Karch R, Pataraia E, Koepp MJ, Abrahim A, Luurtsema G, Brunner M, Sunder-Plassmann R, Zimprich F, Joukhadar C, Gentzsch S, Dudczak R, Kletter K, Muller M, Baumgartner C (2007) Pharmacoresistance in epilepsy: a pilot PET study with the P-glycoprotein substrate R-[11C]verapamil. Epilepsia 48:1774–1784
Laufs et al (2011) Converging PET and fMRI evidence for a common area involved in human focal epilepsies. Neurology 77(9):904–910
Loscher W, Langer O (2010) Imaging of P-glycoprotein function and expression to elucidate mechanisms of pharmacoresistance in epilepsy. Curr Top Med Chem 10(17):1785–1791
Loscher W, Potschka H (2005a) Drug resistance in brain diseases and the role of drug efflux transporters. Nat Rev Neurosci 6:591–602
Loscher W, Potschka H (2005b) Role of drug efflux transporters in the brain for drug disposition and treatment of brain diseases. Prog Neurobiol 76:22–76
Madar I, Lesser RP, Krauss G et al (1997) Imaging of delta- and mu-opioid receptors in temporal lobe epilepsy by positron emission tomography. Ann Neurol 41:358–367
Mayberg HS, Sadzot B, Meltzer CC et al (1991) Quantification of mu and non-mu opiate receptors in temporal lobe epilepsy using positron emission tomography. Ann Neurol 30:3–11
McGinnity CJ, Koepp MJ, Hammers A et al (2015) NMDA receptor binding in focal epilepsies. J Neurol Neurosurg Psychiatry 86(10):1150–1157
Merlet I, Ryvlin P, Costes N et al (2004a) Statistical parametric mapping of 5-HT1A receptor binding in temporal lobe epilepsy with hippocampal ictal onset on intracranial EEG. NeuroImage 22:886–896
Merlet I, Ostrowsky K, Costes N et al (2004b) 5-HT1A receptor binding and intracerebral activity in temporal lobe epilepsy: an [18F]MPPF-PET study. Brain 127:900–913
Muzi M, Mankoff DA, Link JM, Shoner S, Collier AC, Sasongko L, Unadkat JD (2009) Imaging of cyclosporine inhibition of P-glycoprotein activity using 11C-verapamil in the brain: studies of healthy humans. J Nucl Med 50:1267–1275
Muzik O, da Silva EA, Juhasz C et al (2000) Intracranial EEG versus flumazenil and glucose PET in children with extratemporal lobe epilepsy. Neurology 54:171–179
O'Brien TJ et al (2008) The cost-effective use of 18F-FDG PET in the presurgical evaluation of medically refractory focal epilepsy. J Nucl Med 49:931–937
Odano I, Varrone A, Savic I et al (2012) Quantitative PET analyses of regional [11C]PE2I binding to the dopamine transporter--application to juvenile myoclonic epilepsy. NeuroImage 59(4):3582–3593

Piredda S, Gale K (1985) A crucial epileptogenic site in the deep prepiriform cortex. Nature 317:623–625

Ryvlin P et al (1998) Clinical utility of flumazenil-PET versus [18F]fluorodeoxyglucose-PET and MRI in refractory partial epilepsy. A prospective study in 100 patients. Brain 121:2067–2081

Salamon N et al (2008) FDG-PET/MRI coregistration improves detection of cortical dysplasia in patients with epilepsy. Neurology 71:1594–1601

Savic I, Persson A, Roland P, Pauli S, Sedvall G, Widen L (1988) In-vivo demonstration of reduced benzodiazepine receptor binding in human epileptic foci. Lancet 2:863–866

Savic I, Pauli S, Thorell JO, Blomqvist G (1994) In vivo demonstration of altered benzodiazepine receptor density in patients with generalised epilepsy. J Neurol Neurosurg Psychiatry 57:797–804

Savic I, Thorell JO, Roland P (1995) [11C]Flumazenil positron emission tomography visualizes frontal epileptogenic regions. Epilepsia 36:1225–1232

Shin J-W, Chu K, Shin SA, Jung K-H, Lee S-T, Lee Y-S, Moon J et al (2016) Clinical applications of simultaneous PET/MR imaging using (R)-[11 C]-verapamil with Cyclosporin a: preliminary results on a surrogate marker of drug-resistant epilepsy. Am J Neuroradiol 37:600–606

Sisodiya SM, Bates SE (2006) Treatment of drug resistance in epilepsy: one step at a time. Lancet Neurol 5:380–381

Sisodiya SM, Lin WG, Harding BN, Squier MV, Thom M (2002) Drug resistance in epilepsy: expression of drug resistance proteins in common causes of refractory epilepsy. Brain 125:22–31

Theodore WH, Carson RE, Andreasen P et al (1992) PET imaging of opiate receptor binding in human epilepsy using [18F]cyclofoxy. Epilepsy Res 13:129–139

Tishler DM, Weinberg KI, Hinton DR, Barbaro N, Annett GM, Raffel C (1995) MDR1 gene expression in brain of patients with medically intractable epilepsy. Epilepsia 36:1–6

Toczek MT, Carson RE, Lang L et al (2003) PET imaging of 5-HT1A receptor binding in patients with temporal lobe epilepsy. Neurology 60(5):749–756

Vivash L, Gregoire MC, Lau EW, Ware RE, Binns D, Roselt P, Bouilleret V, Myers DE, Cook MJ, Hicks RJ, O'Brien TJ (2013) 18F-flumazenil: a γ-aminobutyric acid A-specific PET radiotracer for the localization of drug-resistant temporal lobe epilepsy. J Nucl Med 54(8):1270–1277

Wagner CC et al (2009) A pilot study to assess the efficacy of tariquidar to inhibit P-glycoprotein at the human blood-brain barrier with (R)–11C-verapamil and PET. J Nucl Med 50:1954–1961

Wakamoto H et al (2008) Alpha-methyl-l-tryptophan positron emission tomography in epilepsy with cortical developmental malformations. Pediatr Neurol 39:181–188

Werhahn KJ, Landvogt C, Klimpe S et al (2006) Decreased dopamine D2/D3-receptor binding in temporal lobe epilepsy: an [18F]fallypride PET study. Epilepsia 47(8):1392–1396

Willmann O, Wennberg R, May T, Woermann FG, Pohlmann-Eden B (2007) The contribution of 18F-FDG PET in preoperative epilepsy surgery evaluation for patients with temporal lobe epilepsy: a meta-analysis. Seizure 16:509–520

Yakushev IY, Dupont E, Buchholz H-G et al (2010) In vivo imaging of dopamine receptors in a model of temporal lobe epilepsy. Epilepsia 51(3):415–422

Imaging Evaluation of Epilepsy: Functional and Structural Approaches

37

Sara K. Inati and William H. Theodore

Contents

Abstract

Carefully selected patients with drug-resistant epilepsy may be candidates for resective surgery. Neuroimaging, including positron emission tomography (PET), magnetic resonance imaging (MRI), and ictal single-photon emission computed tomography (SPECT), are important clinical tools for presurgical seizure focus localization. MRI is an essential part of evaluation for patients with epilepsy. Structural studies may show focal abnormalities such as mesial temporal sclerosis or focal cortical dysplasia, which are the pathological substrates of seizure initiation. Functional localization data from arterial spin labeling for cerebral blood flow and spike-triggered or resting-state signal acquisition are potentially valuable as well. PET and SPECT usually only are performed for patients being considered for surgery. PET may show decreased interictal glu-

S. K. Inati · W. H. Theodore (✉)
National Institute of Neurological Disorders and Stroke, Bethesda, MD, USA
e-mail: Sara.inati@nih.gov; theodorw@ninds.nih.gov

R. A. J. O. Dierckx et al. (eds.), *PET and SPECT in Neurology*,
https://doi.org/10.1007/978-3-030-53168-3_37

cose metabolism in the epileptogenic zone. PET may also contribute to understanding the pathophysiology of epilepsy through the use of ligands for neurotransmitter receptors and neuroinflammation. Reduced benzodiazepine receptor binding may have occasional clinical relevance. Ictal SPECT may show increased blood flow if the tracer is injected soon after seizure onset, particularly if an interictal scan is subtracted and the image co-registered with structural MRI. When interpreting imaging in epilepsy, it is important to consider the clinical context, ictal semiology, and electrographic studies.

37.1 Overview

Positron emission tomography (PET) is relatively unique as a neuroimaging tool given the variety of radioligands that can be used to investigate different aspects of metabolic processes underlying normal brain function and diseases. Since the initial studies in the 1980s, PET using [^{18}F]2-fluoro-2-deoxy-D-glucose ([^{18}F]FDG) for measurement of the cerebral metabolic rate of glucose consumption (CMRglc) has become an established clinical tool for the evaluation of patients with epilepsy. Its most important clinical application is in seizure focus localization to aid with presurgical planning in patients with drug-resistant epilepsy (Fig. 37.1). In addition, FDG-PET can be used to study the pathophysiology of epilepsy and its comorbidities and the effects of antiepileptic drugs and other treatments and may have some diagnostic utility in conditions such as autoimmune encephalitis. PET ligands used

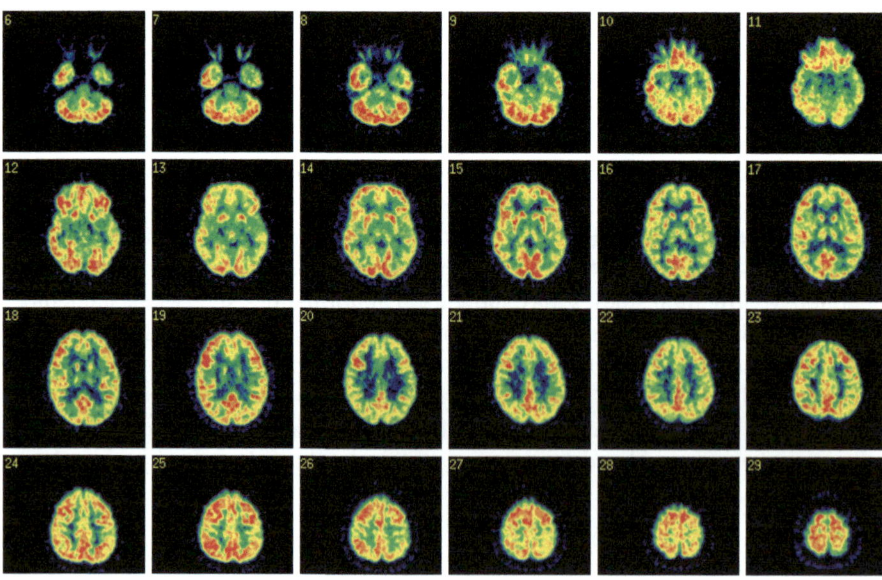

Fig. 37.1 FDG-PET scan showing left temporal hypometabolism in a patient with focal dyscognitive seizures of left mesial temporal onset

to image neuroreceptor binding and inflammation thus far have less clinical importance than FDG but have provided important data on basic mechanisms of epilepsy and can link human epilepsy with experimental models. Recent reviews have summarized the findings to date in the field of PET imaging in epilepsy for [^{18}F]FDG as well as a wide variety of other tracers (Kumar et al. 2012; Theodore 2017; Galovic and Koepp 2016; Juhasz and John 2020; Sidhu et al. 2018).

PET imaging is a fundamentally dynamic process, and there are several aspects of timing that must be taken into account. First, each PET modality involves production of a positron emitter followed by a radiochemistry procedure to bind it to a biologically active molecule. Each of these positron-emitting radioligands has a different half-life, which limits the amount of time available between production of the ligand and the detection of the ligand in a scanner. Since fluorine-18, used in FDG, has a half-life of 110 min, production at a central facility for transport to a scanner is practical. Carbon-11, however, which is used for many neurotransmitter receptor ligands, has a half-life of only 20 min and must be produced onsite; the radiochemistry procedures are thus more time-sensitive than for FDG. Second, uptake of the biologically active molecule that is part of the radioligand is a dynamic functional process. It is thus critical to be aware of the state of the patient during and before scanning. For example, the "metabolic window" measured by FDG lasts 30–40 min after isotope injection; the "time resolution" of PET is therefore significantly wider than for Electroencephalography (EEG) or fMRI. Moreover, there may be effects of recent seizure frequency on hypometabolism, even if no seizure activity occurs during the uptake period. This was demonstrated in a study using the benzodiazepine receptor ligand [11C]flumazenil, in which binding reduction in the seizure focus was partially reversed in the setting of more recent seizures (Bouvard et al. 2005).

Analysis methods for FDG-PET include traditional visual radiologic inspection of the images, region-of-interest-based templates used to measure relative asymmetries in CMRglc, and statistical approaches such as statistical parametric mapping. Some studies suggest that relative measurement of asymmetry indices is superior to pure visual interpretation, but more formal approaches including calculation of FDG kinetic parameters have not shown clear advantages (Theodore et al. 1992; Kim et al. 2003; van't Klooster et al. 2014; Mayoral et al. 2019; Tang et al. 2018). In addition to these analysis approaches, neurotransmitter receptor ligands require more complex tracer kinetic modeling. Some ligands may also be substrates for brain efflux transporters, further complicating binding measurements (Liow et al. 2016). PET imaging has relatively lower spatial resolution than structural MRI (the best current resolution for PET/CT and PET/MRI is ~4.5 mm). This leads to partial volume effects that may be particularly important in analysis of relatively small structures or when neuronal loss is present; these effects can be somewhat reduced by using MRI-based correction procedures (Figs. 37.2 and 37.3).

It is worth noting that many PET studies in epilepsy suffer from small subject numbers as well as methodologic limitations, including insufficient delineation of study populations, retrospective data collection, lack of blinding, and, for surgical outcome studies, inconsistent grading and limited follow-up (Gaillard et al. 2011). Large-scale multicenter studies would be much more efficient and provide a more solid basis for attempting to clarify the uses of PET in epilepsy.

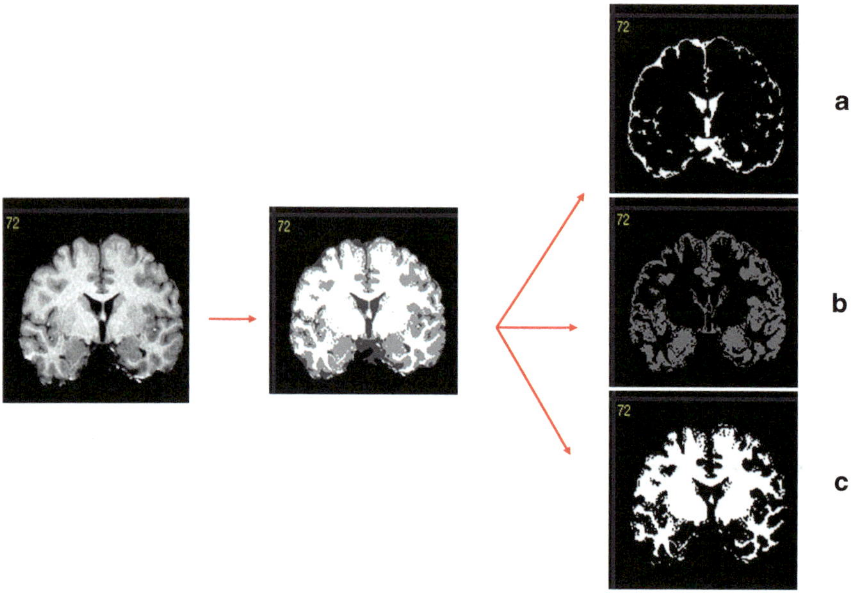

Fig. 37.2 Segmentation for partial volume correction. After skull stripping, the image is parceled into cerebrospinal fluid (**a**), gray matter (**b**), and whiter matter (**c**) spaces

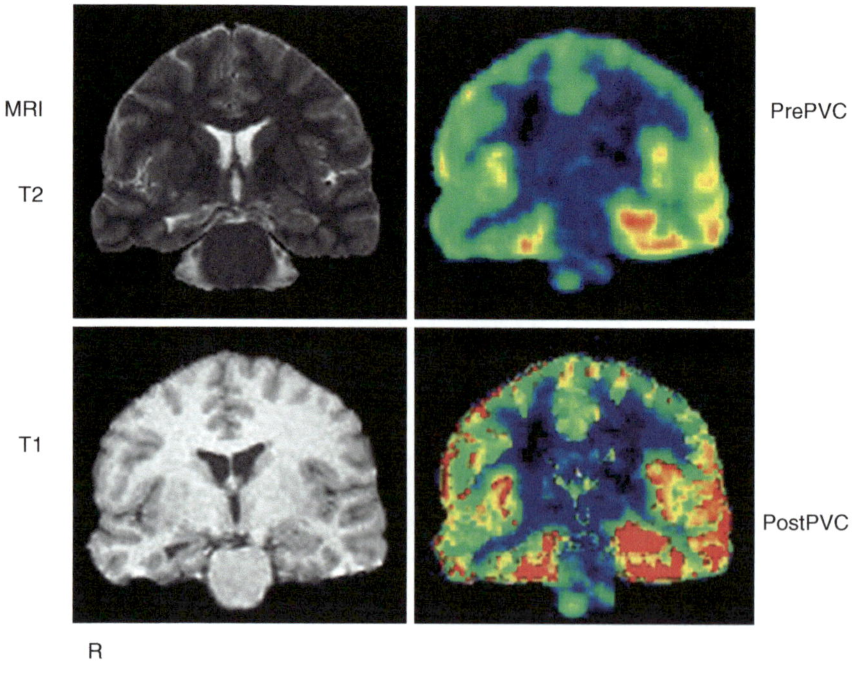

Fig. 37.3 Partial volume correction of FDG-PET scan in a patient with mesial temporal sclerosis. After application of the gray matter mask, apparent glucose metabolism is increased throughout. However, the relative hypometabolism in the right temporal cortex is preserved

37.2 Hypometabolism in Focal Epilepsy Using FDG-PET

FDG-PET has been shown in a large number of studies to detect hypometabolism interictally in patients with focal epilepsy, as well as in some patients with generalized epilepsy. Several factors likely contribute to this finding. The main energy consumption of the brain is dedicated to maintaining ionic gradients such as the Na^+/K^+ pump and neurotransmitter release and reuptake (Bazzigaluppi et al. 2017). Subsidiary uses are related to neurotransmitter synthesis, axonal transport, and biochemical syntheses. During seizures, there appears to be a sudden shift from hypo- to hypermetabolism. Although the mechanisms underlying such shifts are unclear, altered interictal Na^+/K^+ pump activity due to hypometabolism may lead to membrane instability and hyperexcitability. Several studies in experimental animals using the pilocarpine (Guo et al. 2009) and kainic acid models (Jupp et al. 2012) showed that limbic hypometabolism develops in concert with epileptogenesis and precedes the appearance of spontaneous seizures. Several studies suggest that the degree of initial hypometabolism at epilepsy diagnosis may predict prognosis (Gaillard et al. 2007). The extent of hypometabolism may subsequently fluctuate in relation to seizure frequency (Benedek et al. 2006). Over time, hypometabolic regions in children with focal epilepsy may increase in extent and be associated with persistent seizures (Govil-Dalela et al. 2018).

In addition to the mechanisms of neuronal dysfunction and altered metabolism, it appears that neuronal loss also plays a contributing role; it does not, however, account completely for the observations, as shown by studies using partial volume correction. This is also supported by studies in patients with clear unilateral seizure foci, in whom hypometabolism often extends beyond anatomic limits and may be bilateral. Additionally, in focal cortical dysplasia, hypometabolism can extend beyond the observed structural MRI findings and has been hypothesized to reflect reduced mitochondrial complex IV function to a greater degree than the extent of the structural abnormality (Tenney et al. 2014). The extent of seizure spread, in addition to metabolic dysfunction, may also be a contributing factor to the hypometabolism observed in FDG-PET imaging in epilepsy (Chassoux et al. 2016).

37.3 The Role of FDG-PET for Localization in Focal Epilepsy

Accurate identification of seizure foci is critical to the success of epilepsy surgery in treating drug-resistant epilepsy. This can be relatively straightforward in the setting of clear structural lesions on MRI with concordant interictal and ictal EEG findings; patients with lesional epilepsy on MRI have been shown to have improved postoperative seizure outcomes compared to those without lesions (Tellez-Zenteno et al. 2010; Tonini et al. 2004). Mesial temporal lobe epilepsy (mTLE) is one of the most common forms of drug-resistant epilepsy that is treated surgically. In mTLE, a large number of studies have shown that FDG-PET can detect hypometabolism in about 70–80% of patients (Theodore 2017). In these patients, PET hypometabolism appears to be regional, rather than localizing. It is common for patients to have lateral temporal neocortical as well as mesial hypometabolism, and hypometabolism may extend beyond the temporal lobe to include the ipsilateral frontal lobes, insular, and thalamus. These findings, when ipsilateral, do not appear to affect surgical outcome; in a meta-analysis of 46 PET studies from 1992 to 2006, ipsilateral PET hypometabolism was found to have an 86% predictive value for "good" (variably defined in the studies included) surgical outcome (Willmann et al. 2007). While it was unclear whether PET added much of value for patients with lesional MRI, unilateral PET hypometabolism is a favorable prognostic factor in cases in which the MRI is "normal." In a retrospective study of MRI-negative TLE, the presence of focal hypometabolism increased seizure-free outcome from 45 to 82% (Mariani et al. 2019). In contrast, bilateral hypometabolism, associated with bilateral EEG findings, more frequent secondary generalization, and more severe neuropsychological deficits, is associated with worse surgical outcome (Kumar et al. 2012; Cahill et al. 2019).

Results vary more widely for extratemporal epilepsy. In a study of 194 patients, PET was helpful for surgical decision-making in 63% with temporal lobe epilepsy, compared with 38% with frontal lobe epilepsy (Rathore et al. 2014). In a review of 11 studies with normal MRI, reports of localized FDG-PET hypometabolism ranged from 36 to 93% of patients, with a mean of 71% (Juhasz and John 2020). A prospective study of 130 patients found that about 20% of TLE patients had extratemporal, and extratemporal patients temporal, hypometabolism, which was an adverse surgical prognostic factor for both groups (Tomas et al. 2019). Unilobar hypometabolism within the resection zone was a good prognostic factor, with an odds ratio of 5.4 for complete seizure control. For patients with extratemporal seizure foci, hypometabolism that was "remote" from the electrophysiologic seizure focus (contralateral or in a non-contiguous lobe) was an adverse prognostic finding (Wong et al. 2012).

One of the most common causes of non-lesional epilepsy appears to be focal cortical dysplasia (FCD), which is found on pathological examination in approximately 50% of non-lesional epilepsy patients undergoing surgery (Chapman et al. 2005; McGonigal et al. 2007). Conversely, it is estimated that approximately 1/3 of FCDs are not apparent using conventional radiological visual inspection of the MRI (Chassoux et al. 2012). One approach in these cases has been to use quantitative MR image post-processing techniques to aid in identification of subtle FCDs (Adler et al. 2017; Ahmed et al. 2015; Thesen et al. 2011; Wang et al. 2016; Hong et al. 2014). Another approach is to incorporate information from additional imaging modalities, and FDG-PET has been shown to provide additional diagnostic utility in increasing the detection rate or confirming the presence of lesions in apparently MR-negative cases, as well as having some prognostic value in predicting seizure outcomes (Juhasz and John 2020). In some studies, detection of hypometabolism, particularly when co-registered with three-dimensional MRI reconstruction, improved identification of focal cortical dysplasia and surgical outcome. In a study of 48 children, FDG-PET showed a clear advantage over MRI alone in detecting mild malformations of cortical development, which were missed in about 2/3 of the cases using MRI but detected by PET in 77% (Kim et al. 2011). In a study of [18F]FDG-PET scans from 103 consecutive patients with histologically proven FCD type II, visual analysis showed focal or regional hypometabolism corresponding to the FCD in 44%; the main factors influencing positive PET localization were the grade of hypometabolism and the size of the lesion (Desarnaud et al. 2018). MRI was localizing in 59%. However, FDG was able to localize the lesion in 83% of the patients for whom MRI was unrevealing.

37.4 Comparison with Other Imaging Methods in Focal Epilepsy

In non-lesional patients, or in patients with discordant noninvasive studies, invasive electrode studies are often used to identify the seizure-onset zone (SOZ) and currently are the gold standard for seizure focus localization. The presence of focal hypometabolism using FDG-PET is clearly associated with seizure-onset zone localization using invasive electrode studies, at least at the regional level (Montaz-Rosset et al. 2019; Juhasz et al. 2000a, b; Alkonyi et al. 2009). In 16 patients with periventricular nodular heterotopias, there was 84% concordance between hypometabolic and epileptiform nodules on SEEG, and unresected hypometabolic nodules predicted worse surgical outcome (Popescu et al. 2019).

Single-photon emission computed tomography (SPECT) is another tool that has been used for seizure focus localization and will be discussed in detail in this volume in a subsequent chapter. Subtraction ictal SPECT images co-registered to MRI (SISCOM), in which the interictal is subtracted from the ictal SPECT image, was found in a meta-analysis to be localizing in ~50% of FCD-related surgical patients (Lerner et al. 2009) and has been found in multiple studies to predict seizure outcome in both temporal and extratemporal lobe epilepsies (Theodore 2017). In addition to exposure to radiation (as with PET), this modality requires inpatient hospitalization and significant expertise for the injection to occur within 15 s of seizure onset, which is necessary for optimal localization of the seizure focus; late injections can be associated with falsely localizing or non-localizing results (O'Brien et al. 1998). Additionally, other studies have suggested that ictal SPECT may not alter surgical outcomes (Velasco et al. 2011; Noe et al. 2013; Lascano et al. 2016) and can lead to significant additional expense (Sun et al. 2015). In studies directly comparing FDG-PET and SISCOM, these modalities appear overall to be comparable in terms of both localization of the seizure focus and prediction of surgical outcomes, with some studies suggesting that FDG-PET may be more sensitive in TLE, while SPECT may be more sensitive in ETLE (see review in Theodore (2017)). In other multimodality studies, PET hypometabolism was found more frequently than ictal hyperperfusion using SISCOM (Fernandez et al. 2015), and cases with concordance between EEG, MRI, PET, and SISCOM localization had significantly improved seizure outcomes compared to cases with discordant localization results across modalities (Chandra et al. 2014; Perry et al. 2017).

Arterial spin labeling (ASL) is an MRI-based technique that allows for visualization of brain perfusion using magnetically labeled arterial blood water molecules as an endogenous contrast agent. This technique is potentially advantageous in comparison to SISCOM and PET imaging as it does not involve exposure to radioactivity and MRI scanners are widely available. Several studies have reported interictal hypoperfusion in seizure foci, mostly in patients with mesial temporal lobe epilepsy, usually co-localizing with areas of hypometabolism seen using FDG-PET (Lim et al. 2008; Pendse et al. 2010; Pizzini et al. 2013; Wissmeyer et al. 2010; Altrichter et al. 2009; Guo et al. 2015). Several studies have reported hyperperfusion using ASL in the setting of frequent seizures associated with focal cortical dysplasia (Wintermark et al. 2013) or status epilepticus (Matsuura et al. 2015). Other studies have reported variable hypo- and hyperperfusion on ASL in presumed seizure foci, presumably with hypoperfusion seen interictally and hyperperfusion occurring peri-ictally (Storti et al. 2014; Sierra-Marcos et al. 2016; Kim et al. 2016). In total, these findings would be consistent with perfusion changes reported using SPECT, with increased cerebral blood flow seen in ictal in comparison to interictal studies, due either to simple increased blood flow in the setting of increased activity or possibly due to focal inflammation and damage to the blood-brain barrier either due to epileptiform activity or due to epileptogenic lesions such as low-grade tumors (O'Brien et al. 1998; Pizzini et al. 2013; Fabene et al. 2008).

In comparison with other imaging modalities, altered perfusion on ASL tends to co-localize with MRI and PET findings; in a small study of nine children with FCD on MRI, co-localized decreases in cerebral blood flow were observed in all nine children, with PET hypometabolism observed in 5/6 cases (Blauwblomme et al. 2014). In a study of patients with neocortical epilepsy, 15/25 showed alterations in ASL, generally concordant with structural MRI findings (Sierra-Marcos et al. 2016). In this same study, 17/25 patients underwent both ASL and FDG-PET; 9 had PET hypometabolism, of which 5 showed hypoperfusion, 2 hyperperfusion, and 2 no perfusion changes using ASL. In 17/18 patients with hyperperfusion on SISCOM, only 6 showed perfusion abnormalities on ASL. In a study of 20 patients with MR-negative refractory focal epilepsy, PET and ASL were acquired simultaneously using a hybrid PET/MR system, allowing for comparison of the 2 modalities in the identical pathophysiological state. Hypometabolism on PET and hypoperfusion using ASL were found in the same hemisphere in 18/20 patients and were completely concordant in 14/18 (Boscolo Galazzo et al. 2016). In a subsequent study using simultaneous PET and ASL in 12 patients with hippocampal sclerosis and unilateral mTLE based on SEEG, relative hypoperfusion and hypometabolism were seen in all patients in the ipsilateral hippocampus as determined using SEEG, with Engel 1 outcomes in 10/12 patients with 4–13-month follow-up (Wang et al. 2018).

Functional MRI (fMRI) is another technique that has been used to assist with localization of seizure foci and to map epileptogenic networks. Simultaneous EEG-fMRI recordings have been used to detect transient changes in cerebral blood flow (hemodynamic responses) that occur in response to interictal epileptiform discharges (IEDs) on EEG. In focal epilepsy, IED-related blood oxygen level dependent (BOLD) signal changes have been found to be concordant with other metrics of estimating the SOZ, although they are often more widely distributed, with BOLD changes frequently identified in the contralateral homologous cortex and in default mode network areas in temporal lobe epilepsy (see review in Centeno and Carmichael (2014); Pittau et al. (2017)). The cluster with the maximal hemodynamic response has been found to often overlap with intracranial EEG (iEEG) markers of epileptogenicity, including the high-frequency oscillations, the IED spike-onset zone, and the SOZ (Khoo et al. 2018, 2017a; Gonzalez Otarula et al. 2018). Areas demonstrating IED-related hemodynamic responses in the gray matter have also been shown to demonstrate synchronous iEEG IED activity (Khoo et al. 2017b). This suggests that there is consistent spread of epileptiform activity observed using fMRI and iEEG, as is the observation that focal fMRI activations tend to precede more widely distributed network effects associated with the late spike component on EEG (Walz et al. 2017). Propagation of interictal activity may also help to explain the findings of high although not complete concordance between simultaneous intracranial EEG spiking and BOLD responses (Aghakhani et al. 2015). In addition to interictal activity, seizures are occasionally recorded during fMRI-EEG studies. Seizures during EEG-fMRI were described in one study of 20 patients, with significant seizure-related BOLD changes in all patients; in 6 cases that underwent subsequent invasive monitoring, the most significant cluster was found to be within 3.5 cm from the invasively defined SOZ (Chaudhary et al. 2012). Finally, concordance between the maximal IED-related cluster and the area of resection appears to predict a favorable postoperative seizure outcome (PPV 70%), while discordance predicts a poor outcome (NPV 90.95) (An et al. 2013). Similar findings have been described in focal cortical dysplasia, in which discordant or widespread responses were found to be markers of poor prognosis (Thornton et al. 2011; Aubert et al. 2009).

Changes in the underlying patterns of resting-state fMRI activity have also been described in focal epilepsy. Such changes have been most well-described in temporal lobe epilepsy, with altered connectivity found within ipsilateral and contralateral mesial temporal structures and also between medial temporal structures and lateral temporal neocortex, regions involved in the default mode network, and subcortical areas such as the thalamus and brainstem (see reviews in Centeno and Carmichael (2014); Caciagli et al. (2014); Reyes et al. (2016)). These alterations in connectivity appear to change over time, with initial inter-hippocampal disruptions evolving to increased connectivity over years (Morgan et al. 2015). Changes in connectivity have also been described in patients with focal cortical dysplasia, with FCD type IIB lesions appearing to lead to hypo-connectivity and type IIA lesions to hyperconnectivity (Hong et al. 2019). In frontal lobe epilepsy, epileptogenic regions appear to have increased overall functional connections and higher laterality of these connections, with increased local and decreased distant connections (Luo et al. 2014). Changes in dynamic functional connectivity are less well characterized; changes have been described in dynamic regional phase synchrony (Omidvarnia et al. 2017; Pedersen et al. 2017) and in the autocorrelation function, a measure of entropy, with increased local and decreased long-range connectivity in a group of patients with left mesial temporal lobe epilepsy (Nedic et al. 2015).

Some studies have attempted to use these resting-state abnormalities to attempt to identify seizure foci in individual patients with epilepsy. In an early small study, 5/6 patients with focal epilepsy were found to have statistically significant increases in local connectivity compared to 300 control subjects in areas that were later found to be epileptogenic using iEEG (Stufflebeam et al. 2011). Dansereau et al. developed a method to identify abnormal resting-state networks (RSNs) in individual patients and were able to detect abnormalities in 5/6 patients that were "closely related" to the epileptogenic focus as defined by seizure freedom following surgical resection (Dansereau et al. 2014). Lee et al. identified alterations in functional connectivity by measuring differences between intrahemispheric and interhemispheric ICC; concordance was found between the iEEG SOZ and this measure in 21/29 (72.4) of patients, with higher concordance in patients with good surgical outcome (Lee et al. 2014). A different approach is to use visual identification of abnormal independent components obtained from resting-state fMRI data; in 40 evaluated pediatric patients, concordance of these components with the iEEG SOZ was 90%; of 33 patients with at least 1 rs-fMRI EZ concordant with the iEEG SOZ, only 25% with unresected rs-fMRI EZs became seizure-free; in comparison, 76% patients with fully concordant rs-fMRI and iEEG SOZs obtained seizure freedom (Boerwinkle et al. 2017). Additionally, normalization of the identified SOZ resting-state networks (RSNs) postoperatively was found to significantly correlate with seizure outcome, with 97% with SOZ RSN normalization becoming seizure-free, versus 5% seizure freedom in those without SOZ RSN normalization (Boerwinkle et al. 2019).

37.5 FDG-PET in Non-focal Epilepsy Syndromes

Lennox-Gastaut syndrome (LGS) is a rare, severe childhood epilepsy syndrome with a variety of underlying etiologies, characterized by multiple generalized and focal seizure types, cognitive impairment, and characteristic EEG findings. FDG-PET has been shown to have variable patterns of metabolism in LGS, including unilateral focal, unilateral diffuse, and bilateral diffuse hypometabolism and normal metabolism (Kumar et al. 2012). In rare cases, focal hypometabolism can lead to consideration of surgical treatment when consistent with clinical and electrophysiologic data. In children with epileptic spasms, the presence of focal areas of hypometabolism on PET has also helped to provide targets for surgical interventions that can lead to significant improvements in outcome (Chugani et al. 2015; Asarnow et al. 1997). In another rare pediatric epilepsy syndrome caused by mutations in SCN1A, progressive hypometabolism has been reported 1–6 years after diagnosis. Scans were normal initially, followed by development of diffuse cortical hypometabolism (Kumar et al. 2018; Haginoya et al. 2018). Studies of patients with primary generalized epilepsy, which usually has a more benign prognosis, have been reported to have increased ictal with normal interictal metabolism (Kumar et al. 2012).

In autoimmune encephalitis, FDG-PET can identify hypometabolism and may be more sensitive for detection of focal abnormalities than MRI, particularly in early disease stages and for patients with NMDA receptor antibodies (Solnes et al. 2017; Guerin et al. 2019). Occipital hypometabolism has also been reported in these patients (Probasco et al. 2018). A study of 12 patients with new-onset refractory status epilepticus, 9 of whom had antineuronal antibodies, found a combination of hyper- and hypometabolism, predominantly in the mesial temporal region; hypometabolism was predictive of worse outcome (Strohm et al. 2019).

37.6 Neuroinflammation

Neuroinflammation plays a role in epilepsy and can be imaged with PET ligands for translocator protein 18 kDa (TSPO), which is highly expressed in microglia and reactive astrocytes (Alam et al. 2017). An early study using [^{11}C]PK11195 found increased binding in Rasmussen's encephalitis but not in TLE (Banati et al. 1999). [^{11}C]PK11195 binding was also reported to be increased in a patient with presumed focal cortical dysplasia and was greater when a second scan was performed 36 h after a seizure than during a seizure-free period (Butler et al. 2016). Studies in patients with temporal lobe epilepsy using a newer ligand, [^{11}C]PBR28, found increased uptake ipsilateral to seizure foci (Hirvonen et al. 2012; Gershen et al. 2015) (Fig. 37.4). Patients with mesial temporal sclerosis had higher binding

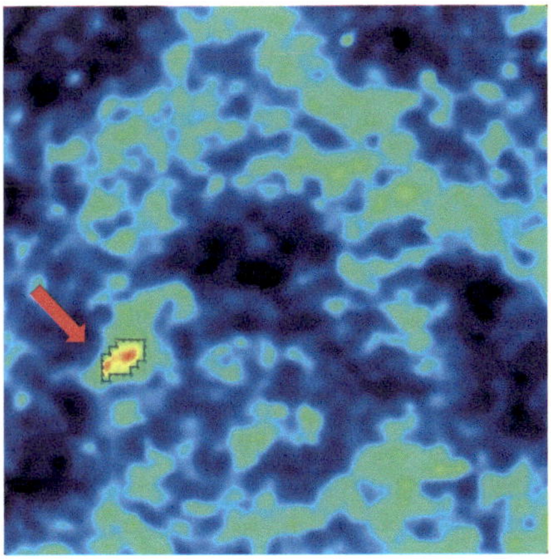

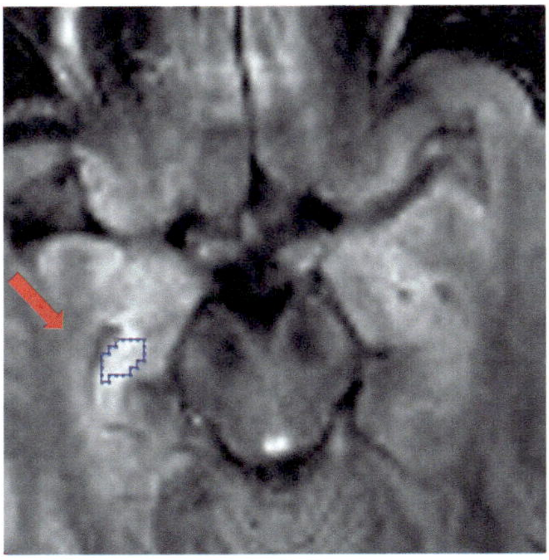

Fig. 37.4 Increased binding of a ligand for the translocator protein 18 kilodalton, expressed in activated microglia and reactive astrocytes, is present in a region of mesial temporal increased flare signal in a patient with mesial temporal sclerosis. This suggests the presence of inflammation

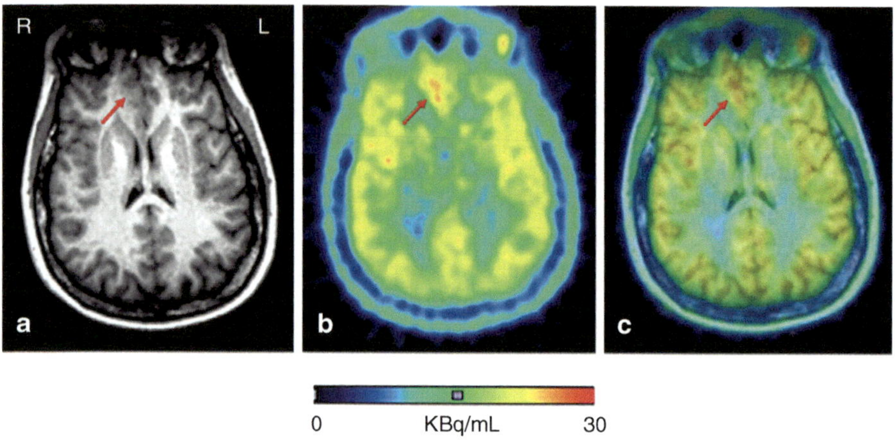

Fig. 37.5 (**a**) Structural MRI showing region of increased right frontal signal suggestive of focal cortical dysplasia. (**b**) TSPO-PET scan showing increased ligand binding. In the same region consistent with inflammation, (**c**) merged images. Reprinted from Dickstein et al. Epilepsia 2019;60:1248–1254

compared to the contralateral hippocampus than those with normal MRI. When full quantitation was carried out, bilateral, although asymmetrical, increases were found compared with healthy volunteers (Gershen et al. 2015). Similarly, in patients with neocortical foci, increased binding was observed ipsilateral to the seizure focus in 9 of 12 patients, 3 with normal MRI and 6 with FCD (Dickstein et al. 2019) (Fig. 37.5).

Inflammation during epileptogenesis has been studied in the mouse unilateral intrahippocampal kainic acid model using PET with another TSPO ligand, [^{18}F]DPA-714, which allowed for tracking of the development of hippocampal sclerosis at 7 days, 14 days, 1 month, and 6 months (Nguyen et al. 2018). PET TSPO binding was observed to peak at 7 days in concert with microglial activation; by 14 days, reactive astrocytes were the main TSPO-expressing cells. Both of these cell types are present in human MTS.

Cannabinoid receptors have also been implicated in inflammatory mechanisms in the hippocampus (Ativie et al. 2018). During electrical amygdala kindling in nonhuman primates, type I cannabinoid receptors (CB1R) were imaged with [^{18}F]MK-9470 PET binding in addition to [^{18}F]FDG-PET. The seizure-onset zone showed increased CB1R binding and decreased glucose metabolism, becoming more marked in extent and intensity during kindling; the ipsilateral thalamus and insula showed transiently increased CB1R binding (Cleeren et al. 2018).

37.7 P-gp Imaging: Mechanisms of Drug Resistance

Several studies have investigated the potential role of P-glycoprotein (P-gp)-mediated drug efflux at the blood-brain barrier in drug-resistant epilepsy using PET imaging with [^{11}C]verapamil. No differences were found between regions ipsilateral and contralateral to the focus in seven patients (Langer et al. 2007). The plasma-to-brain transport rate constant, K1, was investigated before and after administration of the P-glycoprotein inhibitor tariquidar in 16 patients with TLE and 17 healthy controls (Feldmann et al. 2013). Pharmacoresistant epilepsy patients had lower baseline K1 values and lower increases in K1 after administration of tariquidar than healthy controls, suggesting increased P-glycoprotein activity in regions both ipsilateral and contralateral to their seizure foci. Additionally, six patients with drug-resistant epilepsy had increased binding ipsilateral to their temporal lobe seizure focus compared to five patients with drug-responsive epilepsy, as well as eight healthy controls (Shin et al. 2016), supporting a possible role for P-gp-mediated drug efflux in pharmacoresistance in these patients.

37.8 Benzodiazepine Receptors

The benzodiazepine receptor tracer [^{11}C]flumazenil (FMZ) has had more consistent clinical application for epilepsy than any other ligand apart from FDG. Several studies showed that FMZ-PET appeared to have greater sensitivity, but not necessarily specificity, for detecting mesial temporal sclerosis than FDG-PET (Kumar et al. 2012; Komoto et al. 2015). Increased binding reported in some studies may be related to malformations of cortical development and appears to predict poor surgical outcome if these regions are not resected (Yankam Njiwa et al. 2015). FMZ-PET may be more sensitive to seizure recency effects than FDG-PET (Bouvard et al. 2005). An alternative ligand, [^{18}F]flumazenil, may have practical advantages due to its longer half-life (Vivash et al. 2013).

In addition to its use in identification of the seizure focus, [^{11}C]FMZ-PET has been used to investigate the pharmacology of epilepsy. The antiepileptic drug vigabatrin blocks GABA catabolism, increasing synaptic GABA. [^{11}C]FMZ binding volume of distribution was lower in patients taking vigabatrin than other antiepileptic drugs, confirming increased occupation of binding sites due to vigabatrin (Juhasz et al. 2001). Patients with succinic semialdehyde dehydrogenase deficiency, a disorder in which increased GABA is present due to reduced catabolic activity, have also been found to have decreased [^{11}C]FMZ binding due to binding site occupation by GABA, while their parents, obligate heterozygotes, do not (Pearl et al. 2009) (Fig. 37.6).

37.9 Serotonin Receptors

Activation of 5HT1A receptors has been shown to have anti-seizure effects in several animal models. Studies using several 5HT1A receptor ligands have shown reduced binding in mesial temporal seizure foci, including the hippocampus and amygdala, as well as the parahippocampal and fusiform gyri (Kumar et al. 2012) (Fig. 37.7). These findings persisted after MRI-based partial volume correction, suggesting that they are independent of the presence of MRI lesions and related

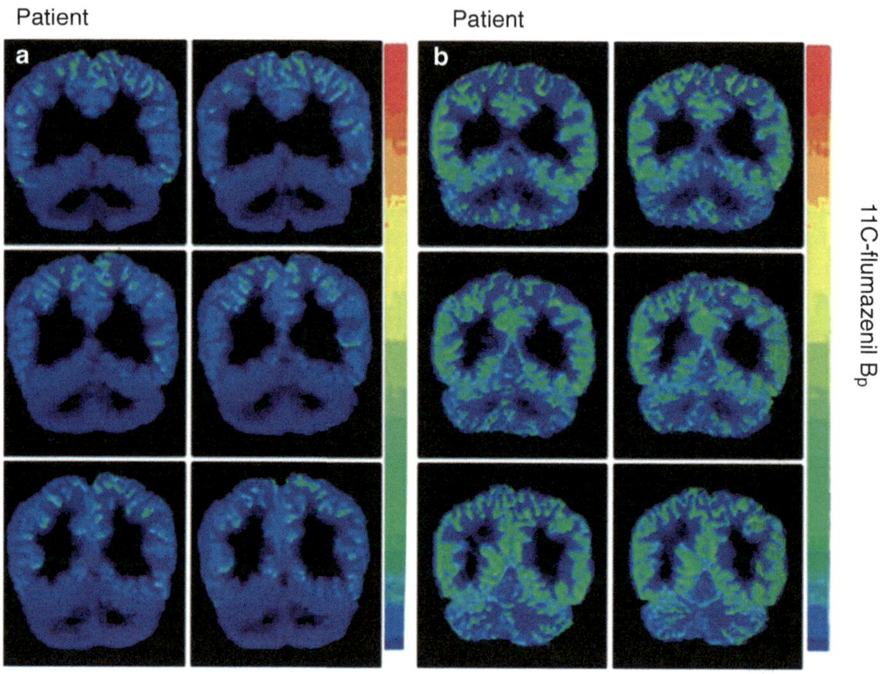

Fig. 37.6 Succinic semialdehyde dehydrogenase deficiency: [^{11}C]flumazenil PET imaging of benzodiazepine receptors. Reduced binding in patients, but normal binding in parents, who are obligate heterozygotes. Reprinted from Pearl et al. Neurology 2009; 73: 423–429

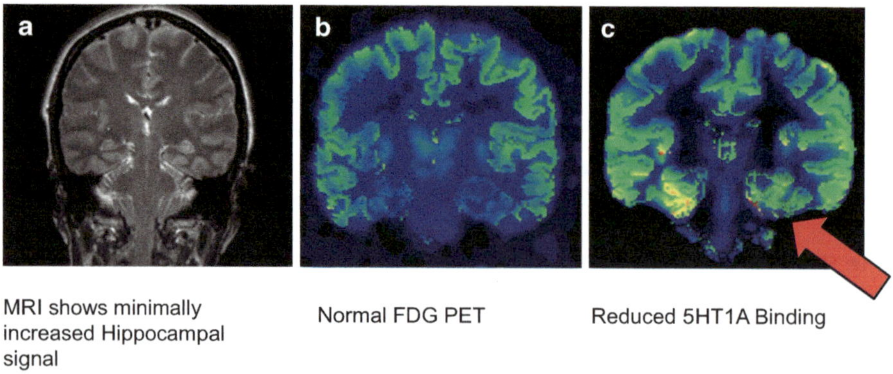

Fig. 37.7 A 44-year-old patient with a history of drug-resistant seizures; surface electroencephalography revealed left temporal seizure onset. (**a**) Normal MRI result. (**b**) Normal [^{18}F]FDG-PET result. (**c**) [^{18}F]FCWAY PET shows relatively decreased left temporal [^{18}]FCWAY binding, indicating reduced 5HT1A receptor availability. Reproduced from Theodore et al. Journal of Nuclear Medicine 2012; 53:1375–1382

neuronal loss. In addition, the combination of [^{18}F]FCWAY 5HT1A receptor imaging and [^{18}F]FDG-PET improved prediction of seizure-free outcome after temporal lobectomy compared with the use of either tracer alone (Theodore et al. 2012). In tuberous sclerosis, a PET ligand for a serotonin precursor, [^{11}C]alpha-methyl tryptophan, has been used to identify epileptogenic tubers (Kumar et al. 2012).

Mood disorders are a frequent and significant comorbidity in patients with drug-resistant focal epilepsy. Reduced 5HT1A receptors have been reported in patients with primary major depressive disorders (Drevets et al. 2007). Studies using [^{11}C]FCWAY and [^{18}F]FCWAY showed correlations between reduced binding and depression rating scales (Savic et al. 2004; Theodore et al. 2007). Patients with a diagnosis of major depressive disorder, based on the Structured Clinical Interview for the Diagnostic and Statistical Manual for Mental Disorders, fourth edition (DSM-IV), had lower binding in limbic regions than those with epilepsy alone (Hasler et al. 2007). In contrast, a study using 2′-methoxyphenyl-(*N*-2′-pyridinyl)-*p*-F-fluoro-benzamidoethylpiperazine ([^{18}F]MPPF) found a positive correlation between Beck Depression Inventory scores and binding in several regions (Lothe et al. 2008). This dichotomy can be explained by the greater sensitivity of MPPF than FCWAY to reduced synaptic serotonin levels, which could lead to apparently increased MPPF binding even in the presence of reduced receptor availability. A study using [^{11}C]DASB, a ligand for serotonin transport, found relatively reduced activity ipsilateral to temporal lobe foci in patients with both seizures and depression compared to subjects with TLE alone, implying additional alteration in synaptic 5HT availability in epilepsy patients in the presence of comorbid depression (Martinez et al. 2013). In kindled rats, [18F]MPPF binding was increased with no change in receptors measured by autoradiography, consistent with the effect of decreased synaptic serotonin (Bascunana et al. 2019). These data underline the importance of understanding the kinetics of specific receptor ligands when interpreting PET neurotransmitter studies.

37.10 Excitatory Amino Acid Receptors

Several recent studies have investigated alterations of excitatory amino acid receptors in epilepsy. The mGLUR5 ligand [^{11}C]ABP688 showed reduced binding in epileptogenic mesial temporal regions after partial volume correction in 31 patients (Lam et al. 2019). The investigators suggested that reductions might be due to receptor internalization or conformational changes in response to excessive extracellular glutamate. Seven of ten patients with FCD studied with [^{11}C]ABP688 had reduced binding in the dysplastic region (DuBois et al. 2016). Balloon cells tended to show lower binding compared with surrounding tissue. Eleven patients had PET with the open-channel *N*-methyl-D-aspartate (NMDA) receptor ligand ([^{18}F]GE-179) (McGinnity et al. 2015). Four had a cluster with increased focal binding, including two with normal MRIs. Interestingly, patients not taking antidepressants had globally increased [^{18}F]GE-179 binding, while three patients taking an antidepressant drug had decreased binding. Taken together, these results could be explained by differences in underlying pathology, in the receptors being imaged, or the vagaries of small PET studies.

This literature continues to grow, with increasing numbers of ligands being investigated. Other tracers studied in patients with epilepsy to date include ligands for several opiate and dopamine receptors, as well as nicotinic acetylcholine receptors (Galovic and Koepp 2016).

37.11 Conclusions

Epilepsy is recognized increasingly as a "spectrum disorder," characterized not only by seizures but neuropsychological and psychiatric comorbidities. Both PET and MRI have made important contributions to evaluation of patients, as well as to our understanding of pathophysiology. Imaging techniques, in concert with genetic and clinical data, may lead to new classification systems based on disease mechanisms that will facilitate more carefully planned and directed treatment.

References

van't Klooster MA, Huiskamp G, Zijlmans M, Debets RM, Comans EF, Bouvard S et al (2014) Can we increase the yield of FDG-PET in the preoperative work-up for epilepsy surgery? Epilepsy Res 108(6):1095–1105

Adler S, Wagstyl K, Gunny R, Ronan L, Carmichael D, Cross JH et al (2017) Novel surface features for automated detection of focal cortical dysplasias in paediatric epilepsy. Neuroimage Clin 14:18–27

Aghakhani Y, Beers CA, Pittman DJ, Gaxiola-Valdez I, Goodyear BG, Federico P (2015) Co-localization between the BOLD response and epileptiform discharges recorded by simultaneous intracranial EEG-fMRI at 3 T. Neuroimage Clin 7:755–763

Ahmed B, Brodley CE, Blackmon KE, Kuzniecky R, Barash G, Carlson C et al (2015) Cortical feature analysis and machine learning improves detection of "MRI-negative" focal cortical dysplasia. Epilepsy Behav 48:21–28

Alam MM, Lee J, Lee SY (2017) Recent progress in the development of TSPO PET ligands for neuroinflammation imaging in neurological diseases. Nucl Med Mol Imaging 51(4):283–296

Alkonyi B, Juhasz C, Muzik O, Asano E, Saporta A, Shah A et al (2009) Quantitative brain surface mapping of an electrophysiologic/metabolic mismatch in human neocortical epilepsy. Epilepsy Res 87(1):77–87

Altrichter S, Pendse N, Wissmeyer M, Jagersberg M, Federspiel A, Viallon M et al (2009) Arterial spin-labeling demonstrates ictal cortical hyperperfusion in epilepsy secondary to hemimegalencephaly. J Neuroradiol 36(5):303–305

An D, Fahoum F, Hall J, Olivier A, Gotman J, Dubeau F (2013) Electroencephalography/functional magnetic resonance imaging responses help predict surgical outcome in focal epilepsy. Epilepsia 54(12):2184–2194

Asarnow RF, LoPresti C, Guthrie D, Elliott T, Cynn V, Shields WD et al (1997) Developmental outcomes in children receiving resection surgery for medically intractable infantile spasms. Dev Med Child Neurol 39(7):430–440

Ativie F, Komorowska JA, Beins E, Albayram O, Zimmer T, Zimmer A et al (2018) Cannabinoid 1 receptor signaling on hippocampal GABAergic neurons influences microglial activity. Front Mol Neurosci 11:295

Aubert S, Wendling F, Regis J, McGonigal A, Figarella-Branger D, Peragut JC et al (2009) Local and remote epileptogenicity in focal cortical dysplasias and neurodevelopmental tumours. Brain 132(pt 11):3072–3086

Banati RB, Goerres GW, Myers R, Gunn RN, Turkheimer FE, Kreutzberg GW et al (1999) [11C](R)-PK11195 positron emission tomography imaging of activated microglia in vivo in Rasmussen's encephalitis. Neurology 53(9):2199–2203

Bascunana P, Garcia-Garcia L, Javela J, Fernandez de la Rosa R, Shiha AA, Kelly J et al (2019) PET neuroimaging reveals serotonergic and metabolic dysfunctions in the hippocampal electrical kindling model of epileptogenesis. Neuroscience 409:101–110

Bazzigaluppi P, Ebrahim Amini A, Weisspapir I, Stefanovic B, Carlen PL (2017) Hungry neurons: metabolic insights on seizure dynamics. Int J Mol Sci 18(11):2269

Benedek K, Juhasz C, Chugani DC, Muzik O, Chugani HT (2006) Longitudinal changes in cortical glucose hypometabolism in children with intractable epilepsy. J Child Neurol 21(1):26–31

Blauwblomme T, Boddaert N, Chemaly N, Chiron C, Pages M, Varlet P et al (2014) Arterial spin Labeling MRI: a step forward in non-invasive delineation of focal cortical dysplasia in children. Epilepsy Res 108(10):1932–1939

Boerwinkle VL, Mohanty D, Foldes ST, Guffey D, Minard CG, Vedantam A et al (2017) Correlating resting-state functional magnetic resonance imaging connectivity by independent component analysis-based epileptogenic zones with intracranial electroencephalogram localized seizure onset zones and surgical outcomes in prospective Pediatric intractable epilepsy study. Brain Connect 7(7):424–442

Boerwinkle VL, Cediel EG, Mirea L, Williams K, Kerrigan JF, Lam S et al (2019) Network-targeted approach and postoperative resting-state functional magnetic resonance imaging are associated with seizure outcome. Ann Neurol 86(3):344–356

Boscolo Galazzo I, Mattoli MV, Pizzini FB, De Vita E, Barnes A, Duncan JS et al (2016) Cerebral metabolism and perfusion in MR-negative individuals with refractory focal epilepsy assessed by simultaneous acquisition of (18)F-FDG PET and arterial spin labeling. Neuroimage Clin 11:648–657

Bouvard S, Costes N, Bonnefoi F, Lavenne F, Mauguiere F, Delforge J et al (2005) Seizure-related short-term plasticity of benzodiazepine receptors in partial epilepsy: a [11C]flumazenil-PET study. Brain 128(pt 6):1330–1343

Butler T, Li Y, Tsui W, Friedman D, Maoz A, Wang X et al (2016) Transient and chronic seizure-induced inflammation in human focal epilepsy. Epilepsia 57(9):e191–e194

Caciagli L, Bernhardt BC, Hong SJ, Bernasconi A, Bernasconi N (2014) Functional network alterations and their structural substrate in drug-resistant epilepsy. Front Neurosci 8:411

Cahill V, Sinclair B, Malpas CB, McIntosh AM, Chen Z, Vivash LE et al (2019) Metabolic patterns and seizure outcomes following anterior temporal lobectomy. Ann Neurol 85(2):241–250

Centeno M, Carmichael DW (2014) Network connectivity in epilepsy: resting state fMRI and EEG-fMRI contributions. Front Neurol 5:93

Chandra PS, Vaghania G, Bal CS, Tripathi M, Kuruwale N, Arora A et al (2014) Role of concordance between ictal-subtracted SPECT and PET in predicting long-term outcomes after epilepsy surgery. Epilepsy Res 108(10):1782–1789

Chapman K, Wyllie E, Najm I, Ruggieri P, Bingaman W, Luders J et al (2005) Seizure outcome after epilepsy surgery in patients with normal preoperative MRI. J Neurol Neurosurg Psychiatry 76(5):710–713

Chassoux F, Landre E, Mellerio C, Turak B, Mann MW, Daumas-Duport C et al (2012) Type II focal cortical dysplasia: electroclinical phenotype and surgical outcome related to imaging. Epilepsia 53(2):349–358

Chassoux F, Artiges E, Semah F, Desarnaud S, Laurent A, Landre E et al (2016) Determinants of brain metabolism changes in mesial temporal lobe epilepsy. Epilepsia 57(6):907–919

Chaudhary UJ, Carmichael DW, Rodionov R, Thornton RC, Bartlett P, Vulliemoz S et al (2012) Mapping preictal and ictal haemodynamic networks using video-electroencephalography and functional imaging. Brain 135(pt 12):3645–3663

Chugani HT, Ilyas M, Kumar A, Juhasz C, Kupsky WJ, Sood S et al (2015) Surgical treatment for refractory epileptic spasms: the Detroit series. Epilepsia 56(12):1941–1949

Cleeren E, Casteels C, Goffin K, Koole M, Van Laere K, Janssen P et al (2018) Positron emission tomography imaging of cerebral glucose metabolism and type 1 cannabinoid receptor availability during temporal lobe epileptogenesis in the amygdala kindling model in rhesus monkeys. Epilepsia 59(5):959–970

Dansereau CL, Bellec P, Lee K, Pittau F, Gotman J, Grova C (2014) Detection of abnormal resting-state networks in individual patients suffering from focal epilepsy: an initial step toward individual connectivity assessment. Front Neurosci 8:419

Desarnaud S, Mellerio C, Semah F, Laurent A, Landre E, Devaux B et al (2018) (18)F-FDG PET in drug-resistant epilepsy due to focal cortical dysplasia type 2: additional value of electroclinical data and coregistration with MRI. Eur J Nucl Med Mol Imaging 45(8):1449–1460

Dickstein LP, Liow JS, Austermuehle A, Zoghbi S, Inati SK, Zaghloul K et al (2019) Neuroinflammation in neocortical epilepsy measured by PET imaging of translocator protein. Epilepsia 60(6):1248–1254

Drevets WC, Thase ME, Moses-Kolko EL, Price J, Frank E, Kupfer DJ et al (2007) Serotonin-1A receptor imaging in recurrent depression: replication and literature review. Nucl Med Biol 34(7):865–877

DuBois JM, Rousset OG, Guiot MC, Hall JA, Reader AJ, Soucy JP et al (2016) Metabotropic glutamate receptor type 5 (mGluR5) cortical abnormalities in focal cortical dysplasia identified in vivo with [11C]ABP688 positron-emission tomography (PET) imaging. Cereb Cortex 26(11):4170–4179

Fabene PF, Navarro Mora G, Martinello M, Rossi B, Merigo F, Ottoboni L et al (2008) A role for leukocyte-endothelial adhesion mechanisms in epilepsy. Nat Med 14(12):1377–1383

Feldmann M, Asselin MC, Liu J, Wang S, McMahon A, Anton-Rodriguez J et al (2013) P-glycoprotein expression and function in patients with temporal lobe epilepsy: a case-control study. Lancet Neurol 12(8):777–785

Fernandez S, Donaire A, Seres E, Setoain X, Bargallo N, Falcon C et al (2015) PET/MRI and PET/MRI/SISCOM coregistration in the presurgical evaluation of refractory focal epilepsy. Epilepsy Res 111:1–9

Gaillard WD, Weinstein S, Conry J, Pearl PL, Fazilat S, Fazilat S et al (2007) Prognosis of children with partial epilepsy: MRI and serial 18FDG-PET. Neurology 68(9):655–659

Gaillard WD, Cross JH, Duncan JS, Stefan H, Theodore WH (2011) Epilepsy imaging study guideline criteria: commentary on diagnostic testing study guidelines and practice parameters. Epilepsia 52(9):1750–1756

Galovic M, Koepp M (2016) Advances of molecular imaging in epilepsy. Curr Neurol Neurosci Rep 16(6):58

Gershen LD, Zanotti-Fregonara P, Dustin IH, Liow JS, Hirvonen J, Kreisl WC et al (2015) Neuroinflammation in temporal lobe epilepsy measured using positron emission tomographic imaging of translocator protein. JAMA Neurol 72(8):882–888

Gonzalez Otarula KA, Khoo HM, von Ellenrieder N, Hall JA, Dubeau F, Gotman J (2018) Spike-related haemodynamic responses overlap with high frequency oscillations in patients with focal epilepsy. Brain 141(3):731–743

Govil-Dalela T, Kumar A, Behen ME, Chugani HT, Juhasz C (2018) Evolution of lobar abnormalities of cerebral glucose metabolism in 41 children with drug-resistant epilepsy. Epilepsia 59(7):1307–1315

Guerin J, Watson RE, Carr CM, Liebo GB, Kotsenas AL (2019) Autoimmune epilepsy: findings on MRI and FDG-PET. Br J Radiol 92(1093):20170869

Guo Y, Gao F, Wang S, Ding Y, Zhang H, Wang J et al (2009) In vivo mapping of temporospatial changes in glucose utilization in rat brain during epileptogenesis: an 18F-fluorodeoxyglucose-small animal positron emission tomography study. Neuroscience 162(4):972–979

Guo X, Xu S, Wang G, Zhang Y, Guo L, Zhao B (2015) Asymmetry of cerebral blood flow measured with three-dimensional pseudocontinuous arterial spin-labeling mr imaging in temporal lobe epilepsy with and without mesial temporal sclerosis. J Magn Reson Imaging 42(5):1386–1397

Haginoya K, Togashi N, Kaneta T, Hino-Fukuyo N, Ishitobi M, Kakisaka Y et al (2018) [(18) F]fluorodeoxyglucose-positron emission tomography study of genetically confirmed patients with Dravet syndrome. Epilepsy Res 147:9–14

Hasler G, Bonwetsch R, Giovacchini G, Toczek MT, Bagic A, Luckenbaugh DA et al (2007) 5-HT1A receptor binding in temporal lobe epilepsy patients with and without major depression. Biol Psychiatry 62(11):1258–1264

Hirvonen J, Kreisl WC, Fujita M, Dustin I, Khan O, Appel S et al (2012) Increased in vivo expression of an inflammatory marker in temporal lobe epilepsy. J Nucl Med 53(2):234–240

Hong SJ, Kim H, Schrader D, Bernasconi N, Bernhardt BC, Bernasconi A (2014) Automated detection of cortical dysplasia type II in MRI-negative epilepsy. Neurology 83(1):48–55

Hong SJ, Lee HM, Gill R, Crane J, Sziklas V, Bernhardt BC et al (2019) A connectome-based mechanistic model of focal cortical dysplasia. Brain 142(3):688–699

Juhasz C, John F (2020) Utility of MRI, PET, and ictal SPECT in presurgical evaluation of non-lesional pediatric epilepsy. Seizure 77:15–28

Juhasz C, Chugani DC, Muzik O, Watson C, Shah J, Shah A et al (2000a) Electroclinical correlates of flumazenil and fluorodeoxyglucose PET abnormalities in lesional epilepsy. Neurology 55(6):825–835

Juhasz C, Chugani DC, Muzik O, Watson C, Shah J, Shah A et al (2000b) Is epileptogenic cortex truly hypometabolic on interictal positron emission tomography? Ann Neurol 48(1):88–96

Juhasz C, Behen ME, Muzik O, Chugani DC, Chugani HT (2001) Bilateral medial prefrontal and temporal neocortical hypometabolism in children with epilepsy and aggression. Epilepsia 42(8):991–1001

Jupp B, Williams J, Binns D, Hicks RJ, Cardamone L, Jones N et al (2012) Hypometabolism precedes limbic atrophy and spontaneous recurrent seizures in a rat model of TLE. Epilepsia 53(7):1233–1244

Khoo HM, Hao Y, von Ellenrieder N, Zazubovits N, Hall J, Olivier A et al (2017a) The hemodynamic response to interictal epileptic discharges localizes the seizure-onset zone. Epilepsia 58(5):811–823

Khoo HM, von Ellenrieder N, Zazubovits N, Dubeau F, Gotman J (2017b) Epileptic networks in action: synchrony between distant hemodynamic responses. Ann Neurol 82(1):57–66

Khoo HM, von Ellenrieder N, Zazubovits N, He D, Dubeau F, Gotman J (2018) The spike onset zone: the region where epileptic spikes start and from where they propagate. Neurology 91(7):e666–ee74

Kim YK, Lee DS, Lee SK, Kim SK, Chung CK, Chang KH et al (2003) Differential features of metabolic abnormalities between medial and lateral temporal lobe epilepsy: quantitative analysis of (18)F-FDG PET using SPM. J Nucl Med 44(7):1006–1012

Kim YH, Kang HC, Kim DS, Kim SH, Shim KW, Kim HD et al (2011) Neuroimaging in identifying focal cortical dysplasia and prognostic factors in pediatric and adolescent epilepsy surgery. Epilepsia 52(4):722–727

Kim BS, Lee ST, Yun TJ, Lee SK, Paeng JC, Jun J et al (2016) Capability of arterial spin labeling MR imaging in localizing seizure focus in clinical seizure activity. Eur J Radiol 85(7):1295–1303

Komoto D, Iida K, Higaki T, Kaichi Y, Takauchi K, Arihiro K et al (2015) Diagnostic performance of positron emission tomography for the presurgical evaluation of patients with non-lesional intractable partial epilepsy: comparison among 18F-FDG, 11C-flumazenil, and 11C-flumazenil binding potential imaging using statistical imaging analysis. Hiroshima J Med Sci 64(4):51–57

Kumar A, Semah F, Chugani HT, Theodore WH (2012) Epilepsy diagnosis: positron emission tomography. Handb Clin Neurol 107:409–424

Kumar A, Juhasz C, Luat A, Govil-Dalela T, Behen ME, Hicks MA et al (2018) Evolution of brain glucose metabolic abnormalities in children with epilepsy and SCN1A gene variants. J Child Neurol 33(13):832–836

Lam J, DuBois JM, Rowley J, Gonzalez-Otarula KA, Soucy JP, Massarweh G et al (2019) In vivo metabotropic glutamate receptor type 5 abnormalities localize the epileptogenic zone in mesial temporal lobe epilepsy. Ann Neurol 85(2):218–228

Langer O, Bauer M, Hammers A, Karch R, Pataraia E, Koepp MJ et al (2007) Pharmacoresistance in epilepsy: a pilot PET study with the P-glycoprotein substrate R-[(11)C]verapamil. Epilepsia 48(9):1774–1784

Lascano AM, Perneger T, Vulliemoz S, Spinelli L, Garibotto V, Korff CM et al (2016) Yield of MRI, high-density electric source imaging (HD-ESI), SPECT and PET in epilepsy surgery candidates. Clin Neurophysiol 127(1):150–155

Lee HW, Arora J, Papademetris X, Tokoglu F, Negishi M, Scheinost D et al (2014) Altered functional connectivity in seizure onset zones revealed by fMRI intrinsic connectivity. Neurology 83(24):2269–2277

Lerner JT, Salamon N, Hauptman JS, Velasco TR, Hemb M, Wu JY et al (2009) Assessment and surgical outcomes for mild type I and severe type II cortical dysplasia: a critical review and the UCLA experience. Epilepsia 50(6):1310–1335

Lim YM, Cho YW, Shamim S, Solomon J, Birn R, Luh WM et al (2008) Usefulness of pulsed arterial spin labeling MR imaging in mesial temporal lobe epilepsy. Epilepsy Res 82(2–3):183–189

Liow JS, Zoghbi SS, Hu S, Hall MD, Hines CS, Shetty HU et al (2016) (18)F-FCWAY, a serotonin 1A receptor radioligand, is a substrate for efflux transport at the human blood-brain barrier. NeuroImage 138:134–140

Lothe A, Didelot A, Hammers A, Costes N, Saoud M, Gilliam F et al (2008) Comorbidity between temporal lobe epilepsy and depression: a [18F]MPPF PET study. Brain 131(pt 10):2765–2782

Luo C, An D, Yao D, Gotman J (2014) Patient-specific connectivity pattern of epileptic network in frontal lobe epilepsy. Neuroimage Clin 4:668–675

Mariani V, Revay M, D'Orio P, Rizzi M, Pelliccia V, Nichelatti M et al (2019) Prognostic factors of postoperative seizure outcome in patients with temporal lobe epilepsy and normal magnetic resonance imaging. J Neurol 266(9):2144–2156

Martinez A, Finegersh A, Cannon DM, Dustin I, Nugent A, Herscovitch P et al (2013) The 5-HT1A receptor and 5-HT transporter in temporal lobe epilepsy. Neurology 80(16):1465–1471

Matsuura K, Maeda M, Okamoto K, Araki T, Miura Y, Hamada K et al (2015) Usefulness of arterial spin-labeling images in periictal state diagnosis of epilepsy. J Neurol Sci 359(1–2):424–429

Mayoral M, Ninerola-Baizan A, Marti-Fuster B, Donaire A, Perissinotti A, Rumia J et al (2019) Epileptogenic zone localization with (18)FDG PET using a new dynamic parametric analysis. Front Neurol 10:380

McGinnity CJ, Koepp MJ, Hammers A, Riano Barros DA, Pressler RM, Luthra S et al (2015) NMDA receptor binding in focal epilepsies. J Neurol Neurosurg Psychiatry 86(10):1150–1157

McGonigal A, Bartolomei F, Regis J, Guye M, Gavaret M, Trebuchon-Da Fonseca A et al (2007) Stereoelectroencephalography in presurgical assessment of MRI-negative epilepsy. Brain 130(pt 12):3169–3183

Montaz-Rosset MS, Scholly J, Voulleminot P, Severac F, Hirsch E, Valenti-Hirsch MP et al (2019) Comparison of functional deficit zone defined by FDG PET to the epileptogenic zones described in stereo-electroencephalograph in drug-resistant epileptic patients treated by surgery. Clin Nucl Med 44(7):526–531

Morgan VL, Abou-Khalil B, Rogers BP (2015) Evolution of functional connectivity of brain networks and their dynamic interaction in temporal lobe epilepsy. Brain Connect 5(1):35–44

Nedic S, Stufflebeam SM, Rondinoni C, Velasco TR, dos Santos AC, Leite JP et al (2015) Using network dynamic fMRI for detection of epileptogenic foci. BMC Neurol 15:262

Nguyen DL, Wimberley C, Truillet C, Jego B, Caille F, Pottier G et al (2018) Longitudinal positron emission tomography imaging of glial cell activation in a mouse model of mesial temporal lobe epilepsy: toward identification of optimal treatment windows. Epilepsia 59(6):1234–1244

Noe K, Sulc V, Wong-Kisiel L, Wirrell E, Van Gompel JJ, Wetjen N et al (2013) Long-term outcomes after nonlesional extratemporal lobe epilepsy surgery. JAMA Neurol 70(8):1003–1008

O'Brien TJ, So EL, Mullan BP, Hauser MF, Brinkmann BH, Bohnen NI et al (1998) Subtraction ictal SPECT co-registered to MRI improves clinical usefulness of SPECT in localizing the surgical seizure focus. Neurology 50(2):445–454

Omidvarnia A, Pedersen M, Vaughan DN, Walz JM, Abbott DF, Zalesky A et al (2017) Dynamic coupling between fMRI local connectivity and interictal EEG in focal epilepsy: a wavelet analysis approach. Hum Brain Mapp 38(11):5356–5374

Pearl PL, Gibson KM, Quezado Z, Dustin I, Taylor J, Trzcinski S et al (2009) Decreased GABA-A binding on FMZ-PET in succinic semialdehyde dehydrogenase deficiency. Neurology 73(6):423–429

Pedersen M, Omidvarnia A, Curwood EK, Walz JM, Rayner G, Jackson GD (2017) The dynamics of functional connectivity in neocortical focal epilepsy. Neuroimage Clin 15:209–214

Pendse N, Wissmeyer M, Altrichter S, Vargas M, Delavelle J, Viallon M et al (2010) Interictal arterial spin-labeling MRI perfusion in intractable epilepsy. J Neuroradiol 37(1):60–63

Perry MS, Bailey L, Freedman D, Donahue D, Malik S, Head H et al (2017) Coregistration of multimodal imaging is associated with favourable two-year seizure outcome after paediatric epilepsy surgery. Epileptic Disord 19(1):40–48

Pittau F, Ferri L, Fahoum F, Dubeau F, Gotman J (2017) Contributions of EEG-fMRI to assessing the Epileptogenicity of focal cortical dysplasia. Front Comput Neurosci 11:8

Pizzini FB, Farace P, Manganotti P, Zoccatelli G, Bongiovanni LG, Golay X et al (2013) Cerebral perfusion alterations in epileptic patients during peri-ictal and post-ictal phase: PASL vs DSC-MRI. Magn Reson Imaging 31(6):1001–1005

Popescu CE, Mai R, Sara R, Lizio D, Zanni D, Rossetti C et al (2019) The role of FDG-PET in patients with epilepsy related to periventricular nodular heterotopias: diagnostic features and Long-term outcome. J Neuroimaging 29(4):512–520

Probasco JC, Solnes L, Nalluri A, Cohen J, Jones KM, Zan E et al (2018) Decreased occipital lobe metabolism by FDG-PET/CT: an anti-NMDA receptor encephalitis biomarker. Neurol Neuroimmunol Neuroinflamm 5(1):e413

Rathore C, Dickson JC, Teotonio R, Ell P, Duncan JS (2014) The utility of 18F-fluorodeoxyglucose PET (FDG PET) in epilepsy surgery. Epilepsy Res 108(8):1306–1314

Reyes A, Thesen T, Wang X, Hahn D, Yoo D, Kuzniecky R et al (2016) Resting-state functional MRI distinguishes temporal lobe epilepsy subtypes. Epilepsia 57(9):1475–1484

Savic I, Lindstrom P, Gulyas B, Halldin C, Andree B, Farde L (2004) Limbic reductions of 5-HT1A receptor binding in human temporal lobe epilepsy. Neurology 62(8):1343–1351

Shin JW, Chu K, Shin SA, Jung KH, Lee ST, Lee YS et al (2016) Clinical applications of simultaneous PET/MR imaging using (R)-[11C]-verapamil with Cyclosporin A: preliminary results on a surrogate marker of drug-resistant epilepsy. AJNR Am J Neuroradiol 37(4):600–606

Sidhu MK, Duncan JS, Sander JW (2018) Neuroimaging in epilepsy. Curr Opin Neurol 31(4):371–378

Sierra-Marcos A, Carreno M, Setoain X, Lopez-Rueda A, Aparicio J, Donaire A et al (2016) Accuracy of arterial spin labeling magnetic resonance imaging (MRI) perfusion in detecting the epileptogenic zone in patients with drug-resistant neocortical epilepsy: comparison with electrophysiological data, structural MRI, SISCOM and FDG-PET. Eur J Neurol 23(1):160–167

Solnes LB, Jones KM, Rowe SP, Pattanayak P, Nalluri A, Venkatesan A et al (2017) Diagnostic value of (18)F-FDG PET/CT versus MRI in the setting of antibody-specific autoimmune encephalitis. J Nucl Med 58(8):1307–1313

Storti SF, Boscolo Galazzo I, Del Felice A, Pizzini FB, Arcaro C, Formaggio E et al (2014) Combining ESI, ASL and PET for quantitative assessment of drug-resistant focal epilepsy. NeuroImage 102(pt 1):49–59

Strohm T, Steriade C, Wu G, Hantus S, Rae-Grant A, Larvie M (2019) FDG-PET and MRI in the evolution of new-onset refractory status epilepticus. AJNR Am J Neuroradiol 40(2):238–244

Stufflebeam SM, Liu H, Sepulcre J, Tanaka N, Buckner RL, Madsen JR (2011) Localization of focal epileptic discharges using functional connectivity magnetic resonance imaging. J Neurosurg 114(6):1693–1697

Sun PY, Wyatt K, Nickels KC, Wong-Kisiel LC, Mandrekar J, Wirrell E (2015) Predictors of length of stay in children admitted for presurgical evaluation for epilepsy surgery. Pediatr Neurol 53(3):207–210

Tang Y, Liow JS, Zhang Z, Li J, Long T, Li Y et al (2018) The evaluation of dynamic FDG-PET for detecting epileptic foci and Analyzing reduced glucose phosphorylation in refractory epilepsy. Front Neurosci 12:993

Tellez-Zenteno JF, Hernandez Ronquillo L, Moien-Afshari F, Wiebe S (2010) Surgical outcomes in lesional and non-lesional epilepsy: a systematic review and meta-analysis. Epilepsy Res 89(2–3):310–318

Tenney JR, Rozhkov L, Horn P, Miles L, Miles MV (2014) Cerebral glucose hypometabolism is associated with mitochondrial dysfunction in patients with intractable epilepsy and cortical dysplasia. Epilepsia 55(9):1415–1422

Theodore WH (2017) Presurgical focus localization in epilepsy: PET and SPECT. Semin Nucl Med 47(1):44–53

Theodore WH, Sato S, Kufta C, Balish MB, Bromfield EB, Leiderman DB (1992) Temporal lobectomy for uncontrolled seizures: the role of positron emission tomography. Ann Neurol 32(6):789–794

Theodore WH, Hasler G, Giovacchini G, Kelley K, Reeves-Tyer P, Herscovitch P et al (2007) Reduced hippocampal 5HT1A PET receptor binding and depression in temporal lobe epilepsy. Epilepsia 48(8):1526–1530

Theodore WH, Martinez AR, Khan OI, Liew CJ, Auh S, Dustin IM et al (2012) PET of serotonin 1A receptors and cerebral glucose metabolism for temporal lobectomy. J Nucl Med 53(9):1375–1382

Thesen T, Quinn BT, Carlson C, Devinsky O, DuBois J, McDonald CR et al (2011) Detection of epileptogenic cortical malformations with surface-based MRI morphometry. PLoS One 6(2):e16430

Thornton R, Vulliemoz S, Rodionov R, Carmichael DW, Chaudhary UJ, Diehl B et al (2011) Epileptic networks in focal cortical dysplasia revealed using electroencephalography-functional magnetic resonance imaging. Ann Neurol 70(5):822–837

Tomas J, Pittau F, Hammers A, Bouvard S, Picard F, Vargas MI et al (2019) The predictive value of hypometabolism in focal epilepsy: a prospective study in surgical candidates. Eur J Nucl Med Mol Imaging 46(9):1806–1816

Tonini C, Beghi E, Berg AT, Bogliun G, Giordano L, Newton RW et al (2004) Predictors of epilepsy surgery outcome: a meta-analysis. Epilepsy Res 62(1):75–87

Velasco TR, Wichert-Ana L, Mathern GW, Araujo D, Walz R, Bianchin MM et al (2011) Utility of ictal single photon emission computed tomography in mesial temporal lobe epilepsy with hippocampal atrophy: a randomized trial. Neurosurgery 68(2):431–436; discussion 436

Vivash L, Gregoire MC, Lau EW, Ware RE, Binns D, Roselt P et al (2013) 18F-flumazenil: a gamma-aminobutyric acid A-specific PET radiotracer for the localization of drug-resistant temporal lobe epilepsy. J Nucl Med 54(8):1270–1277

Walz JM, Pedersen M, Omidvarnia A, Semmelroch M, Jackson GD (2017) Spatiotemporal mapping of epileptic spikes using simultaneous EEG-functional MRI. Brain 140(4):998–1010

Wang ZI, Suwanpakdee P, Jones SE, Jaisani Z, Moosa AN, Najm IM et al (2016) Re-review of MRI with post-processing in nonlesional patients in whom epilepsy surgery has failed. J Neurol 263(9):1736–1745

Wang YH, An Y, Fan XT, Lu J, Ren LK, Wei PH et al (2018) Comparison between simultaneously acquired arterial spin labeling and (18)F-FDG PET in mesial temporal lobe epilepsy assisted by a PET/MR system and SEEG. Neuroimage Clin 19:824–830

Willmann O, Wennberg R, May T, Woermann FG, Pohlmann-Eden B (2007) The contribution of 18F-FDG PET in preoperative epilepsy surgery evaluation for patients with temporal lobe epilepsy a meta-analysis. Seizure 16(6):509–520

Wintermark P, Lechpammer M, Warfield SK, Kosaras B, Takeoka M, Poduri A et al (2013) Perfusion imaging of focal cortical dysplasia using arterial spin Labeling: correlation with histopathological vascular density. J Child Neurol 28(11):1474–1482

Wissmeyer M, Altrichter S, Pereira VM, Viallon M, Federspiel A, Seeck M et al (2010) Arterial spin-labeling MRI perfusion in tuberous sclerosis: correlation with PET. J Neuroradiol 37(2):127–130

Wong CH, Bleasel A, Wen L, Eberl S, Byth K, Fulham M et al (2012) Relationship between preoperative hypometabolism and surgical outcome in neocortical epilepsy surgery. Epilepsia 53(8):1333–1340

Yankam Njiwa J, Gray KR, Costes N, Mauguiere F, Ryvlin P, Hammers A (2015) Advanced [(18) F]FDG and [(11)C]flumazenil PET analysis for individual outcome prediction after temporal lobe epilepsy surgery for hippocampal sclerosis. Neuroimage Clin 7:122–131

SISCOM (Subtraction Ictal SPECT with Coregistration to MRI) 38

Hwareung Lee, Jung Sik Kim, Ji Hyun Kim, and Seung Bong Hong

Contents

Abstract

Brain single-photon emission computed tomography (SPECT) is a functional nuclear imaging technique that can provide a regional map of cerebral blood flow (CBF) changes during the interictal or ictal period in patients with epilepsy and other neurological disorders. The radiotracer for brain SPECT is rapidly taken up by the brain within 30–60 s after its injection. The radiotracer injection during

H. Lee
Department of Neurology, Samsung Medical Center, Samsung Biomedical Research Institute, Sungkyunkwan University, Seoul, Republic of Korea

Severnace Hospital, Yonsei University, Seoul, South Korea

J. S. Kim · S. B. Hong (✉)
Department of Neurology, Samsung Medical Center, Samsung Biomedical Research Institute, Sungkyunkwan University, Seoul, Republic of Korea
e-mail: sbhong@skku.edu

J. H. Kim
The David S. Olton Behavioral Biology Program, Krieger School of Arts and Sciences, Johns Hopkins University, Baltimore, MD, USA

R. A. J. O. Dierckx et al. (eds.), *PET and SPECT in Neurology*,
https://doi.org/10.1007/978-3-030-53168-3_38

seizure activity (ictal SPECT) can show a snapshot of regional CBF (rCBF) changes during seizure. The sensitivity of ictal SPECT is high in temporal lobe epilepsy but relatively lower in extratemporal epilepsy. SISCOM is an imaging technique to subtract ictal and interictal SPECT images and to coregister them on brain MRI. SISCOM significantly improves the sensitivity of ictal SPECT and can further localize epileptic focus. But the successful localization of epileptic focus can be affected by the time of radiotracer injection, seizure duration, and propagation pattern of ictal EEG. Ictal hypoperfusion as well as ictal hyperperfusion is an important finding. Thus, ictal SPECT and SISCOM should be carefully interpreted by simultaneous review with seizure semiology, clinical information, features, injection time, duration of seizure, and ictal EEG pattern at the injection times. SISCOM is also useful for localizing brain structure generating specific feature of seizures and studying propagation pathways of epileptic seizures and pathomechanism of other neurological disorders and sleep disorders.

38.1 Introduction

Ictal SPECT (single-photon emission computed tomography) has been used successfully for localizing mesial temporal lobe epilepsy and has been reported to be less sensitive but more specific in extratemporal lobe epilepsy (O'Brien et al. 1998a; Spanaki et al. 1999; Lee et al. 2000; Valenti et al. 2002; Kaiboriboon et al. 2005). The low sensitivity of ictal SPECT in neocortical epilepsy may be related to various clinical factors such as inhomogeneous and various perfusion patterns in brain regions, difficulty in detection of subtle perfusion changes, differences in the amount of radioisotope delivered to the brain and time taken to inject radioisotope, different slice levels and orientation arising from different patient positioning during the interictal and ictal SPECT scans, and lack of quantitative assessment of the difference between interictal and ictal SPECT images. To solve these problems arising from qualitative analysis, quantitative analysis methods were developed by calculating the perfusion difference between ictal and interictal SPECTs. SPECT difference images can be calculated by subtraction of ictal and interictal SPECT scans (Zubal et al. 1995) or subtraction ictal SPECT with coregistration to MRI (SISCOM) (O'Brien et al. 1998a).

38.2 Image Processing for SISCOM

Subtraction ictal SPECT with coregistration to MRI (SISCOM) procedure consists of the following steps (Fig. 38.1):

Ictal–interictal SPECT registration: Before subtracting each voxel value of the ictal and interictal SPECT images, three-dimensional position of the interictal SPECT is transformed to the ictal SPECT using a chamfer surface matching algorithm. In all cases, root mean square distance is within one voxel. It is crucial to

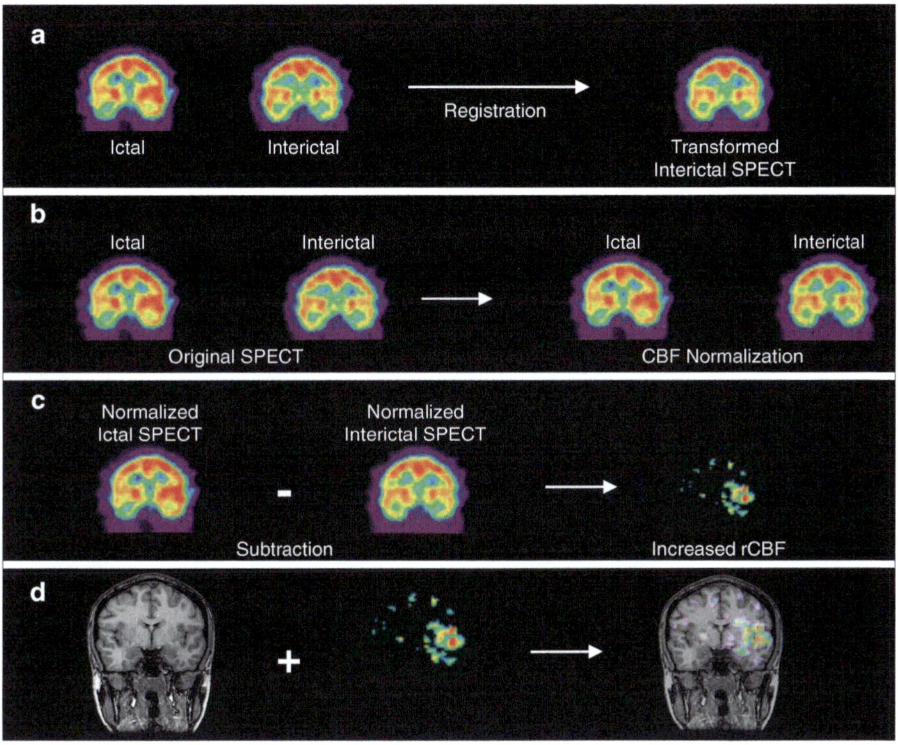

Fig. 38.1 The process of subtraction ictal SPECT with coregistration to MRI. Interictal SPECT is linearly transformed to the same patient's ictal SPECT using chamfer surface matching algorithm (**a**). The total intensity levels of ictal and transformed interictal SPECTs are normalized (**b**). The difference of two corresponding pixel values of ictal and interictal SPECTs is calculated and separated into positive (increased rCBF) and negative difference (decreased rCBF) images (**c**). Finally, subtracted SPECT is overlaid to MRI for anatomical localization (**d**)

make an accurate interictal-to-ictal SPECT registration both for improving the sensitivity of the SPECT subtraction and for preventing false-negative or false-positive perfusion differences.

Normalization of differences in pixel intensities: Ictal and interictal cerebral pixel intensities are rescaled to constant mean pixel intensities to normalize different levels of radioisotope uptake, retention, and decay. A normalization factor is calculated based on total pixel counts in the whole brain (global normalization), but sometimes this method can produce false-positive or false-negative findings especially when the areas of perfusion changes are extensive. In that case, regional normalization using the cerebellum, white matter, non-epileptic hemisphere, or brain stem may be a better normalization scheme (Zubal et al. 1995).

Ictal-transformed interictal SPECT subtraction: To obtain the cerebral perfusion difference, transformed and normalized interictal SPECT is subtracted from ictal SPECT pixel by pixel. Thus, brain regions of increased rCBF (with positive pixel values) and regions of decreased rCBF (with negative pixel values) are separately identified.

Intensity thresholding: To eliminate scattered and non-interest region from the subtracted images, it is required to calculate the standard deviation (SD) of subtracted SPECT pixels. It may be possible to use varying thresholds (1.0–3.0 SD) according to SISCOM results. In clinical purpose, it is commonly used for 2 SD to localize seizure-onset zone. Placing the significance level at 3 SD increases specificity, but decreases sensitivity. If no significant rCBF change is observed in subtracted SPECT, one can consider reducing the threshold to 1 SD and searching for (nonsignificant) tendencies of ictal rCBF changes.

MRI-subtracted SPECT registration: For the localization of difference images, the subtracted SPECT is coregistered with a structural brain MRI. In most cases, the error ranges of SPECT–MRI registration for clinical use are within 5 mm (O'Brien et al. 1998a).

38.3 Interpretation of SISCOM

Ictal hyperperfusion and hypoperfusion in subtracted SPECT are generally considered significant when the difference of rCBF in each pixel is greater than 2 SD. The location of significant ictal hyperperfusion is visually decided on MRI by SPECT–MRI coregistration. For the determination of significant rCBF changes, only brain regions showing three and more voxels (3.56 mm × 3 = 10.68 mm) with significantly different intensity values between ictal and interictal SPECT images are included. Because the subtracted SPECT may reflect the peri-ictal or postictal state when the injection of radioisotope was delayed or seizures were very short-lasting, the subtracted SPECT should be interpreted with considering the interval between radioisotope injection and seizure onset, duration of seizure, and time of seizure end. The propagation pattern of ictal EEG discharges at the time of radiotracer injection is also very important because it may affect the final result of subtracted SPECT. Frontal lobe seizures show a tendency of more rapid propagation compared to temporal lobe seizures. The interpretation of SISCOM should include careful simultaneous review of seizure semiology, sequences of ictal EEG patterns, injection time in relation to seizure duration, structural lesion, and other clinical information. SISCOM reflects only cerebral perfusion changes (significantly different from the interictal state) at the time of tracer injection, not always the zone of seizure onset.

Recent two studies assessed the optimal *z*-score threshold of SISCOM to localize seizure-onset zone (Newey et al. 2013; Coster et al. 2018). One study (2013) examined 4 thresholding values (1, 1.5, 2, and 2.5) for the optimal SISCOM analysis to localize a seizure-onset zone in 26 epilepsy patients who underwent epilepsy surgery with at least 6-month seizure-free after surgery and found a slightly improved localization accuracy with a *z*-score threshold of 1.5 compared to evaluation at the *z*-score threshold of 1 and 2. Other study (2018) investigated the robustness of *z*-score threshold in 80 patients with drug-resistant epilepsy in whom the exact location of the ictal-onset zone was known after successful epilepsy surgery. This study showed no difference in correct seizure localization between the two thresholds (1.5 SD, 70%; 2 SD, 72%). They suggested that the z-score threshold of 2 SD should be used in a routine clinical setting since 2 SD threshold shows higher inter-rater agreement and observer confidence rates than 1.5 SD threshold.

38.4 Clinical Significance and Research Applications of SISCOM

The first study using subtracted SPECT was published by Zubal et al. (1995). From this difference image technique, the epileptic focus was localized in five of six temporal lobe focus patients and in four of six for extratemporal seizure patients. This result was superior to visual analysis, and the difference images provided more precise information regarding location of seizure focus.

Subtraction of interictal from ictal SPECT coregistered to three-dimensional MRI (SISCOM) is an improved and better validated technique for ictal and interictal SPECT subtraction. Various clinical studies have been performed using this SISCOM technique in the field of epilepsy (O'Brien et al. 1998a, b, 1999; Lee et al. 2000). In the first study on patients with intractable partial epilepsy (O'Brien et al. 1998a), SISCOM was able to localize the epileptic focus in 45 out of 51 (88.2%) patients, while the traditional side-by-side inspection of ictal and interictal SPECT images localized 20 out of 51 (39.2%). However, late injection of the radiotracer (>45 s after seizure onset) but not secondary generalization was associated with a falsely localizing or non-localizing SISCOM. To overcome the problem of delayed injection, automated equipment for self-injection was developed which improved the sensitivity of ictal SPECT (Van Paesschen et al. 2000). To circumvent the difficulty of early injection during seizures, a postictal SPECT study was performed (O'Brien et al. 1999). The combined interpretation of hyperperfusion (positive values) and hypoperfusion (negative values) of SISCOM showed a better concordance rate with the final diagnosis than the analysis of either the hyperperfusion or hypoperfusion SISCOM image alone. In a similar study (Lee et al. 2000), the sensitivity of the combined hyperperfusion and hypoperfusion SISCOM (91.8%) was superior to only hyperperfusion SISCOM (85.2%) and visual inspection of ictal SPECT (68.9%). Ictal hypoperfusion at the epileptic focus was first reported in that study. Figure 38.2e demonstrated that a patient with an epileptic focus at the left posterior lateral temporal cortex showed ictal hypoperfusion at the epileptic focus, while ictal hyperperfusion was seen at the left anterior temporal region where ictal discharges propagated rapidly at the time of radiotracer injection. Rapid propagation of ictal discharges to other brain regions with early postictal state of the epileptic focus despite persistence of clinical seizures is the probable explanation for ictal hypoperfusion. In cases where early radiotracer injection is difficult, postictal SPECT subtraction can also be helpful in the evaluation and localization of the epileptic focus (Zubal et al. 1999).

Other study compared the ability of MSI, FDG-PET, and ictal SPECT to predict seizure-free outcome after epilepsy surgery with intracranial EEG monitoring. The odds ratios of MSI (magnetic source imaging), FDG-PET, and ictal SPECT for prediction of seizure outcome were 4.4, 7.1, and 9.1, respectively, although the number of patients who had MSI, FDG-PET, or ictal SPECT was different (Knowlton et al. 2008).

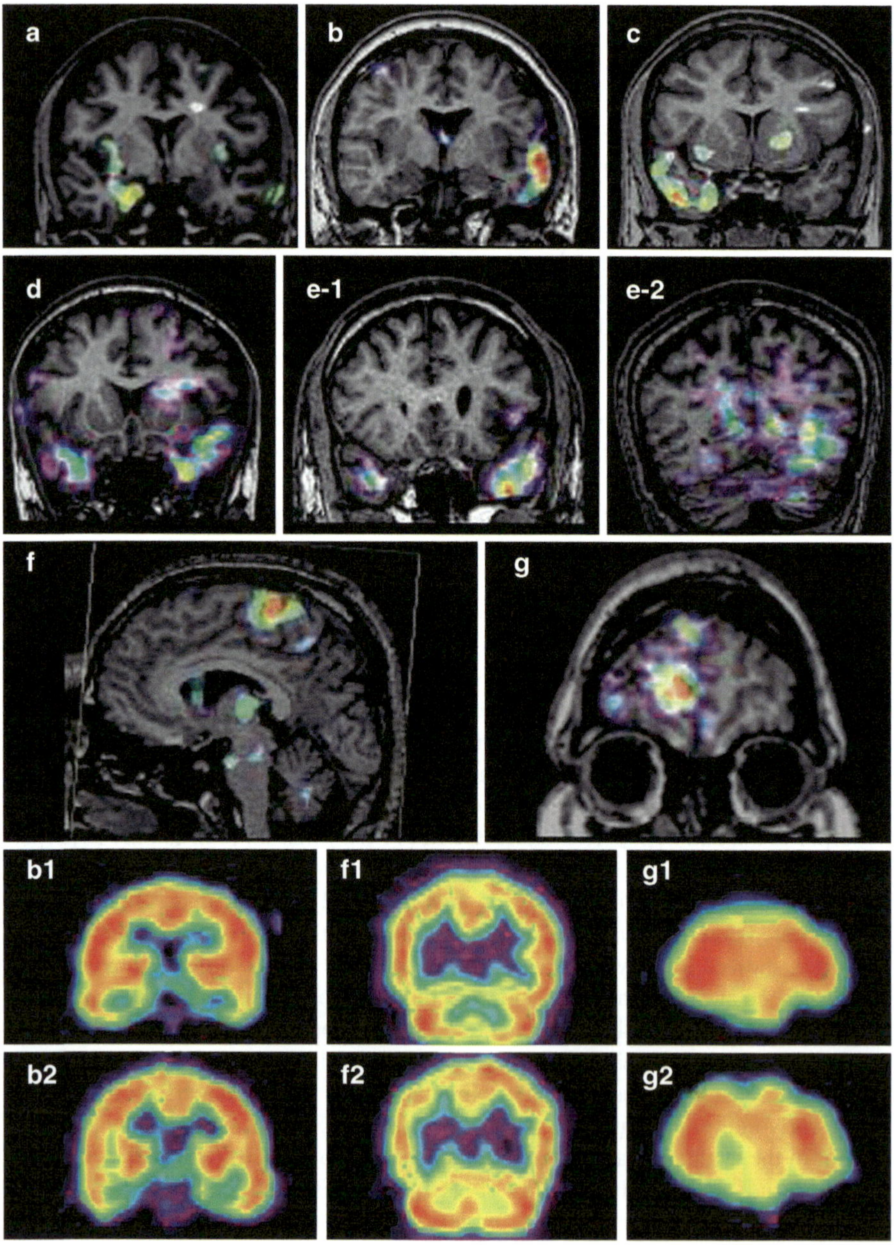

Another study compared different diagnostic tools in the prognostic factors for surgical outcome in neocortical epilepsy patients. Diagnostic sensitivities of interictal EEG, ictal scalp EEG, FDG-PET, and subtraction ictal single-photon emission computed tomography were 37.1%, 70.8%, 44.3%, and 41.1%, respectively. Localization by FDG-PET and interictal EEG was correlated with a seizure-free outcome. Concordance with two or more presurgical evaluations was significantly related to a seizure-free outcome. But this study showed lower sensitivity of SISCOM compared to other studies (Lee et al. 2005). So there are many factors affecting the result of ictal SPECT and SISCOM including seizure type and duration, radiotracer type, injection time, epilepsy monitoring unit setting, experience of technicians, and the method of SISCOM.

Ahnlide et al. (2007) analyzed SISCOM in 26 patients who had intracranial EEG monitoring and epilepsy surgery. SISCOM findings altered and extended the strategy for electrode placement at invasive recording in 15 patients. In this study, SISCOM was a prerequisite for seizure outcome in all six patients with favorable outcomes, and SISCOM is valuable for the identification of the epileptogenic zone in patients with drug-resistant epilepsy scheduled for invasive video-EEG.

Other two studies also indicated that SISCOM may have an impact on surgical decision (Tan et al. 2008; von Oertzen et al. 2011) (Fig. 38.3).

A previous study with 95 pediatric epilepsy patients investigated impact of timing of radiotracer injection, MRI findings, and seizure characteristics on SISCOM results (Stamoulis et al. 2017). This study showed that the SISCOM results were correlated with the radioisotope injection delay ($p < 0.01$) and cerebral lobe of seizure onset (specifically frontal vs. temporal, $p = 0.02$) but not with MRI findings ($p = 0.33$), epilepsy etiology ($p = 0.27$), or seizure duration ($p = 0.20$).

Repeated ictal SPECTs ictal SPECT with SISCOM analysis was shown to be helpful for localizing an epileptic focus in patients with partial epilepsy who had a non-localized first ictal SPECT and SISCOM (Lee et al. 2011). The SISCOM results of the second ictal SPECT were further localized in 43 (62.3%) patients. In the second ictal SPECT, radiotracer injection time from seizure onset was significantly

Fig. 38.2 Various perfusion patterns of subtracted SPECT in TLE (temporal lobe epilepsy) and ETLE (extratemporal lobe epilepsy) patients. The perfusion patterns of subtracted SPECT in TLE are (**a**) hyperperfusion in only mesial temporal region of the right mesial TLE, (**b**) hyperperfusion in lateral temporal region of the left neocortical TLE, (**c**) hyperperfusion in both mesial and lateral temporal areas in the right mesial TLE, and (**d**) hyperperfusion-plus pattern of subtracted SPECT: bilateral temporal hyperperfusion with left predominance in the left neocortical TLE. (*e-1* and *e-2*) Combined hyperperfusion–hypoperfusion pattern of subtracted SPECT in a patient with an epileptic focus at the left posterior lateral temporal cortex; *e-1* is a positive image showing hyperperfusion in the left anterior temporal region, and *e-2* is a negative image showing hypoperfusion in the left posterior lateral and basal temporal cortex from the same interictal and ictal SPECT images. (**f** and **g**) Perfusion patterns of subtracted SPECT in ETLE patients: (**f**) focal hyperperfusion in a left supplementary motor area seizure and (**g**) focal hypoperfusion in the right frontal lobe epilepsy. *b-2*, *f-2*, and *g-2* are conventional ictal SPECT of patients *b*, *f*, and *g*, while *b-1*, *f-1*, and *g-1* are conventional interictal SPECT of patients *b*, *f*, and *g*. All images are presented in radiological view

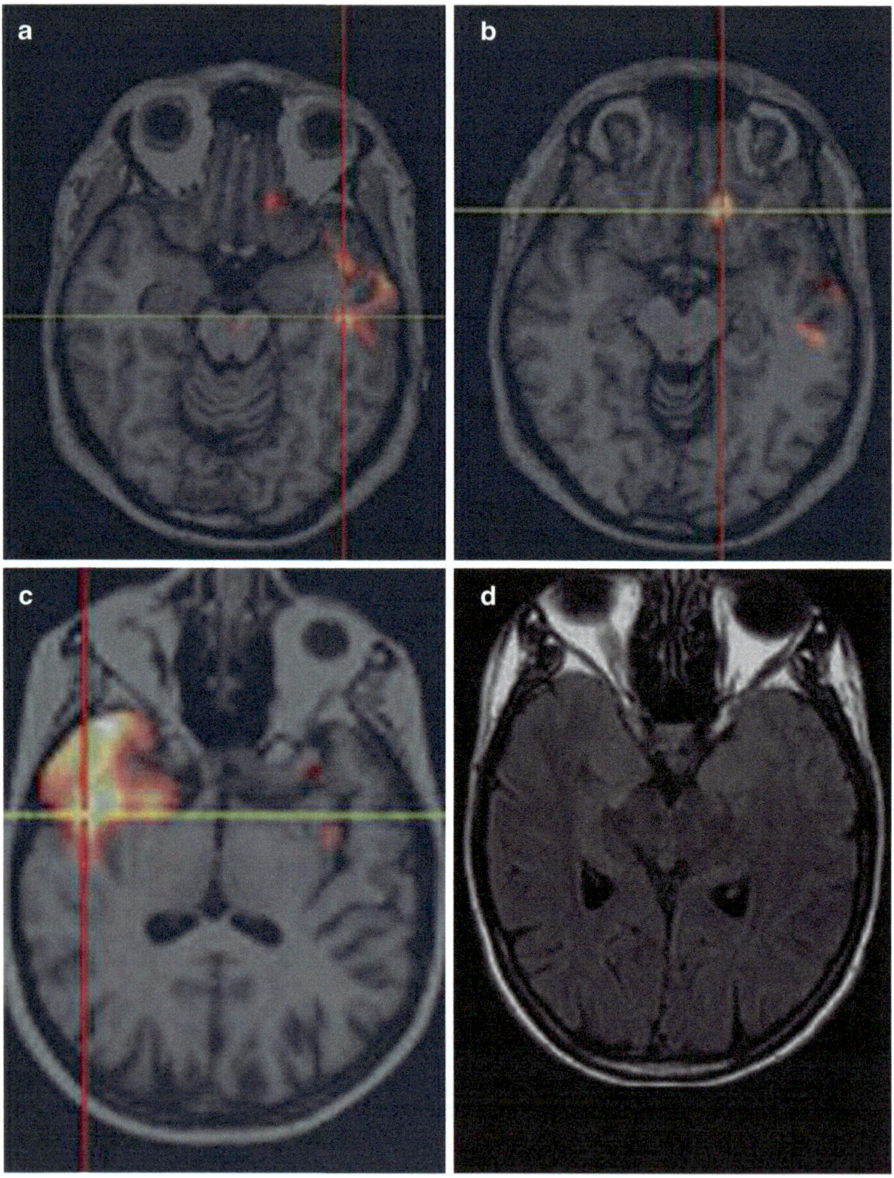

Fig. 38.3 (**a**, **b**) Example of multiple SISCOM hyperperfusions which are concordant to multifocal ECoG (electrocorticography) seizure onsets: a 22-year-old male patient with drug-refractory epilepsy had two types of seizures. (**c**, **d**) Example of nonlesional MRI with SISCOM concordant to site of surgery and seizure-free outcome

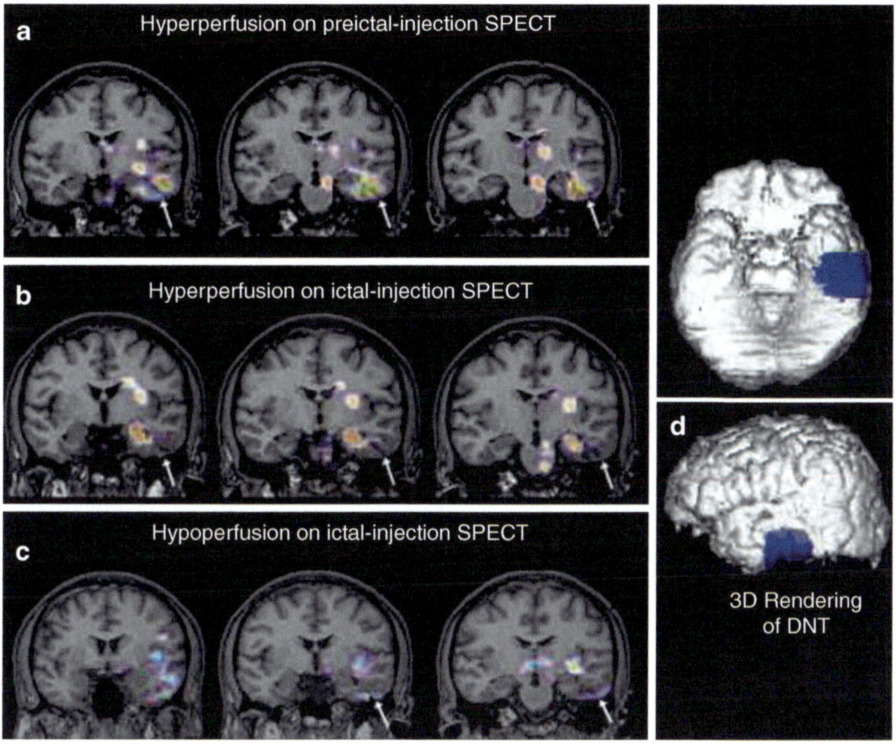

Fig. 38.4 Preictal SISCOM results. (**a**) SISCOM with preictal-injection SPECT shows hyperperfusion on the tumor lesion located at the left inferior–basal temporal area, ipsilateral midbrain, and thalamus. ^{99m}Tc-ECD injection was completed 11 s before the seizure began. (**b**) SISCOM with ictal-injection SPECT shows hyperperfusion at the ipsilateral amygdala–hippocampus, basal ganglia, and pons. The ^{99m}Tc-ECD injection was completed after 25 s (out of a 47 s seizure duration). (**c**) SISCOM with ictal-injection SPECT shows hypoperfusion at the tumor lesion and adjacent temporal lobe tissue. (**d**) A three-dimensional rendering view of the patient's brain MRI and tumor (*blue color*). **White arrows* indicate the location of the tumor

shorter in the localized group (25.1 ± 8.9 s) than the non-localized group (49.2 ± 55.8 s) ($p = 0.008$).

Since the time of radiotracer injection greatly affects ictal SPECT and SISCOM, preictal SPECT has been reported (Hong et al. 2008). We injected the radiotracer for SPECT study two times (one was injected during seizure and the other was 11 s prior to clinical seizure). While SISCOM with ictal SPECT showed focal hyperperfusion in ipsilateral hippocampus, SISCOM with preictal SPECT revealed early ictal hyperperfusion in an ipsilateral tumor located in the inferior temporal lobe (Fig. 38.4). So we presumed seizure started from the tumor itself and then rapidly propagated to the hippocampus. The patient had a resection of the tumor with preservation of the hippocampus and became seizure-free without memory deficit postsurgically. Indeed, if we are able to inject radiotracer preictally, SISCOM will theoretically show early changes of CBF during seizures.

SISCOM is also useful in guiding the location and extent of resection in the surgery of intractable extratemporal lobe epilepsy. The extent of resection according to the cortical region of the SISCOM focus is significantly associated with the rate of excellent outcome (100% with complete resection, 60% with partial resection, and 20% with non-resection) (O'Brien et al. 2000). But another study reported inferior sensitivity of subtracted SPECT compared to visual inspection of ictal and interictal SPECT (Koh et al. 1998). The reasons for this difference of sensitivity may be the differences in study design, the technical method of SPECT subtraction, the rapidity of radiotracer injection in each laboratory, and the way of subtracted SPECT interpretation.

In 2016, Jalota et al. (2016) assessed the positive predictive value of surgical outcomes obtained by presurgical SISCOM in 44 patients with lesional (MRI-positive) and nonlesional (MRI-negative) refractory ETLE and TLE (Jalota et al. 2016). Concordance between one or more regions of SISCOM hyperperfusion with ECoG and at least partial resection of the dominant SISCOM signal provided additional useful information for predicting long-term surgical outcomes. The authors suggested that such regions are likely critical nodes in more extensive, active, epileptogenic circuits.

A meta-analysis study demonstrated the role of SISCOM in presurgical evaluation for patients who had epilepsy surgery in 11 SISCOM studies (Chen and Guo 2016). The authors assessed the value of SISCOM in identifying the epileptogenic zone and predicting postoperative outcomes. This study indicates that SISCOM has moderate sensitivity in localizing the epileptogenic zone and can provide complementary information when MRI is negative.

SISCOM is useful not only for localizing an epileptic focus but also for localizing the brain structure producing specific features of seizures or other paroxysmal neurological disorders. TLE seizure associated with or without contralateral dystonia showed different CBF changes during seizures (Joo et al. 2004). SISCOM showed that TLE seizures with dystonia were associated with significantly higher incidences of ictal hyperperfusion in the caudate nucleus, putamen, and thalamus compared to those without dystonia (Fig. 38.5). Other study showed that temporal lobe seizure presenting dystonic posturing are associated with ictal hyperperfusion on contralateral basal ganglia (Shin et al. 2002).

SISCOM revealed ictal hyperperfusion in the right amygdala, hippocampus, insula, and anterior temporal lobe during musicogenic seizures, which was concordant to the brain regions with hypometabolism in FDG-PET (Fig. 38.6) (Cho et al. 2007). Two complex partial seizures were provoked by listening to a ballad.

The patient experienced palpitation and an unpleasant feeling 1–2 min after listening to a song and then progressed to a complex partial seizure.

A SISCOM of apneic seizures showed ictal hyperperfusion in the left, posterior, mid-lateral temporal cortex. This finding supports the previous theory that apneic

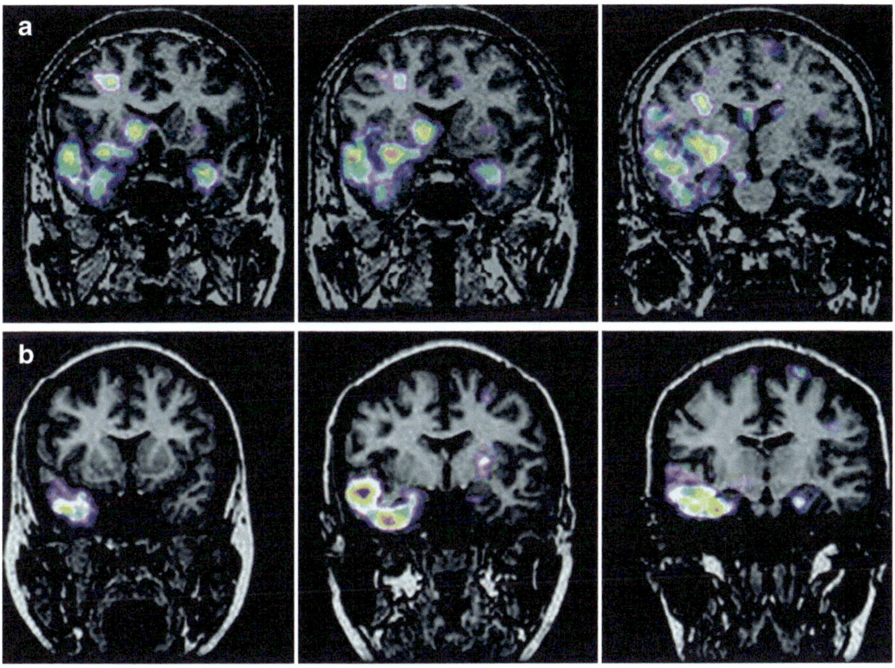

Fig. 38.5 (**a**) SISCOM of a patient with dystonic posturing during seizure. Ictal hyperperfusion on the right temporal lobe with ipsilateral caudate nucleus and putamen in a 24-year-old woman with right mesial temporal lobe epilepsy (TLE). (**b**) SISCOM of a patient without dystonic posturing. Ictal hyperperfusion on the right temporal lobe without basal ganglia hyperperfusion in a 31-year-old man with right mesial TLE

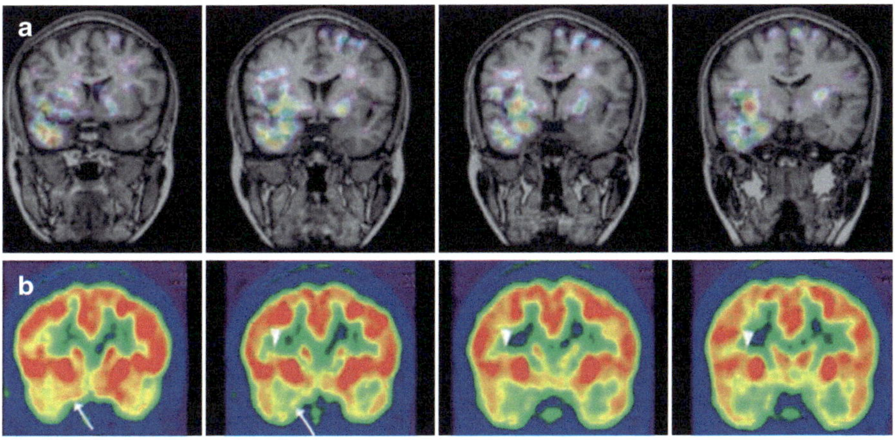

Fig. 38.6 SISCOM and FDG-PET. SISCOM images show the hyperperfusion in the right anterior mesial temporal regions, amygdala, hippocampal head, and insula (**a**). FDG-PET demonstrates interictal hypometabolism in the right amygdala (*arrow*), hippocampal head, and insula (*arrow heads*) (**b**)

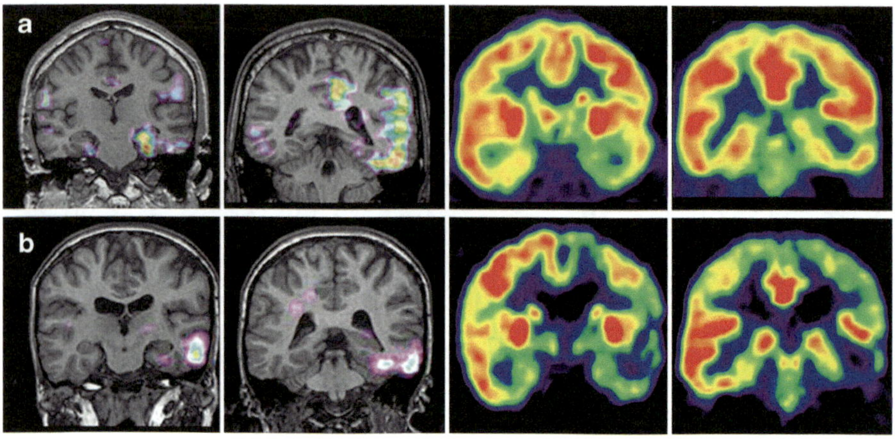

Fig. 38.7 SISCOM and FDG-PET findings in a MLTLE and a LTLE patient. (**a**) Left upper two SISCOM images show ictal hyperperfusion in left mesial and lateral temporal regions during seizure, and right upper two FDG-PET images depict interictal hypometabolism in the left mesial and lateral temporal regions in a MLTLE patient. (**b**) Lower row shows ictal hyperperfusion in left middle–inferior temporal gyrus and posterior basal temporal regions (left two SISCOM images) and interictal hypometabolism in the left hemisphere, especially in the lateral and basal temporal and frontoparietal regions (right two FDG-PET images) in a LTLE patient

seizures might be mediated through the limbic and associated cortical systems (Lee et al. 1999).

Our study demonstrated the usefulness of SISCOM and FDG-PET analyses for differentiating between two subtypes of TLE (mesio-lateral TLE (MLTLE) and lateral TLE (LTLE)) (Joo et al. 2015). We investigated the differences of the functional neuroimaging features (FDG-PET hypometabolism and ictal SPECT hyperperfusion) in addition to clinical, electrophysiological, and neuropsychological findings between MLTLE ($n = 31$) and LTLE ($n = 41$) groups. Our study showed that MLTLE group was more likely to have FDG-PET hypometabolism and SISCOM hyperperfusion restricted to the temporal areas, compared to the LTLE group (Fig. 38.7). Interestingly, no significant differences were found in scalp EEG, MRI, and Wada asymmetry between the two groups. The overall seizure-free rate was good (73.8%, mean follow-up = 9.7 years), which was not different in MLTLE (Engel class I, 74.3%) vs. LTLE (73.6%). Memory function after surgery was spared in LTLE patients, while visual memory was impaired in MLTLE patients when their mesial temporal structures were sufficiently resected.

SISCOM can be very helpful in refractory epilepsy patients with a normal MRI for intracranial electrode implantation to map a seizure-onset zone. In 26 MRI-negative refractory TLE or ETLE patients, SISCOM images in 92% of the patients had a focus of abnormal perfusion detected by blinded reviewers (O'Brien et al. 1998a). They also evaluated the usefulness of SISCOM in the presurgical evaluation of 17 patients with MRI-negative ETLE (O'Brien et al. 2000). Seventy-seven percent of them showed a correct localization in SISCOM results by blinded reviewers.

Concordance of the SISCOM localization with the site of surgical resection was associated with a significantly better chance of excellent surgery outcome than those in whom the SISCOM results were either non-concordant or non-localizing (55% vs. 0%, $p < 0.05$). In 33 MRI-negative TLE patients who underwent SISCOM studies and surgery (Bell et al. 2009), the SISCOM abnormality localized to the resection site was found to be significantly associated with postsurgical seizure-free outcome. Another study in 85 patients with MRI-negative ETLE showed that SISCOM was localizing in 68% (58/85) of the patients (Noe et al. 2013). However, 38% of only 24 patients who had a resective surgery were seizure-free after 10 more years after surgery.

SISCOM can be used for studies of propagation pathways of epileptic seizures in human brain. To investigate ictal hyperperfusion patterns during semiologic progression of seizures, we performed ictal SPECT and SISCOM in 50 patients with mesial TLE (Shin et al. 2002). The patients were categorized into five groups according to semiologic progression during ictal SPECT (Group 1 had aura only; Group 2 had motionless staring with or without aura; Group 3 had motionless staring and then automatism with or without aura; Group 4 had motionless staring and then dystonic posturing with or without aura and automatism; and Group 5 had motionless staring, automatism, and then head version and generalized seizures with or without aura and dystonic posturing). The semiologic progression in TLE seizures were related to the propagation of hyperperfusion from ipsilateral temporal lobe to contralateral temporal lobe, insula, basal ganglia, and frontal lobe (Fig. 38.8).

By SISCOM analysis, we studied ictal hyperperfusion in the cerebellum and basal ganglia in TLE (Shin et al. 2001). During TLE seizures, hemispheric cerebellar hyperperfusion occurred not only in contralateral but also in ipsilateral or bilateral cerebellar hemispheres to the side of seizure origin. Although temporal lobe origin seizures associated with additional frontal hyperperfusion produced more frequent hemispheric cerebellar hyperperfusion, seizures showing only temporal hyperperfusion without frontal hyperperfusion could produce hyperperfusion of the basal ganglia and cerebellar hyperperfusion.

Another study showed that impairment of consciousness showed a strong association with secondary hyperperfusion in the thalamic/upper brain stem region. The authors suggest that the spread of epileptic discharges or a transsynaptic activation (diaschisis) of these structures is an important mechanism in the alteration of consciousness during seizures (Lee et al. 2002).

A recent SISCOM study in 31 consecutive focal epilepsy patients who underwent an intracranial electrode implantation investigated whether ictal perfusion changes correspond to electrically connected brain networks (Tousseyn et al. 2017). In all patients, cortico-cortical evoked potential examinations were performed after repetitive electrical stimulation of an ictal-onset zone. The authors concluded that strong connectivity was demonstrated between the ictal-onset zone and hyperperfused SISCOM regions, while connectivity was weaker in the direction of baseline-perfused or hypoperfused SISCOM areas, and suggested that one should consider the contribution of all hyperperfused regions, as these are likely not random but represent an electrically connected epileptic network.

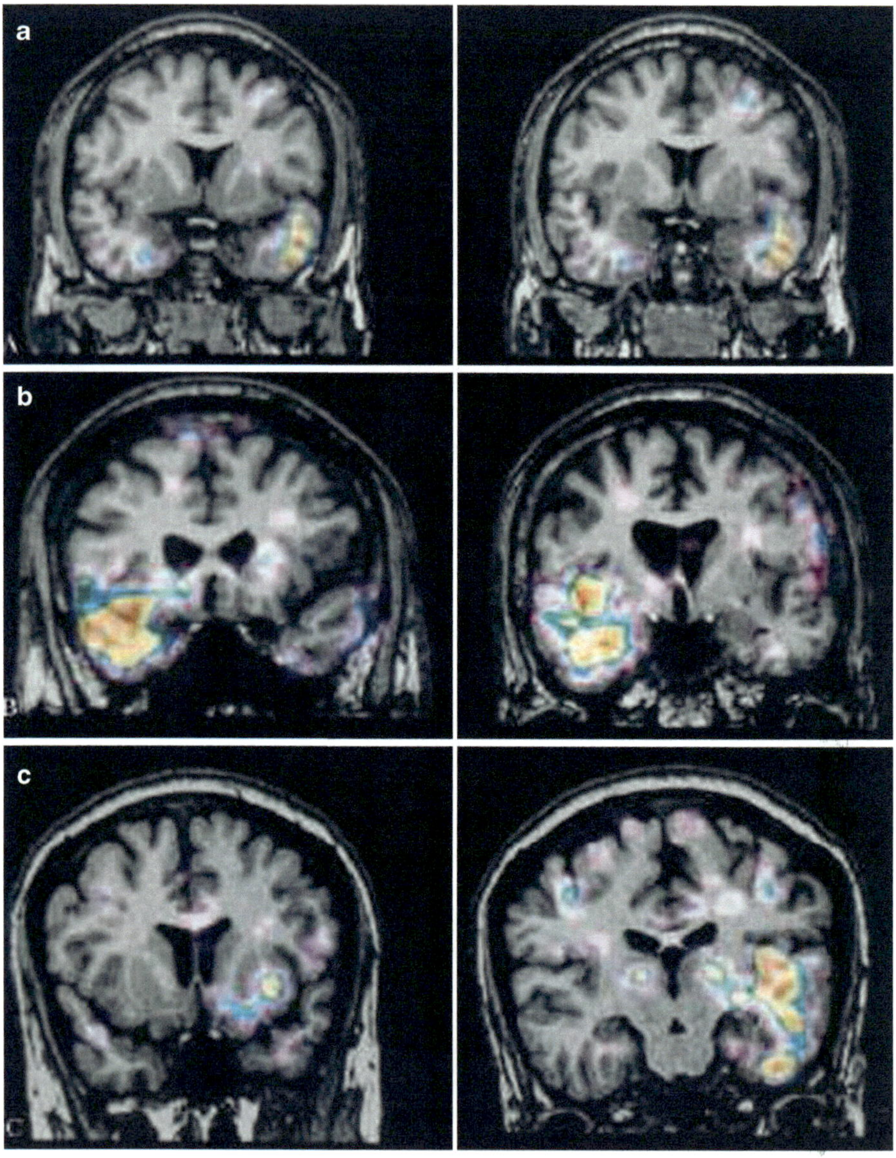

Fig. 38.8 Images of subtracted SPECT with MRI coregistration in each group. (**a**) Ictal hyperperfusion on the left temporal lobe with subtle right temporal change in a 37-year-old woman with left temporal lobe epilepsy (Group 1). (**b**) Ictal hyperperfusion on the right temporal lobe and ipsilateral insular cortex in a 25-year-old man with right temporal lobe epilepsy (Group 2). (**c**) A 42-year-old man with left temporal lobe epilepsy showing ictal hyperperfusion of the left temporal lobe, its adjacent insula, and small portions of basal ganglia (Group 3). (**d**) Ictal hyperperfusion on the left temporal lobe, basal ganglia, and insula in a 34-year-old man with left temporal lobe epilepsy (Group 4). (**e**) A 28-year-old man with right temporal lobe epilepsy showing ictal hyperperfusion on bilateral multiple brain regions with right temporal predominance (Group 5)

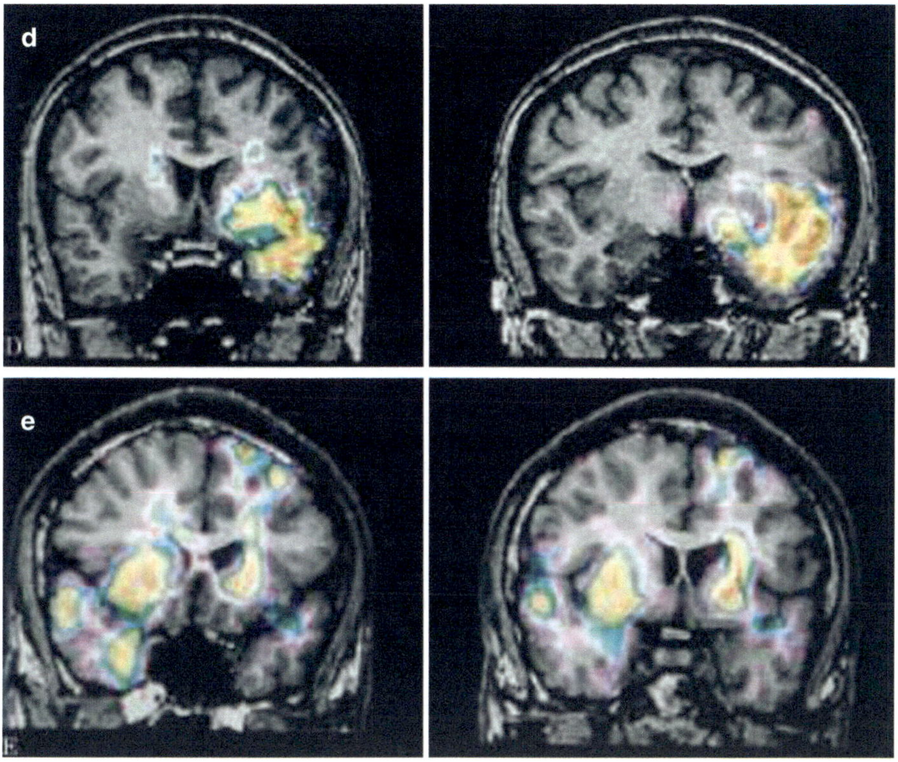

Fig. 38.8 (continued)

SISCOM can be used for the study of other paroxysmal neurological disorders. SISCOM with ictal SPECT during cataplectic attack in a narcolepsy patient showed ictal hyperperfusion in the right amygdala, bilateral cingulate gyri, basal ganglia, thalami, premotor cortices, sensorimotor cortices, right insula, and brain stem and hypoperfusion in the prefrontal cortex and occipital lobe (Hong et al. 2006a). A SISCOM study during the symptomatic period of Kleine–Levin syndrome revealed significant hypoperfusion in the left hypothalamus, bilateral thalami, basal ganglia, bilateral medial and dorsolateral frontal regions, and left temporal lobe during the hypersomnia period compared to the asymptomatic period (Hong et al. 2006b).

In summary, SISCOM is a useful tool for presurgical evaluation of patients with drug-resistant partial epilepsy. SISCOM improves the sensitivity of ictal SPECT for localizing an epileptic focus, but the time of radiotracer injection, seizure semiology and duration, and ictal EEG pattern at injection time may affect the result. SISCOM is also useful for clinical research aimed at examining the brain structure–semiology relationship, seizure propagation pathways, and brain pathomechanisms of other neurological disorders and sleep disorders.

References

Ahnlide JA, Rosén I, Lindén-Mickelsson Tech P, Källén K (2007) Does SISCOM contribute to favorable seizure outcome after epilepsy surgery? Epilepsia 48(3):579–588

Bell M, Rao S, So E et al (2009) Epilepsy surgery outcomes in temporal lobe epilepsy with a normal MRI. Epilepsia 50:2053–2060

Chen T, Guo L (2016) The role of SISCOM in preoperative evaluation for patients with epilepsy surgery: a meta-analysis. Seizure 41:43–50

Cho JW, Seo DW, Joo EY et al (2007) Neural correlates of musicogenic epilepsy: SISCOM and FDG-PET. Epilepsy Res 77(2–3):169–173

Coster LD, Laere KV, Cleeren E et al (2018) On the optimal z-score threshold for SISCOM analysis to localize the ictal onset zone. EJNMMI Res 8(1):34

Hong SB, Tae WS, Joo EY (2006a) Cerebral perfusion changes during cataplexy in narcolepsy patients. Neurology 66(11):1747–1749

Hong SB, Joo EY, Tae WS et al (2006b) Episodic diencephalic hypoperfusion in Kleine-Levin syndrome. Sleep 29(8):1091–1093

Hong SB, Joo EY, Tae WS et al (2008) Preictal versus ictal injection of radiotracer for SPECT study in partial epilepsy: SISCOM. Seizure 17(4):383–386

Jalota A, Rossi MA, Pylypyuk V et al (2016) Resecting critical nodes from an epileptogenic circuit in refractory focal-onset epilepsy patients using subtraction ictal SPEC coregistered to MRI. J Neurosurg 125:1565–1576

Joo YE, Hong SB, Lee EK et al (2004) Regional cerebral hyperperfusion with ictal dystonic posturing: ictal-interictal SPECT subtraction. Epilepsia 45(6):686–689

Joo EY, Seo DW, Hong SC et al (2015) Functional neuroimaging findings in patients with lateral and mesio-lateral temporal lobe epilepsy; FDG-PET and ictal SPECT studies. J Neurol 262:1120–1129

Kaiboriboon K, Bertrand ME, Osman MM, Hogan RE (2005) Quantitative analysis of cerebral blood flow patterns in mesial temporal lobe epilepsy using composite SISCOM. J Nucl Med 46:38–43

Knowlton RC, Elgavish RA, Bartolucci A, Ojha B, Limdi N, Blount J, Burneo JG, Ver Hoef L, Paige L, Faught E, Kankirawatana P, Riley K, Kuzniecky R (2008) Functional imaging: II. Prediction of epilepsy surgery outcome. Ann Neurol 64(1):35

Koh CS, Lee MC, Chung JK, Lee DS, Lee SK, Seo JM, Lee JS, Kim HJ (1998) Diagnosis of ictal hyperperfusion using subtraction image of ictal and interictal brain perfusion SPECT. Korean J Nucl Med 32(1):20–31

Lee HW, Hong SB, Tae WS et al (1999) Partial seizures manifesting as apnea only in an adult. Epilepsia 40:1828–1831

Lee HW, Hong SB, Tae WS (2000) Opposite ictal perfusion patterns of subtracted SPECT. Hyperperfusion and hypoperfusion. Brain 123:2150–2159

Lee KH, Meador KJ, Park YD et al (2002) Pathophysiology of altered consciousness during seizures: subtraction SPECT study. Neurology 59:841–846

Lee SK, Lee SY, Kim KK, Hong KS, Lee DS, Chung CK (2005) Surgical outcome and prognostic factors of cryptogenic neocortical epilepsy. Ann Neurol 58(4):525–532

Lee JY, Joo EY, Park HS et al (2011) Repeated ictal SPECT in partial epilepsy patients: SISCOM analysis. Epilepsia 52(12):2249–2256

Newey CR, Wong C, Wang ZI et al (2013) Optimizing SPECT SISCOM analysis to localize seizure-onset zone by using varying z scores. Epilepsia 54(5):793–800

Noe K, Sulc V, Wong-Kisiel L et al (2013) Long-term outcomes after nonlesional extratemporal lobe epilepsy surgery. JAMA Neurol 70:1003–1008

O'Brien TJ, So EL, Mullan BP et al (1998a) Subtraction ictal SPECT co-registered to MRI improves clinical usefulness of SPECT in localizing the surgical seizure focus. Neurology 50:445–454

O'Brien TJ, O'Connor MK, Mullan BP et al (1998b) Subtraction ictal SPET co-registered to MRI in partial epilepsy: description and technical validation of the method with phantom and patient studies. Nucl Med Commun 19:31–45

O'Brien TJ, So EL, Mullan BP et al (1999) Subtraction SPECT co-registered to MRI improves postictal SPECT localization of seizure foci. Neurology 52:137–146

O'Brien TJ, So EL, Mullan BP et al (2000) Subtraction peri-ictal SPECT is predictive of extratemporal epilepsy surgery outcome. Neurology 55:1668–1677

von Oertzen TJ, Mormann F, Urbach H, Reichmann K, Koenig R, Clusmann H, Biersack HJ, Elger CE (2011) Prospective use of subtraction ictal SPECT coregistered to MRI (SISCOM) in presurgical evaluation of epilepsy. Epilepsia 52(12):2239–2248

Shin WC, Hong SB, Tae WS et al (2001) Ictal hyperperfusion of cerebellum and basal ganglia in temporal lobe epilepsy: SPECT subtraction with MRI coregistration. J Nucl Med 42:853–858

Shin WC, Hong SB, Tae WS et al (2002) Ictal hyperperfusion patterns according to the progression of temporal lobe seizures. Neurology 58:373–380

Spanaki MV, Spencer SS, Corsi M et al (1999) Sensitivity and specificity of quantitative difference SPECT analysis in seizure localization. J Nucl Med 40:730–736

Stamoulis C, Verma N, Kaulas H et al (2017) The promise of subtraction ictal SPECT co-registered to MRI for improved seizure localization in pediatric epilepsies: affecting factors and relationship to the surgical outcome. Epilepsy Res 129:59–66

Tan KM, Britton JW, Buchhalter JR, Worrell GA, Lagerlund TD, Shin C, Cascino GD, Meyer FB, So EL (2008) Influence of subtraction ictal SPECT on surgical management in focal epilepsy of indeterminate localization: a prospective study. Epilepsy Res 82(2–3):190–193

Tousseyn S, Krishnan B, Wang ZI et al (2017) Connectivity in ictal single photon emission computed tomography perfusion: a cortico-cortical evoked potential study. Brain 140:1872–1884

Valenti MP, Froelich S, Armspach JP et al (2002) Contribution of SISCOM imaging in the presurgical evaluation of temporal lobe epilepsy related to dysembryoplastic neuroepithelial tumors. J Nucl Med 43:991–998

Van Paesschen W, Dupont P, Van Heerden B et al (2000) Self-injection ictal SPECT during partial seizures. Neurology 54:1994–1997

Zubal IG, Spencer SS, Imam K et al (1995) Difference images calculated from ictal and interictal technetium-99 m-HMPAO SPECT scans of epilepsy. J Nucl Med 36:684–689

Zubal IG, Spanaki MV, MacMullan J et al (1999) Influence of technetium-99m-hexamethylpropylene amine oxime injection time on single-photon emission tomography perfusion changes in epilepsy. Eur J Nucl Med 26:12–17

Part VII

Tumors of the Nervous System

Gliomas

39

Karl Herholz

Contents

Abstract

Positron emission tomography (PET) is increasingly contributing to diagnosis and management decision in patients with brain tumours and especially gliomas. Through the use of FDG, amino acid tracers ([^{11}C]-methionine, [^{18}F]-fluoro-ethyl-tyrosine and [^{18}F]-fluorodopa) and [^{18}F]-fluorothymidine, PET contributes to diagnosis as well as planning and monitoring of therapy. Amino acid tracers are particularly sensitive for delineating the extent of gliomas and detection of recurrence. They are also being investigated for planning of resection and conformal radiation therapy. Further PET applications include the monitoring and outcome prediction in radiotherapy and chemotherapy and the identification of hypoxic tissue.

K. Herholz (✉)
The University of Manchester, Division of Neuroscience and Experimental Psychology, Manchester, UK
e-mail: karl.herholz@manchester.ac.uk

R. A. J. O. Dierckx et al. (eds.), *PET and SPECT in Neurology*,
https://doi.org/10.1007/978-3-030-53168-3_39

39.1 Introduction

Imaging methods have made enormous progress in the past decades. For instance, magnetic resonance imaging (MRI) provides excellent sensitivity for detection of brain tumours, even for low-grade gliomas that do not exhibit enhancement after application of contrast material. However, even though detection is no longer a major issue, many other problems of diagnosis and management remain unresolved. This is particularly true for gliomas as the most frequent type of intrinsic brain tumours.

Gliomas occur in a wide range of malignancy grades (1–4; see Table 39.1) and different histological subtypes, which are associated with substantial differences in prognosis and require different therapeutic strategies. The recent revision of the WHO histopathological classification (Louis et al. 2016) now also includes molecular markers. Gliomas with the wild-type isocitrate dehydrogenase (IDH) gene are most aggressive. They typically progress to the most malignant type, glioblastoma, even when initially presenting as grade 2 or 3 astrocytomas. IDH-mutant astrocytomas have longer survival times but ultimately also mostly recur and progress. In contrast to astrocytomas, oligodendrogliomas are characterised by 1p19q codeletion.

Gliomas of grade 1, such as pilocytic astrocytoma, most frequently occur in children. Their imaging features, biological characteristics and treatment options are different in many respects from gliomas of grades 2–4 (Galldiks et al. 2010a, Kumar et al. 2010, Dunkl et al. 2015). Therefore, pilocytic astrocytoma and other childhood brain tumours have not been included in this review.

PET and SPECT as imaging techniques in brain tumours have been reviewed recently (Herholz et al. 2012, Herholz 2017), and PET guidelines have been published by a joint working group for the European Associations of Nuclear Medicine and Neuro-Oncology (Law et al. 2019). Therefore, I will concentrate this review on the potential and perspectives of these methods to address frequent clinical questions in the diagnosis and treatment of gliomas.

Table 39.1 Glioma grades

<table>
<tr><th>WHO grade</th><th>Mean age</th><th>Typical survival time</th><th>Main histological types</th><th>Surgical therapy</th><th>Medical therapy</th></tr>
<tr><td>1</td><td>Children</td><td>Cure possible</td><td>Pilocytic astrocytoma</td><td>Total resection</td><td>Not required (if resected)</td></tr>
<tr><td rowspan="2">2</td><td>35</td><td>10–16 years</td><td>Oligodendroglioma</td><td rowspan="4">Gross total resection (when possible)</td><td rowspan="2">Individual decision</td></tr>
<tr><td>35</td><td>6–8 years</td><td>Astrocytoma</td></tr>
<tr><td>3</td><td>50</td><td>3 years</td><td>Anaplastic astrocytoma or oligodendroglioma</td><td rowspan="2">Radiotherapy and chemotherapy</td></tr>
<tr><td>4</td><td>>60</td><td>3–24 months</td><td>Glioblastoma</td></tr>
</table>

39.2 Glioma Grading and Detection of Malignant Transformation

Grading and classification of gliomas have been improved substantially in recent years by use of molecular markers (Louis et al. 2016). Still, imaging is essential for treatment planning. Tumour heterogeneity is a big challenge, as different parts of gliomas frequently exhibit different degrees of malignancy, and for correct grading of the tumour, the most malignant part is relevant. However, if only parts of the tumour were accessible to surgical intervention or only few small tumour samples have been taken, as in stereotactic biopsies, the most malignant part may not even be available for histological examination.

Grade 2 gliomas pose a particular therapeutic dilemma, as aggressive therapy may do more harm than good (Douw et al. 2009), while a "wait-and-see" strategy may allow progression and malignant degeneration of the tumour that could possibly be prevented by earlier intervention. Also, recurrent tumours may present with a more malignant grade than seen in the original histopathologic sample. Therefore, imaging techniques are often required for accurate grading of gliomas and detection of areas progressing to a higher grade.

Malignant transformation of gliomas is associated with many changes that are accessible to imaging (Table 39.2). This provides many diagnostic possibilities but

Table 39.2 Aspects of malignant degeneration and associated imaging techniques in brain tumours

• Vascular changes
– Increase of blood volume and blood flow
Dynamic CT, perfusion-/diffusion-weighted MRI
Perfusion PET and SPECT ([^{15}O]-water, [^{99m}Tc]-HMPAO, [^{99m}Tc]-ECD)
– Endothelial activation and proliferation
Amino acid PET/SPECT (MET, FET, FDOPA and others)
PET of endothelial markers (e.g., [^{18}F]-galacto-RGD: αVβ3-integrin)
– BBB breakdown
MRI/CT contrast enhancement
PET and SPECT (^{201}Tl, ^{82}Rb, [^{68}Ga]-EDTA, FLT)
• Cellular changes
– Increase of glycolysis
FDG PET
MRS (lactate)
– Increase of proliferation
FLT (also requiring BBB breakdown)
– Changes of lipid metabolism
[^{11}C]-choline (possibly also [^{18}F]-fluorocholine)
MRS (choline, phospholipids)

is also a source of considerable uncertainty about their relative merits as only few of these imaging techniques have been directly compared with each other in large and representative samples. Most likely malignant degeneration is the consequence of cumulative genetic and biochemical changes that facilitate each other but do not necessarily occur in a regular order (Masui et al. 2012).

39.3 Vascular and Blood-Brain Barrier Changes

39.3.1 Vascular Proliferation

Gliomas show multiple alterations of vasculature and blood-brain barrier (BBB). Malignant transformation is associated with vascular proliferation, which may result in an increase in blood volume and blood flow, while it is also associated with tissue hypoxia. Cerebral blood flow (CBF) has been studied mostly by SPECT and PET, but the impact has been limited by variability of results and poor relation to tumour grade (Langen et al. 1988). The advent of functional MRI techniques to measure blood volume and perfusion (Waldman et al. 2009) has renewed the interest in this topic. Apparently, blood volume is subject to less physiological variability than blood flow and may thus provide a more reliable diagnostic marker. Several studies indicate that an increase in blood volume is related to expression of endothelial growth factor (Maia et al. 2005, Ludemann et al. 2006, Kapoor et al. 2009).

Imaging molecular markers of vascular proliferation directly has been the goal of several research studies. For instance, [^{18}F]-galacto-RGD images correlated with immunohistochemical alpha(v)beta(3) integrin expression of corresponding tumour samples in glioblastoma (Schnell et al. 2009). This receptor has also been targeted in experimental studies by other tracers labelled with ^{18}F, ^{68}Ga or ^{64}Cu. However, a multicentre clinical trial of [^{18}F]-fluciclatide (GE-135-03) showed only weak correlation with expression of alpha(v)beta(3) integrin in glioma (Sharma et al. 2015). Studies often were motivated by the advent of antiangiogenic therapy with bevacizumab, which even has been labelled with ^{89}Zr to identify patients who would most likely benefit from that therapy (Jansen et al. 2017).

39.3.2 Blood-Brain Barrier

The BBB prevents the transfer of many drugs, including radiopharmaceuticals, from blood to brain. It is modified in glioma, most prominently in the most malignant manifestation as glioblastoma (Dimberg 2014), but more subtle changes are also present at lower grades.

The standard techniques for imaging of BBB breakdown, allowing leakage of large molecules, in malignant gliomas and most other brain tumours are contrast-enhanced CT and MRI. By dynamic scanning, these techniques also allow quantitation of BBB permeability (Haroon et al. 2004, Herholz et al. 2007). Corresponding nuclear medicine techniques, such as 201Tl SPECT (Dierckx et al. 1994), have attracted only limited interest because of their relatively low resolution, even though the sensitivity of the potassium analogue 201Tl for BBB changes may be higher than the large inert molecules used as contrast agents with CT and MRI (Gomez-Rio et al. 2008).

The main motivation for imaging of BBB permeability with PET is investigating functional BBB alterations, which may be present already in low-grade gliomas, and to assess the transfer of labelled therapeutic drugs (van Tellingen et al. 2015). There is an increased transport of amino acids by specific transporter enzymes, which is widely utilised with PET for imaging gliomas (Herholz et al. 2012) as described in subsequent sections.

In relation to therapeutic drugs, studies have been performed to assess the activity of enzymes that may help in delivering drugs or reducing efflux. These include studies of ABCB1 and ABCG2 transporters with [^{11}C]-erlotinib (Verheijen et al. 2018) and p-glycoprotein activity (Hendrikse et al. 1999).

Imaging with PET and SPECT tracers in the brain generally depends on tracer delivery to tissue. Blood flow is the limiting factor for freely diffusible tracers, which are rarely used in brain tumours. FDG uptake is provided by a high-capacity glucose transporter, while uptake of other tracers depends to some degree on BBB alterations. Thus, it is often difficult to demonstrate that in vivo uptake is related to specific binding in gliomas, especially for tracers which do not pass the intact BBB. For instance, the capacity of their transporters at the BBB is very limited for [^{18}F]-fluorothymidine (FLT), and tumours without substantial BBB damage are negative on a FLT scan (Tripathi et al. 2009). Dependency of tracer uptake on BBB damage but lack of correlation with somatostatin receptor expression was also observed in glioblastoma with ^{68}Ga-DOTA-peptides (Kiviniemi et al. 2015). Unfortunately, this problem is also largely preventing clinical translation of experimental PET studies using labelled macromolecules.

39.3.2.1 Amino Acid Tracers

An essential function of the endothelial cells in the cerebral vasculature is the active transport of amino acids from blood to tissue, and endothelial proliferation is associated with an increase of transporter expression and activity (Verrey et al. 2004). Several amino acids are being used as PET tracers, and increased uptake in gliomas has been demonstrated clinically (see reviews by Herholz et al. 2012, Herholz 2017 and Parent et al. 2019) and in experimental studies (Miyagawa et al. 1998, Viel et al. 2012). When compared to FDG, amino acid tracers provide higher sensitivity for tumour detection (Dunet et al. 2015).

For many years since 1980, [^{11}C]-methionine (MET) has been the most widely used amino acid tracer. Compared to normal brain, the uptake is increased in most gliomas, including the majority of low-grade gliomas with intact blood-brain barrier (BBB) (Herholz et al. 1998). On average, uptake is higher in high-grade than in low-grade gliomas, but the difference is quantitatively less pronounced than with tracers and contrast agents that depend on BBB breakdown, which is present in the majority of high-grade but absent in the majority of low-grade gliomas. In cross-sectional studies, there is no consensus about the utility of MET for glioma grading

(Moulin-Romsee et al. 2007). This may partially be due to the quantitatively small mean difference between grades and is potentially confounded by the fact that oligodendrogliomas have significantly higher uptake than astrocytomas of the same WHO grade (Derlon et al. 1997, Herholz et al. 1998, Ribom and Smits 2005, Shinozaki et al. 2011), even though they tend to have longer survival times. Nevertheless, longitudinal studies demonstrate that malignant progression of gliomas is associated with a significant increase of MET uptake that is absent in non-progressing tumours (Ullrich et al. 2009).

The very short physical half-life of carbon-11 (20 min) restricts the application of MET to PET research centres with own cyclotron and thus prevents wider clinical use. Therefore, fluorine-18-labelled amino acid tracers have found broad interest for clinical application. In recent years, [^{18}F]-fluoro-ethyl-tyrosine (FET) has been used by many clinical research groups and has been included in multiple clinical trials. Similar to MET, it is also a substrate for large neutral amino acid transporters LAT1 (Habermeier et al. 2015) and LAT2 (Langen et al. 2006), while, in contrast to MET, it is not incorporated into proteins. Interestingly, studies comparing the clinical properties of these two tracers directly (Weber et al. 2000) found similar tumour-to-background ratios (while overall tissue uptake of FET is somewhat lower than MET), suggesting that the activated transport is the process that dominates the signal (rather than further metabolism and protein synthesis) even for MET. Correspondingly, it was also found that the magnitude of FET uptake is not a particularly strong indicator of tumour grade. This limitation can be overcome by dynamic FET scans, because the early phase of tracer uptake provides a better differentiation between high- and low-grade gliomas than late uptake (Popperl et al. 2007, Jansen et al. 2012).

As an alternative to FET, FDOPA has also been used for imaging of gliomas (Heiss et al. 1996, Ledezma et al. 2009, Tripathi et al. 2009, Walter et al. 2012, Nioche et al. 2013, Villani et al. 2015, Chiaravalloti et al. 2019). Clinical results are similar to FET, while there is more variable background than with FET because of the high physiological accumulation of FDOPA in the basal ganglia. Another alternative is [^{11}C]-alpha-methyltryptophan, which also relates to the kynurenic pathway and has been used in promising clinical research studies (Juhasz et al. 2011, 2014, Bosnyak et al. 2016).

Cyclic amino acids, most notably anti-[^{18}F]FACBC ([^{18}F]-fluciclovine), accumulate in tumours by Na^+-dependent transporters, while there is little uptake in normal brain. Few studies have been performed in glioma, demonstrating even better tumour-to-background contrast in recurrent glioma than MET (Michaud et al. 2019) and good discrimination between low- and high-grade glioma (Parent et al. 2018).

39.3.3 Metabolic Changes

Malignant degeneration of gliomas is associated with many changes in their metabolism. Imaging these changes is particularly attractive if it can be done without interference by BBB damage. The situation in that respect is best for FDG, because of the relatively rapid kinetics and large capacity of the glucose transporter. Freely diffusible tracers, the uptake of which also does not depend on BBB disruption, are not available for targeting metabolic processes. An exception may be the blood flow marker [^{13}N]-NH_3, which is trapped in tissue by glutamine synthase and has successfully been used in glioma (Shi et al. 2013, Khangembam et al. 2014).

39.3.3.1 FDG

Several studies demonstrated that FDG uptake in gliomas is related to prognosis (Patronas et al. 1985, Holzer et al. 1993, Kaschten et al. 1998, De Witte et al. 2001, Padma et al. 2003, Pardo et al. 2004, Van Laere et al. 2005, Pauleit et al. 2009, Colavolpe, Metellus, Mancini, Barrie, Bequet-Boucard, Figarella-Branger, Mundler, Chinot, and Guedj 2012b). The main limitation for putting that into broader clinical use has probably been the difficulty to identify gliomas on FDG PET scans. FDG uptake in normal grey matter is similar to that of malignant gliomas, resulting in poor contrast. White matter FDG uptake is lower (typically about 40–50% of grey matter on a FDG PET scan), and FDG uptake of low-grade gliomas is usually only slightly higher than white matter uptake. Thus, the regional heterogeneity of normal brain metabolism is comparable to the difference between low- and high-grade gliomas. Thus, in most studies comparing FDG with amino acid tracers (Fig. 39.1), the latter appear to provide the more sensitive and distinct signal (Derlon et al. 2000, Kim et al. 2005, Van Laere et al. 2005, Potzi et al. 2007, Pauleit et al. 2009, Li et al. 2012).

The limitations caused by poor image contrast can be overcome by PET-MRI coregistration (Padma et al. 2003, Leiva-Salinas et al. 2017), which achieves an accuracy of 1–2 mm and thus considerably better than actual PET scan spatial resolution (Cizek et al. 2004). On hybrid PET/MRI scanners, PET can even be combined directly with multiparametric MRI assessment of glioma (Sacconi et al. 2016). Reliable classification of FDG uptake in tumour, as localised on the coregistered MRI, can be achieved by a grading scale in relation to normal brain tissue, e.g. 0 = no uptake; 1 = uptake less or equal to contralateral white matter; 2 = uptake greater than contralateral white matter and less than grey matter; and 3 = equal to or greater than contralateral grey matter (Padma et al. 2003). Rather than relying on a plain SUV only, semiquantitative assessment of lesion uptake should be done in the tissue volume that is suspect of tumour on the MRI scan and divided by uptake in a contralateral mirror region, providing a SUV ratio (SUVR) which is equivalent to a simple activity ratio. Normal brain glucose metabolism is reduced in patients with aggressive tumours (DeLaPaz et al. 1983, Holzer et al. 1993), thus enhancing the contrast between malignant gliomas with high FDG uptake and normal brain background. An improvement of the contrast can also be achieved by delayed scanning, which may demonstrate continuing accumulation of FDG in the tumour (Spence et al. 2004, Prieto et al. 2011).

39.3.3.2 Proliferation

The most important factors being considered in histological grading of gliomas are the degree of cellular anaplasia and indicators of cellular proliferation. Initial work

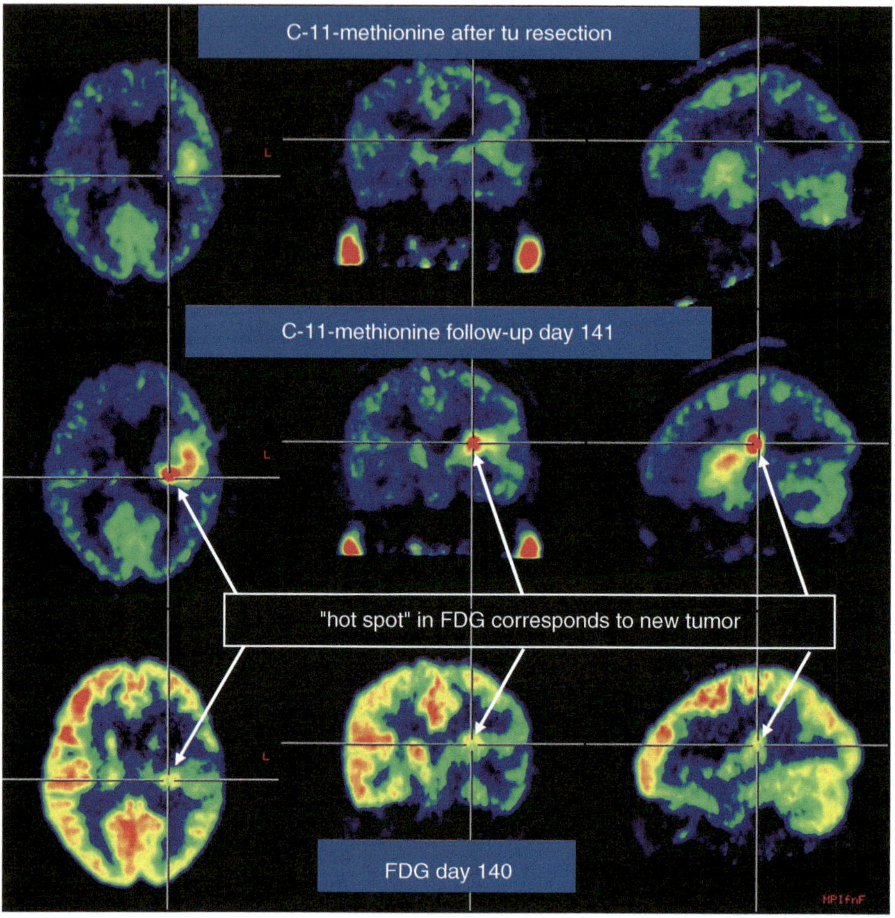

Fig. 39.1 Comparison of MET PET and FDG in recurrent glioblastoma. Within a few weeks after macroscopically complete tumour resection, MET PET is already showing increased uptake in the resection area (top row), which increases in intensity during the next 3 months (middle row), when the recurrence is also identified with less signal intensity on FDG PET (bottom row)

with [^{11}C]-thymidine demonstrated in vitro and in vivo that the activity of thymidine kinase 1 (TK-1) is associated with cellular accumulation of the tracer and tumour proliferation (Eary et al. 1999). To facilitate more widespread applicability, the fluorine-18-labelled thymidine analogue FLT has been developed for imaging of tumour proliferation (Shields et al. 1998). Although its affinity to cellular nucleoside transporters and TK-1 is less than that of thymidine (Krohn et al. 2005), a correlation between tracer uptake kinetics and proliferation markers has been demonstrated in malignant glioma (Ullrich et al. 2008, Price et al. 2009). Volume and intensity of FLT uptake predicted survival in patients with recurrent malignant glioma (Zhao et al. 2014). FLT does not cross the intact BBB (at least not at an amount that would allow clinical PET imaging); thus it provides a negative finding in most low-grade gliomas (Chen et al. 2005) and is not suitable for measuring proliferation rates in this tumour group (Tripathi et al. 2009).

Another potential proliferation marker is choline. Magnetic resonance spectroscopy has demonstrated significant differences with respect to the phospholipid and choline signal between low- and high-grade gliomas (Tedeschi et al. 1997). Correspondingly, there is also interest whether this could also be achieved by [^{11}C]-choline (Shinoura et al. 1997). Ohtani et al. (2001) demonstrated increased uptake in high-grade gliomas and extra-axial tumours lacking the BBB, while uptake in most low-grade gliomas was comparable to background. While initial experience with [^{18}F]-fluorocholine was limited (Lam et al. 2011) and tracer uptake is affected by BBB disruption, a subsequent study indicated high sensitivity for detection of recurrent glioma (Gomez-Rio et al. 2015).

Recently, expression of the mitochondrial translocator protein (TSPO) by glioma cells has been identified as a potential proliferation marker (Janczar et al. 2015). It has been imaged using [^{11}C]-PK11195 (Su et al. 2015), demonstrating increased binding to TSPO in high-grade glioma, and with [^{18}F]-GE180 (Unterrainer et al. 2019) which, however, does not cross the intact BBB in normal brain.

39.4 Biopsy Targeting

Unfortunately, none of the currently available PET tracers are absolutely specific for tumours. For instance, FDG uptake is also increased in inflammation, and increased amino acid uptake has been observed in various acute brain lesions (Floeth et al. 2006). Thus histological tissue examination remains the ultimate tool for accurate diagnosis, and PET can contribute to accurate diagnosis by guiding neurosurgeons towards the most active glioma parts (Pirotte et al. 2004a, b, Kunz et al. 2011). Areas of increased FDG and methionine uptake tend to correspond with each other (Pirotte et al. 2004a, b). There is also some correlation with increased CBV in gliomas, but focal increases of tracer uptake and CBF are often not co-localised (Fig. 39.2) (Filss et al. 2017).

39.5 Guiding and Monitoring Therapy

There is currently no definitive therapy for gliomas in adults. Diffuse tissue infiltration is the primary reason for glioma recurrence (Scherer 1940), preventing curative resection (with the exception of pilocytic astrocytoma) and probably also contributing to ultimate failure of regional radiotherapy. Furthermore, at recurrence, gliomas often progress to a higher grade. Imaging is essential to tailor therapy individually for each patient at each stage of progression.

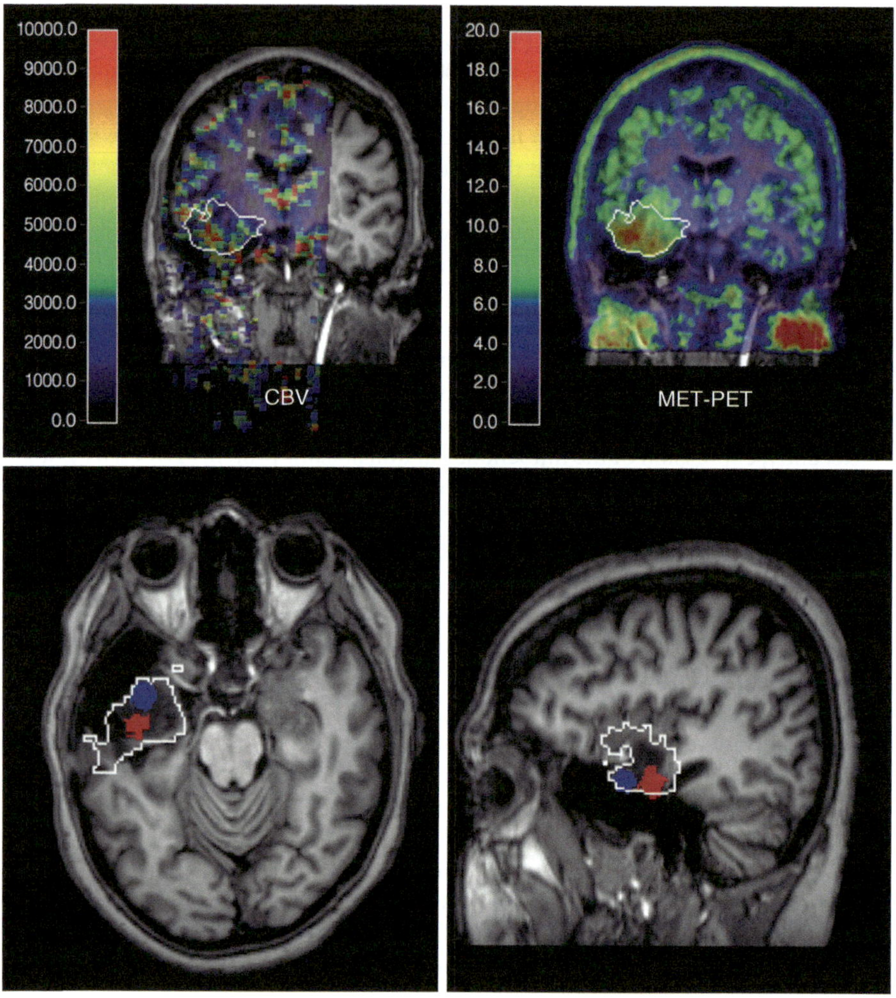

Fig. 39.2 Low-grade glioma with focal increases of CBV (Dynamic susceptibility contrast-enhanced MRI) and amino acid uptake (MET PET) indicating beginning focal dedifferentiation. Images are shown in coregistration and fusion with T1-weighted contrast-enhanced MRI; the white outline indicates the extent of the lesion on FLAIR MRI. On the coronal cuts (top row), there is some correspondence between CBV and MET PET within the tumour, while the transaxial and sagittal slices (bottom row) demonstrate that peaks are actually not in the same position (peak MET uptake marked blue, peak CBV red)

39.5.1 Planning Surgical Resection

There are some issues that need to be considered when using PET for therapy planning. Diffuse infiltration does not have sharp borders, and in order to prevent recurrence, one would rather treat as large a volume as possible, in principle irrespective of any imaging guidance. The very narrow limit to that approach is the need to minimise treatment side effects and especially treatment-induced neurological deficits. Therefore "eloquent areas", i.e. brain areas that are crucial for particular neurological function, need to be excluded from resection or intense irradiation. The individual location of these areas can vary considerably, and therefore functional imaging methods to localise eloquent areas are increasingly being used for therapy planning. This work has initially been pioneered with ^{15}O-water PET (Herholz et al. 1997) and has been continued and expanded with functional MRI techniques. Coregistration of structural, functional and molecular images can then provide the comprehensive information delineating macroscopic anatomy, eloquent brain areas and tumour extent to maximise the radicality of intervention to improve prognosis while minimising side effects and maintaining neurological function.

Amino acid tracers are prime candidates for guiding resection because of their excellent sensitivity for delineation of glioma including parts that do not take up contrast material (Galldiks et al. 2010b). Studies have demonstrated that radiolabelled amino acids detect the solid mass of gliomas and metabolically active tumour areas more reliably than either CT or MRI (Mosskin et al. 1989, Goldman et al. 1997, Kracht et al. 2004, Pirotte et al. 2004a, b, Pauleit et al. 2005). Pirotte et al. (2009) demonstrated that total resection of tumour guided by amino acid tracer uptake was associated with a significantly longer survival in patients with malignant gliomas.

39.5.2 Planning Radiotherapy

While surgery is aiming at removal of solid tumour, radiotherapy also is also aiming at stopping tumour infiltration of healthy tissue. Thus, irradiation fields typically include a "safety margin" around resected and solid tumour. Studies have been initiated to clarify whether amino acid PET can improve radiation planning and ultimate outcome of radiotherapy (Piroth et al. 2016, Oehlke and Grosu 2017, Poulsen et al. 2017, Hirata et al. 2019). However, there is no clear limit of infiltration, and there is also some variation of the background signal with lower normal uptake of amino acids in white than in grey matter (Coope et al. 2007). Depending on the chosen thresholds, resulting target volumes for conformal radiotherapy may vary considerably, and there is a need for standardisation based on proven improvement of outcome.

Hypoxic tumour tissue is relatively resistant to irradiation, asking for individual adjustment of radiotherapy protocols to overcome resistance while keeping side effects under control. Macroscopic and microscopic heterogeneity of vascular proliferation and hypoxia pose substantial challenges to imaging. Imaging of hypoxic tissue can be provided by [^{18}F]-fluoromisonidazole (FMISO) (Valk et al. 1992) and related tracers (Koch et al. 2010, Shibahara et al. 2010, Mapelli et al. 2017). Several recent studies indicate that this may provide a clinically useful tool for detection of hypoxia (Spence et al. 2008) and diagnosis of glioblastoma (Hirata et al. 2012). Increased binding of hypoxia markers is often found close to areas with BBB damage and contrast enhancement (Swanson et al. 2009, Kawai et al. 2011) but does not correspond to areas with vascular deoxygenation, as measured by MRI oxygen imaging (Preibisch et al. 2017).

39.5.3 Monitoring of Therapy

There is a clinical need for monitoring of therapy in gliomas. As with most tumours, a definitive assessment of response based on clinical symptoms or structural imaging is possible only after several months, and it is even more difficult for low-grade gliomas because of their slow natural progression (Reardon et al. 2011). Furthermore, there is the problem with possible pseudoprogression and pseudoresponse on CT and standard MRI (Brandsma and van den Bent 2009), and there is considerable interindividual variability of gliomas in the response to therapy. Especially with the rapidly progressing glioblastomas, one would want to leave any inefficient chemotherapy as soon as possible and switch to an alternative regimen to avoid unnecessary side effects and loss of the bone marrow reserve that is needed for more intense protocols. Thus, reliable early response markers are needed.

Consistent early responses to radiotherapy and chemotherapy have been observed with amino acid tracers (Galldiks et al. 2006, 2012, Wyss et al. 2009, Hutterer et al. 2011). The critical distinction between tumour progression and pseudoprogression with necrosis has also been addressed by amino acid PET, most successfully with more than 80% accuracy by dynamic imaging or combination with perfusion MRI (Galldiks et al. 2017). FET PET has been used for evaluation of emerging new therapies, such as TTFields (Ceccon et al. 2018), and detailed recommendations for amino acid PET in clinical oncology have been published (Albert et al. 2016).

While FDG may also serve as a response marker in radiotherapy (Tralins et al. 2002) and chemotherapy (Charnley et al. 2006, Colavolpe et al. 2012a), it is potentially complicated by the "flare" effect (Trigonis and Jackson 2010), which has been observed as an initial response to radiotherapy before ultimately FDG uptake declines as the viability of tumour cells decreases. Its clinical significance is not clear, and it may be associated with radiological pseudoprogression (Hygino da Cruz et al. 2011).

Expectations have been high for FLT as an early response marker, and indeed a study by Chen et al. (2007) demonstrated a large and early reduction of uptake after therapy that included the antiangiogenic drug bevacizumab, predicting later response on structural imaging. However, a subsequent study demonstrated that FLT did not predict overall survival, while this was achieved by FDOPA (Harris et al. 2012).

39.5.4 Detection of Recurrent Glioma

Recurrent glioma poses specific diagnostic problems because treatment, especially surgery and radiotherapy, can induce alterations in non-tumour tissue that can be indistinguishable from recurrent tumour using standard contrast-enhanced CT and MRI (Rachinger et al. 2005). In particular, radiation-induced necrosis needs to be distinguished from recurrent tumour, while both lesions may show contrast enhancement. Studies demonstrate that FDG, FLT and amino acid tracers have the potential to provide that differentiation (see Table 39.3 and de Zwart et al. (2019) for

Table 39.3 Discrimination between recurrent glioma and necrosis (modified from Herholz et al. (2012))

Tracer	*n*	Sensitivity	Specificity	Lesion type	References
FDG	47	75% (21/28)	81% (13/16)	Malignant tumour	Chao et al. (2001)
FDG	15	43% (6/14)	100% (1/1)	Glioma	Thompson et al. (1999)
FDG	84	73%	56%	Malignant tumour	Ricci et al. (1998)
FDG	38	88% (15/17)	81% (17/21)	Glioma	Valk et al. (1988)
FDG	21	81% (13/16)	40% (2/5)	Tumour	Kahn et al. (1994)
FDG	9	80% (4/5)	100% (4/4)	Tumour[a]	Ogawa et al. (1991)
FDG	30	95%	50%	Glioma	Van Laere et al. (2005)
MET	30	75%	70%	Glioma	Van Laere et al. (2005)
MET	12	100% (5/5)	86% (6/7)	Glioma[a]	Sonoda et al. (1998)
MET	32	75%	75%	Glioma[a]	Terakawa et al. (2008)
MET	11	100% (6/6)	60% (3/5)	Glioma[a]	Tsuyuguchi et al. (2004)
FET	53	100% (42/42)	100% (11/11)	Glioma	Popperl et al. (2004)
FET	127	70%	71%	Glioma	Maurer et al. (2020)
FLT[b]	19	100% (15/15)	100% (4/4)	Glioma	Spence et al. (2009)

[a]With histopathological verification in all tumour cases
[b]Dynamic scans with tracer kinetic analysis

overview). There are also reports that assessments of CBV by dynamic MRI (Kim et al. 2010) or measures derived from MRS (Smith et al. 2009) may provide similar information, but interpretation of amino acid PET is easier due to better separation of tumour from background (Cicone et al. 2015). Amino acid PET also provides very high sensitivity to detect recurrent or residual glioma (Galldiks et al. 2015). Patient survival with recurrent malignant glioma can also be predicted by FLT (Zhao et al. 2014).

39.6 Summary and Conclusion

PET can make major contributions to management of glioma patients (Table 39.4). Of the most frequently used tracer types, the amino acids (mainly MET, FET and FDOPA) are most versatile because they show better tumour-to-background contrast than FDG and uptake is increased even in most low-grade gliomas, whereas FLT uptake depends on BBB damage. Thus, amino acid PET is increasingly recognised in clinical guidelines as a sensitive and relatively specific marker for planning and monitoring of glioma therapy. It is also useful for distinction between gliomas and benign brain lesions. Oligodendrogliomas show higher amino acid uptake than astrocytomas of the same grade, which needs to be kept in mind when using amino acid PET for tumour grading. Multiple radiopharmaceuticals and dynamic contrast-enhanced MRI techniques are being used to assess changes in tumour vasculature, which are also related to tumour malignancy and progression. More research is needed to evaluate the potential of nucleoside, choline and hypoxia markers in clinical glioma management.

Table 39.4 Contribution of PET tracers to management of gliomas

Management issue	FDG	AA	FLT
Grading	x	(1)	x
Targeting biopsy	x	x	(2)
Determining extent and infiltration		x	
Detecting residual/recurrent tumour		x	
Monitoring therapy		x	(2)

AA amino acids (MET, FET, FDOPA)
(1) Low grading accuracy with static scanning
(2) Contrast enhancing tumours only; dynamic data analysis may be required

References

Albert NL, Weller M, Suchorska B, Galldiks N, Soffietti R, Kim MM, la Fougere C, Pope W, Law I, Arbizu J, Chamberlain MC, Vogelbaum M, Ellingson BM, Tonn JC (2016) Response assessment in Neuro-Oncology working group and European Association for Neuro-Oncology recommendations for the clinical use of PET imaging in gliomas. Neuro-Oncology 18(9):1199–1208

Bosnyak E, Kamson DO, Robinette NL, Barger GR, Mittal S, Juhasz C (2016) Tryptophan PET predicts spatial and temporal patterns of post-treatment glioblastoma progression detected by contrast-enhanced MRI. J Neuro-Oncol 126(2):317–325

Brandsma D, van den Bent MJ (2009) Pseudoprogression and pseudoresponse in the treatment of gliomas. Curr Opin Neurol 22(6):633–638

Ceccon G, Lazaridis L, Stoffels G, Rapp M, Weber M, Blau T, Lohmann P, Kebir S, Herrmann K, Fink GR, Langen K-J, Glas M, Galldiks N (2018) Use of FET PET in glioblastoma patients undergoing neurooncological treatment including tumour-treating fields: initial experience. Eur J Nucl Med Mol Imaging 45(9):1626–1635

Chao ST, Suh JH, Raja S, Lee SY, Barnett G (2001) The sensitivity and specificity of FDG PET in distinguishing recurrent brain tumor from radionecrosis in patients treated with stereotactic radiosurgery. Int J Cancer 96(3):191–197

Charnley N, West CM, Barnett CM, Brock C, Bydder GM, Glaser M, Newlands ES, Swindell R, Matthews J, Price P (2006) Early change in glucose metabolic rate measured using FDG-PET in patients with high-grade glioma predicts response to temozolomide but not temozolomide plus radiotherapy. Int J Radiat Oncol Biol Phys 66(2):331–338

Chen W, Cloughesy T, Kamdar N, Satyamurthy N, Bergsneider M, Liau L, Mischel P, Czernin J, Phelps ME, Silverman DH (2005) Imaging proliferation in brain tumors with 18F-FLT PET: comparison with 18F-FDG. J Nucl Med 46(6):945–952

Chen W, Delaloye S, Silverman DH, Geist C, Czernin J, Sayre J, Satyamurthy N, Pope W, Lai A, Phelps ME, Cloughesy T (2007) Predicting treatment response of malignant gliomas to bevacizumab and irinotecan by imaging proliferation with [18F] fluorothymidine positron emission tomography: a pilot study. J Clin Oncol 25(30):4714–4721

Chiaravalloti A, Esposito V, Ursini F, Di Giorgio E, Zinzi M, Calabria F, Cimini A, Schillaci O (2019) Overall survival and progression-free survival in patients with primary brain tumors after treatment: is the outcome of [^{18}F] FDOPA PET a prognostic factor in these patients? Ann Nucl Med 33(7):471–480

Cicone F, Filss CP, Minniti G, Rossi-Espagnet C, Papa A, Scaringi C, Galldiks N, Bozzao A, Shah NJ, Scopinaro F, Langen KJ (2015) Volumetric assessment of recurrent or progressive gliomas: comparison between F-DOPA PET and perfusion-weighted MRI. Eur J Nucl Med Mol Imaging 42(6):905–915

Cizek J, Herholz K, Vollmar S, Schrader R, Klein J, Heiss WD (2004) Fast and robust registration of PET and MR images of human brain. NeuroImage 22(1):434–442

Colavolpe C, Chinot O, Metellus P, Mancini J, Barrie M, Bequet-Boucard C, Tabouret E, Mundler O, Figarella-Branger D, Guedj E (2012a) FDG-PET predicts survival in recurrent high-grade gliomas treated with bevacizumab and irinotecan. Neuro-Oncology 14(5):649–657

Colavolpe C, Metellus P, Mancini J, Barrie M, Bequet-Boucard C, Figarella-Branger D, Mundler O, Chinot O, Guedj E (2012b) Independent prognostic value of pre-treatment 18-FDG-PET in high-grade gliomas. J Neuro-Oncol 107(3):527–535

Coope DJ, Cizek J, Eggers C, Vollmar S, Heiss W-D, Herholz K (2007) Evaluation of primary brain tumors using 11C-methionine PET with reference to a normal methionine uptake map. J Nucl Med 48:1971–1980

De Witte O, Lefranc F, Levivier M, Salmon I, Brotchi J, Goldman S (2001) FDG-PET as a prognostic factor in high-grade astrocytoma. JNeurooncol 49(2):157–163

DeLaPaz RL, Patronas NJ, Brooks RA, Smith BH, Kornblith PL, Milam H, Di Chiro G (1983) Positron emission tomographic study of suppression of gray-matter glucose utilization by brain tumors. AJNR Am J Neuroradiol 4(3):826–829

Derlon JM, Petit-Taboue MC, Chapon F, Beaudouin V, Noel MH, Creveuil C, Courtheoux P, Houtteville JP (1997) The in vivo metabolic pattern of low-grade brain gliomas: a positron emission tomographic study using 18F-fluorodeoxyglucose and 11C-L-methylmethionine. Neurosurgery 40(2):276–288

Derlon JM, Chapon F, Noel MH, Khouri S, Benali K, Petit-Taboue MC, Houtteville JP, Chajari MH, Bouvard G (2000) Non-invasive grading of oligodendrogliomas: correlation between in vivo metabolic pattern and histopathology. Eur J Nucl Med 27(7):778–787

Dierckx RA, Martin JJ, Dobbeleir A, Crols R, Neetens I, De Deyn PP (1994) Sensitivity and specificity of thallium-201 single-photon emission tomography in the functional detection and differential diagnosis of brain tumours. Eur J Nucl Med 21(7):621–633

Dimberg A (2014) The glioblastoma vasculature as a target for cancer therapy. Portland Press, London

Douw L, Klein M, Fagel SS, van den Heuvel J, Taphoorn MJ, Aaronson NK, Postma TJ, Vandertop WP, Mooij JJ, Boerman RH, Beute GN, Sluimer JD, Slotman BJ, Reijneveld JC, Heimans JJ (2009) Cognitive and radiological effects of radiotherapy in patients with low-grade glioma: long-term follow-up. Lancet Neurol 8(9):810–818

Dunet V, Pomoni A, Hottinger A, Nicod-Lalonde M, Prior JO (2015) Performance of 18F-FET versus 18F-FDG-PET for the diagnosis and grading of brain tumors: systematic review and meta-analysis. Neuro-Oncology 18(3):426–434

Dunkl V, Cleff C, Stoffels G, Judov N, Sarikaya-Seiwert S, Law I, Bogeskov L, Nysom K, Andersen SB, Steiger HJ, Fink GR, Reifenberger G, Shah NJ, Coenen HH, Langen KJ, Galldiks N (2015) The usefulness of dynamic O-(2-18F-fluoroethyl)-L-tyrosine PET in the clinical evaluation of brain tumors in children and adolescents. J Nucl Med 56(1):88–92

Eary JF, Mankoff DA, Spence AM, Berger MS, Olshen A, Link JM, O'Sullivan F, Krohn KA (1999) 2-[C-11]thymidine imaging of malignant brain tumors. Cancer Res 59(3):615–621

Filss CP, Cicone F, Shah NJ, Galldiks N, Langen K-J (2017) Amino acid PET and MR perfusion imaging in brain tumours. Clin Transl Imaging 3(5):209–223

Floeth FW, Pauleit D, Sabel M, Reifenberger G, Stoffels G, Stummer W, Rommel F, Hamacher K, Langen KJ (2006) 18F-FET PET differentiation of ring-enhancing brain lesions. J Nucl Med 47(5):776–782

Galldiks N, Kracht LW, Burghaus L, Thomas A, Jacobs AH, Heiss WD, Herholz K (2006) Use of 11C-methionine PET to monitor the effects of temozolomide chemotherapy in malignant gliomas. Eur J Nucl Med Mol Imaging 33(5):516–524

Galldiks N, Kracht LW, Berthold F, Miletic H, Klein JC, Herholz K, Jacobs AH, Heiss WD (2010a) [11C]-L-methionine positron emission tomography in the management of children and young adults with brain tumors. J Neuro-Oncol 96(2):231–239

Galldiks N, Ullrich R, Schroeter M, Fink G, Kracht L (2010b) Volumetry of [11C]-methionine PET uptake and MRI contrast enhancement in patients with recurrent glioblastoma multiforme. Eur J Nucl Med Mol Imaging 37(1):84–92

Galldiks N, Langen KJ, Holy R, Pinkawa M, Stoffels G, Nolte KW, Kaiser HJ, Filss CP, Fink GR, Coenen HH, Eble MJ, Piroth MD (2012) Assessment of treatment response in patients with glioblastoma using O-(2-18F-fluoroethyl)-L-tyrosine PET in comparison to MRI. J Nucl Med 53(7):1048–1057

Galldiks N, Stoffels G, Filss C, Rapp M, Blau T, Tscherpel C, Ceccon G, Dunkl V, Weinzierl M, Stoffel M, Sabel M, Fink GR, Shah NJ, Langen KJ (2015) The use of dynamic O-(2-18F-fluoroethyl)-l-tyrosine PET in the diagnosis of patients with progressive and recurrent glioma. Neuro-Oncology 17(9):1293–1300

Galldiks N, Law I, Pope WB, Arbizu J, Langen K-J (2017) The use of amino acid PET and conventional MRI for monitoring of brain tumor therapy. NeuroImage Clin 13:386–394

Goldman S, Levivier M, Pirotte B, Brucher JM, Wikler D, Damhaut P, Dethy S, Brotchi J, Hildebrand J (1997) Regional methionine and glucose uptake in high-grade gliomas: a comparative study on PET-guided stereotactic biopsy. J Nucl Med 38(9):1459–1462

Gomez-Rio M, Rodriguez-Fernandez A, Ramos-Font C, Lopez-Ramirez E, Llamas-Elvira JM (2008) Diagnostic accuracy of 201Thallium-SPECT and 18F-FDG-PET in the clinical assessment of glioma recurrence. Eur J Nucl Med Mol Imaging 35(5):966–975

Gomez-Rio M, Testart Dardel N, Santiago Chinchilla A, Rodriguez-Fernandez A, Olivares Granados G, Luque Caro R, Zurita Herrera M, Chamorro Santos CE, Lardelli-Claret P, Llamas-Elvira JM (2015) 18F-Fluorocholine PET/CT as a complementary tool in the follow-up of low-grade glioma: diagnostic accuracy and clinical utility. Eur J Nucl Med Mol Imaging 42(6):886–895

Habermeier A, Graf J, Sandhofer BF, Boissel JP, Roesch F, Closs EI (2015) System L amino acid transporter LAT1 accumulates O-(2-fluoroethyl)-L-tyrosine (FET). Amino Acids 47(2):335–344

Haroon HA, Buckley DL, Patankar TA, Dow GR, Rutherford SA, Baleriaux D, Jackson A (2004) A comparison of Ktrans measurements obtained with conventional and first pass pharmacokinetic models in human gliomas. J Magn Reson Imaging 19(5):527–536

Harris RJ, Cloughesy TF, Pope WB, Nghiemphu PL, Lai A, Zaw T, Czernin J, Phelps ME, Chen W, Ellingson BM (2012) 18F-FDOPA and 18F-FLT positron emission tomography parametric response maps predict response in recurrent malignant gliomas treated with bevacizumab. Neuro-Oncology 14(8):1079–1089

Heiss WD, Wienhard K, Wagner R, Lanfermann H, Thiel A, Herholz K, Pietrzyk U (1996) F-Dopa as an amino acid tracer to detect brain tumors. J Nucl Med 37:1180–1182

Hendrikse NH, de Vries EG, Eriks-Fluks L, van der Graaf WT, Hospers GA, Willemsen AT, Vaalburg W, Franssen EJ (1999) A new in vivo method to study P-glycoprotein transport in tumors and the blood-brain barrier. Cancer Res 59(10):2411–2416

Herholz K (2017) Brain tumors: an update on clinical PET research in gliomas. Semin Nucl Med 47(1):5–17

Herholz K, Reulen HJ, von Stockhausen HM, Thiel A, Ilmberger J, Kessler J, Eisner W, Yousry TA, Heiss WD (1997) Preoperative activation and intraoperative stimulation of language-related areas in glioma patients. Neurosurgery 41:1253–1262

Herholz K, Holzer T, Bauer B, Schroder R, Voges J, Ernestus RI, Mendoza G, Weber-Luxenburger G, Lottgen J, Thiel A, Wienhard K, Heiss WD (1998) 11C-Methionine PET for differential diagnosis of low-grade gliomas. Neurology 50(5):1316–1322

Herholz K, Coope D, Jackson A (2007) Metabolic and molecular imaging in neuro-oncology. Lancet Neurol 6(8):711–724

Herholz K, Langen KJ, Schiepers C, Mountz JM (2012) Brain tumors. Semin Nucl Med 42(6):356–370

Hirata K, Terasaka S, Shiga T, Hattori N, Magota K, Kobayashi H, Yamaguchi S, Houkin K, Tanaka S, Kuge Y, Tamaki N (2012) (18)F-Fluoromisonidazole positron emission tomography may differentiate glioblastoma multiforme from less malignant gliomas. Eur J Nucl Med Mol Imaging 39(5):760–770

Hirata T, Kinoshita M, Tamari K, Seo Y, Suzuki O, Wakai N, Achiha T, Umehara T, Arita H, Kagawa N, Kanemura Y, Shimosegawa E, Hashimoto N, Hatazawa J, Kishima H, Teshima T,

Ogawa K (2019) 11C-methionine-18F-FDG dual-PET-tracer-based target delineation of malignant glioma: evaluation of its geometrical and clinical features for planning radiation therapy. J Neurosurg 131:676–686

Holzer T, Herholz K, Jeske J, Heiss WD (1993) FDG-PET as a prognostic indicator in radiochemotherapy of glioblastoma. J Comput Assist Tomogr 17(5):681–687

Hutterer M, Nowosielski M, Putzer D, Waitz D, Tinkhauser G, Kostron H, Muigg A, Virgolini IJ, Staffen W, Trinka E, Gotwald T, Jacobs AH, Stockhammer G (2011) O-(2-18F-fluoroethyl)-L-tyrosine PET predicts failure of antiangiogenic treatment in patients with recurrent high-grade glioma. J Nucl Med 52(6):856–864

Hygino da Cruz LC Jr, Rodriguez I, Domingues RC, Gasparetto EL, Sorensen AG (2011) Pseudoprogression and pseudoresponse: imaging challenges in the assessment of posttreatment glioma. AJNR Am J Neuroradiol 32(11):1978–1985

Janczar K, Su Z, Raccagni I, Anfosso A, Kelly C, Durrenberger PF, Gerhard A, Roncaroli F (2015) The 18-kDa mitochondrial translocator protein in gliomas: from the bench to bedside. Biochem Soc Trans 43(4):579–585

Jansen NL, Graute V, Armbruster L, Suchorska B, Lutz J, Eigenbrod S, Cumming P, Bartenstein P, Tonn JC, Kreth FW, la Fougere C (2012) MRI-suspected low-grade glioma: is there a need to perform dynamic FET PET? Eur J Nucl Med Mol Imaging 39(6):1021–1029

Jansen MH, van Zanten SEMV, Van Vuurden DG, Huisman MC, Vugts DJ, Hoekstra OS, van Dongen GA, Kaspers G-JL (2017) Molecular drug imaging: 89Zr-bevacizumab PET in children with diffuse intrinsic pontine glioma. J Nucl Med 58(5):711–716

Juhasz C, Muzik O, Chugani DC, Chugani HT, Sood S, Chakraborty PK, Barger GR, Mittal S (2011) Differential kinetics of alpha-[(11)C]methyl-L-tryptophan on PET in low-grade brain tumors. J Neuro-Oncol 102(3):409–415

Juhasz C, Dwivedi S, Kamson DO, Michelhaugh SK, Mittal S (2014) Comparison of amino acid positron emission tomographic radiotracers for molecular imaging of primary and metastatic brain tumors. Mol Imaging 13. https://doi.org/10.2310/7290.2014.00015

Kahn D, Follett KA, Bushnell DL, Nathan MA, Piper JG, Madsen M, Kirchner PT (1994) Diagnosis of recurrent brain tumor: value of 201Tl SPECT vs 18F- fluorodeoxyglucose PET. AJR 163(6):1459–1465

Kapoor GS, Gocke TA, Chawla S, Whitmore RG, Nabavizadeh A, Krejza J, Lopinto J, Plaum J, Maloney-Wilensky E, Poptani H, Melhem ER, Judy KD, O'Rourke DM (2009) Magnetic resonance perfusion-weighted imaging defines angiogenic subtypes of oligodendroglioma according to 1p19q and EGFR status. J Neuro-Oncol 92(3):373–386

Kaschten B, Stevenaert A, Sadzot B, Deprez M, Degueldre C, Del FG, Luxen A, Reznik M (1998) Preoperative evaluation of 54 gliomas by PET with fluorine-18-fluorodeoxyglucose and/or carbon-11-methionine. J Nucl Med 39(5):778–785

Kawai N, Maeda Y, Kudomi N, Miyake K, Okada M, Yamamoto Y, Nishiyama Y, Tamiya T (2011) Correlation of biological aggressiveness assessed by 11C-methionine PET and hypoxic burden assessed by 18F-fluoromisonidazole PET in newly diagnosed glioblastoma. Eur J Nucl Med Mol Imaging 38(3):441–450

Khangembam BC, Karunanithi S, Sharma P, Kc SS, Kumar R, Julka PK, Bal C (2014) Perfusion-metabolism coupling in recurrent gliomas: a prospective validation study with 13N-ammonia and 18F-fluorodeoxyglucose PET/CT. Neuroradiology 56(10):893–902

Kim S, Chung JK, Im SH, Jeong JM, Lee DS, Kim DG, Jung HW, Lee MC (2005) 11C-methionine PET as a prognostic marker in patients with glioma: comparison with 18F-FDG PET. Eur J Nucl Med Mol Imaging 32(1):52–59

Kim YH, Oh SW, Lim YJ, Park CK, Lee SH, Kang KW, Jung HW, Chang KH (2010) Differentiating radiation necrosis from tumor recurrence in high-grade gliomas: assessing the efficacy of 18F-FDG PET, 11C-methionine PET and perfusion MRI. Clin Neurol Neurosurg 112(9):758–765

Kiviniemi A, Gardberg M, Frantzen J, Pesola M, Vuorinen V, Parkkola R, Tolvanen T, Suilamo S, Johansson J, Luoto P, Kemppainen J, Roivainen A, Minn H (2015) Somatostatin receptor subtype 2 in high-grade gliomas: PET/CT with (68)Ga-DOTA-peptides, correlation to prognostic markers, and implications for targeted radiotherapy. EJNMMI Res 5:25

Koch CJ, Scheuermann JS, Divgi C, Judy KD, Kachur AV, Freifelder R, Reddin JS, Karp J, Stubbs JB, Hahn SM, Driesbaugh J, Smith D, Prendergast S, Evans SM (2010) Biodistribution and dosimetry of (18)F-EF5 in cancer patients with preliminary comparison of (18)F-EF5 uptake versus EF5 binding in human glioblastoma. Eur J Nucl Med Mol Imaging 37(11):2048–2059

Kracht LW, Miletic H, Busch S, Jacobs AH, Voges J, Hoevels M, Klein JC, Herholz K, Heiss WD (2004) Delineation of brain tumor extent with [11C]L-methionine positron emission tomography: local comparison with stereotactic histopathology. Clin Cancer Res 10(21):7163–7170

Krohn KA, Mankoff DA, Muzi M, Link JM, Spence AM (2005) True tracers: comparing FDG with glucose and FLT with thymidine. Nucl Med Biol 32(7):663–671

Kumar AJ, Leeds NE, Kumar VA, Fuller GN, Lang FF, Milas Z, Weinberg JS, Ater JL, Sawaya R (2010) Magnetic resonance imaging features of pilocytic astrocytoma of the brain mimicking high-grade gliomas. J Comput Assist Tomogr 34(4):601–611

Kunz M, Thon N, Eigenbrod S, Hartmann C, Egensperger R, Herms J, Geisler J, la Fougere C, Lutz J, Linn J, Kreth S, von Deimling A, Tonn JC, Kretzschmar HA, Popperl G, Kreth FW (2011) Hot spots in dynamic (18)FET-PET delineate malignant tumor parts within suspected WHO grade II gliomas. Neuro-Oncology 13(3):307–316

Lam WW, Ng DC, Wong WY, Ong SC, Yu SW, See SJ (2011) Promising role of [18F] fluorocholine PET/CT vs [18F] fluorodeoxyglucose PET/CT in primary brain tumors-early experience. Clin Neurol Neurosurg 113(2):156–161

Langen KJ, Herzog H, Kuwert T, Roosen N, Rota E, Kiwit JC, Bock WJ, Feinendegen LE (1988) Tomographic studies of rCBF with [99mTc]-HM-PAO SPECT in patients with brain tumors: comparison with C15O2 continuous inhalation technique and PET. J Cereb Blood Flow Metab 8(6):S90–S94

Langen KJ, Hamacher K, Weckesser M, Floeth F, Stoffels G, Bauer D, Coenen HH, Pauleit D (2006) O-(2-[18F]fluoroethyl)-L-tyrosine: uptake mechanisms and clinical applications. Nucl Med Biol 33(3):287–294

Law I, Albert NL, Arbizu J, Boellaard R, Drzezga A, Galldiks N, la Fougere C, Langen KJ, Lopci E, Lowe V, McConathy J, Quick HH, Sattler B, Schuster DM, Tonn JC, Weller M (2019) Joint EANM/EANO/RANO practice guidelines/SNMMI procedure standards for imaging of gliomas using PET with radiolabelled amino acids and [(18)F]FDG: version 1.0. Eur J Nucl Med Mol Imaging 46(3):540–557

Ledezma CJ, Chen W, Sai V, Freitas B, Cloughesy T, Czernin J, Pope W (2009) 18F-FDOPA PET/MRI fusion in patients with primary/recurrent gliomas: initial experience. Eur J Radiol 71(2):242–248

Leiva-Salinas C, Schiff D, Flors L, Patrie JT, Rehm PK (2017) FDG PET/MR imaging coregistration helps predict survival in patients with glioblastoma and radiologic progression after standard of care treatment. Radiology 283(2):508–514

Li DL, Xu YK, Wang QS, Wu HB, Li HS (2012) 11C-methionine and 18F-fluorodeoxyglucose positron emission tomography/CT in the evaluation of patients with suspected primary and residual/recurrent gliomas. Chin Med J 125(1):91–96

Louis DN, Perry A, Reifenberger G, Von Deimling A, Figarella-Branger D, Cavenee WK, Ohgaki H, Wiestler OD, Kleihues P, Ellison DW (2016) The 2016 World Health Organization classification of tumors of the central nervous system: a summary. Acta Neuropathol 131(6):803–820

Ludemann L, Grieger W, Wurm R, Wust P, Zimmer C (2006) Glioma assessment using quantitative blood volume maps generated by T1-weighted dynamic contrast-enhanced magnetic resonance imaging: a receiver operating characteristic study. Acta Radiol 47(3):303–310

Maia AC Jr, Malheiros SM, da Rocha AJ, da Silva CJ, Gabbai AA, Ferraz FA, Stavale JN (2005) MR cerebral blood volume maps correlated with vascular endothelial growth factor expression and tumor grade in nonenhancing gliomas. AJNR Am J Neuroradiol 26(4):777–783

Mapelli P, Incerti E, Bettinardi V, Conte GM, Fallanca F, Bailo M, Vuozzo M, Callea M, Gianolli L, Picchio M (2017) Hypoxia 18F-FAZA PET/CT imaging in lung cancer and high-grade glioma: open issues in clinical application. Clin Transl Imaging 4(5):389–397

Masui K, Cloughesy TF, Mischel PS (2012) Review: molecular pathology in adult high-grade gliomas: from molecular diagnostics to target therapies. Neuropathol Appl Neurobiol 38(3):271–291

Maurer GD, Brucker DP, Stoffels G, Filipski K, Filss CP, Mottaghy FM, Langen KJ (2020) ^{18}F-FET PET Imaging in differentiating glioma progression from treatment-related changes: a single-center experience. J Nucl Med. 61(4):505–511

Michaud L, Beattie BJ, Akhurst T, Dunphy M, Zanzonico P, Finn R, Mauguen A, Schöder H, Weber WA, Lassman AB, Blasberg R (2019) 18F-Fluciclovine (^{18}F-FACBC) PET imaging of recurrent brain tumors. Eur J Nucl Med Mol Imaging 47(6):1353–1367

Miyagawa T, Oku T, Uehara H, Desai R, Beattie B, Tjuvajev J, Blasberg R (1998) "Facilitated" amino acid transport is upregulated in brain tumors. J Cereb Blood Flow Metab 18(5):500–509

Mosskin M, Ericson K, Hindmarsh T, von Holst H, Collins VP, Bergstrom M, Eriksson L, Johnstrom P (1989) Positron emission tomography compared with magnetic resonance imaging and computed tomography in supratentorial gliomas using multiple stereotactic biopsies as reference. Acta Radiol 30(3):225–232

Moulin-Romsee G, D'Hondt E, de Groot T, Goffin J, Sciot R, Mortelmans L, Menten J, Bormans G, Van Laere K (2007) Non-invasive grading of brain tumours using dynamic amino acid PET imaging: does it work for 11C-methionine? Eur J Nucl Med Mol Imaging 34(12):2082–2087

Nioche C, Soret M, Gontier E, Lahutte M, Dutertre G, Dulou R, Capelle L, Guillevin R, Foehrenbach H, Buvat I (2013) Evaluation of quantitative criteria for glioma grading with static and dynamic 18F-FDopa PET/CT. Clin Nucl Med 38(2):81–87

Oehlke O, Grosu A-L (2017) PET/MRI and brain tumors: focus on radiation oncology treatment planning. Clin Transl Imaging 5(2):159–167

Ogawa T, Kanno I, Shishido F, Inugami A, Higano S, Fujita H, Murakami M, Uemura K, Yasui N, Mineura K, Kowada M (1991) Clinical value of PET with 18F-fluorodeoxyglucose and L-methyl- 11C-methionine for diagnosis of recurrent brain tumor and radiation injury. Acta Radiol 32(3):197–202

Ohtani T, Kurihara H, Ishiuchi S, Saito N, Oriuchi N, Inoue T, Sasaki T (2001) Brain tumour imaging with carbon-11 choline: comparison with FDG PET and gadolinium-enhanced MR imaging. Eur J Nucl Med 28(11):1664–1670

Padma MV, Said S, Jacobs M, Hwang DR, Dunigan K, Satter M, Christian B, Ruppert J, Bernstein T, Kraus G, Mantil JC (2003) Prediction of pathology and survival by FDG PET in gliomas. J Neuro-Oncol 64(3):227–237

Pardo FS, Aronen HJ, Fitzek M, Kennedy DN, Efird J, Rosen BR, Fischman AJ (2004) Correlation of FDG-PET interpretation with survival in a cohort of glioma patients. Anticancer Res 24(4):2359–2365

Parent EE, Benayoun M, Ibeanu I, Olson JJ, Hadjipanayis CG, Brat DJ, Adhikarla V, Nye J, Schuster DM, Goodman MM (2018) [18 F]-Fluciclovine PET discrimination between high- and low-grade gliomas. EJNMMI Res 8(1):67

Parent EE, Sharma A, Jain M (2019) Amino acid PET imaging of glioma. Curr Radiol Rep 7(5):14

Patronas NJ, Di Chiro G, Kufta C, Bairamian D, Kornblith PL, Simon R, Larson SM (1985) Prediction of survival in glioma patients by means of positron emission tomography. J Neurosurg 62(6):816–822

Pauleit D, Floeth F, Hamacher K, Riemenschneider MJ, Reifenberger G, Muller HW, Zilles K, Coenen HH, Langen KJ (2005) O-(2-[18F]fluoroethyl)-L-tyrosine PET combined with MRI improves the diagnostic assessment of cerebral gliomas. Brain 128(pt 3):678–687

Pauleit D, Stoffels G, Bachofner A, Floeth FW, Sabel M, Herzog H, Tellmann L, Jansen P, Reifenberger G, Hamacher K, Coenen HH, Langen KJ (2009) Comparison of (18)F-FET and (18)F-FDG PET in brain tumors. Nucl Med Biol 36(7):779–787

Piroth MD, Galldiks N, Pinkawa M, Holy R, Stoffels G, Ermert J, Mottaghy FM, Shah NJ, Langen KJ, Eble MJ (2016) Relapse patterns after radiochemotherapy of glioblastoma with FET PET-guided boost irradiation and simulation to optimize radiation target volume. Radiat Oncol 11:87

Pirotte B, Goldman S, Massager N, David P, Wikler D, Lipszyc M, Salmon I, Brotchi J, Levivier M (2004a) Combined use of 18F-fluorodeoxyglucose and 11C-methionine in 45 positron emission tomography-guided stereotactic brain biopsies. J Neurosurg 101(3):476–483

Pirotte B, Goldman S, Massager N, David P, Wikler D, Vandesteene A, Salmon I, Brotchi J, Levivier M (2004b) Comparison of 18F-FDG and 11C-methionine for PET-guided stereotactic brain biopsy of gliomas. J Nucl Med 45(8):1293–1298

Pirotte BJ, Levivier M, Goldman S, Massager N, Wikler D, Dewitte O, Bruneau M, Rorive S, David P, Brotchi J (2009) Positron emission tomography-guided volumetric resection of supratentorial high-grade gliomas: a survival analysis in 66 consecutive patients. Neurosurgery 64(3):471–481, discussion 481

Popperl G, Gotz C, Rachinger W, Gildehaus FJ, Tonn JC, Tatsch K (2004) Value of O-(2-[18F]fluoroethyl)- L-tyrosine PET for the diagnosis of recurrent glioma. Eur J Nucl Med Mol Imaging 31(11):1464–1470

Popperl G, Kreth FW, Mehrkens JH, Herms J, Seelos K, Koch W, Gildehaus FJ, Kretzschmar HA, Tonn JC, Tatsch K (2007) FET PET for the evaluation of untreated gliomas: correlation of FET uptake and uptake kinetics with tumour grading. Eur J Nucl Med Mol Imaging 34(12):1933–1942

Potzi C, Becherer A, Marosi C, Karanikas G, Szabo M, Dudczak R, Kletter K, Asenbaum S (2007) [11C] methionine and [18F] fluorodeoxyglucose PET in the follow-up of glioblastoma multiforme. J Neuro-Oncol 84(3):305–314

Poulsen SH, Urup T, Grunnet K, Christensen IJ, Larsen VA, Jensen ML, Af Rosenschold PM, Poulsen HS, Law I (2017) The prognostic value of FET PET at radiotherapy planning in newly diagnosed glioblastoma. Eur J Nucl Med Mol Imaging 44(3):373–381

Preibisch C, Shi K, Kluge A, Lukas M, Wiestler B, Göttler J, Gempt J, Ringel F, Al Jaberi M, Schlegel J, Meyer B, Zimmer C, Pyka T, Förster S (2017) Characterizing hypoxia in human glioma: a simultaneous multimodal MRI and PET study. NMR Biomed 30(11). https://doi.org/10.1002/nbm.3775

Price SJ, Fryer TD, Cleij MC, Dean AF, Joseph J, Salvador R, Wang DD, Hutchinson PJ, Clark JC, Burnet NG, Pickard JD, Aigbirhio FI, Gillard JH (2009) Imaging regional variation of cellular proliferation in gliomas using 3′-deoxy-3′-[18F]fluorothymidine positron-emission tomography: an image-guided biopsy study. Clin Radiol 64(1):52–63

Prieto E, Marti-Climent JM, Dominguez-Prado I, Garrastachu P, Diez-Valle R, Tejada S, Aristu JJ, Penuelas I, Arbizu J (2011) Voxel-based analysis of dual-time-point 18F-FDG PET images for brain tumor identification and delineation. J Nucl Med 52(6):865–872

Rachinger W, Goetz C, Popperl G, Gildehaus FJ, Kreth FW, Holtmannspotter M, Herms J, Koch W, Tatsch K, Tonn JC (2005) Positron emission tomography with O-(2-[18F]fluoroethyl)-l-tyrosine versus magnetic resonance imaging in the diagnosis of recurrent gliomas. Neurosurgery 57(3):505–511, discussion 505–511

Reardon DA, Galanis E, DeGroot JF, Cloughesy TF, Wefel JS, Lamborn KR, Lassman AB, Gilbert MR, Sampson JH, Wick W, Chamberlain MC, Macdonald DR, Mehta MP, Vogelbaum MA, Chang SM, Van den Bent MJ, Wen PY (2011) Clinical trial end points for high-grade glioma: the evolving landscape. Neuro-Oncology 13(3):353–361

Ribom D, Smits A (2005) Baseline 11C-methionine PET reflects the natural course of grade 2 oligodendrogliomas. Neurol Res 27(5):516–521

Ricci PE, Karis JP, Heiserman JE, Fram EK, Bice AN, Drayer BP (1998) Differentiating recurrent tumor from radiation necrosis: time for re-evaluation of positron emission tomography? [see comments]. AJNR Am J Neuroradiol 19(3):407–413

Sacconi B, Raad RA, Lee J, Fine H, Kondziolka D, Golfinos JG, Babb JS, Jain R (2016) Concurrent functional and metabolic assessment of brain tumors using hybrid PET/MR imaging. J Neuro-Oncol 127(2):287–293

Scherer HJ (1940) The forms of growth in gliomas and their practical significance. Brain 63(1):1–35

Schnell O, Krebs B, Carlsen J, Miederer I, Goetz C, Goldbrunner RH, Wester HJ, Haubner R, Popperl G, Holtmannspotter M, Kretzschmar HA, Kessler H, Tonn JC, Schwaiger M, Beer AJ

(2009) Imaging of integrin {alpha}v{beta}3 expression in patients with malignant glioma by [18F]galacto-RGD positron emission tomography. Neuro Oncol 11(6):861–870

Sharma R, Kallur KG, Ryu JS, Parameswaran RV, Lindman H, Avril N, Gleeson FV, Lee JD, Lee KH, O'Doherty MJ, Groves AM, Miller MP, Somer EJ, Coombes CR, Aboagye EO (2015) Multicenter reproducibility of 18F-fluciclatide PET imaging in subjects with solid tumors. J Nucl Med 56(12):1855–1861

Shi X, Liu Y, Zhang X, Yi C, Wang X, Chen Z, Zhang B (2013) The comparison of 13N-ammonia and 18F-FDG in the evaluation of untreated gliomas. Clin Nucl Med 38(7):522–526

Shibahara I, Kumabe T, Kanamori M, Saito R, Sonoda Y, Watanabe M, Iwata R, Higano S, Takanami K, Takai Y, Tominaga T (2010) Imaging of hypoxic lesions in patients with gliomas by using positron emission tomography with 1-(2-[18F] fluoro-1-[hydroxymethyl]ethoxy)methyl-2-nitroimidazole, a new 18F-labeled 2-nitroimidazole analog. J Neurosurg 113(2):358–368

Shields AF, Grierson JR, Dohmen BM, Machulla HJ, Stayanoff JC, Lawhorn-Crews JM, Obradovich JE, Muzik O, Mangner TJ (1998) Imaging proliferation in vivo with [F-18]FLT and positron emission tomography. Nat Med 4(11):1334–1336

Shinoura N, Nishijima M, Hara T, Haisa T, Yamamoto H, Fujii K, Mitsui I, Kosaka N, Kondo T, Hara T (1997) Brain tumors: detection with C-11 choline PET. Radiology 202(2):497–503

Shinozaki N, Uchino Y, Yoshikawa K, Matsutani T, Hasegawa A, Saeki N, Iwadate Y (2011) Discrimination between low-grade oligodendrogliomas and diffuse astrocytoma with the aid of 11C-methionine positron emission tomography. J Neurosurg 114(6):1640–1647

Smith EA, Carlos RC, Junck LR, Tsien CI, Elias A, Sundgren PC (2009) Developing a clinical decision model: MR spectroscopy to differentiate between recurrent tumor and radiation change in patients with new contrast-enhancing lesions. AJR Am J Roentgenol 192(2):W45–W52

Sonoda Y, Kumabe T, Takahashi T, Shirane R, Yoshimoto T (1998) Clinical usefulness of 11C-MET PET and 201T1 SPECT for differentiation of recurrent glioma from radiation necrosis. Neurol Med Chir (Tokyo) 38(6):342–347

Spence AM, Muzi M, Mankoff DA, O'Sullivan SF, Link JM, Lewellen TK, Lewellen B, Pham P, Minoshima S, Swanson K, Krohn KA (2004) 18F-FDG PET of gliomas at delayed intervals: improved distinction between tumor and normal gray matter. J Nucl Med 45(10):1653–1659

Spence AM, Muzi M, Swanson KR, O'Sullivan F, Rockhill JK, Rajendran JG, Adamsen TC, Link JM, Swanson PE, Yagle KJ, Rostomily RC, Silbergeld DL, Krohn KA (2008) Regional hypoxia in glioblastoma multiforme quantified with [18F]fluoromisonidazole positron emission tomography before radiotherapy: correlation with time to progression and survival. Clin Cancer Res 14(9):2623–2630

Spence AM, Muzi M, Link JM, O'Sullivan F, Eary JF, Hoffman JM, Shankar LK, Krohn KA (2009) NCI-sponsored trial for the evaluation of safety and preliminary efficacy of 3′-deoxy-3′-[18F]fluorothymidine (FLT) as a marker of proliferation in patients with recurrent gliomas: preliminary efficacy studies. Mol Imaging Biol 11(5):343–355

Su Z, Roncaroli F, Durrenberger PF, Coope DJ, Karabatsou K, Hinz R, Thompson G, Turkheimer FE, Janczar K, Du Plessis D, Brodbelt A, Jackson A, Gerhard A, Herholz K (2015) The 18-kDa mitochondrial translocator protein in human gliomas: an 11C-(R)PK11195 PET imaging and neuropathology study. J Nucl Med 56(4):512–517

Swanson KR, Chakraborty G, Wang CH, Rockne R, Harpold HL, Muzi M, Adamsen TC, Krohn KA, Spence AM (2009) Complementary but distinct roles for MRI and 18F-fluoromisonidazole PET in the assessment of human glioblastomas. J Nucl Med 50(1):36–44

Tedeschi G, Lundbom N, Raman R, Bonavita S, Duyn JH, Alger JR, Di Chiro G (1997) Increased choline signal coinciding with malignant degeneration of cerebral gliomas: a serial proton magnetic resonance spectroscopy imaging study. J Neurosurg 87(4):516–524

van Tellingen O, Yetkin-Arik B, de Gooijer MC, Wesseling P, Wurdinger T, de Vries HE (2015) Overcoming the blood-brain tumor barrier for effective glioblastoma treatment. Drug Resist Updat 19:1–12

Terakawa Y, Tsuyuguchi N, Iwai Y, Yamanaka K, Higashiyama S, Takami T, Ohata K (2008) Diagnostic accuracy of 11C-methionine PET for differentiation of recurrent brain tumors from radiation necrosis after radiotherapy. J Nucl Med 49(5):694–699

Thompson TP, Lunsford LD, Kondziolka D (1999) Distinguishing recurrent tumor and radiation necrosis with positron emission tomography versus stereotactic biopsy. StereotactFunctNeurosurg 73(1–4):9–14

Tralins KS, Douglas JG, Stelzer KJ, Mankoff DA, Silbergeld DL, Rostomily RC, Hummel S, Scharnhorst J, Krohn KA, Spence AM (2002) Volumetric analysis of 18F-FDG PET in glioblastoma multiforme: prognostic information and possible role in definition of target volumes in radiation dose escalation. J Nucl Med 43(12):1667–1673

Trigonis I, Jackson A (2010) Imaging pharmacodynamics in oncology: the potential significance of "flares". Ann Nucl Med 24(3):137–147

Tripathi M, Sharma R, D'Souza M, Jaimini A, Panwar P, Varshney R, Datta A, Kumar N, Garg G, Singh D, Grover RK, Mishra AK, Mondal A (2009) Comparative evaluation of F-18 FDOPA, F-18 FDG, and F-18 FLT-PET/CT for metabolic imaging of low grade gliomas. Clin Nucl Med 34(12):878–883

Tsuyuguchi N, Takami T, Sunada I, Iwai Y, Yamanaka K, Tanaka K, Nishikawa M, Ohata K, Torii K, Morino M, Nishio A, Hara M (2004) Methionine positron emission tomography for differentiation of recurrent brain tumor and radiation necrosis after stereotactic radiosurgery--in malignant glioma. Ann Nucl Med 18(4):291–296

Ullrich R, Backes H, Li H, Kracht L, Miletic H, Kesper K, Neumaier B, Heiss WD, Wienhard K, Jacobs AH (2008) Glioma proliferation as assessed by 3′-fluoro-3′-deoxy-L-thymidine positron emission tomography in patients with newly diagnosed high-grade glioma. Clin Cancer Res 14(7):2049–2055

Ullrich RT, Kracht L, Brunn A, Herholz K, Frommolt P, Miletic H, Deckert M, Heiss WD, Jacobs AH (2009) Methyl-L-11C-methionine PET as a diagnostic marker for malignant progression in patients with glioma. J Nucl Med 50(12):1962–1968

Unterrainer M, Fleischmann DF, Diekmann C, Vomacka L, Lindner S, Vettermann F, Brendel M, Wenter V, Ertl-Wagner B, Herms J, Wetzel C, Rupprecht R, Tonn JC, Belka C, Bartenstein P, Niyazi M, Albert NL (2019) Comparison of (18)F-GE-180 and dynamic (18)F-FET PET in high grade glioma: a double-tracer pilot study. Eur J Nucl Med Mol Imaging 46(3):580–590

Valk PE, Budinger TF, Levin VA, Silver P, Gutin PH, Doyle WK (1988) PET of malignant cerebral tumors after interstitial brachytherapy. Demonstration of metabolic activity and correlation with clinical outcome. J Neurosurg 69(6):830–838

Valk PE, Mathis CA, Prados MD, Gilbert JC, Budinger TF (1992) Hypoxia in human gliomas: demonstration by PET with fluorine-18-fluoromisonidazole. J Nucl Med 33(12):2133–2137

Van Laere K, Ceyssens S, Van Calenbergh F, de Groot T, Menten J, Flamen P, Bormans G, Mortelmans L (2005) Direct comparison of 18F-FDG and 11C-methionine PET in suspected recurrence of glioma: sensitivity, inter-observer variability and prognostic value. Eur J Nucl Med Mol Imaging 32(1):39–51

Verheijen RB, Yaqub M, Sawicki E, van Tellingen O, Lammertsma AA, Nuijen B, Schellens JHM, Beijnen JH, Huitema ADR, Hendrikse NH (2018) Molecular imaging of ABCB1 and ABCG2 inhibition at the human blood–brain barrier using Elacridar and 11C-Erlotinib PET. J Nucl Med 59(6):973–979

Verrey F, Closs EI, Wagner CA, Palacin M, Endou H, Kanai Y (2004) CATs and HATs: the SLC7 family of amino acid transporters. Pflugers Arch 447(5):532–542

Viel T, Talasila KM, Monfared P, Wang J, Jikeli JF, Waerzeggers Y, Neumaier B, Backes H, Brekka N, Thorsen F, Stieber D, Niclou SP, Winkeler A, Tavitian B, Hoehn M, Bjerkvig R, Miletic H, Jacobs AH (2012) Analysis of the growth dynamics of angiogenesis-dependent and -independent experimental glioblastomas by multimodal small-animal PET and MRI. J Nucl Med 53(7):1135–1145

Villani V, Carapella CM, Chiaravalloti A, Terrenato I, Piludu F, Vidiri A, Schillaci O, Floris R, Marzi S, Fabi A, Pace A (2015) The role of PET [18F]FDOPA in evaluating low-grade glioma. Anticancer Res 35(9):5117–5122

Waldman AD, Jackson A, Price SJ, Clark CA, Booth TC, Auer DP, Tofts PS, Collins DJ, Leach MO, Rees JH (2009) Quantitative imaging biomarkers in neuro-oncology. Nat Rev Clin Oncol 6(8):445–454

Walter F, Cloughesy T, Walter MA, Lai A, Nghiemphu P, Wagle N, Fueger B, Satyamurthy N, Phelps ME, Czernin J (2012) Impact of 3,4-dihydroxy-6-18F-fluoro-L-phenylalanine PET/CT on managing patients with brain tumors: the referring physician's perspective. J Nucl Med 53(3):393–398

Weber WA, Wester HJ, Grosu AL, Herz M, Dzewas B, Feldmann HJ, Molls M, Stocklin G, Schwaiger M (2000) O-(2-[18F]fluoroethyl)-L-tyrosine and L-[methyl-11C]methionine uptake in brain tumours: initial results of a comparative study. Eur J Nucl Med 27(5):542–549

Wyss M, Hofer S, Bruehlmeier M, Hefti M, Uhlmann C, Bartschi E, Buettner UW, Roelcke U (2009) Early metabolic responses in temozolomide treated low-grade glioma patients. J Neuro-Oncol 95(1):87–93

Zhao F, Cui Y, Li M, Fu Z, Chen Z, Kong L, Yang G, Yu J (2014) Prognostic value of 3′-deoxy-3′-18F-fluorothymidine ([(18)F] FLT PET) in patients with recurrent malignant gliomas. Nucl Med Biol 41(8):710–715

de Zwart PL, van Dijken BRJ, Holtman GA, Stormezand GN, Dierckx RA, van Laar PJ, van der Hoorn A (2019) Diagnostic accuracy of positron emission tomography tracers for the differentiation of tumor progression from treatment-related changes in high-grade glioma: a systematic review and meta-analysis. J Nucl Med 61(4):498–504

Single-Photon Emission Computed Tomography [Neuro-SPECT] Imaging of Brain Tumors

40

George A. Alexiou, Spyridon Tsiouris, and Andreas D. Fotopoulos

Contents

Abstract

Primary brain tumors have an annual incidence rate of 7–19.1 cases per 100,000 population. Metastatic tumors to the brain are more common with more than 100,000 patients per year in the United States. Gliomas are the most common primary brain tumor. CT and MRI are necessary to characterize the tumor type, size, and extension. Nevertheless, in patients with brain lesions, it is not uncommon for CT and MRI to provide nonspecific information, even after contrast or gadolinium infusion. Imaging of intracranial space-occupying lesions by nuclear medicine techniques such as SPECT and PET has also been introduced as a method providing information about the metabolic status of various brain tumors. Although PET constitutes the most sophisticated modality of nuclear medicine

G. A. Alexiou (✉)
Department of Neurosurgery, University of Ioannina Medical School, Ioannina, Greece

S. Tsiouris · A. D. Fotopoulos
Department of Nuclear Medicine, University of Ioannina, Medical School, Ioannina, Greece

R. A. J. O. Dierckx et al. (eds.), *PET and SPECT in Neurology*,
https://doi.org/10.1007/978-3-030-53168-3_40

imaging, SPECT has a lower cost, worldwide availability, and gained practical experience. The primary role of SPECT in brain tumor patients lies on the non-invasive assessment of tumor aggressiveness, differentiation of treatment-induced necrosis from tumor recurrence, assessment of response to treatment, and estimation of overall prognosis.

40.1 Introduction

The incidence rate of primary brain tumors is ranging between 7 and 19 cases per 100,000 person-years. In persons over 40 years, the annual average age-adjusted incidence for brain and other central nervous system tumors (CNS) was 40.82 per 100,000 population, and the median age at diagnosis was 59 years. Nearly 42% of all brain and CNS tumors occur in males and 58% in females. These malignancies are more common in the white race (Ostrom et al. 2017). Brain metastases from systemic cancer are up to ten times more common than primary brain malignancies (Figs. 40.1, 40.2, 40.3, and 40.4).

Primary brain tumors can be benign or malignant. According to the World Health Organization (WHO) grading system, they are classified into four grades (I–IV). The latest WHO 2016 CNS tumor classification uses molecular parameters in addition to histology to define several tumor entities (Louis et al. 2016). There are many types of primary intracranial tumors; meningiomas are the most common, accounting for 34% of all, followed by gliomas (32%). Glioblastoma (WHO Grade IV) is the most malignant primary brain tumor, accounting for 14.9% of all CNS tumors.

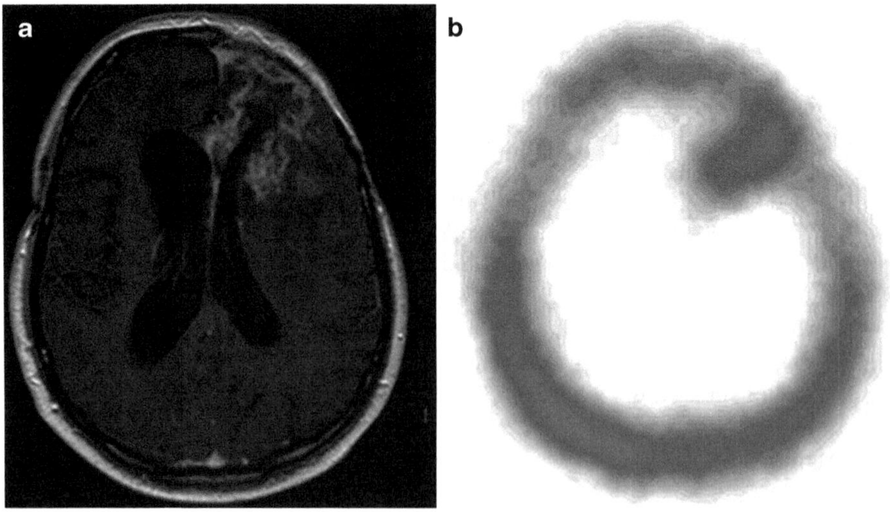

Fig. 40.1 (**a**) Gadolinium-enhanced T1-weighted MRI revealing recurrence of an anaplastic oligoastrocytoma. (**b**) ^{99m}Tc-tetrofosmin brain SPECT revealing increased tracer uptake in the corresponding area

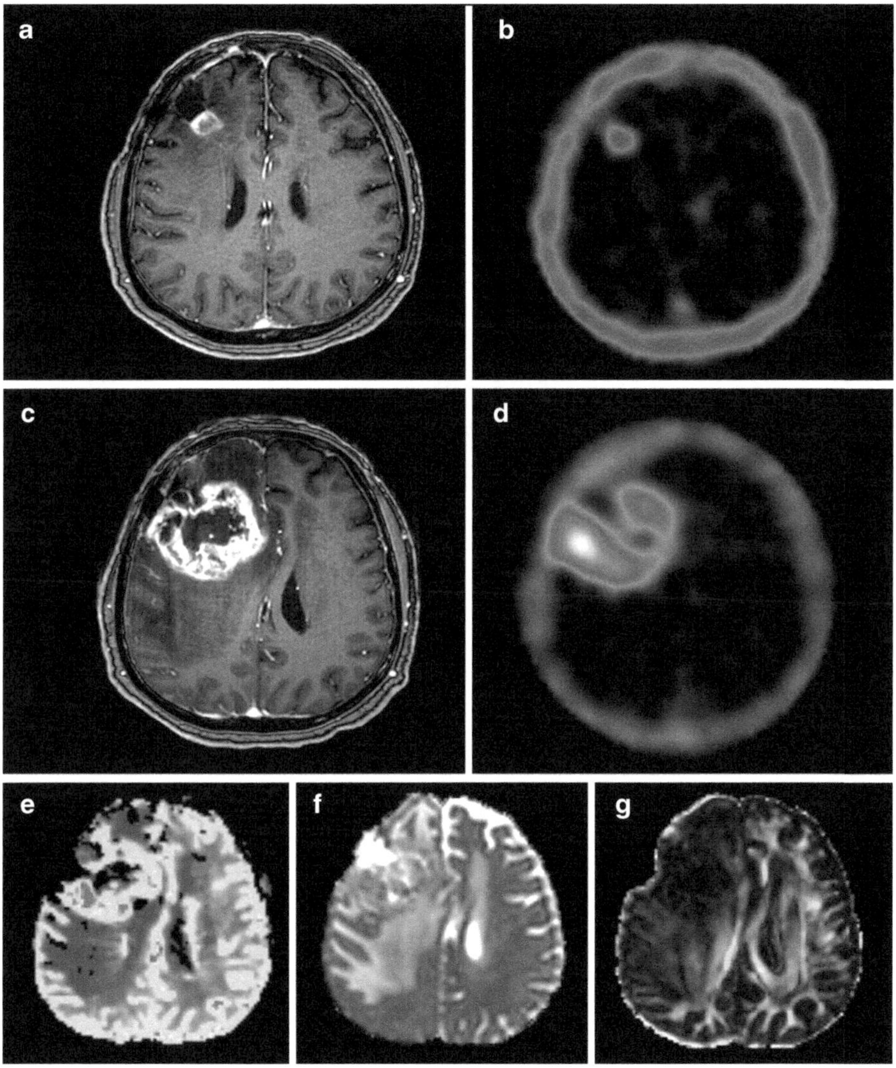

Fig. 40.2 A 66-year-old male with glioblastoma of the right frontal lobe diagnosed 21 months earlier and treated by surgery and radiochemotherapy (temozolomide). (**a**) Gadolinium-enhanced T1-weighted MRI revealed a postsurgical cavity with an adjacent enhancing dense area that raised the question of tumor recurrence versus radiation necrosis. (**b**) A few days later, ^{99m}Tc-tetrofosmin SPECT revealed intense tracer uptake (tumor-to-background ratio [TBR] = 11) in the corresponding area of gadolinium enhancement suggesting recurrence. (**c**) Eight months later—a new surgery in the meantime verified recurrent glioblastoma—Gd-T1w MRI revealed tumor progression. (**d**) The corresponding SPECT image at the time was also typical of tumor progression (TBR > 20) with a central photopenic necrotic area. (**e**) Further investigation by advanced MRI techniques showed an increased relative cerebral blood volume (rCBV) in the corresponding areas of profound radiotracer uptake, indicating intense angiogenesis. (**f**) The apparent diffusion coefficient (ADC) map showed highly irregular water diffusivity throughout the lesion that was surrounded by extensive edema. (**g**) Diffusion tensor imaging (DTI) with fractional anisotropy (FA) mapping revealed abrupt white matter fiber disruption by the lesion consistent with a high-grade recurrent tumor

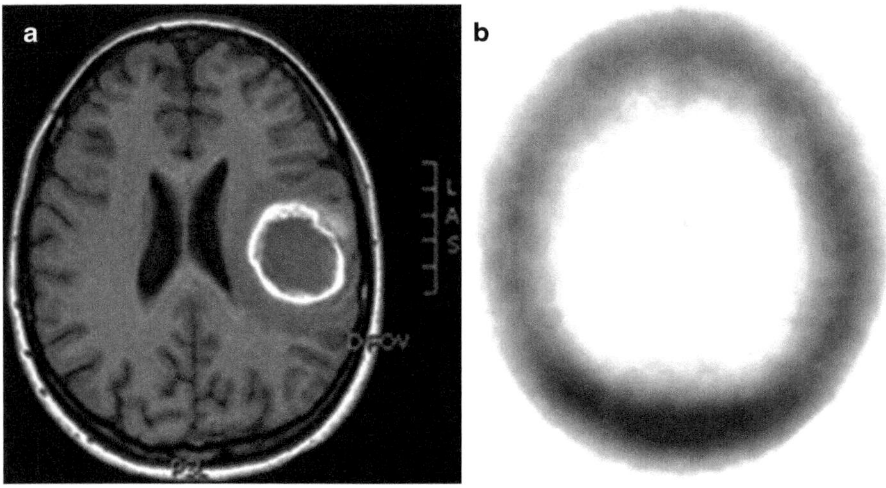

Fig. 40.3 (**a**) T1-weighted MRI in a patient with an intracerebral hemorrhage. The neoplastic hemorrhagic origin could not be ruled out. (**b**) Brain SPECT demonstrating no tracer uptake suggesting nonneoplastic hemorrhagic origin

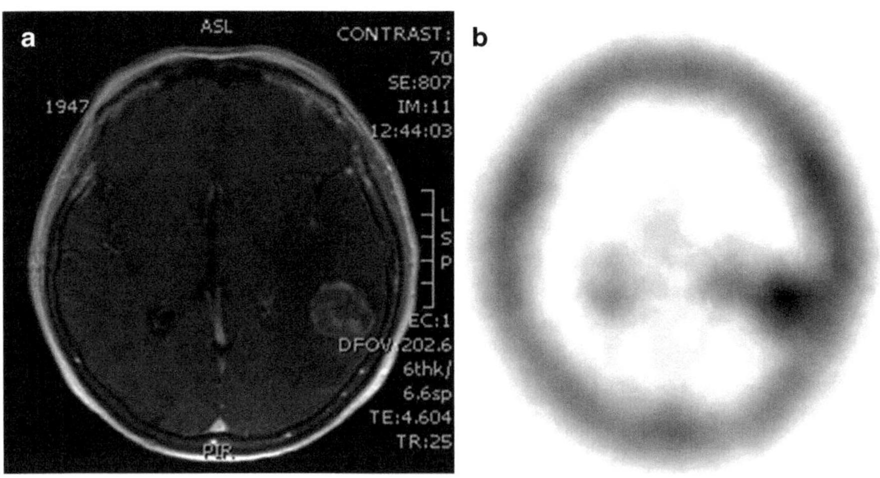

Fig. 40.4 (**a**) T1-weighted MRI after gadolinium infusion in a patient with a metastatic lesion. (**b**) ^{99m}Tc-tetrofosmin brain SPECT revealing increased tracer uptake in the corresponding area

Other types are pituitary adenomas (13.1%), neuroepithelial tumors (5.1%), lymphoma (2.4%), oligodendrogliomas (2%), ependymomas (1.8%), embryonal tumors (1%), and craniopharyngioma (0.7%).

Causes and risk factors can be environmental and genetic. The most common presenting symptoms of brain tumors are due to increased intracranial pressure (headache, nausea, vomiting), seizures, focal neurological deficits, and possibly cognitive deterioration (Perry and Schmidt 2006). Treatment depends on tumor aggressiveness. Radical surgical excision is usually curative in benign tumor. Treatment options for high-grade lesions are surgery, radiation therapy, and chemotherapy. The majority of patients get a combination of treatments (Alexiou et al. 2009).

With regard to imaging, the most commonly used method for diagnosis and follow-up is magnetic resonance imaging (MRI). Nevertheless, in patients with brain lesions, it is not uncommon for MRI to provide nonspecific information, even after contrast administration. Advanced MRI techniques, including diffusion, perfusion (dynamic susceptibility contrast, dynamic contrast enhanced, and arterial spin labeling), and spectroscopy, offer important diagnostic advantages over conventional imaging in the assessment of patients with brain tumors. Imaging modalities used in nuclear medicine, namely, positron emission tomography (PET) and single-photon emission computed tomography (SPECT), have also been employed toward the evaluation of brain tumors. At present, PET constitutes the most sophisticated modality of nuclear medicine imaging for brain tumor evaluation, owing to higher resolution compared to SPECT. Nevertheless, SPECT has a lower cost, worldwide availability, and gained practical experience. The more sophisticated hybrid SPECT-CT scanners provide both functional and anatomic imaging to be acquired simultaneously (Hasegawa et al. 2002). Various SPECT radiotracers have been used to date and are presented in detail.

40.2 SPECT Radiotracers

Various SPECT radiotracers have been evaluated toward noninvasive assessment of brain lesions, with image acquisition usually performed 20 min after intravenous radiotracer administration. Among them, thallium-201 (^{201}Tl) was one of the first tracers that were widely employed (physical half-life 73 h, emitting γ-rays at 135 and 167 keV, and X-rays at ~70–80 keV, administered activity 148 MBq). The precise cellular uptake process is still questioned, but the sodium-potassium ATPase pump is probably involved, at least in part.

Technetium-99m-labeled compounds (physical half-life 6 h, emitting γ-rays at 140 keV) have also been studied and were proven advantageous over ^{201}Tl due to higher photon flux, better spatial resolution, and less radiation burden to the patient (Benard et al. 2002; Soler et al. 1998). Among them, ^{99m}Tc-hexamethypropyleneamine oxime (HMPAO) (administered activity 1110 MBq) and more extensively ^{99m}Tc-hexakis-2-methoxy isobutyl isonitrile (^{99m}Tc-sestamibi or ^{99m}Tc-MIBI) and ^{99m}Tc-tetrofosmin (^{99m}Tc-TF) (administered activity 700 MBq for both) have also been studied. ^{99m}Tc-MIBI diffuses passively into the cell through the intact cellular membrane, driven by the membrane negative electric potential, and an estimated 95% of the tracer is localized in the mitochondria. ^{99m}Tc-TF enters viable cells similar to sestamibi, and mostly localizes within the cytosol, with only a small fraction passing into the mitochondria. Although both ^{99m}Tc-TF and ^{99m}Tc-MIBI have been found in vitro to be substrates of P-gp, the fact that ^{99m}Tc-TF uptake in glioma cells is not particularly influenced by the expression of their multidrug resistance proteins (MDR) protein genotype substantiates a plausible clinical superiority over ^{99m}Tc-MIBI, which is prone to extracellular excretion by P-gp. Pentavalent Tc-99m dimercaptosuccinic acid (^{99m}Tc-(V) DMSA) (administered activity 700 MBq) is another tumor-seeking SPECT tracer, being a possible $PO4^{3-}$ anion analogue. Its proliferative imaging potential in gliomas has been suggested in vitro and sporadically reported in vivo. Tsiouris et al. stated that mounting evidence indicates that ^{99m}Tc-(V)DMSA is a credible noninvasive proliferation depicter and its cellular accumulation linked closely to phosphate uptake and kinase pathway activation (Denoyer et al. 2004, 2005; Tsiouris et al. 2007; Amin et al. 2012). ^{99m}Tc-methionine and ^{99m}Tc-glucoheptonate have also been utilized, but are not easily available and not commonly used.

Radiolabeled amino acids have been evaluated and proved tracers for the delineation of tumors, particularly brain neoplasms. These tracers are not taken up by normal brain and provide a greater target-to-background contrast, thus allowing better characterization and differentiation of the tumor from the normal brain. L-3-[Iodine-123]-iodo-alpha-methyl-L-tyrosine (^{123}I-IMT) is well established for SPECT imaging of gliomas, and p-[iodine-123]-iodo-L-phenylalanine (^{123}I-IPA) has been also used. The latter may prove promising for therapeutic use in gliomas after labeling with iodine-131 (Hellwig et al. 2008).

40.3 Clinical Applications

The primary role of SPECT in brain tumor patients lies on the noninvasive assessment of tumor's aggressiveness, differentiation of treatment-induced necrosis from tumor recurrence, assessment of response to treatment, and estimation of overall prognosis.

40.3.1 Characterization of Intracranial Masses: Differentiation of Brain Tumors from Nonneoplastic Lesions

The noninvasive assessment of the nature of an intracranial lesion is of paramount importance for patient's management. Differentiation of high-grade from low-grade gliomas may not be always possible on conventional MRI, since non-enhancing high-grade gliomas exist. Furthermore, a ring-enhanced lesion may be a brain tumor, an abscess, tumefactive multiple sclerosis, or other nonneoplastic pathologies such as an intracerebral hemorrhage. The above problems are encountered in everyday practice.

^{99m}Tc-TF brain SPECT was evaluated in 106 patients with intracranial lesion suspicious of tumor on conventional radiological imaging. Ninety patients suffered from neoplastic lesions, and 16 harbored nonneoplastic pathologies (abscesses, nonmalignant hemorrhages, radiation necroses). A lesion-to-normal (L/N) tracer uptake ratio of 2.8 could differentiate high-grade gliomas from low-grade lesions

(Fotopoulos et al. 2011). Similar findings have been reported by other authors (Choi et al. 2000). Furthermore, ^{99m}Tc-TF differentiated effectively high- and low-grade gliomas from nonneoplastic lesions. Nonetheless, differentiation between primary gliomas (low or high grade) and metastases was not feasible on the basis of quantitative scintigraphic criteria.

Thallium-201, one of the most commonly used tracers for brain tumor imaging, showed promise for the differentiation of malignant from benign brain tumors. ^{201}Tl brain SPECT could increase confidence in the diagnosis of intracranial lesions with ring-like contrast enhancement when conventional MRI was not able to differentiate between benign and malignant disease. A brain tumor would show avid tracer uptake compared to the low uptake of a brain abscess (Kita et al. 2007). Another important issue that has been addressed is the optimal lesion size for an accurate diagnosis. In a study comparing ^{201}Tl uptake between primary CNS lymphoma and abscess, the authors reported that lesion size is a significant determinant of the accuracy of this tracer, which should be the initial diagnostic tool for lesions over 2 cm (Young et al. 2005). Furthermore, the location of a lesion is important, since infratentorial lesions may tend to display lower tracer uptake (Scott et al. 1994).

^{99m}Tc-(V)DMSA has been proven valuable for brain tumor characterization. Hirano et al. compared ^{99m}Tc-(V)DMSA and ^{201}Tl in 100 patients with various brain pathologies. They found that early uptake ratios of both radiopharmaceuticals were closely related to tumor vascularity, but could not differentiate benign from malignant disease. The delayed tracer uptake ratio, retention ratio, and retention index were higher in malignant tumors than benign ones on ^{99m}Tc(V)-DMSA; however, there was no statistically significant difference between benign and malignant tumors on ^{201}Tl. They concluded that ^{99m}Tc(V)DMSA is superior in imaging primary and metastatic brain tumors and differentiating their histological malignancy grade noninvasively (Hirano et al. 1997a).

^{99m}Tc-MIBI has been evaluated in various brain pathologies. If performed within 5 days of symptom onset, it has been found capable to differentiate neoplastic from nonneoplastic intracerebral hematomas (Minutoli et al. 2005). When compared to ^{201}Tl, it proved superior for differentiating intracranial lymphoma from nonmalignant lesions, exhibiting similar sensitivity but higher specificity (Naddaf et al. 1998).

Somatostatin receptors (SSRs) are expressed in 70–100% of meningiomas and can be used to image the radiolabeled tumors for maximizing resection, detection of residual, or early recurrent tumors or for therapeutic purposes (Dammers et al. 2009). Brain SPECT by the radiolabeled SSR-agonist peptide indium-111 (^{111}In)-pentetreotide (^{111}In-DTPA-octreotide) may provide important information for the noninvasive differentiation of meningiomas from other cranial dural-based pathology in conjugation with conventional MRI. This method provided high-negative predictive value (100%) for the diagnosis of meningiomas (Nathoo et al. 2007). Yttrium-90 (^{90}Y)-DOTA-Phe1-Tyr3-octreotide (^{90}Y-SMT 487, OctreoTher™) has shown potential for effectively treating patients with neuroendocrine tumors (Bushnell et al. 2004).

40.3.2 Differentiate Glioma Recurrence from Treatment-Induced Necrosis (TIN)

Malignant gliomas are the most common type of primary brain tumors and carry a dismal prognosis. Glioblastoma multiforme (GBM) usually has a rapid and fatal clinical course. The standard of care for newly diagnosed GBM includes maximal surgical resection when possible, followed by radiotherapy and concomitant and adjuvant temozolomide. Nevertheless, high-grade gliomas usually recur despite treatment, whereas radiotherapy may cause post-radiation damage (Alexiou et al. 2009). The incidence of treatment-related necrosis in GBM patients treated with concomitant temozolomide and radiotherapy reaches 30%. Furthermore, apart from radiation necrosis, new posttreatment entities such as pseudoprogression and pseudoresponse have been recognized (Zikou et al. 2018). Differentiation between TIN and recurrent glioma on the basis of CT and conventional MRI is not always possible. Nuclear medicine/molecular imaging has also been actively implicated in the detection of recurrent tumor by SPECT and PET. Among the SPECT tracers, the most extensively studied are ^{201}Tl and ^{99m}Tc-MIBI.

Recurrent disease exhibits increased ^{201}Tl uptake compared to necrosis. Early and delayed postinjection imaging has been used to calculate the radiotracer retention index (RI) (i.e., the ratio of delayed L/N uptake ratio to early L/N uptake ratio); RI has been suggested as a significant diagnostic marker by Matsunaga et al. (2013). Even in the follow-up of low-grade gliomas by ^{201}Tl, a tracer uptake index value of 1.25 as cutoff for detecting recurrent tumor activity resulted in 90% sensitivity and 80% specificity (Gómez-Río et al. 2004).

^{99m}Tc-MIBI has also been extensively evaluated, with good reported results and a significant diagnostic advantage over contrast-enhanced MRI (Soler et al. 1998). In a study that included 81 patients, the sensitivity for tumor recurrence was 90%, specificity 91.5%, and accuracy 90.5% (Le Jeune et al. 2006a). H-MRS proved equal to ^{99m}Tc-MIBI SPECT with 90% sensitivity, 100% specificity, 93% accuracy, 83% negative predictive value, and 100% positive predictive value (Palumbo et al. 2006).

Apart from ^{201}Tl and ^{99m}Tc-MIBI, ^{99m}Tc-TF has been also evaluated toward the detection of recurrent tumor, having the advantage of not being influenced by glioma MDR phenotype (P-gp expression). A cutoff L/N value of 4.8 was found as the most accurately discriminating recurrence from postirradiation damage (Alexiou et al. 2007). In a comparative study between relative cerebral blood volume (rCBV) by perfusion MRI and ^{99m}Tc-TF brain SPECT, they were found of similar diagnostic accuracy. Furthermore, a significant correlation between tracer uptake ratio and rCBV was verified (Alexiou et al. 2014). However, it must be kept in mind that ^{99m}Tc-TF SPECT exhibits suboptimal sensitivity in the detection of recurrent tumors located supratentorially in the posterior fossa (Barai et al. 2003).

^{99m}Tc-(V)DMSA also proved useful for the detection of glioma recurrence. In a comparative study between ^{99m}Tc-(V)DMSA SPECT and H-MRS, the first was more accurate for the detection of tumor residual tissues or recurrence in glioma patients with previous radiotherapy. ^{99m}Tc-(V)DMSA allowed an early and noninvasive differentiation of residual tumor or recurrence from TIN (Amin et al. 2012).

Imaging protein synthesis with the use of radiolabeled amino acids is another approach that has been employed toward the noninvasive detection of tumor recurrence. Amino acid uptake in normal brain tissue is low; thus recurrent gliomas can be readily distinguished from their surrounding normal tissue. The majority of labeled amino acid tracers have been developed for PET imaging; however, SPECT tracers may be a cost-effective alternative. ^{99m}Tc-methionine can be a possible substitute to ^{11}C-MET PET and was compared to F-FDG PET/CT and contrast-enhanced MRI for the detection of recurrent glioma. The specificity of ^{99m}Tc-methionine SPECT/CT proved to be higher than MRI but not of F-FDG PET/CT (Arora et al. 2018).

^{99m}Tc DTPA-bismethionine (^{99m}Tc-MDM) has been also evaluated for the detection of recurrent/residual glioma. This tracer was found comparable to contrast-enhanced MRI and ^{18F}FLT-PET for the postsurgical follow-up period (Singh et al. 2015). ^{123}I-IMT has been validated in SPECT studies. Samnick et al. studied 78 glioma patients after primary therapy and possible tumor recurrence and found that ^{123}I-IMT had 100% sensitivity for the detection of high-grade glioma recurrence and 84% and 92% for Grade II and Grade III glioma recurrence, respectively (Samnick et al. 2002). In a comparative study between single-voxel H-MRS at 3.0 T and ^{123}I-IMT SPECT, a tracer uptake cutoff value of 1.62 proved superior to MRS (sensitivity 95%, specificity 100%, and accuracy 96% vs. 89%, 83%, and 88%, respectively) (Plotkin et al. 2004).

40.3.3 Assessment of Glioma Aggressiveness

Assessing the proliferative potential of tumor cells is of paramount importance for predicting their biological behavior, response to therapy, and prognosis. Noninvasive imaging modalities that could reliably assess the proliferative potential of intracranial space-occupying lesions in vivo would be of obvious significance (Alexiou et al. 2010a). Various methods have been proposed to estimate proliferation in tissue samples. The most extensively studied are flow cytometry, bromodeoxyuridine (BrdU) labeling index, MIB-1 antibody staining to the nuclear antigen Ki-67, staining to the proliferating cell nuclear antigen (PCNA), and argyrophilic staining to nucleolar organizing regions (AgNOR) (Prayson 2005). Among these, the MIB-1/Ki-67 assay can be easily applied, is considered as the most reliable method, and is performed routinely.

A significant correlation between L/N ^{201}Tl uptake and BrdU labeling index in glioma was first reported by Oriuchi et al. (1993). Subsequent studies using the PCNA as proliferation marker also reported a positive correlation. Both ^{99m}Tc-MIBI and ^{99m}Tc-TF depicted a significant positive correlation with both Ki-67 index and S-phase estimated by flow cytometry cell-cycle analysis. ^{99m}Tc-(V)DMSA enters cancer cells via the Na^+-Pi co-transporter like the phosphate ion, this uptake being directly linked to the cellular levels of phosphorylated (activated) focal adhesion kinase protein, a keypoint of increased proliferation. In a study of glioma cell lines, 99mTc-(V)DMSA reflected Pi3-K and protein kinase C (PKC) activity and correlated with tumor aggressiveness (Le Jeune et al. 2006b). In the clinical setting of primary brain tumors, ^{99m}Tc-(V)DMSA SPECT could noninvasively differentiate histological malignancy and tumor grade (Hirano et al. 1997b). With regard to amino acid imaging, a study with ^{123}I-IMT in 27 glioma patients revealed a significant correlation between tracer uptake and Ki-67 (Kuwert et al. 1997).

40.3.4 Assessment of Meningioma Aggressiveness

Meningiomas are the most common benign intracranial tumors arising from the dural coverings of the brain at any site, most commonly the skull vault and the skull base. Although meningiomas typically exhibit benign histological features and total resection is associated with favorable prognosis, atypical (WHO Grade II) or anaplastic (WHO Grade III) tumors can be found in 6% of cases and are associated with increased risk of recurrence (Alexiou et al. 2010b).

^{201}Tl uptake in meningiomas was thought mainly to be related to lesional vascularity. Tracer RI may provide clues to differentiate meningothelial from transitional or fibroplastic tumors. Although these meningioma subtypes are benign variants, transitional and fibrous meningiomas have different chromosomal abnormalities (Maillo et al. 2001). The delayed ^{201}Tl uptake index of atypical meningiomas is significantly higher than that of the benign subtypes. A significant correlation between delayed ^{201}Tl uptake index, MIB-1/Ki-67 labeling index, and vascular endothelial growth factor (VEGF) expression has been described (Takeda et al. 2011).

^{99m}Tc-MIBI has not been extensively evaluated in meningiomas and few reports exist. A small-scale study found no correlation between Ki-67 index and tracer uptake; still ^{99m}Tc-MIBI could predict anticancer drug resistance related to the expression of MDR-1 mRNA and its gene product P-gp (Kunishio et al. 2003). Tumor ^{99m}Tc-TF uptake is not influenced by MDR phenotype expression and has been proven suitable for discriminating malignant from benign meningiomas, with an L/N tracer uptake value of 9.6 being the optimal threshold (Fotopoulos et al. 2008). Furthermore, L/N correlated significantly with both meningioma grade and Ki-67 expression. These initial results were supported by a subsequent study that aimed to correlate meningioma ^{99m}Tc-TF uptake with its proliferative profile, as assessed by cell-cycle analysis with flow cytometry. This study revealed a significant correlation of radiotracer uptake with both the S-phase fraction and the level of DNA aneuploidy (Alexiou et al. 2008). DNA ploidy and S-phase, as assessed by flow cytometry, are useful indicators of tumors with different biological behavior. Nuclear DNA content has been reported to predict risk of recurrence and clinical outcome for several brain tumors (Alexiou et al. 2008; Coons et al. 1994). Coons et al. found three groups of astrocytoma patients with significantly different survival, based on S-phase fraction ranges of $<3.0\%$, 3.0–5.9%, and $\geq 6\%$ (Coons et al. 1994).

40.3.5 Assessment of Patient Prognosis

Assessing prognosis and predicting patient outcome is of paramount importance in gliomas and more notably in GBM. Although the mean survival of GBM is 15 months, a subset of patients demonstrate long-term survival that may exceed 3 years (Liu et al. 2010). Thus, the identification of prognostic variables is important to identify patients that could benefit from more aggressive treatment schemes.

The prognostic value of tumoral ^{201}Tl uptake has been evaluated in glioma patients and was found associated with worse survival for lesions located supratentorially (Oriuchi et al. 1993). Recently, Vos et al. (2012) reported that ^{201}Tl uptake correlated with overall survival in glioma patients treated with temozolomide. Even in low-grade glioma, ^{201}Tl SPECT is useful for the prediction of early tumor progression, not only in resected low-grade astrocytomas (LGAs) but also in biopsy-proven lesions. Thus, patients with biopsy-proven LGAs should be considered as high-risk groups for early progression, if the tumor exhibits a high ^{201}Tl uptake (Park et al. 2012).

Postirradiation ^{99m}Tc-MIBI uptake has also been described to comprise prognostic implications in high-grade gliomas, and similar results have been reported for ^{123}I-IMT (Beauchesne et al. 2004; Weber et al. 2001). Pretreatment ^{99m}Tc-TF uptake was well correlated with overall survival in patients with glioblastoma. Patients with an L/N index exceeding 4.7 bore significantly worse survival than those with lower uptake values (Alexiou et al. 2010c). ^{99m}Tc-(V)DMSA also showed promise for the evaluation of glioblastoma patients' prognosis in a study of 40 patients. In the multivariate analysis, ^{99m}Tc-(V)DMSA SPECT was an independent prognostic factor for survival (Amin et al. 2015).

40.4 Conclusion

Although brain imaging by conventional MRI and CT is of paramount importance in identifying structural abnormalities secondary to the development of space-occupying lesions, especially when those pathologies disrupt the blood-brain barrier and give rise to contrast enhancement, edema, and mass effects, the true nature of each visible lesion may lie well beyond gross structural patterns, down in the cellular and molecular level. It is therefore of paramount importance to identify noninvasively the true nature of any visible lesion, and this is where functional metabolic imaging by SPECT, PET, and modern MRI techniques come into play and excel their role.

SPECT can provide accurate and important information for proper patient management, having the advantages of lower cost and excellent availability compared to PET. Various radiotracers are available in clinical practice that can accurately characterize brain tumor metabolism. The results of several studies thus far justify further research on the clinical utility of this imaging modality, entailing additional comparative studies with PET and functional MR techniques.

References

Alexiou GA, Fotopoulos AD, Papadopoulos A, Kyritsis AP, Polyzoidis KS, Tsiouris S (2007) Evaluation of brain tumor recurrence by ^{99m}Tc-tetrofosmin SPECT: a prospective pilot study. Ann Nucl Med 21:293–298

Alexiou GA, Tsiouris S, Goussia A, Papadopoulos A, Kyritsis AP, Polyzoidis KS, Fotopoulos AD (2008) Evaluation of glioma proliferation by ^{99m}Tc-Tetrofosmin. Neuro-Oncology 10:104–105

Alexiou GA, Tsiouris S, Kyritsis AP, Voulgaris S, Argyropoulou MI, Fotopoulos AD (2009) Glioma recurrence versus radiation necrosis: accuracy of current imaging modalities. J Neuro-Oncol 95:1–11

Alexiou GA, Tsiouris S, Kyritsis AP, Argyropoulou MI, Voulgaris S, Fotopoulos AD (2010a) Assessment of glioma proliferation using imaging modalities. J Clin Neurosci 17:1233–1238

Alexiou GA, Gogou P, Markoula S, Kyritsis AP (2010b) Management of meningiomas. Clin Neurol Neurosurg 112:177–182

Alexiou GA, Tsiouris S, Kyritsis AP, Fotakopoulos G, Goussia A, Voulgaris S, Fotopoulos AD (2010c) The value of ^{99m}Tc-tetrofosmin brain SPECT in predicting survival in patients with glioblastoma multiforme. J Nucl Med 51:1923–1926

Alexiou GA, Zikou A, Tsiouris S et al (2014) Comparison of diffusion tensor, dynamic susceptibility contrast MRI and (99m)Tc-Tetrofosmin brain SPECT for the detection of recurrent high-grade glioma. Magn Reson Imaging 32:854–859

Amin A, Moustafa H, Ahmed E, El-Toukhy M (2012) Glioma residual or recurrence versus radiation necrosis: accuracy of pentavalent technetium-99 m-dimercaptosuccinic acid [Tc-99 m (V) DMSA] brain SPECT compared to proton magnetic resonance spectroscopy (1H-MRS): initial results. J Neuro-Oncol 106:579–587

Amin A, Mustafa M, Abd El-Hadi E, Monier A, Badwey A, Saad E (2015) Pentavalent technetium-99m-dimercaptosuccinic acid [Tc-99m (V) DMSA] brain SPECT: does it have a place in predicting survival in patients with glioblastoma multiforme? J Neuro-Oncol 121:303–309

Arora G, Sharma P, Sharma A et al (2018) 99mTc-methionine hybrid SPECT/CT for detection of recurrent glioma: comparison with 18F-FDG PET/CT and contrast-enhanced MRI. Clin Nucl Med 43:e132–e138

Barai S, Bandopadhayaya GP, Julka PK, Haloi AK, Seith A, Malhotra A (2003) Evaluation of single photon emission computerised tomography (SPECT) using Tc99m-tetrofosmin as a diagnostic modality for recurrent posterior fossa tumours. J Postgrad Med 49:316–320

Beauchesne P, Pedeux R, Boniol M, Soler C (2004) ^{99m}Tc-sestamibi brain SPECT after chemoradiotherapy is prognostic of survival in patients with high-grade glioma. J Nucl Med 3:409–413

Benard F, Romsa J, Hustinx R (2002) Imaging gliomas with positron emission tomography and single-photon emission computed tomography. Semin Nucl Med 33:148–162

Bushnell D, Menda Y, O'Dorisio T, Madsen M, Miller S, Carlisle T, Squires S, Kahn D, Walkner W, Connolly M, O'Dorisio S, Karwal M, Ponto J, Bouterfa H (2004) Effects of intravenous amino acid administration with Y-90 DOTA-Phe1-Tyr3-Octreotide [SMT487(OctreoTher)] treatment. Cancer Biother Radiopharm 19:35–41

Choi JY, Kim SE, Shin HJ, Kim BT, Kim JH (2000) Brain tumor imaging with 99mTc-tetrofosmin: comparison with 201Tl, 99mTc-MIBI, and 18F-fluorodeoxyglucose. J Neuro-Oncol 46:63–70

Coons SW, Johnson PC, Pearl DK (1994) Prognostic significance of flow cytometry deoxyribonucleic acid analysis of human astrocytomas. Neurosurgery 35:119–125

Dammers R, Hsu SP, Krisht AF (2009) Radioguided improved resection of a cranial base meningioma. Neurosurgery 64:84–85

Denoyer D, Perek N, Le Jeune N, Frere D, Dubois F (2004) Evidence that 99mTc-(V)- DMSA uptake is mediated by NaPi cotransporter type III in tumour cell lines. Eur J Nucl Med Mol Imaging 31:77–84

Denoyer D, Perek N, Le Jeune N, Cornillon J, Dubois F (2005) Correlation between 99mTc-(V)-DMSA uptake and constitutive level of phosphorylated focal adhesion kinase in an in vitro model of cancer cell lines. Eur J Nucl Med Mol Imaging 32:820–827

Fotopoulos AD, Alexiou GA, Goussia A, Papadopoulos A, Kyritsis AP, Polyzoidis KS, Voulgaris S, Tsiouris S (2008) ^{99m}Tc-Tetrofosmin brain SPECT in the assessment of meningiomas-correlation with histological grade and proliferation index. J Neuro-Oncol 89:225–230

Fotopoulos AD, Kyritsis AP, Tsiouris S, Al-Boucharali J, Papadopoulos A, Voulgaris S, Alexiou GA (2011) Characterization of intracranial space-occupying lesions by ^{99m}Tc-Tetrofosmin SPECT. J Neuro-Oncol 101:83–89

Gómez-Río M, Martínez Del Valle Torres D, Rodríguez-Fernández A, Llamas-Elvira JM, Lozano SO, Font CR, López Ramírez E, Katati M (2004) (201)Tl-SPECT in low-grade gliomas: diagnostic accuracy in differential diagnosis between tumour recurrence and radionecrosis. Eur J Nucl Med Mol Imaging 31:1237–1243

Hasegawa BH et al (2002) Dual-modality imaging of cancer with SPECT/CT. Technol Cancer Res Treat 1:449–458

Hellwig D, Romeike BF, Ketter R, Moringlane JR, Kirsch CM, Samnick S (2008) Intra-individual comparison of p-[123I]-iodo-L-phenylalanine and L-3-[123I]-iodo-alpha-methyl-tyrosine for SPECT imaging of gliomas. Eur J Nucl Med Mol Imaging 35:24–31

Hirano T, Otake H, Kazama K, Wakabayashi K, Zama A, Shibasaki T, Tamura M, Endo K (1997a) Technetium-99 m(V)-DMSA and thallium-201 in brain tumor imaging: correlation with histology and malignant grade. J Nucl Med 38:1741–1749

Hirano T, Otake H, Shibasaki T, Tamura M, Endo K (1997b) Differentiating histologic malignancy of primary brain tumors: pentavalent technetium-99 m-DMSA. J Nucl Med 38:20–26

Kita T, Hayashi K, Yamamoto M, Kawauchi T, Sakata I, Iwasaki Y, Kosuda S (2007) Does supplementation of contrast MR imaging with thallium-201 brain SPECT improve differentiation between benign and malignant ring-like contrast-enhanced cerebral lesions? Ann Nucl Med 21:251–256

Kunishio K, Morisaki K, Matsumoto Y, Nagao S, Nishiyama Y (2003) Technetium-99m sestamibi single photon emission computed tomography findings correlated with P-glycoprotein expression, encoded by the multidrug resistance gene-1 messenger ribonucleic acid, in intracranial meningiomas. Neurol Med Chir (Tokyo) 43:573–580

Kuwert T, Probst-Cousin S, Woesler B et al (1997) Iodine-123-alpha-methyl tyrosine in gliomas: correlation with cellular density and proliferative activity. J Nucl Med 38:1551–1555

Le Jeune FP, Dubois F, Blond S, Steinling M (2006a) Sestamibi technetium-99 m brain single-photon emission computed tomography to identify recurrent glioma in adults: 201 studies. J Neuro-Oncol 77:177–183

Le Jeune N, Perek N, Dubois F (2006b) Influence of Pi3-K and PKC activity on 99mTc-(V)-DMSA uptake: correlation with tumour aggressiveness in an in vitro malignant glioblastoma cell line model. Eur J Nucl Med Mol Imaging 33:1206–1213

Liu Y, Shete S, Etzel CJ et al (2010) Polymorphisms of LIG4, BTBD2, HMGA2, and RTEL1 genes involved in the double-strand break repair pathway predict glioblastoma survival. J Clin Oncol 28:2467–2474

Louis DN, Perry A, Reifenberger G et al (2016) The 2016 World Health Organization classification of tumors of the central nervous system: a summary. Acta Neuropathol 131:803–820

Maillo A, Diaz P, Sayagues JM, Blanco A, Tabernero MD, Ciudad J, Lopez A, Goncalves JM, Orfao A (2001) Gains of chromosome 22 by fluorescence in situ hybridization in the context of an hyperdiploid karyotype are associated with aggressive clinical features in meningioma patients. Cancer 92:377–385

Matsunaga S, Shuto T, Takase H, Ohtake M, Tomura N, Tanaka T, Sonoda M (2013) Semiquantitative analysis using thallium-201 SPECT for differential diagnosis between tumor recurrence and radiation necrosis after gamma knife surgery for malignant brain tumors. Int J Radiat Oncol Biol Phys 85(1):47–52

Minutoli F, Angileri FF, Conti A, Herberg A, Aricò D, Baldari S, Cardali S, de Divitiis O, Germanò A, Baldari S (2005) Timing of examination affects reliability of 99mTc-methoxyisobutylisonitrile SPECT in distinguishing neoplastic from nonneoplastic brain hematomas. J Nucl Med 46:574–579

Naddaf SY, Akisik MF, Aziz M, Omar WS, Hirschfeld A, Masdeu J, Donnenfeld H, Abdel-Dayem HM (1998) Comparison between 201Tl-chloride and 99Tc(m)-sestamibi SPET brain imaging for differentiating intracranial lymphoma from non-malignant lesions in AIDS patients. Nucl Med Commun 19:47–53

Nathoo N, Ugokwe K, Chang AS, Li L, Ross J, Suh JH, Vogelbaum MA, Barnett GH (2007) The role of 111indium-octreotide brain scintigraphy in the diagnosis of cranial, dural-based meningiomas. J Neuro-Oncol 81:167–174

Oriuchi N, Tamura M, Shibazaki T et al (1993) Clinical evaluation of thallium-201 SPECT in supratentorial gliomas: relationship to histologic grade, prognosis and proliferative activities. J Nucl Med 34:2085–2089

Ostrom QT, Gittleman H, Liao P et al (2017) CBTRUS statistical report: primary brain and other central nervous system tumors diagnosed in the United States in 2010-2014. Neuro-Oncology 6:v1–v88

Palumbo B, Lupattelli M, Pelliccioli GP, Chiarini P, Moschini TO, Palumbo I, Siepi D, Buoncristiani P, Nardi M, Giovenali P, Palumbo R (2006) Association of 99mTc-MIBI brain SPECT and proton magnetic resonance spectroscopy (1H-MRS) to assess glioma recurrence after radiotherapy. Q J Nucl Med Mol Imaging 50:88–93

Park KJ, Kang SH, Park DH, Cho TH, Choe JG, Chung YG (2012) Usefulness of thallium-201 SPECT for prediction of early progression in low-grade astrocytomas diagnosed by stereotactic biopsy. Clin Neurol Neurosurg 114:223–229

Perry A, Schmidt RE (2006) Cancer therapy-associated CNS neuropathology: an update and review of the literature. Acta Neuropathol 111:197–212

Plotkin M, Eisenacher J, Bruhn H, Wurm R, Michel R, Stockhammer F, Feussner A, Dudeck O, Wust P, Felix R, Amthauer H (2004) 123I-IMT SPECT and 1H MR-spectroscopy at 3.0 T in the differential diagnosis of recurrent or residual gliomas: a comparative study. J Neuro-Oncol 70:49–58

Prayson R (2005) The utility of MIB-1/Ki-67 immunostaining in the evaluation of central nervous system neoplasms. Adv Anat Pathol 12:144–148

Samnick S, Bader JB, Hellwig D, Moringlane JR, Alexander C, Romeike BF, Feiden W, Kirsch CM (2002) Clinical value of iodine-123-alpha-methyl-L-tyrosine single-photon emission tomography in the differential diagnosis of recurrent brain tumor in patients pretreated for glioma at follow-up. J Clin Oncol 20:396–404

Scott AM, Macapinlac H, Zhang JJ et al (1994) Clinical applications of fusion imaging in oncology. Nucl Med Biol 21:775–784

Singh B, Kumar N, Sharma S et al (2015) 99mTc-MDM brain SPECT for the detection of recurrent/remnant glioma-comparison with ceMRI and 18F-FLT PET imaging: initial results. Clin Nucl Med 40:e475–e479

Soler C, Beauchesne P, Maatougui K, Schmitt T, Barral FG, Michel D, Dubois F, Brunon J (1998) Technetium-99 m sestamibi brain single-photon emission tomography for detection of recurrent gliomas after radiation therapy. Eur J Nucl Med 25:1649–1657

Takeda T, Nakano T, Asano K, Shimamura N, Ohkuma H (2011) Usefulness of thallium-201 SPECT in the evaluation of tumor natures in intracranial meningiomas. Neuroradiology 53:867–873

Tsiouris S, Pirmettis I, Chatzipanagiotou T, Ptohis N, Papantoniou V (2007) Pentavalent technetium-99 m dimercaptosuccinic acid 99mTc-(V) DMSA brain scintitomography a plausible non-invasive depicter of glioblastoma proliferation and therapy response. J Neuro-Oncol 85:291–295

Vos MJ, Berkhof J, Hoekstra OS, Bosma I, Sizoo EM, Heimans JJ, Reijneveld JC, Sanchez E, Lagerwaard FJ, Buter J, Noske DP, Postma TJ (2012) MRI and thallium-201 SPECT in the prediction of survival in glioma. Neuroradiology 54:539–546

Weber WA, Dick S, Reidl G et al (2001) Correlation between postoperative 3-[(123)I]iodo-L-alpha-methyltyrosine uptake and survival in patients with gliomas. J Nucl Med 8:1144–1150

Young RJ, Ghesani MV, Kagetsu NJ, Derogatis AJ (2005) Lesion size determines accuracy of thallium-201 brain single-photon emission tomography in differentiating between intracranial malignancy and infection in AIDS patients. AJNR Am J Neuroradiol 26:1973–1979

Zikou A, Sioka C, Alexiou GA, Fotopoulos A, Voulgaris S, Argyropoulou MI (2018) Radiation necrosis, pseudoprogression, pseudoresponse, and tumor recurrence: imaging challenges for the evaluation of treated gliomas. contrast media. Mol Imaging 2018:6828396

The Value of Positron Emission Tomography for Differentiating Brain Tumor Progression and Treatment-Induced Changes

41

Bart R. J. van Dijken, Roelien H. Enting, Hanne-Rinck Jeltema, Miranda C. A. Kramer, Rudi A. J. O. Dierckx, and Anouk van der Hoorn

Contents

B. R. J. van Dijken (✉) · A. van der Hoorn
Department of Radiology, Medical Imaging Center (MIC), University Medical Center Groningen, University of Groningen, RB, Groningen, The Netherlands
e-mail: b.r.j.van.dijken@umcg.nl

R. H. Enting
Department of Neurology, University Medical Center Groningen, University of Groningen, RB, Groningen, The Netherlands

H.-R. Jeltema
Department of Neurosurgery, University Medical Center Groningen, University of Groningen, RB, Groningen, The Netherlands

M. C. A. Kramer
Department of Radiotherapy, University Medical Center Groningen, University of Groningen, RB, Groningen, The Netherlands

R. A. J. O. Dierckx
Department of Nuclear Medicine and Molecular Imaging, Medical Imaging Center (MIC), University Medical Center Groningen, University of Groningen, RB, Groningen, The Netherlands

R. A. J. O. Dierckx et al. (eds.), *PET and SPECT in Neurology*,
https://doi.org/10.1007/978-3-030-53168-3_41

Abstract

Accurate differentiation of tumor progression and treatment-induced changes is the key to treatment decision in brain tumors. Several new tracer options are promising, of which [^{11}C]-methyl-L-methionine (MET) and O-(2-[^{18}F]-fluoroethyl)-L-tyrosine (FET) positron emission tomography (PET) are the most used. This chapter provides a clinical overview of important issues of treatment evaluation in primary brain tumors and brain metastases. The role and dilemmas in neuroimaging, including magnetic resonance imaging (MRI) and PET, are discussed. An overview is given of the role of MRI and PET in brain tumor follow-up with special focus on available literature in the role of amino acid PET to differentiate between tumor progression and treatment-induced changes.

41.1 Introduction

Malignant brain tumors are relatively uncommon tumors in adults, making up less than 2% of all cancer cases (DeAngelis 2001; Miranda-Filho et al. 2017). The two major groups are a heterogeneous group of primary brain tumors and cerebral metastases from systemic cancer, with the latter being more common (DeAngelis 2001). Brain tumors are responsible for a significant loss of healthy life years and impaired quality of life. Treatment is often aggressive trying to improve this outcome. During and after treatment, patients are monitored with imaging to assess treatment response and to decide whether the current treatment should be continued or not.

41.1.1 Primary Brain Tumors

Primary intra-axial brain tumors are most commonly gliomas (in approximately 80% of the cases), with the majority being grade IV glioblastoma (Ostrom et al. 2019). Less frequent intra-axial primary brain tumors are lymphomas (6% of cases) and embryonal tumors (in about 3%) (Ostrom et al. 2019; Louis et al. 2016). In this chapter, we focus on gliomas.

To determine the tumor grade of gliomas, historically, the WHO grading system is used, representing a malignancy scale varying from I to IV. Grade I lesions are regarded as benign tumors due to their low proliferative potential and curative intent of surgical resection alone. Grade II tumors represent low-grade tumors, and grade III and IV tumors are high-grade tumors, often associated with rapid disease evolution and a dismal survival.

Recently, the WHO grading system for brain tumors has been revised. Genetic and molecular markers have now become integral to the grading (Louis et al. 2016). Survival has been shown to be greatly dependent upon these molecular markers (Rogers et al. 2018; Bell et al. 2018; Binabaj et al. 2018). Diffuse gliomas, being astrocytomas and oligodendrogliomas, are defined based on their molecular profile. Currently, the most important molecular markers are mutations in the isocitrate dehydrogenase (IDH) genes, most often IDH-1 and sometimes IDH-2. They are associated with a better prognosis in lower-grade gliomas or secondary glioblastomas (Rogers et al. 2018). Low-grade gliomas are diffusely infiltrating and slow-growing. Low-grade astrocytomas are currently defined as IDH-1- or IDH-2-mutated tumors without a 1p/19q co-deletion (Louis et al. 2016). Oligodendrogliomas are both IDH-mutant and 1p/19q-co-deleted (Louis et al. 2016).

High-grade gliomas usually lack the aforementioned IDH mutations. Another important prognostic marker for high-grade gliomas is O6-methylguanine methyltransferase (MGMT) gene methylation status. Patients with an MGMT-methylated tumor are more susceptible to alkalizing chemotherapy such as temozolomide and thus have a better survival (Bell et al. 2018; Binabaj et al. 2018).

Patients with IDH-mutant grade II tumors or co-deleted gliomas have a median survival of 10+ years, and patients with a non-co-deleted WHO grade III tumor have a median survival of 5 years (van den Bent et al. 2017), in contrast with patients with IDH wild-type grade IV tumors with a median survival of 1 year. Unfortunately, high-grade gliomas account for over 70% of newly diagnosed gliomas (Ostrom et al. 2019).

Peak incidence of low-grade gliomas occurs in patients aged between 35 and 45 years (Weller et al. 2017). It is assumed that all low-grade gliomas will transform into high-grade gliomas. Current clinical practice of low-grade gliomas recommends early surgical resection when safely possible. This is followed by both radiotherapy and chemotherapy or a wait-and-scan policy. The latter is usually chosen in completely resected young patients (Weller et al. 2017).

Patients with glioblastoma have a median age of onset of approximately 60 years. Prognosis of patients with high-grade gliomas has remained poor for the last decades. Glioblastomas, as all gliomas, are infiltrating in nature, often involving eloquent structures, and extend beyond visual borders on imaging, making complete resection without unacceptable damage impossible (Boonzaier et al. 2017; Yan et al. 2019). Nevertheless, surgery remains the cornerstone in glioblastoma treatment. Patients with high-grade gliomas benefit from a greater extent of resection in terms of survival (Sanai and Berger 2008; Yan et al. 2017). The standard adjuvant treatment in patients in good general and neurological condition, aged up to 70 years, is 60 Gy radiotherapy with concomitant temozolomide chemotherapy followed by a six-course regimen of maintenance temozolomide chemotherapy (Stupp et al. 2005). Recurrence, however, is inevitable due to the inability of radical resection and subsequent resistance to chemoradiation therapy. Currently the median survival after standard treatment of chemoradiation is 14.9 months, with the biggest gain for patients with a methylated MGMT tumor (Stupp et al. 2005). A lack of standard of care for patients with recurrent glioblastoma further contributes to the poor prognosis for these patients.

41.1.2 Brain Metastases

In adults, brain metastases are by far the most common cause of intracranial neoplasms. Brain metastases occur in approximately 20% of the patients with systemic cancer (Achrol et al. 2019). The incidence of brain metastases has increased over the years due to therapeutic advances for patients with metastatic cancer that are associated with prolonged survival.

Brain metastases originate most commonly, in order of cumulative incidence, from lung, breast, and skin (melanoma) cancers (Tabouret et al. 2012). Although the highest numbers of brain metastases arise from the lung, melanoma has the highest propensity to metastasize to the brain (Tabouret et al. 2012).

The distribution of brain metastases correlates with blood flow and tissue volume, with 80% detected in the cerebral hemispheres, 15% in the cerebellum, and 5% in the brain stem (Delattre et al. 1988). Often, brain metastases are asymptomatic and are seen on staging brain scans. Most patients (80%) present with multiple brain metastases, and only a minority of patients (10–20%) have a solitary metastasis (Tabouret et al. 2012).

Therapeutic approaches for brain metastases are resection, radiotherapy, and systemic treatment, including immunotherapy (Hardesty and Nakaji 2016; Soffietti et al. 2017; Chen et al. 2018). Radiotherapy options can be differentiated into whole-brain radiation therapy (WBRT), which is used less frequently in recent years, and stereotactic radiotherapy (SRT), the primary choice if possible.

41.2 Imaging: Role and Dilemma

Neuroimaging is essential in the follow-up and treatment evaluation in brain tumors. Regular follow-up through neuroimaging aids clinical decision-making (Dhermain et al. 2010). Treatment is continued in patients responsive to treatment. For patient unresponsive to treatment, the treatment should be stopped. However, (beneficial) treatment reaction may appear similar to recurrent disease on conventional imaging, greatly complicating treatment decisions.

41.2.1 Role of Magnetic Resonance Imaging

41.2.1.1 Conventional MRI

Magnetic resonance imaging (MRI) is the gold standard for treatment response imaging due to its high spatial resolution, allowing detailed visualization of lesions in relation to brain anatomy. Low-grade gliomas (>90%) usually demonstrate no or limited contrast enhancement on T1-weighted imaging after gadolinium administration and are best evaluated on fluid-attenuated inversion recovery (FLAIR) and T2-weighted MRI; on the contrary, high-grade gliomas usually have contrast enhancement and are surrounded by extensive vasogenic edema (Dhermain et al. 2010). Brain metastases usually present as contrast-enhancing lesion on T1-weighted

MRI with peritumoral edema visualized on FLAIR/T2-weighted MRI. Microlesions <5 mm can already be detected with the current 1.5 and 3.0 T MRI scanners.

41.2.1.2 Advanced MRI

The rationale behind advanced MRI sequences is a better visualization of biological processes (Dhermain et al. 2010; van Dijken et al. 2017). The increased cellularity of brain tumors causes impaired diffusivity of water molecules, which is detectable by diffusion-weighted imaging. Tissue perfusion is measurable with perfusion-weighted imaging through means of detectable cerebral blood flow and volume parameters (van Dijken et al. 2019). Neovascularization, which is a hallmark of neoplasms, generally causes a measurable increase in blood flow and volume on perfusion-weighted imaging. Finally, concentrations of specific metabolites can be calculated with MR spectroscopy. Detectable metabolites include N-acetylaspartate (NAA), a marker of neuronal viability and thus intact brain tissue, choline which marks increased cellular proliferation, and lactate which demonstrates anaerobic metabolism and cell death. Increases in choline and lactate with simultaneous decrease in NAA are suggestive of tumor.

41.2.2 Role of Positron Emission Tomography

Positron emission tomography (PET) has recently been recommended by the Response Assessment in Neuro-oncology (RANO) working group to be of added value in oncological neuroimaging, thereby complementing MRI (Albert et al. 2016; Langen et al. 2017; Galldiks et al. 2019; Law et al. 2019).

41.2.2.1 FDG PET

[^{18}F]-2-fluoro-2-deoxy-D-glucose (FDG) is glucose-based and to date remains the most widely employed tracer in oncology based on an increased glucose consumption of tumors. Despite the fact that FDG is the most available tracer worldwide, its use in oncological neuroimaging is limited due to the relatively high physiological glucose metabolism of normal brain tissue (Fig. 41.1).

41.2.2.2 Amino Acid PET

Cellular proliferation associated with malignant tumors activates increased protein synthesis. Amino acids function as essential compounds of proteins, and thus amino acid transport and protein synthesis are vastly increased in malignant proliferating cells and higher compared to normal healthy tissue. Radiolabeled amino acids and amino acid analogs have different metabolic fates depending on their chemical structures (van Waarde and Elsinga 2008). Amino acid tracers are predominantly based on L-type amino acid transporters (LAT), LAT-1 and LAT-2. The most frequently used radiolabeled amino acids are [^{11}C]-methyl-L-methionine (MET) (Figs. 41.2 and 41.3), O-(2-[^{18}F]-fluoroethyl)-L-tyrosine (FET), and 3,4-dihydroxy-6-[^{18}F]-fluoro-L-phenylalanine (FDOPA) (Fig. 41.4) (Glaudemans et al. 2013; de Zwart et al. 2019).

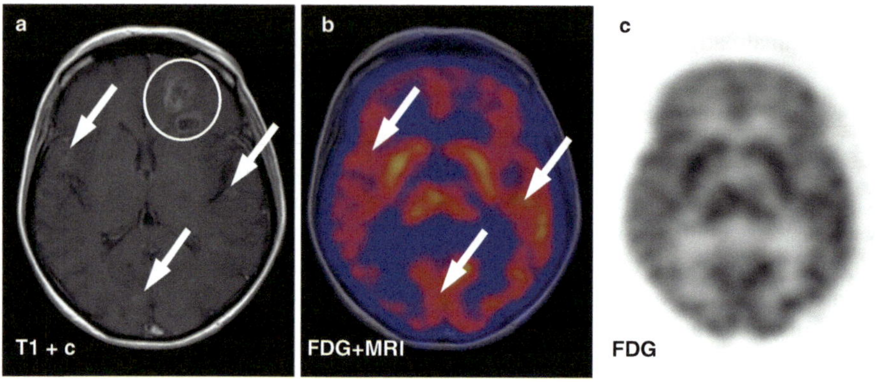

Fig. 41.1 Treatment follow-up with FDG PET in a patient with multiple brain metastases. A 62-year-old female patient with multiple brain metastases of a small cell lung cancer. Gadolinium-enhanced MRI (**a**) was performed after WBRT and demonstrated multiple contrast-enhancing lesions, with two larger lesions frontally on the left side (white circle) and several smaller lesions (white arrows). FDG PET (**b**, **c**) demonstrated high physiological uptake throughout the brain but failed to clearly localize most contrast-enhancing MRI lesions as demonstrated by the white arrows on co-registration of FDG PET images with MRI (**b**). This case demonstrates the lack of diagnostic sensitivity of FDG PET for treatment response evaluation in brain tumors

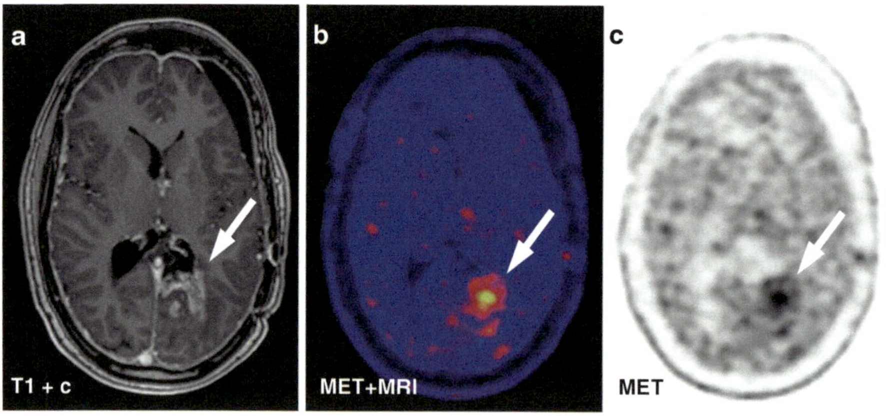

Fig. 41.2 Example of MET PET follow-up in a patient with an anaplastic astrocytoma. Case of a 49-year-old patient with an anaplastic astrocytoma (WHO grade III) after treatment with surgical resection followed by radiotherapy and temozolomide chemotherapy. One year after surgery, follow-up gadolinium-enhanced MRI (**a**) showed new contrast enhancement (white arrow). The differentiation between tumor progression and radionecrosis could not be made, and MET PET was performed (**b**, **c**). MET PET (**c**) demonstrated high tracer uptake (white arrow) suggestive of tumor progression. Co-registration of MET PET images with MRI (**b**) shows good agreement of the contrast-enhancing lesion and increased tracer uptake

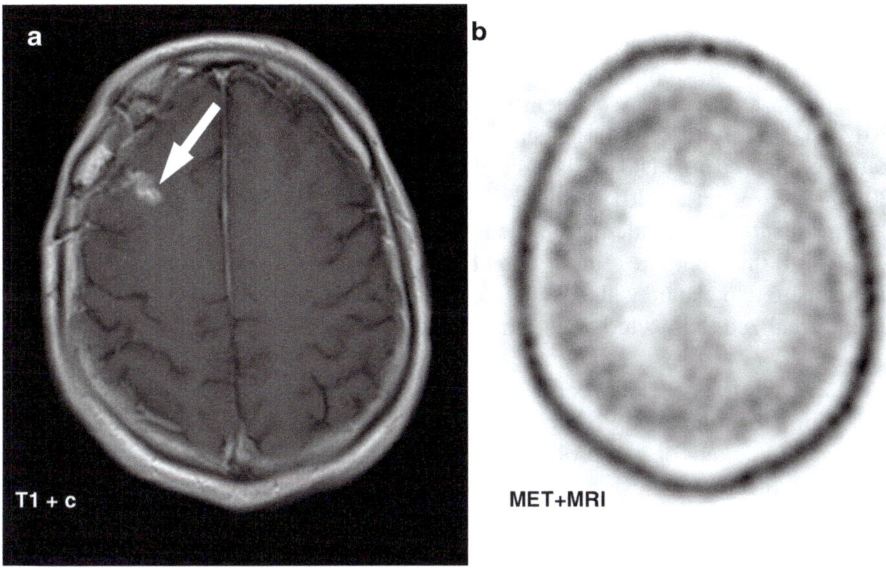

Fig. 41.3 Example of MET PET follow-up in a patient with a brain metastasis. Case of a 54-year-old male with right frontal solitary brain metastasis from a fibrosarcoma. The patient was treated with surgical resection and stereotactic radiosurgery. After treatment, follow-up gadolinium-enhanced MRI showed a new contrast-enhancing lesion (white arrow). MET PET was performed which did not demonstrate increased tracer uptake at the lesion site. The contrast enhancement was in this case shown to be due to treatment-induced changes

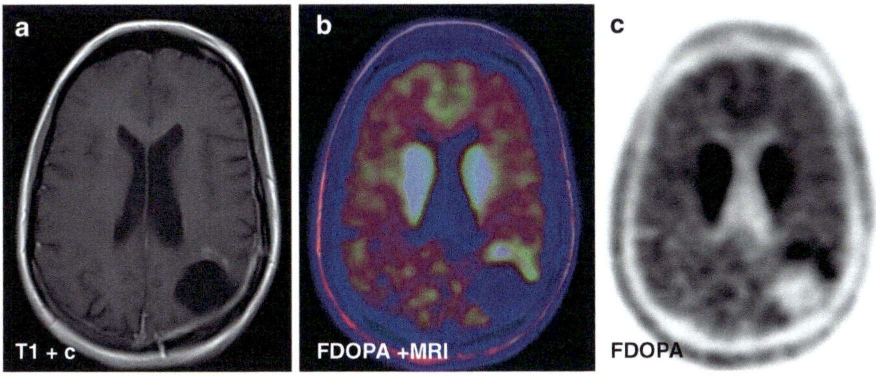

Fig. 41.4 Example of FDOPA PET follow-up in a patient with a glioblastoma. Follow-up imaging of a 26-year-old female glioblastoma patient, after surgical resection and chemoradiotherapy. Gadolinium-enhanced T1-weighted MRI (left image) 5 months after surgery was suggestive of tumor progression (white arrow). FDOPA PET was performed for other reasons (middle and right images) and demonstrated increased uptake (white arrows), also suggesting tumor progression. Co-registration of FDOPA PET and MRI (middle image) showed increased uptake at the site of enhancement on MRI. Subsequent follow-up MRI later showed further growth, confirming this case of tumor progression. The patient deceased within a year after the FDOPA PET scan

Physiological uptake of amino acid tracers in the brain is generally low, depending on anatomical region and age (Coope et al. 2007; Nagata et al. 2011). The high tumor uptake in combination with low background uptake is associated with straightforward visual assessment of amino acid PET tracers (Glaudemans et al. 2013). Therefore, the tumor detection rate and tumor delineation are thought to be better compared to FDG (Albert et al. 2016; Langen et al. 2017; Galldiks et al. 2019; de Zwart et al. 2019). Images can be interpreted visually or quantitatively. The most often used calculation method is the tumor-to-normal background ratio (T/N ratio) that compares tumor uptake to physiological uptake in the contralateral hemisphere. Uptake may also be defined by the standardized uptake value (SUV), a unit normalized to injected tracer dose per kilogram of body weight.

41.2.2.3 Other PET Tracers

In addition to amino acid PET tracers, other tracers have also been advanced. These tracers are markers of cell proliferation, such as 3′-deoxy-3′-[^{18}F]-fluorothymidine (FLT), or of the synthesis of membrane phospholipids, such as [^{11}C]-choline or [^{18}F]-fluorocholine (de Zwart et al. 2019). Both processes displayed by these tracers are active in brain tumors, thus leading to increased tracer uptake. However, these tracers are not capable of crossing an intact blood-brain barrier (BBB) (Galldiks et al. 2019). Although the BBB is usually disrupted in tumors, this is not always the case for the full extent of the tumor. To this end, only limited literature exists on these tracers. In this chapter, we will focus on amino acid PET only.

41.2.3 Dilemma of Treatment-Induced Changes

The extensive treatment regimen of malignant brain tumors, especially high-dose radiotherapy with or without concomitant chemotherapy, can produce adverse events. Damage to healthy brain tissue may lead to radiological suspicion of tumor progression (Fig. 41.3) which can even be accompanied by clinical symptoms indistinguishable from tumor progression (Brandsma et al. 2008; Thust et al. 2018). It is important to timely identify the nature of the radiological changes. True progression is indicative of failing treatment, while treatment-induced changes in fact conform with a desired response to the given treatment.

These treatment-induced changes, often called pseudoprogression in literature, are resulting from blood-brain barrier dysfunction, vasodilation, and subsequent vasogenic edema due to damage from given radiotherapy with or without chemotherapy (Brandsma et al. 2008; Thust et al. 2018). Typically, these changes occur within 3 months after treatment and will ultimately stabilize or decrease in size (Brandsma et al. 2008). Therefore, early posttreatment progression should not automatically lead to interruption of current treatment and start of second-line regimens. Delayed and longer-lasting effects, 6 months to several years after treatment, can sometimes also be seen and are then referred to as radiation necrosis.

Pseudoprogression and radiation necrosis are different clinical entities, although within the same pathological spectrum.

In high-grade gliomas, the incidence of treatment-induced changes is as high as 36% (Abbasi et al. 2018). Advances in radiotherapy planning techniques enable a high conformal dose distribution around the target volume; however, radiation dose to healthy brain tissue is unavoidable due to the infiltrative behavior of gliomas. Furthermore, treatment-induced changes are more frequent in IDH wild-type and MGMT-methylated tumors (van Dijken et al. 2019).

The incidence of treatment-induced changes in brain metastases after hypofractionated stereotactic radiotherapy (HFSRT) or stereotactic radiosurgery (SRS) is approximately 15% (Sneed et al. 2015), but some studies have suggested higher percentages (Donovan et al. 2019). Factors related to the development of radiation necrosis, especially after SRS, include dose, treated volume, and volume of the brain receiving a specific dose. An increase in the occurrence of treatment-induced changes is also expected with immunotherapy. The first studies have shown that immunotherapy alone or in addition to radiotherapy can lead to pseudoprogression and pose a new challenge for follow-up of brain metastases (Galldiks et al. 2020).

Conventional MRI cannot reliably differentiate between tumor recurrence and treatment-induced changes (van Dijken et al. 2017). Both tumor progression (Figs. 41.2 and 41.4) and treatment-induced changes (Fig. 41.3) demonstrate contrast enhancement on T1-weighted MRI with surrounding FLAIR/T2 hyperintensities. Conventional MRI, to date still the gold standard for brain tumor treatment response imaging, reached a pooled sensitivity and specificity of 68% (95% CI 51–81) and 77% (95% CI 45–93), respectively, for the detection of tumor progression in a recent meta-analysis for gliomas (van Dijken et al. 2017). Robust meta-analyses similar to those for gliomas are currently lacking for MRI in brain metastases.

To assist the clinician in the problematic differentiation of tumor progression and treatment-induced changes, the RANO criteria for gliomas and for brain metastases have been established (Wen et al. 2010; Lin et al. 2015). According to the RANO criteria, progression on conventional imaging within 3 months after chemoradiotherapy is only certain if there is new enhancement outside of the radiation field or after pathological confirmation (Wen et al. 2010). These criteria are similar for gliomas and metastases (Wen et al. 2010; Lin et al. 2015). However, in clinical practice, pathological confirmation is often not acquired in asymptomatic patients since this requires a neurosurgical intervention with a chance of morbidity. As a consequence, follow-up with imaging is usually chosen. However, this is time-consuming and can potentially expose a patient to a failing, but possibly toxic, treatment or delay the start of a second-line treatment. More advanced MRI sequences and PET tracers have therefore extensively been studied to overcome the limitations of conventional MRI (Dhermain et al. 2010; van Dijken et al. 2017, 2019; Langen et al. 2017; Galldiks et al. 2019; de Zwart et al. 2019).

41.3 Opportunities of Neuroimaging in Differentiating Tumor Progression and Treatment-Induced Changes

41.3.1 Advanced MRI

Advanced MRI sequences that have been studied for the aforementioned differentiation include diffusion-weighted imaging, detecting changes in cellular density; perfusion-weighted imaging, visualizing increased blood flow and neovascularization; and MR spectroscopy, an imaging technique capable of detecting changes in metabolites. All these advanced MRI techniques outperformed conventional MRI. Meta-analysis in high-grade gliomas showed a sensitivity and specificity for diffusion-weighted imaging of 71% (95% CI 60–80) and 86% (95% CI 76–92), respectively (van Dijken et al. 2017). For perfusion-weighted imaging, this was 87% (95% CI 82–91) and 86% (95% CI 77–91) (van Dijken et al. 2017). MR spectroscopy demonstrated the highest diagnostic accuracy with a sensitivity of 91% (95% CI 79–97) and specificity of 95% (95% CI 65–99) (van Dijken et al. 2017). As MR spectroscopy is time-consuming, with risk of movement artifacts, diffusion-weighted imaging and perfusion-weighted imaging are most often used to aid in the differentiation of tumor progression from treatment-induced changes.

Studies on the diagnostic value of advanced MRI in brain metastases after treatment are limited. Perfusion-weighted imaging and MR spectroscopy demonstrate the most promising results thus far (Chuang et al. 2016). Diagnostic accuracy seems to be in a similar good range as seen for gliomas. However, a drawback of MR spectroscopy is the relatively large voxel size, making differentiation of tumor progression from treatment-induced changes in smaller metastases difficult.

41.3.2 PET

The uptake of PET tracers is physiologically different in tumor progression and treatment-induced changes. In progressive tumors, the uptake is caused by active uptake of tracer in the tumor cells (Figs. 41.2 and 41.4). On the other hand, in treatment-induced changes, uptake is caused by passive diffusion across a disrupted BBB (Fig. 41.3). Theoretically, the uptake in tumor cells should thus exceed the uptake after radiation injury; however, there is an overlap between these uptakes. The value of PET for differentiating tumor progression from treatment-induced changes has been extensively studied in high-grade gliomas (de Zwart et al. 2019).

Recently, a meta-analysis has been conducted (de Zwart et al. 2019). This meta-analysis included 39 studies and confirmed a lower diagnostic accuracy for FDG (Fig. 41.1) than for the two most common amino acid tracers. FDG reached a sensitivity of 84% (95%CI 72–92) and specificity of 84% (95%CI 69–93), while FET, with a sensitivity of 90% (95%CI 81–95) and a specificity of 85% (95%CI 71–93), and MET (Figs. 41.2 and 41.3), with a sensitivity and specificity of 93% (95%CI 80-98) and 82% (95%CI 68-91), respectively, performed significantly better (de Zwart et al. 2019). FDOPA is a less studied tracer (Fig. 41.4), with only four known studies being published, but demonstrates comparable diagnostic accuracy with a sensitivity ranging from 85% to 100% and specificity ranging from 72% to 100% (Lapa et al. 2014; Karunanithi et al. 2013; Paquet et al. 2017; Herrmann et al. 2014).

The usefulness of FDG PET is very limited in brain metastases (Fig. 41.1). Studies have shown that FDG PET only marginally improves accurate differentiation between tumor progression and treatment-induced changes after ambiguous MRI (Chao et al. 2001; Belohlávek et al. 2003). As expected, the accuracy of amino acid PET is superior to FDG PET.

Several studies have confirmed that a difference in FET T/N ratios can quantitatively distinguish metastatic progression from treatment-induced changes (Galldiks et al. 2012; Romagna et al. 2016; Ceccon et al. 2017). However, the number of patients studied with FET PET ($N = 126$) is much smaller than for MET PET.

For MET PET, most studies had a relatively high sensitivity, specificity, and diagnostic accuracy (>85%) in common, with advantages over conventional imaging (Figs. 41.2 and 41.3) (Terakawa et al. 2008; Yomo and Oguchi 2017; Okamoto et al. 2010; Yamane et al. 2010; Tsuyuguchi et al. 2003). However, a considerable overlap in the uptake values of methionine in progressing tumor and treatment-induced change occurs (Minamimoto et al. 2015).

A visual analysis of 83 lesions in 32 patients also demonstrated positive results for FDOPA (Lizarraga et al. 2014). In another study, among 13 patients of whom 3 had histologically confirmed treatment-induced changes, there was a visual difference in FDOPA uptake between recurrent or progressive metastases and treatment-induced changes (Papin-Michault et al. 2016). This study additionally demonstrated a difference in LAT-1 expression between tumor progression cases and treatment-induced changes, explaining the difference in FDOPA uptake (Papin-Michault et al. 2016). Interestingly, FDOPA outperformed perfusion-weighted imaging in a study among 42 patients with brain metastases after SRS (Cicone et al. 2015).

41.4 Limitations and Future Perspectives of MRI and PET

MRI and PET seem to perform similar in the differentiation of treatment-induced changes from tumor progression. However, only few studies have compared MRI and PET directly.

A study by Kim et al. (2010) stated that perfusion-weighted MRI is superior in distinguishing a recurrence of high-grade glioma from radiation necrosis compared to MET. Dandois et al. (2010) also found that perfusion-weighted MRI had an at least similar diagnostic accuracy to MET in differentiating tumor recurrence and treatment-induced changes. However, FDOPA was suggested to outperform perfusion-weighted MRI (Cicone et al. 2015), and another study also demonstrated that amino acid PET is possibly superior over perfusion-weighted MRI (Tomura et al. 2017).

The diagnostic accuracy of the different amino acid PET tracers seems comparable, although FDOPA is somewhat understudied compared to MET and FET PET. Most experience is gathered with MET. However, MET is impractical since it demands a cyclotron due to its very short half-life (20 min). Fluorine-18-labeled FET has gained ground due to its longer half-life (109.7 min).

There is an urgent need for uniform scanning protocols and quantification methods for both advanced MRI and amino acid PET. Furthermore, few data are available on interobserver agreement in the interpretation of these advanced MRI sequences and PET studies. Amino acid PET can usually relatively easily be interpreted visually, but there is a lack of consensus on the used reference region for calculation of T/N ratios. Local variations in tracer uptake between different reference regions may significantly alter results. With T/N ratios still being the most reported quantitative parameter, this is troublesome. Future studies should thus focus on establishing robust guidelines for analysis and quantification methods for amino acid PET in brain tumors.

It has been suggested that the recent development of hybrid PET/MRI cameras could lead to a jump forward in the imaging of brain tumors. Combining both modalities might overcome a number of individual limitations and avoids the necessity of additional scanning. This would enable an absolute match between tissue information of both modalities under the same physiological conditions and may thus lead to better localization of the PET signal within the soft tissues. However, the economic cost of hybrid PET/MRI scanners is substantial. The first studies have been published and indeed demonstrate the feasibility of using combined PET/MRI machines (Hojjati et al. 2018; Deuschl et al. 2018). However, these studies are limited to FDG PET (Hojjati et al. 2018), which has insufficient value in brain tumor imaging, and carbon-bound MET PET (Deuschl et al. 2018), which is not feasible in many centers. Therefore, more PET/MRI studies with emphasis on treatment evaluation of gliomas and brain metastases using fluorine-bound amino tracers are desired.

41.5 Summary

Treatment-induced changes are a common phenomenon among both treated gliomas and brain metastases. Conventional MRI is not able to differentiate tumor progression and treatment-induced changes. Both advanced MRI techniques and amino acid PET provide additional information that can aid the clinician in decision-making following treatment. Combining all evidence that we presented in this chapter, there does not seem to be a preferred advanced MRI or PET imaging method to differentiate tumor progression from treatment-induced changes.

References

Abbasi AW, Westerlaan HE, Holtman GA, Aden KM, van Laar PJ, van der Hoorn A (2018) Incidence of tumour progression and pseudoprogression in high-grade gliomas: a systematic review and meta- analysis. Clin Neuroradiol 28:401–411

Achrol A, Rennert R, Anders C et al (2019) Brain metastases. Nat Rev Dis Primers 5(1):5

Albert NL, Weller M, Suchorska B et al (2016) Response assessment in neuro-oncology working group and european association for neuro-oncology recommendations for the clinical use of PET imaging in gliomas. Neuro-Oncology 18:1199–1208

Bell EH, Zhang P, Fisher BJ et al (2018) Association of MGMT promoter methylation status with survival outcomes in patients with high-risk glioma treated with radiotherapy and temozolomide: an analysis from the NRG oncology/RTOG 0424 trial. JAMA Oncol 4(10):1405–1409

Belohlávek O, Simonová G, Kantorová I, Novotný J Jr, Liscák R (2003) Brain metastases after stereotactic radiosurgery using the leksell gamma knife: can FDG PET help to differentiate radionecrosis from tumour progression? Eur J Nucl Med Mol Imaging 30(1):96–100

Binabaj MM, Bahrami A, ShahidSales S et al (2018) The prognostic value of MGMT promoter methylation in glioblastoma: a meta-analysis of clinical trials. J Cell Physiol 233(1):378–386

Boonzaier NR, Larkin TJ, Matys T et al (2017) Multiparametric MR imaging of diffusion and perfusion in contrast-enhancing and nonenhancing components in patients with glioblastoma. Radiology 284(1):180–190

Brandsma D, Stalpers L, Taal W, Sminia P, van den Bent MJ (2008) Clinical features, mechanisms, and management of pseudoprogression in malignant gliomas. Lancet Oncol 9:453–461

Ceccon G, Lohmann P, Stoffels G et al (2017) Dynamic O-(2-18F-fluoroethyl)-L-tyrosine positron emission tomography differentiates brain metastasis recurrence from radiation injury after radiotherapy. Neuro-Oncology 19(2):281–288

Chao ST, Suh JH, Raja S, Lee SY, Barnett G (2001) The sensitivity and specificity of FDG PET in distinguishing recurrent brain tumor from radionecrosis in patients treated with stereotactic radiosurgery. Int J Cancer 96(3):191–197

Chen L, Douglass J, Kleinberg L et al (2018) Concurrent immune checkpoint inhibitors and stereotactic radiosurgery for brain metastases in non-small cell lung cancer, melanoma, and renal cell carcinoma. Int J Radiat Oncol Biol Phys 100(4):916–925

Chuang MT, Liu YS, Tsai YS, Chen YC, Wang CK (2016) Differentiating radiation-induced necrosis from recurrent brain tumor using MR perfusion and spectroscopy: a meta-analysis. PLoS One 11(1):e0141438

Cicone F, Minniti G, Romano A et al (2015) Accuracy of F-DOPA PET and perfusion-MRI for differentiating radionecrotic from progressive brain metastases after radiosurgery. Eur J Nucl Med Mol Imaging 42(1):103–111

Coope DJ, Cizek J, Eggers C et al (2007) Evaluation of primary brain tumors using 11C-methionine PET with reference to a normal methionine uptake map. J Nucl Med 48(12):1971–1980

Dandois V, Rommel D, Renard L, Jamart J, Cosnard G (2010) Substitution of 11C-methionine PET by perfusion MRI during the follow-up of treated high-grade gliomas: preliminary results in clinical practice. Neuroradiology 37:89–97

de Zwart PL, van Dijken BRJ, Holtman GA et al (2019) Diagnostic accuracy of positron emission tomography tracers for the differentiation of tumor progression from treatment-related changes in high-grade glioma: a systematic review and meta-analysis. J Nucl Med 119:233809

DeAngelis LM (2001) Brain tumors. N Engl J Med 344:114–123

Delattre JY, Krol G, Thaler HT, Posner JB (1988) Distribution of brain metastases. Arch Neurol 45(7):741–744

Deuschl C, Kirchner J, Poeppel TD et al (2018) 11C-MET PET/MRI for detection of recurrent glioma. Eur J Nucl Med Mol Imaging 45(4):593–601

Dhermain FG, Hau P, Lanfermann H, Jacobs AH, van den Bent MJ (2010) Advanced MRI and PET imaging for assessment of treatment response in patients with gliomas. Lancet Neurol 9:906–920

Donovan EK, Parpia S, Greenspoon JN (2019) Incidence of radionecrosis in single-fraction radiosurgery compared with fractionated radiotherapy in the treatment of brain metastasis. Curr Oncol 26(3):e328–e333

Galldiks N, Stoffels G, Fills CP et al (2012) Role of O-(2-(18)F-fluoroethyl)-L-tyrosine PET for differentiation of local recurrent brain metastasis from radiation necrosis. J Nucl Med 53(9):1367–1374

Galldiks N, Lohmann P, Albert NL et al (2019) Current status of PET imaging in neuro-oncology. Neuro-Oncol Adv 1(1):vdz010

Galldiks N, Kocher M, Ceccon G et al (2020) Imaging challenges of immunotherapy and targeted therapy in patients with brain metastases: response, progression, and pseudoprogression. Neuro-Oncology 22(1):17–30

Glaudemans AWJM, Enting RH, Heesters MAAM et al (2013) Value of 11C-methionine PET in imaging brain tumours and metastases. Eur J Nucl Med Mol Imaging 40:615–635

Hardesty D, Nakaji P (2016) The current and future treatment of brain metastases. Front Surg 3(30):1–7

Herrmann K, Czernin J, Cloughesy T et al (2014) Comparison of visual and semiquantitative analysis of 18F-FDOPA- PET/CT for recurrence detection in glioblastoma patients. Neuro-Oncology 16:603–609

Hojjati M, Badve C, Garg V et al (2018) Role of FDG-PET/MRI, FDG-PET/CT, and dynamic susceptibility contrast perfusion mri in differentiating radiation necrosis from tumor recurrence in glioblastomas. J Neuroimaging 28:118–125

Karunanithi S, Sharma P, Kumar A et al (2013) Comparative diagnostic accuracy of contrast-enhanced MRI and 18F-FDOPA PET-CT in recurrent glioma. Eur Radiol 23:2628–2635

Kim YH, Oh SW, Lim YJ et al (2010) Differentiating radiation necrosis from tumor recurrence in high-grade gliomas: assessing the efficacy of 18F-FDG PET, 11C-methionine PET and perfusion MRI. Clin Neurol Neurosurg 112(9):758–765

Langen KJ, Galldiks N, Hattingen E, Shah NJ (2017) Advances in neuro-oncology imaging. Nat Rev Neurol 13:279–289

Lapa C, Linsenmann T, Monoranu CM et al (2014) Comparison of the amino acid tracers 18F-FET and 18F-DOPA in high-grade glioma patients. J Nucl Med 55:1611–1616

Law I, Albert NL, Arbizu J et al (2019) Joint EANM/EANO/RANO practice guidelines/SNMMI procedure standards for imaging of gliomas using PET with radiolabelled amino acids and [18F]FDG: version 1.0. Eur J Nucl Med Mol Imaging 46:540–557

Lin NU, Lee EQ, Aoyama H et al (2015) Response assessment criteria for brain metastases: proposal from the RANO group. Lancet Oncol 16(6):e270–e278. https://doi.org/10.1016/S1470-2045(15)70057-4

Lizarraga KJ, Allen-Auerbach M, Czernin J et al (2014) (18)F-FDOPA PET for differentiating recurrent or progressive brain metastatic tumors from late or delayed radiation injury after radiation treatment. J Nucl Med 55(1):30–36

Louis DN, Perry A, Reifenberger G et al (2016) The 2016 World Health Organization classification of tumors of the central nervous system: a summary. Acta Neuropathol 131:803–820

Minamimoto R, Saginoya T, Kondo C, Tomura N, Ito K, Matsuo Y et al (2015) Differentiation of brain tumor recurrence from post-radiotherapy necrosis with 11C-methionine PET: visual assessment versus quantitative assessment. PLoS One 10(7):e0132515

Miranda-Filho A, Pineros M, Soerjomataram I et al (2017) Cancers of the brain and CNS: global patterns and trends in incidence. Neuro-Oncology 19(2):270–280

Nagata T, Tsuyuguchi N, Uda T et al (2011) Examination of 11C-methionine metabolism by the standardized uptake value in the normal brain of children. J Nucl Med 52:201–205

Okamoto S, Shiga T, Hattori N, Kubo N, Takei T, Katoh N et al (2010) Semiquantitative analysis of C-11 methionine PET may distinguish brain tumor recurrence from radiation necrosis even in small lesions. Ann Nucl Med 25(3):213–220

Ostrom QT, Cioffi G, Gittleman H et al (2019) BTRUS statistical report: primary brain and other central nervous system tumors diagnosed in the United States in 2012–2016. Neuro Oncol 21(Suppl 5):v1–v100

Papin-Michault C, Bonnetaud C, Dufour M et al (2016) Study of LAT1 expression in brain metastases: towards a better understanding of the results of positron emission tomography using amino acid tracers. PLoS One 11(6):e0157139

Paquet M, Doyen J, Mondot L et al (2017) Value of early and delayed imaging for 18F-FDOPA PET high grade gliomas evaluation [abstract]. Eur J Nucl Med Mol Imaging 44:S642–S643

Rogers TW, Toor G, Drummond K et al (2018) The 2016 revision of the WHO classification of central nervous system tumours: retrospective application to a cohort of diffuse gliomas. J Neuro-Oncol 137(1):181–189

Romagna A, Unterrainer M, Schmid-Tannwald C et al (2016) Suspected recurrence of brain metastases after focused high dose radiotherapy: can [18F]FET- PET overcome diagnostic uncertainties? Radiat Oncol 11(1):139

Sanai N, Berger MS (2008) Glioma extent of resection and its impact on patient outcome. Neurosurgery 62(4):753–764

Sneed P, Mendez J, Vemer-van den Hoek J et al (2015) Adverse radiation effect after stereotactic radiosurgery for brain metastases: incidence, time course, and risk factors. J Neurosurg 123(2):373–386

Soffietti R, Abacioglu U, Baumert B et al (2017) Diagnosis and treatment of brain metastases from solid tumors: guidelines from the European Association of Neuro-Oncology (EANO). Neuro-Oncology 19(2):162–174

Stupp R, Mason WP, van den Bent MJ et al (2005) Radiotherapy plus concomitant and adjuvant temozolomide for glioblastoma. N Engl J Med 352:987–996

Tabouret E et al (2012) Recent trends in epidemiology of brain metastases: an overview. Anticancer Res 32:4655–4662

Terakawa Y, Tsuyuguchi N, Iwai Y, Yamanaka K, Higashiyama S, Takami T et al (2008) Diagnostic accuracy of 11C-methionine PET for differentiation of recurrent brain tumors from radiation necrosis after radiotherapy. J Nucl Med 49(5):694–699

Thust SC, Van Den Bent MJ, Smits M (2018) Pseudoprogression of brain tumors. J Magn Reson Imaging 48:571–589

Tomura N, Kokubun M, Saginoya T et al (2017) Differentiation between treatment-induced necrosis and recurrent tumors in patients with metastatic brain tumors: comparison among 11C-methionine-PET, FDG-PET, MR permeability imaging, and MRI-ADC—preliminary results. AJNR 38(8):1520–1527

Tsuyuguchi N, Sunada I, Iwai Y et al (2003) Methionine positron emission tomography of recurrent metastatic brain tumor and radiation necrosis after stereotactic radiosurgery: is a differential diagnosis possible? J Neurosurg 98(5):1056–1064

van den Bent MJ, Baumert B, Erridge SC et al (2017) Interim results from the CATNON trial (EORTC study 26053-22054) of treatment with concurrent and adjuvant temozolomide for 1p/19q non-co-deleted anaplastic glioma: a phase 3, randomised, open-label intergroup study. Lancet 390(10103):1645–1653

van Dijken BRJ, van Laar PJ, Holtman GA, van der Hoorn A (2017) Diagnostic accuracy of magnetic resonance imaging techniques for treatment response evaluation in patients with high-grade glioma, a systematic review and meta-analysis. Eur Radiol 27:4129–4144

van Dijken BRJ, van Laar PJ, Smits M et al (2019) Perfusion MRI in treatment evaluation of glioblastomas: clinical relevance of current and future techniques. J Magn Reson Imaging 49:11–22

van Waarde A, Elsinga PH (2008) Proliferation markers for the differential diagnosis of tumor and inflammation. Curr Pharm Des 14(31):3326–3339

Weller M, van den Bent MJ, Tonn JC et al (2017) European Association for Neuro-Oncology (EANO) guideline on the diagnosis and treatment of adult astrocytic and oligodendroglial gliomas. Lancet Oncol 18(6):e315–e329

Wen PY, Macdonald DR, Reardon DA et al (2010) Updated response assessment criteria for high-grade gliomas: response assessment in neuro-oncology working group. J Clin Oncol 28:1963–1972

Yamane T, Sakamoto S, Senda M (2010) Clinical impact of 11C-methionine PET on expected management of patients with brain neoplasm. Eur J Nucl Med Mol Imaging 37(4):685–690

Yan JL, van der Hoorn A, Larkin TTJ et al (2017) Extent of resection of peritumoral diffusion tensor imaging-detected abnormality as a predictor of survival in adult glioblastoma patients. J Neurosurg 126(1):234–241

Yan JL, Li C, Boonzaier NR et al (2019) Multimodal MRI characteristics of the glioblastoma infiltration beyond contrast enhancement. Ther Adv Neurol Disord 12:1756286419844664

Yomo S, Oguchi K (2017) Prospective study of 11C-methionine PET for distinguishing between recurrent brain metastases and radiation necrosis: limitations of diagnostic accuracy and long-term results of salvage treatment. BMC Cancer 17(1):713

Imaging Brain Metastases of Neuroendocrine Tumors

42

Klaas Pieter Koopmans and A. H. Brouwers

Contents

Abstract

Neuroendocrine tumors (NETs) are rare tumors with a low incidence, characterized by a slow growth with often an indolent course. These tumors can arise in nearly all organs, with gastrointestinal and bronchopulmonary sites being the most common primary sites. The occurrence of primary neuroendocrine brain tumors is very rare, but metastases of NET to the brain are more common. The incidence of brain metastasis in patients with NET is approximately 1.5–5% with a median age of diagnosis of 60 years. Detection of NET brain metastases occurs

K. P. Koopmans (✉)
Department of Radiology and Nuclear Medicine, Martini Hospital Groningen, Groningen, The Netherlands
e-mail: k.koopmans@mzh.nl

A. H. Brouwers
Department of Nuclear Medicine and Molecular Imaging,
University of Groningen, University Medical Center Groningen, Groningen, The Netherlands

R. A. J. O. Dierckx et al. (eds.), *PET and SPECT in Neurology*,
https://doi.org/10.1007/978-3-030-53168-3_42

with a median of 1.5 years after diagnosis of primary NET with a likely underdiagnosis. Brain metastases most commonly develop in patients with bronchopulmonary NET. Brain metastases grow globoid with a microglial boundary and are often surrounded by vasogenic edema. Metastatic brain lesions are made up of a subgroup of cells with a different biological behavior compared to the primary NET and other metastases which can be explained by the difficulties these cells have to face before being able to successfully grow within the brain. These patients suffer from a more aggressive NET behavior, and in many patients, carcinoid syndrome is also present. Clinical presentation is mostly characterized by headaches, personality changes, and gait disturbances.

According to the European Neuroendocrine Tumor Society (ENETS) consensus guidelines, MRI is the preferred modality for detection of NET brain metastases. However, PET has gained a very important role in the staging of NET, and it is likely that PET will become very helpful for the detection of neuroendocrine brain tumors and metastases. Several tracers are available at this moment, of which somatostatin receptor PET and 18F-DOPA PET seem the most promising at this moment. Due to the high background uptake in the brain and the relatively low glucose metabolism in NET cells, the indication of 18F-FDG PET seems very limited for the detection of neuroendocrine brain tumors.

However, due to the rarity of NET overall and thus especially for NET brain metastases, data on these tumors is limited, and additional research is warranted.

42.1 Introduction

Neuroendocrine tumors are a unique group of slow-growing tumors arising from neuroendocrine cells. Neuroendocrine cells are widely dispersed within the body. These neuroendocrine cells are characterized by a common phenotype which consists of the expression of hormonal products and general protein markers which are specific for each cell type (Reubi 1995). Neuroendocrine cells regulate many different body functions through paracrine signalling with dedicated amines and peptides. The most commonly produced are the biogenic amines, of which serotonin and catecholamines are the most prominent. Other well-known biogenic amines produced by neuroendocrine cells are, for example, adrenocorticotropic hormone, growth hormone, neuropeptide K, substance P, bradykinin, kallikrein, and prostaglandins (Kloppel et al. 1996; Schnirer et al. 2003). Neuroendocrine tumors have a low incidence, which has been estimated to be approximately 1–2 cases per 100,000 individuals in the United States (Godwin 1975; Modlin et al. 2003). Although these tumors can arise in nearly all organs, the most common primary sites are the gastrointestinal (56–64%) and bronchopulmonary tracts (12–20%) (Modlin et al. 2003; Soga 2003). Generally, neuroendocrine tumors are characterized by a slow growth, which accounts for the long time span before these tumors become symptomatic. Although neuroendocrine tumors often follow an indolent course, in 12–69% of patients, dependent on tumor differentiation, metastatic disease was already evident at first diagnosis (Lepage et al. 2013; Modlin et al. 2003). Generally neuroendocrine tumors metastasize to the liver, lungs, and bone. Other sites, such as the brain, are much rarer.

42.2 Incidence

Metastases of neuroendocrine tumors to the central nervous system constitute approximately 1.3–1.4% of all patients presenting with brain metastases (Cho et al. 1998; Maiuri et al. 2004). Conversely, it is estimated that the incidence of brain metastases in patients with neuroendocrine tumors is approximately 1.5–5% (Hlatky et al. 2004; Krug et al. 2019; Patchell and Posner 1986; Pavel et al. 2010). The median age at the time of diagnosis of brain metastasis is 60 years, but the time course after which these brain metastases occur varies. The time between detection of the primary site and brain metastases ranges from 0 months to 16.3 years from a median of 1.5 years (Hlatky et al. 2004; Patchell and Posner 1986). However, data on brain metastases of neuroendocrine tumors are rare. Consequently, it is likely that the reported incidence is an underestimation of the true incidence of neuroendocrine tumor brain metastases, since dedicated brain imaging is not routinely performed to assess metastatic spread in these patients (Pavel et al. 2010). Additional imaging of the brain is usually only performed when patients present with neurological symptoms caused by the intracranial mass.

42.3 Origin of Neuroendocrine Brain Metastases

Brain metastases of neuroendocrine tumors have been reported with several neuroendocrine primary tumor locations. Most commonly primary neuroendocrine tumors of the lungs give brain metastasis (Hlatky et al. 2004; Krug et al. 2019; Pavel et al. 2010). The development of brain metastasis of neuroendocrine tumors can be explained by two separate mechanisms. The first is direct hematogenous spread from lung tumors/metastases, and the second is spread from pelvic neuroendocrine tumor metastases via Batson's venous plexus. Batson's venous plexus is a venous plexus system, which directly connects pelvic structures with the brain via valveless veins running in the spinal epidural space (Batson 1940; Hlatky et al. 2004).

42.4 Growth Patterns of Neuroendocrine Brain Metastases

Generally, brain metastases grow as well-circumscribed globoid lesions. Activated microglial cells form a distinct boundary between the tumor mass and brain tissue (He et al. 2006; Sul and Posner 2007). This boundary may account for the well-circumscribed appearance of brain metastases. Vasogenic edema often surrounds metastatic brain lesions. This edema is caused by intratumoral leakage of protein-rich fluids through the disrupted blood-brain barrier. These fluids then diffuse into the surrounding brain, increasing the local fluid content of the brain.

Brain metastases are formed by a subset of cells which have detached from the primary tumor. During their passage through the extracellular environment, into the bloodstream, and finally to their place of growth, these metastatic cells will have encountered and successfully counteracted or "fooled" a huge number of host defense mechanisms. Hence, this collection of cells must have specific properties which make them suitable for metastasizing. Especially metastatic tumor cells in the brain, which is a difficult environment for free circulating tumor cells to successfully grow out to a metastatic lesion, can have a greatly different biological behavior as compared to the cells constituting the primary lesion. Additionally, brain tumor lesions may be constituted from different subsets of tumor cells. This also explains why several brain lesions can differ in behavior from each other (Klein et al. 2002; Sul and Posner 2007). Unfortunately, only series with small numbers of patients with neuroendocrine tumor metastasis to the brain have been described. From the available literature, it has become clear that both well- and poorly differentiated neuroendocrine tumors can give rise to metastatic brain lesions. From data limited to pulmonary neuroendocrine tumors, it has been reported that typical carcinoids (Granberg et al. 2000), atypical carcinoids (Nakamura et al. 2001), and large cell neuroendocrine tumors (Doddoli et al. 2004) can all lead to metastatic brain lesions. Only 1.3–1.4% of patients with neuroendocrine tumors present with neurological symptoms caused by brain lesions as first presentation of their disease (Maiuri et al. 2004; Nakamura et al. 2001; Porter et al. 2000).

42.5 Clinical Presentation

Hlatky et al. found in their series of 24 patients with brain metastases from carcinoid tumors that most patients with neuroendocrine brain metastases experience symptoms directly related to the brain metastases (96%). These symptoms consisted of headaches (96%), personality changes (25%), gait disturbances (21%), cranial nerve deficits (13%), seizures (8%), nausea (8%), motor deficits (4%), and memory deficits (4%) (Hlatky et al. 2004). In their patient group, only one patient (4%) was asymptomatic, and the metastatic brain lesion was found during a regular metastatic work-up. In 50% of these patients, carcinoid syndrome was present.

From the data of the study of Krug et al. in a retrospective study comprising 51 patients with brain metastasis from NET, it appeared that most patients suffered from a more aggressive behavior of the NET. These patients also showed a shorter overall median survival compared to patients without brain metastases with a median survival time of 11 months (Krug et al. 2019).

42.6 Imaging

Generally, due to the low incidence of brain metastases from neuroendocrine tumors, patients with neuroendocrine tumors are not routinely screened for brain metastases during the metastatic work-up. The European Neuroendocrine Tumor Society (ENETS) published a consensus guideline for brain metastases in neuroendocrine tumors which dates from 2010, titled "ENETS consensus guidelines for the management of brain, cardiac and ovarian metastases from neuroendocrine tumors" (Pavel et al. 2010). In these guidelines, they also described the position of the currently used nuclear medicine imaging techniques. They stated that, due to the inadequate data on nuclear imaging techniques for the detection of neuroendocrine brain metastasis, MRI thus far has the highest sensitivity for the detection of single and multiple brain metastases and should be recommended as part of the diagnostic work-up in patients with neuroendocrine carcinoma of the lung.

It is unfortunate that there is inadequate data to support clinical applicability of nuclear medicine imaging techniques for the detection of neuroendocrine brain metastases. However, from evidence from case reports and on metastases outside the brain, it can be argued that nuclear medicine techniques may be applicable for the detection of neuroendocrine brain metastases. Much research on the position of nuclear medicine imaging techniques for neuroendocrine brain metastases is however warranted.

42.7 Somatostatin Receptor Imaging

For the regulation of several functions in both body and brain, regulatory peptides play an important role. Several receptors for regulatory peptides are overexpressed on the cellular membranes of neuroendocrine tumors and their metastases with an increased density as compared with normal tissue. Somatostatin (SST) is a cyclic hormone, of which two forms have been identified, SST-14 and SST-28. SST acts as an inhibitor for the release of many hormones by neuroendocrine cells in the body and brain, such as growth hormone, glucagon, and insulin, by binding to G-coupled SST receptors (SSTr) (Weckbecker et al. 2003). Five different subtypes of these receptors have thus far been identified in humans, named SSTr1–SSTr5. Generally, neuroendocrine tumor cells express the highest density of the SSTr2 subtype (Khan and Beck-Sickinger 2008). Somatostatin binds to SSTr and is subsequently transported to the intracellular environment where these hormone-receptor complexes are metabolized in lysosomes (Hofland and Lamberts 2003). Historically somatostatin receptor scintigraphy has played a very important role in the staging of neuroendocrine tumors for the last 20 years (Koopmans et al. 2009; Krenning et al. 1992; Lamberts et al. 1993). In 2001, somatostatin analogues have been coupled to positron-emitting isotopes, enabling the use of PET camera systems (Henze et al. 2001; Hofmann et al. 2001). Provided that the primary neuroendocrine tumor is

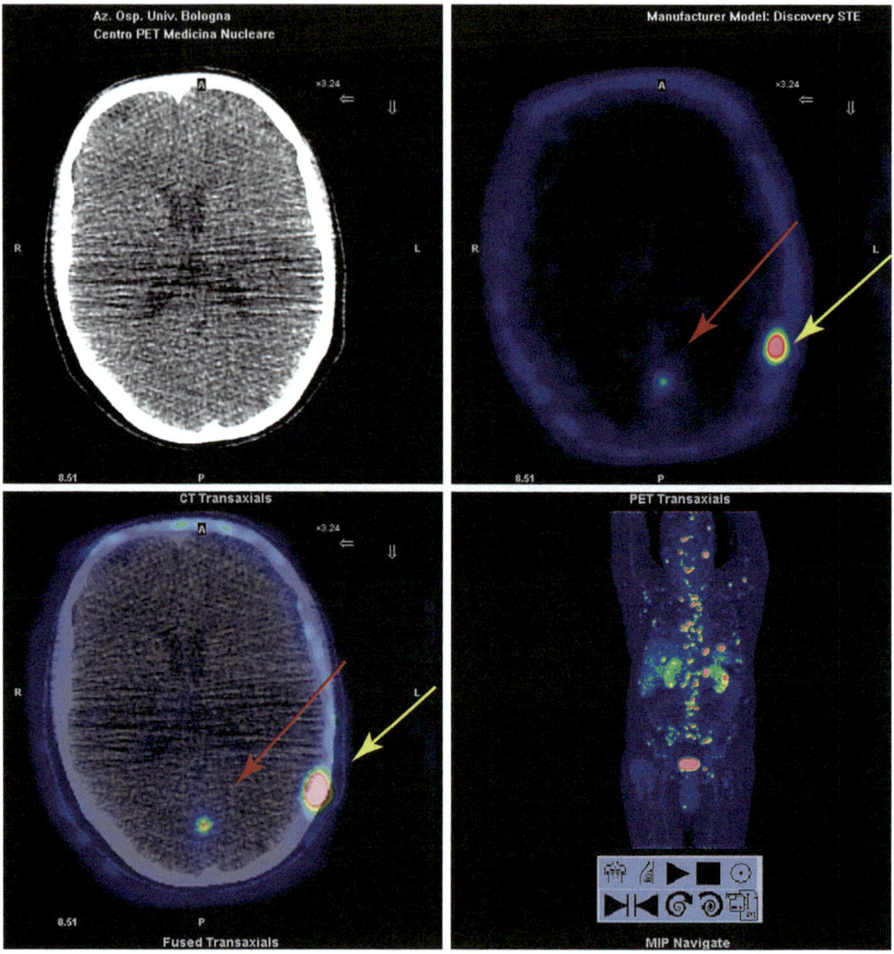

Fig. 42.1 ^{68}Ga-DOTATOC PET scan of a patient with extensively metastasized neuroendocrine lung tumor, who also had a small brain metastasis (red arrow) as well as an ossal lesion in the skull (yellow arrow). (Courtesy of Valentina Ambrosini, Nuclear Medicine, Azienda Ospedaliero-Universitaria di Bologna, Policlinico S. Orsola-Malpighi, Bologna, Italy)

well differentiated and has shown pathologically increased tracer uptake of ^{111}Indium somatostatin analogues or ^{68}Ga-labelled somatostatin analogues, these tracers might be helpful for the diagnosis of neuroendocrine brain metastasis. An example of ^{68}Ga-somatostatin PET is provided in Fig. 42.1. In a publication, ^{68}Ga-somatostatin receptor PET/CT was able to identify 6 metastatic brain lesions in 4210 scans in patients with neuroendocrine tumors (Carreras et al. 2013). Many case reports have been published in the last 10 years, in which the role of PET imaging with somatostatin analogues seems to perform a pivotal role. However, false-positive ^{68}Ga-SSTr uptake can be caused by other tumors such as non-Hodgkin lymphoma, metastatic meningioma, breast cancer, thyroid adenoma, and papillary carcinoma resulting in a positive PET/CT scan (Yamagi et al. 2017).

42.8 Metabolic Imaging

^{18}F-Fluorodeoxyglucose (^{18}FDG), which is important in oncology, has a limited role for the detection of brain metastasis due to the high glucose metabolism of the brain (Kruger et al. 2011). The potential role of ^{18}FDG PET scanning for the detection of neuroendocrine brain metastasis will very likely be even more limited. In contrast to many other malignancies, well-differentiated gastroenteropancreatic (GEP neuroendocrine tumors (NETs) generally have a low glucose metabolism (Adams et al. 1998; Belhocine et al. 2002). For the primary staging of neuroendocrine tumors, ^{18}F-fluorodeoxyglucose (^{18}FDG) PET scanning has limited value due to the only moderately increased glucose metabolism of most GEP NET. Therefore, as a staging tool, ^{18}FDG PET is most likely not suited for the detection of suspected brain metastasis in patients with neuroendocrine tumors (Adams et al. 1998; Pasquali et al. 1998).

Many neuroendocrine tumors and their metastasis have an increased synthesis and secretion of hormones and neurotransmitters. Serotonin, catecholamine, and histamine are the most common examples of secreted hormones by these tumors (Jager et al. 2008). The increased biosynthesis of catecholamines and serotonin in neuroendocrine tumors enables imaging with specific amine precursors. In this chapter, we will shortly discuss 6-^{18}F-L-3,4-dihydroxyphenylalanine (^{18}F-DOPA), a PET tracer for the catecholamine pathway, and β-[^{11}C]-5-hydroxy-L-tryptophan (^{11}C-5-HTP), a PET tracer for the serotonin pathway.

42.8.1 Catecholamine Pathway

In the brain, catecholamines, such as adrenaline, act as neurotransmitters or as hormones, via α- and β-adrenergic receptors located on vessels and internal organs.

For the synthesis of catecholamines, phenylalanine and intermediate products such as L-3,4-dihydroxyphenylalanine (L-DOPA) are taken up via system L large amino acid transporters (LAT). These precursors are decarboxylated to dopamine intracytoplasmatically via the enzyme aromatic amino acid decarboxylase (AADC). The resulting products are then taken up by vesicular monoamine transporters (VMAT) for intravesicular storage. Intravesicularly, dopamine can, depending on the activity of specific enzymes, be further metabolized to noradrenaline and adrenaline. These vesicles are capable to release the end products dopamine, noradrenaline, and adrenaline in the extracellular environment. Selective re-uptake transporter systems, e.g., dopamine and noradrenaline transporters, are capable to transport these hormones back into the cell.

For the catecholamine pathway, both 6-^{18}F-L-3,4-dihydroxyphenylalanine (^{18}F-DOPA) and 6-^{18}F-dopamine are available as tracers. However, currently no data exist on the use of 6-^{18}F-dopamine for brain tumors or metastases in general, so this chapter will be limited to ^{18}F-DOPA.

^{18}F-DOPA can be produced via two different synthesis routes: regioselective fluorodestannylation (electrophilic fluorination) and nucleophilic fluorination, which is a multistep procedure. This last synthesis procedure is more time-consuming but has the advantage of having readily available large quantities of no-carrier-added ^{18}F-fluoride (Jager et al. 2008; Lemaire et al. 1994).

The tracer ^{18}F-DOPA was developed and first studied in men at McMaster University, Hamilton, Canada, during the 1970s and 1980s of the last century (Garnett et al. 1983). In the first years after development of this tracer, it was solely used for imaging of the dopaminergic system of the brain. Several years later, the first whole-body scans in patients with NETs and other brain tumors were published (Heiss et al. 1996; Hoegerle et al. 2001).

Although data on the performance of ^{18}F-DOPA PET(/CT) imaging for the detection of neuroendocrine metastases outside the brain shows a high potential, unfortunately, no data are reported on the use of ^{18}F-DOPA for the detection of brain metastases of these tumors (Koopmans et al. 2008). For other brain tumors, like glioma, ^{18}F-DOPA has proven to be of value (Chen et al. 2006).

Since ^{18}F-DOPA is already commercially available in many countries, the increased availability may lead to a better understanding of the place of ^{18}F-DOPA PET in clinical decision-making for brain metastases of NETs.

42.8.2 Serotonin Pathway

Serotonin is a monoamine neurotransmitter present in the brain, blood platelets, and intestinal wall. In the brain, it acts as a neurotransmitter and plays a role in feelings of well-being.

The serotonin pathway shares the LAT and VMAT systems with the catecholamine pathway for transport and synthesis. In both pathways, the enzyme AADC plays a key role in the final step for the synthesis to a functional hormone, which is serotonin in the serotonin pathway.

After uptake via the LAT system, the amino acid tryptophan and the intermediate product 5-hydroxytryptophan (5-HTP) are used as precursors for the serotonin pathway. These precursors are decarboxylated to serotonin via the enzyme AADC. Serotonin is taken up via VMAT transporters into storage vesicles for future extracellular release. After release, serotonin is eventually metabolized to 5-hydroxyindole acetic acid (5-HIAA) which is secreted in the urine. The serotonin pathway is overactive in many NETs, which makes this pathway a good candidate for imaging with PET tracers (Koopmans et al. 2009).

The carbon-11-labelled tracer β-[^{11}C]-5-hydroxy-L-tryptophan (^{11}C-5-HTP) has been developed in the 1980s in the last century in Uppsala, Sweden, and is thus far the only suitable tracer for the serotonin pathway. The synthesis of this tracer is complex, demanding an on-site cyclotron for the production of the ^{11}C isotope which has a half-life of only 20 min. The synthesis requires two multi-enzyme steps (Bjurling et al. 1989; Neels et al. 2006). ^{11}C-5-HTP is therefore only produced by a few centers in the world. Image interpretation in the brain is mostly easy due to a very low background uptake and, at least in extracranial tumor localizations, a high tumor tracer uptake (Koopmans et al. 2008).

Due to the low worldwide tracer availability of ^{11}C-5-HTP, and the limited number of patients scanned with this tracer, no published data exist on the efficacy of ^{11}C-5-HTP PET for the detection of neuroendocrine tumor metastasis to the brain. Due to the biodistribution, however, it can be expected that this tracer likely results in good uptake in brain metastasis. Synthesis of this tracer is very difficult, which hampers widespread use and experience.

42.9 Conclusion

Due to the low incidence of neuroendocrine tumors and metastatic brain lesions of neuroendocrine tumors, inadequate data is available to determine the relative efficacy of nuclear medicine imaging techniques such as ^{68}Ga-DOTATOC PET, ^{18}F-DOPA PET, or, for example, ^{11}C-HTP for the detection of brain metastasis of neuroendocrine tumors. Although the incidence of brain metastasis in NET is rare, it appears that these patients show a worse survival compared to patients without brain metastases. More and more case reports published thus far mention the accidental finding of brain metastasis with PET techniques. From the data available and these case reports, it can be argued that it could be worthwhile to screen for brain metastases in patients conforming to the ENETS guidelines, to start appropriate treatment early. Nevertheless, MRI is still the recommended imaging modality for the detection of neuroendocrine brain metastasis. Research is warranted, although due to the low incidence, we can only hope for better data.

References

Adams S, Baum R, Rink T, Schumm-Drager PM, Usadel KH, Hor G (1998) Limited value of fluorine-18 fluorodeoxyglucose positron emission tomography for the imaging of neuroendocrine tumours. Eur J Nucl Med 25(1):79–83

Batson OV (1940) The function of the vertebral veins and their role in the spread of metastases. Ann Surg 112(1):138–149

Belhocine T, Foidart J, Rigo P, Najjar F, Thiry A, Quatresooz P, Hustinx R (2002) Fluorodeoxyglucose positron emission tomography and somatostatin receptor scintigraphy for diagnosing and staging carcinoid tumours: correlations with the pathological indexes p53 and Ki-67. Nucl Med Commun 23(8):727–734

Bjurling P, Watanabe Y, Tokushige M, Oda T, Långström B (1989) Syntheses of β-11C-labelled L-tryptophan and 5-hydroxy-L-tryptophan using a multi-enzymatic reaction route. J Chem Soc Perkin Trans 1(7):1331–1334

Carreras C, Kulkarni HR, Baum RP (2013) Rare metastases detected by (68)Ga-somatostatin receptor PET/CT in patients with neuroendocrine tumors. Recent Results Cancer Res 194:379–384. https://doi.org/10.1007/978-3-642-27994-2_20

Chen W, Silverman DH, Delaloye S, Czernin J, Kamdar N, Pope W et al (2006) 18F-FDOPA PET imaging of brain tumors: comparison study with 18F-FDG PET and evaluation of diagnostic accuracy. J Nucl Med 47(6):904–911

Cho KH, Hall WA, Gerbi BJ, Higgins PD, Bohen M, Clark HB (1998) Patient selection criteria for the treatment of brain metastases with stereotactic radiosurgery. J Neurooncol 40(1):73–86

Doddoli C, Barlesi F, Chetaille B, Garbe L, Thomas P, Giudicelli R, Fuentes P (2004) Large cell neuroendocrine carcinoma of the lung: an aggressive disease potentially treatable with surgery. Ann Thorac Surg 77(4):1168–1172. https://doi.org/10.1016/j.athoracsur.2003.09.049

Garnett ES, Firnau G, Nahmias C (1983) Dopamine visualized in the basal ganglia of living man. Nature 305(5930):137–138

Godwin JD II (1975) Carcinoid tumors. An analysis of 2,837 cases. Cancer 36(2):560–569

Granberg D, Wilander E, Oberg K, Skogseid B (2000) Prognostic markers in patients with typical bronchial carcinoid tumors. J Clin Endocrinol Metab 85(9):3425–3430

He BP, Wang JJ, Zhang X, Wu Y, Wang M, Bay BH, Chang AY (2006) Differential reactions of microglia to brain metastasis of lung cancer. Mol Med 12(7–8):161–170. https://doi.org/10.2119/2006-00033.He

Heiss WD, Wienhard K, Wagner R, Lanfermann H, Thiel A, Herholz K, Pietrzyk U (1996) F-Dopa as an amino acid tracer to detect brain tumors. J Nucl Med 37(7):1180–1182

Henze M, Schuhmacher J, Hipp P, Kowalski J, Becker DW, Doll J et al (2001) PET imaging of somatostatin receptors using [68GA]DOTA-D-Phe1-Tyr3-octreotide: first results in patients with meningiomas. J Nucl Med 42(7):1053–1056

Hlatky R, Suki D, Sawaya R (2004) Carcinoid metastasis to the brain. Cancer 101(11):2605–2613. https://doi.org/10.1002/cncr.20659

Hoegerle S, Altehoefer C, Ghanem N, Koehler G, Waller CF, Scheruebl H et al (2001) Whole-body 18F dopa PET for detection of gastrointestinal carcinoid tumors. Radiology 220(2):373–380

Hofland LJ, Lamberts SW (2003) The pathophysiological consequences of somatostatin receptor internalization and resistance. Endocr Rev 24(1):28–47

Hofmann M, Maecke H, Borner R, Weckesser E, Schoffski P, Oei L et al (2001) Biokinetics and imaging with the somatostatin receptor PET radioligand (68)Ga-DOTATOC: preliminary data. Eur J Nucl Med 28(12):1751–1757. https://doi.org/10.1007/s002590100639

Jager PL, Chirakal R, Marriott CJ, Brouwers AH, Koopmans KP, Gulenchyn KY (2008) 6-L-18F-fluorodihydroxyphenylalanine PET in neuroendocrine tumors: basic aspects and emerging clinical applications. J Nucl Med 49(4):573–586. https://doi.org/10.2967/jnumed.107.045708

Khan IU, Beck-Sickinger AG (2008) Targeted tumor diagnosis and therapy with peptide hormones as radiopharmaceuticals. Anti Cancer Agents Med Chem 8(2):186–199

Klein CA, Blankenstein TJ, Schmidt-Kittler O, Petronio M, Polzer B, Stoecklein NH, Riethmuller G (2002) Genetic heterogeneity of single disseminated tumour cells in minimal residual cancer. Lancet 360(9334):683–689. https://doi.org/10.1016/S0140-6736(02)09838-0

Kloppel G, Heitz PU, Capella C, Solcia E (1996) Pathology and nomenclature of human gastro-intestinal neuroendocrine (carcinoid) tumors and related lesions. World J Surg 20(2):132–141

Koopmans KP, Neels OC, Kema IP, Elsinga PH, Sluiter WJ, Vanghillewe K et al (2008) Improved staging of patients with carcinoid and islet cell tumors with 18F-dihydroxy-phenyl-alanine and 11C-5-hydroxy-tryptophan positron emission tomography. J Clin Oncol 26(9):1489–1495. https://doi.org/10.1200/JCO.2007.15.1126

Koopmans KP, Neels ON, Kema IP, Elsinga PH, Links TP, de Vries EG, Jager PL (2009) Molecular imaging in neuroendocrine tumors: molecular uptake mechanisms and clinical results. Crit Rev Oncol Hematol 71(3):199–213. https://doi.org/10.1016/j.critrevonc.2009.02.009

Krenning EP, Bakker WH, Kooij PP, Breeman WA, Oei HY, de Jong M et al (1992) Somatostatin receptor scintigraphy with indium-111-DTPA-D-Phe-1-octreotide in man: metabolism, dosimetry and comparison with iodine-123-Tyr-3-octreotide. J Nucl Med 33(5):652–658

Krug S, Teupe F, Michl P, Gress TM, Rinke A (2019) Brain metastases in patients with neuroendocrine neoplasms: risk factors and outcome. BMC Cancer 19(1):362. https://doi.org/10.1186/s12885-019-5559-7

Kruger S, Mottaghy FM, Buck AK, Maschke S, Kley H, Frechen D et al (2011) Brain metastasis in lung cancer. Comparison of cerebral MRI and 18F-FDG-PET/CT for diagnosis in the initial staging. Nuklearmedizin 50(3):101–106. https://doi.org/10.3413/Nukmed-0338-10-07

Lamberts SW, Reubi JC, Krenning EP (1993) Validation of somatostatin receptor scintigraphy in the localization of neuroendocrine tumors. Acta Oncol 32(2):167–170

Lemaire C, Damhaut P, Plenevaux A, Comar D (1994) Enantioselective synthesis of 6-[fluorine-18]-fluoro-L-dopa from no-carrier-added fluorine-18-fluoride. J Nucl Med 35(12):1996–2002
Lepage C, Bouvier AM, Faivre J (2013) Endocrine tumours: epidemiology of malignant digestive neuroendocrine tumours. Eur J Endocrinol 168(4):R77–R83. https://doi.org/10.1530/EJE-12-0418
Maiuri F, Cappabianca P, Del Basso De Caro M, Esposito F (2004) Single brain metastases of carcinoid tumors. J Neurooncol 66(3):327–332
Modlin IM, Lye KD, Kidd M (2003) A 5-decade analysis of 13,715 carcinoid tumors. Cancer 97(4):934–959. https://doi.org/10.1002/cncr.11105
Nakamura Y, Shimokawa S, Ishibe R, Ikee T, Taira A (2001) Pulmonary carcinoid found in a patient who presented with initial symptoms of brain metastasis: report of a case. Surg Today 31(6):510–512
Neels OC, Jager PL, Koopmans KP, Eriks E, de Vries EGE, Kema IP, Elsinga PL (2006) Development of a reliable remote-controlled synthesis of β-[11C]-5-hydroxy-L-tryptophan on a Zymark robotic system. J Label Compd Radiopharm 49:889–895
Pasquali C, Rubello D, Sperti C, Gasparoni P, Liessi G, Chierichetti F et al (1998) Neuroendocrine tumor imaging: can 18F-fluorodeoxyglucose positron emission tomography detect tumors with poor prognosis and aggressive behavior? World J Surg 22(6):588–592
Patchell RA, Posner JB (1986) Neurologic complications of carcinoid. Neurology 36(6):745–749
Pavel M, Grossman A, Arnold R, Perren A, Kaltsas G, Steinmuller T et al (2010) ENETS consensus guidelines for the management of brain, cardiac and ovarian metastases from neuroendocrine tumors. Neuroendocrinology 91(4):326–332. https://doi.org/10.1159/000287277
Porter DG, Chakrabarty A, McEvoy A, Bradford R (2000) Intracranial carcinoid without evidence of extracranial disease. Neuropathol Appl Neurobiol 26(3):298–300
Reubi JC (1995) Neuropeptide receptors in health and disease: the molecular basis for in vivo imaging. J Nucl Med 36(10):1825–1835
Schnirer II, Yao JC, Ajani JA (2003) Carcinoid—a comprehensive review. Acta Oncol 42(7):672–692
Soga J (2003) Carcinoids and their variant endocrinomas. An analysis of 11842 reported cases. J Exp Clin Cancer Res 22(4):517–530
Sul J, Posner JB (2007) Brain metastases: epidemiology and pathophysiology. Cancer Treat Res 136:1–21
Weckbecker G, Lewis I, Albert R, Schmid HA, Hoyer D, Bruns C (2003) Opportunities in somatostatin research: biological, chemical and therapeutic aspects. Nat Rev Drug Discov 2(12):999–1017. https://doi.org/10.1038/nrd1255
Yamagi, L.Y.I., Wagner, J., Funari M.B.G. (2017)68Ga-DOTATATE PET/CT in nonneuroendocrine tumors: a pictorial essay. Clin Nucl Med 42(6):e313-e316

Traumatic Brain Injury: Nuclear Medicine Neuroimaging

43

Carlos A. Sanchez-Catasus, Gilles N. Stormezand, David Vállez García, Eloísa Le Riverend Morales, Reinaldo Galvizu Sánchez, and Rudi A. J. O. Dierckx

Contents

C. A. Sanchez-Catasus (✉)
Division of Nuclear Medicine, Department of Radiology, University of Michigan, Ann Arbor, MI, USA

Department of Nuclear Medicine and Molecular Imaging, University Medical Center Groningen, Groningen, The Netherlands
e-mail: carlosas@umich.edu

G. N. Stormezand · D. Vállez García
Department of Nuclear Medicine and Molecular Imaging, University Medical Center Groningen, Groningen, The Netherlands
e-mail: g.n.stormezand01@umcg.nl; d.vallez-garcia@umcg.nl

E. Le Riverend Morales
Department of Vaccine Regulation, Finlay Institute, Havana, Cuba
e-mail: lochy@infomed.sld.cu

R. Galvizu Sánchez
Department of Nuclear Medicine, Center for Neurological Restoration (CIREN), Havana, Cuba
e-mail: rgalvizu@neuro.ciren.cu

R. A. J. O. Dierckx
Department of Nuclear Medicine and Molecular Imaging, University Medical Center Groningen, Groningen, The Netherlands

Department of Radiology and Nuclear Medicine, Ghent University, Ghent, Belgium
e-mail: r.a.dierckx@umcg.nl

R. A. J. O. Dierckx et al. (eds.), *PET and SPECT in Neurology*,
https://doi.org/10.1007/978-3-030-53168-3_43

Abstract

This chapter provides an up-to-date review of nuclear medicine neuroimaging in traumatic brain injury (TBI). Although the role of FDG PET may be limited in the acute phase due to the more rapid availability of CT or MRI, ^{18}F-FDG PET could remain a valuable tool in researching complex mechanisms associated with early metabolic dysfunction in TBI, particularly in the absence of structurally apparent brain damage. $^{15}O_2$-PET is also a solid technique for research in acute TBI, but in contrast to ^{18}F-FDG PET, it is not widely available due to its high cost. In the chronic TBI phase, most ^{18}F-FDG PET studies converge to identify a diffuse cortical–subcortical hypometabolism involving key regions for cognitive function. In these cases, FDG PET may also be used for the evaluation of therapeutic interventions. More recently, research has focused on the imaging of specific pathological processes, such as neuroinflammation and accumulation of tau, as well as on distinct entities as chronic traumatic encephalopathy and the post-concussion syndrome. In this light, the in vivo demonstration of tau deposits in athletes exposed to repetitive head injury has gained special interest. These techniques may provide useful information, especially in situations where structural damage typically fails to show a pathologic substrate. Despite a paucity of recent research publications, SPECT may still be regarded a valid alternative for the study of TBI.

Abbreviations

AChE	Acetylcholinesterase
BP	Binding potential
BP_{ND}	Non-displaceable binding potential
BZR	Central-type benzodiazepine receptor
C-(R)-PK11195	1-[2-Chlorophenyl]-*N*-methyl-*N*-[1-methylpropyl]-3-isoquinoline carboxamide
CBF	Cerebral blood flow
C-MP4A	[Methyl-^{11}C]*N*-methylpiperidyl-4-acetate
CMRFDG	Cerebral metabolic rate of FDG
CMRglc	Cerebral metabolic rate of glucose
$CMRO_2$	Cerebral metabolic rate of oxygen
C-NMSP	^{11}C-*N*-methylspiperone
CT	Computed tomography
CTE	Chronic traumatic encephalopathy
D_2	Dopamine receptor type 2
DAI	Diffuse axonal injury

DTI	Diffusion tensor imaging
FIQ	Full-scale intelligence quotient
FMZ	Flumazenil
GCS	Glasgow Coma Scale
GM	Gray matter
GOS	Glasgow Outcome Scale
L/N ratio	Lesion-to-normal contralateral ratio
MRI	Magnetic resonance imaging
NSC	Neural stem cell
OEF	Oxygen extraction fraction
OGR	Oxygen-to-glucose metabolic ratio
ROI	Regions of interest
SPM	Statistical parametric mapping
TBI	Traumatic brain injury
TSPO	Translocator protein
V/C ratio	Vermis-to-cerebellum ratio
WM	White matter

43.1 Introduction

Traumatic brain injury (TBI) is described as a traumatically induced disruption of the brain, in the presence of one of the following symptoms: loss of consciousness, anterograde or retrograde memory loss, alterations of the mental state at the time of the incident, or focal neurological deficits. The worldwide prevalence of TBI demands global attention and effective actions involving all levels of society. The annual incidence of TBI has been estimated to be up to 500 per 100,000 inhabitants in the European Union and the United States, causing 200 out of every 100,000 hospital admissions (Faul et al. 2010; Stryke et al. 2007; Tagliaferri et al. 2006). Worldwide incidence is growing mainly due to traffic accidents, with a higher increase in developing countries (WHO/OMS 2009). Not less important is the rise of the social and economic TBI burden because of military conflicts and civilian exposure in war zones. TBI as a consequence of sports practice and recreational activities should not be underestimated either. TBI has devastating effects on patients and their families due to death or chronic disabilities, with high socioeconomic cost throughout the world. Therefore, a widespread international effort is necessary to reduce TBI causes as much as possible and at the same time to increase knowledge on this complex disease that will allow mitigating or reverting short- and long-term outcomes.

TBI includes a wide and heterogeneous spectrum of pathologies ranging from focal damage caused by contusion (with or without cranial fracture) to diffuse axonal injury (DAI), including complex secondary pathophysiological processes (Zasler et al. 2007), which could be aggravated by systemic events, patient age, or preexisting chronic disease. In many cases, TBI may secondarily lead to epilepsy

(Frey 2003), and after aging, it is the most important nongenetic factor that increases the risk of dementia (McKee et al. 2009), including chronic traumatic encephalopathy.

Immediate clinical TBI consequences are directly related to the severity, mechanism, location, and duration of the impact (Maas et al. 2008). Conventional computed tomography (CT) is the technique of choice for the initial evaluation of TBI patients because it enables detection of fractures and helps to decide whether the patient requires an immediate surgical intervention, when focal injury with hematomas is suspected (Kubal 2012). When results on CT are unclear or negative, MRI may be performed to demonstrate occult traumatically induced injury, such as microhemorrhages (Haller et al. 2018). After the initial examination, secondary damage—indirect consequences of trauma—may contribute significantly to short- and long-term impairment, which is especially due to cell and inflammatory damage (Park et al. 2008). Secondary damage is a key concept, since it opens doors to treatment methods for preventing and limiting secondary injury. Neuroimaging using nuclear medicine techniques also has great potential for studying secondary damage and may serve as a guide to evaluate several therapeutic approaches.

In this chapter, a review of several relevant contributions of nuclear medicine neuroimaging toward improved understanding of TBI is presented, using both positron emission tomography (PET) and single-photon emission computed tomography (SPECT). Various articles published in the last years, which summarize current knowledge on the roles of PET and SPECT, could be considered starting points for new research and clinical applications. The molecular basis of both techniques, especially PET, provides unique possibilities for studying complex cellular processes that take place in TBI, which are not yet fully understood.

43.2 PET

Despite the large number of studies using PET in TBI, in which the usefulness of this technique was shown in several clinical settings, there is no meta-analysis clarifying the importance of this technique either by itself or by complementary to structural neuroimaging. This is mostly due to the clinical heterogeneity and complexity of TBI, reflected in the diversity of studies published with regard to several aspects: first, differences in the time elapsed between the moment of injury and image acquisition; second, differences in patient characteristics with respect to TBI severity; third, differences in PET radiotracers; fourth, differences in methodological designs; and fifth, the use of different image analysis methodologies. In addition, no prospective randomized, blinded clinical trials have been conducted for obtaining major evidence, which can partly be explained by the high cost of such studies that require several years of follow-up. It is not surprising that such studies are scarce in medical imaging, including conventional CT and MRI (Medina et al. 2011).

43.2.1 ^{18}F-FDG PET in the Acute Phase of Brain Trauma

The first ^{18}F-FDG PET studies in TBI patients appeared in the 1980s and 1990s (Rao et al. 1984; Langfitt et al. 1986; Alavi 1989; Alavi et al. 1997; Tenjin et al. 1990; Yamaki et al. 1996; Fontaine et al. 1999). They pointed out that abnormalities detected by ^{18}F-FDG PET were more extensive than those observed by CT and that it was possible to detect them very early when structural modalities could still be negative. In those years, PET was still restricted to very few centers in the world. This situation began to change after the beginning of the present century. One of the predominant issues from the 1990s to date has been the study of brain metabolism in the acute phase of TBI. Findings of Bergsneider et al. (1997, 2000, 2001) suggested the existence of a triphasic pattern in the cerebral metabolic rate of glucose (CMRglc) measured by ^{18}F-FDG PET. This pattern had been previously observed in animal models. The first and brief hyperacute phase is characterized by an increase of metabolic activity and followed by a second, relatively prolonged, period of reduced metabolism (for a month approximately), until a stable level within normal limits is achieved again. However, later studies have found that regional diffuse deficits may persist chronically (this will be discussed in Sect. 43.2). These studies also suggested that during the intermediate phase, there was disassociation between the global CMRglc and the level of consciousness measured by the Glasgow Coma Scale (GCS) (Bergsneider et al. 2000). The paper published by this group in 2001 is particularly interesting (Bergsneider et al. 2001). Fifty-four patients in acute phase (2–39 days post onset), with the three degrees of severity defined by the GCS (34 severe and 20 moderate or mild), were studied. ^{18}F-FDG PET scan was repeated in 13 patients during trauma evolution (6–15 months after the onset of injury). In the whole sample, the authors found the previously mentioned triphasic pattern, independent of the degree of TBI severity, suggesting that the degree of TBI severity does not affect the time course of CMRglc changes. In a follow-up study on 13 patients with ^{18}F-FDG PET, no relationship was found between CMRglc changes and neurological state changes measured by the disability rating scale. The authors concluded that ^{18}F-FDG PET should not be used as a surrogate marker to estimate the degree of functional recovery following TBI.

On the other hand, Hattori et al. (2003) using a new generation of PET scanners with better spatial resolution, capable of identifying smaller brain regions, demonstrated in 23 acute-phase patients (5 days post onset) that, unlike global CMRglc, there was a direct association between level of consciousness measured by GCS and CMRglc values for the thalamus, brain stem, and cerebellum. This study significantly contributed to a better understanding of how the level of consciousness and brain glucose metabolism measured by ^{18}F-FDG PET are related.

Three articles published by the UCLA group in 2004 made the role of ^{18}F-FDG PET in the acute phase of TBI even clearer (Hattori et al. 2004; Wu et al. 2004a, b). The first of these papers was a thorough characterization of brain tissue ^{18}F-FDG kinetics during the acute phase (Hattori et al. 2004). In this study, the authors characterized ^{18}F-FDG uptake, transport, and hexokinase activity using kinetic modeling. The study group comprised 21 TBI patients with cerebral contusions. Cerebral blood flow (CBF) was also evaluated by dynamic $H_2{}^{15}O$-PET. Results demonstrated that hexokinase activity was reduced in the entire brain, including apparently undamaged brain cortex, while glucose transport and CBF were reduced only in pericontusional areas. Seven patients showed regionally increased ^{18}F-FDG uptake in pericontusional areas, probably associated with residual regional increase of hexokinase activity during the hyperacute phase (first phase of the triphasic pattern).

Hypotheses taken into account to explain focal pericontusional hyperglycolysis were anaerobic glycolysis, ionic disturbance, release of excitatory amino acids, and glycolysis due to increased glutamate activity. Bearing in mind that glycolysis takes place mainly in glial cells, authors suggested that an increase in glial metabolic activity was a possible cause of hyperglycolysis.

The following study was inspired by an important observation (Wu et al. 2004a) concerning the fact that gray matter (GM) to white matter (WM) contrast in ^{18}F-FDG PET images is reduced in patients with acute TBI, with or without focal damage, compared to normal healthy controls. Interestingly, this reduction was not observed in $H_2{}^{15}O$-PET of CBF in the same patients. For this reason, the authors hypothesized that changes of glucose metabolism in the acute phase were different in GM and WM. They studied 14 patients with severe to moderate TBI (0–4 days post onset), all with structural focal abnormalities by CT. In all subjects, ^{18}F-FDG PET, triple dynamic ^{15}O-PET ($C^{15}O$, $O^{15}O$, $H_2{}^{15}O$), and MRI were carried out. Initial GCS at onset and the Glasgow Outcome Scale (GOS) 12 months post onset were also evaluated. Peri-hemorrhagic regions were excluded from the analysis. For comparison, a control group of 18 healthy subjects was studied. The results showed that the GM-to-WM ratio in ^{18}F-FDG PET images was significantly reduced in the TBI group. Although a global reduction of CMRglc was observed in the patients, as expected from the previous study (Hattori et al. 2004), CMRglc and hexokinase activity were selectively reduced in the GM and not in the WM. Significant changes of global CBF were not found in GM or in WM, corroborating that glucose supply to the brain was not limited. Even more interesting was the finding that the GM-to-WM ratio was positively correlated with the initial GCS and patients with higher GM-to-WM ratio showed better recovery (GOS) after 12 months. Before this study, physiological changes occurring in WM after TBI had received less attention compared to changes in GM. Based on prior observations in animal models, the authors considered several hypotheses to explain the unexpected finding that there were no significant changes in CMRglc in WM (or that it was increased with respect to the global CMRglc). One of these hypotheses is that in WM there was a combination of infiltration of inflammatory cells and reactive gliosis after TBI, which was probably associated with DAI.

The third article of the UCLA group (Wu et al. 2004b) was a direct consequence of the aforementioned study. The authors examined the relationship between glucose and oxygen metabolism in WM in the acute phase to determine the nature, extension, and degree of abnormalities in regions remote from hemorrhagic lesions. The study sample was essentially the previous one and using the same image acquisitions (PET and MRI). Five types of quantitative images were generated: CMRglc, CBF, cerebral metabolic rate of oxygen ($CMRO_2$), oxygen extraction fraction (OEF), and oxygen-to-glucose metabolic ratio (OGR). The results corroborated that CMRglc was reduced only in GM. CBF and OEF were preserved, while $CMRO_2$ was reduced in both GM and WM. The main result was that OGR was selectively reduced in WM. Thus, this study showed that acute metabolic changes in WM had a particular feature, characterized by $CMRO_2$ depression, without parallel depression of CMRglc, suggesting a nonoxidative use of glucose in this region during the acute phase. These findings were present throughout WM, even in regions without evidence of DAI based on conventional MRI images, thus suggesting that DAI detected by multimodal PET was much more extensive and subtle than that detected by conventional MRI. As possible explanations for these findings, authors indicated an increase in inflammatory cells during the acute phase, especially in the WM, which are more prone to anaerobic glycolytic metabolism. Combining results published by the UCLA group between 2003 and 2004 (Hattori et al. 2003, 2004; Wu et al. 2004a, b), the state of coma was shown to involve a thalamocortical disconnection with a clearly defined metabolic substrate, and a prognostic value of ^{18}F-FDG PET was suggested (Wu et al. 2004a).

Complexity of metabolic dysfunction during the acute phase continues to be the object of current research and debate. Findings from the Cambridge University group, combining microdialysis and ^{18}F-FDG PET studies, did not support the hypothesis of nonoxidative metabolism associated with an increase in glucose cerebral metabolism in the acute phase (Hutchinson et al. 2009; O'Connell et al. 2005).

On the other hand, another study indicated that early dysfunction of nonischemic oxidative metabolism in the acute phase leads to chronic brain atrophy in TBI patients (Xu et al. 2010). This study showed that both cortical CMRglc and $CMRO_2$ were reduced in the acute phase, even in apparently normal areas by MRI. However, the extent of regional brain atrophy 6 months after TBI correlated better with $CMRO_2$ and CBF, particularly in the frontal and temporal lobes ($N = 32$). CMRglc correlated with atrophy only in the frontal lobe. They also found that OEF was not in the ischemic range and did not correlate with chronic brain atrophy. These results emphasized the fact that chronic brain atrophy is related with early metabolic changes, especially in brain areas not directly damaged during TBI.

Another work carried out a longitudinal study in vivo that identified and traced the spatial and temporal metabolic and structural changes in an experimental TBI model in rats (Liu et al. 2010). Images were acquired 1 week and 1, 3, and 6 months post TBI by micro^{18}F-FDG PET and microMRI in 16 rats with lateral fluid percussion injury and 11 control rats (sham procedure). Using several methods of image analysis, including statistical parametric mapping (SPM), the authors found that regions with hypometabolism at 1 week and 1 month after TBI were essentially the same that subsequently showed progressive atrophy by microMRI. Hypometabolism was highest at 1 month but persisted in the study at 6 months in the ipsilateral amygdala. Disagreement was also found between structural and metabolic changes. Hypometabolism decreased or resolved at 6 months and preceded atrophy. Atrophy continued progressing for up to 6 months. Hippocampi changed shape with reduction in volume, and both sides showed different patterns of change. The most interesting observation in this study was that both structural and functional changes seemed to consolidate between 3 and 6 months, suggesting that the temporal window to intervene and limit secondary neurodegenerative damage (atrophy) may be wider than expected.

In our view, ^{18}F-FDG PET will remain a valuable tool in researching complex mechanisms associated with early metabolic dysfunction in TBI, presently not well understood. Future research may benefit from more stringent inclusion of patients based on the timing and the type of trauma. From a clinical point of view, although appropriate clinical trials are still needed to provide more evidence, ^{18}F-FDG PET in the TBI acute phase appeared to be more useful and to show incremental validity (prognostic information) in those patients in whom CT (or MRI) failed to show damage explaining their neurological state. Of note, as has been addressed in a critical review in 2014, CMRglc values may be less reproducible in patients with traumatic brain injury, as the lumped constant—CMRFDG divided by CMRglc—could be altered after traumatic brain injury (Byrnes et al. 2014). With the growing number of hybrid PET–CT and PET/MRI systems and ^{18}F-FDG availability, combined studies of both structural and functional damage are now more feasible. This could facilitate acquisition of multicenter databases to carry out evidence-based imaging studies that enable demonstration of incremental validity of ^{18}F-FDG PET. Cost-effectiveness analysis is also necessary to compare ^{18}F-FDG PET with MRI-based techniques, such as diffusion tensor imaging (DTI), magnetization transfer imaging, magnetic resonance spectroscopy, and functional magnetic resonance (Hunter et al. 2012).

43.2.1.1 $^{15}O_2$-PET

TBI consequences are not only determined by primary injury but also by subsequent neuronal death due to secondary damage, which already starts during the acute phase. For this reason, the main strategy in TBI patient management, especially those in critical neurological state, is to prevent or limit secondary damage as much as possible (Park et al. 2008). Secondary damage can be initiated or aggravated by hypoperfusion, arterial hypotension, hypoxemia, autoregulation failure, as well as metabolic, immunologic, and biochemical changes. Although delayed ischemia is one of the routes of secondary damage, reperfusion can also take place, elevating intracranial pressure, reducing perfusion pressure, and finally reducing CBF again.

Triple dynamic $^{15}O_2$-PET is the best technique for determining true ischemia because it is the only one that can simultaneously measure CBF, $CMRO_2$, and OEF globally and regionally. To demonstrate true ischemia, it is not enough to demonstrate that CBF is reduced, since this could be a response to $CMRO_2$ decrease (flow metabolism coupling). Therefore, it is essential to demonstrate that CBF is also inadequate for the oxygen demand, which means confirming a significant OEF increase in the ischemic range.

Since the beginning of this century, several articles have been published about triple $^{15}O_2$-PET studies that have allowed a deepened understanding of regional ischemia mechanisms in acute TBI. Some studies have demonstrated significant regional ischemia in the first hours after TBI (Coles et al. 2004a; Coles and Fryer 2004; Abate et al. 2008), while in other studies, ischemia has been less evident (Wu et al. 2004b; Vespa et al. 2005; Kawai et al. 2008; Xu et al. 2010). This apparent contradiction could be due to the heterogeneity and complexity of TBI. Another explanation for these contradictory results has been provided by triple $^{15}O_2$-PET studies (Cunningham et al. 2005). The authors found that unlike classical acute ischemia (stroke), the quantitative CBF threshold that defines irreversible ischemia did not discriminate correctly between surviving and irreversibly damaged tissue acutely post TBI ($N = 14$). Although the quantitative $CMRO_2$ threshold was comparable to the threshold reported for brain infarction, extensive overlapping was found for both tissues. From this study, the hypothesis emerged that selective neuronal death could be present in apparently surviving regions, which are not visible in conventional MR images that better identify regions with pan-necrosis. Studies using ^{11}C-flumazenil (FMZ) seem to corroborate this idea. ^{11}C-FMZ PET studies in TBI patients are examined in the next subsection of this chapter.

Other $^{15}O_2$-PET studies have allowed examination of new hypotheses about additional mechanisms of hypoxia and energetic failure, such as metabolic suppression, mitochondrial dysfunction, and microvascular disease in the acute phase of TBI (Menon et al. 2004; Vespa et al. 2005; Robertson 2004). Other studies have proven useful to evaluate the impact of therapeutic interventions in critical state patients (Coles et al. 2004b, 2006; Johnston et al. 2005; Diringer et al. 2007, 2011; Nortje et al. 2008) and in animal models of TBI (Ley et al. 2009; Ley and Park 2010). $^{15}O_2$-PET studies also validated and refined bedside monitoring technologies, which facilitate continuous monitoring of cerebrovascular physiology (Hutchinson et al. 2002; Gupta et al. 2002; Coles et al. 2004b). Bedside monitoring has the advantage of continuous temporal monitoring of CBF, autoregulation, and metabolic state of the patient (Dagal and Lam 2011). The main difficulty is that it can only monitor a small area of the brain, unlike $^{15}O_2$-PET which allows studying the whole brain in a more quantitative way. The main disadvantages of $^{15}O_2$-PET are that continuous monitoring is not possible and the patient must be moved from the intensive care unit to the scanner and the high cost of the cyclotron. In our opinion, $^{15}O_2$-PET is a solid technique for research into the complex pathophysiology of acute TBI, but in contrast to ^{18}F-FDG PET, it is not widely available due to its high cost. Also it presents a more logistical challenge, when compared to perfusion CT or MRI. Therefore, it is used mainly in research and less in clinical practice.

43.2.2 ^{18}F-FDG PET in the Chronic Phase of Brain Trauma

In the last years, there have been important advances in the care of neurocritical patients after TBI, resulting in a significant decrease of mortality (Bullock et al. 2007). However, TBI survivors frequently suffer from a wide variety of chronic cognitive, emotional, and behavioral disorders that hinder return to normal social and work life. Persistent vegetative state is the worst final outcome.

Neural networks connecting brain cortical and subcortical regions are crucial to maintain normal cognitive function (Bassett and Bullmore 2009). TBI damages, both primary and secondary, can impair not only particular nodes of these networks (focal damage) but also the wiring (DAI). Focal damage is easily identifiable both in structural and functional neuroimages, unlike DAI which can be underestimated by routine structural imaging in many patients.

Findings of the UCLA group in acute TBI using ^{18}F-FDG PET already suggested a thalamocortical disconnection as the cause of coma (Hattori et al. 2004; Wu et al. 2004a, b). Cortical–subcortical disconnection may persist to a larger or lesser extent in many patients in the chronic phase after TBI. ^{18}F-FDG PET studies in chronic TBI patients have allowed characterization and unveiling of many aspects of this cortical–subcortical disconnection. The use of voxel-based image analysis methods, especially SPM (Friston 1994), is common in several of these studies. Unlike the methods based on regions of interest (ROI), SPM enables analysis of the whole-brain volume voxel by voxel, without prior spatial hypothesis. In this regard, the exploration range is considerably broadened, giving in many cases unexpected results that reveal subtle information contained in the images, which are very difficult to extract using the visual qualitative method or ROI analysis. Table 43.1 summarizes the findings of FDG PET in the chronic phase of traumatic brain injury. Taken together, studies point toward the presence of corticothalamic deficits which carry an association with the neurological outcome, even without structural abnormalities. In addition to neuronal loss, altered ionic states, protein synthesis inhibition, CBF reduction, and alterations of the neurotransmitter systems could be involved to explain these findings (Marklund et al. 2009). Preliminary studies indicated that abnormalities at baseline may be monitored using FDG PET to evaluate the effectivity of treatment regimens. Kraus et al. (2005) evaluated the effects of amantadine. Amantadine is a dopaminergic agent and *N*-methyl-D-aspartate (NMDA) receptor antagonist. The results showed significant improvement of the executive function in a group of patients after amantadine therapy ($N = 22$). Analysis of ^{18}F-FDG PET images also showed a significant increase in the metabolism of the left prefrontal cortex. This region correlated positively with the executive function in the patient group.

Two more recent studies evaluated the effects of donepezil, an acetylcholinesterase inhibitor, and memantine, a noncompetitive NMDA receptor antagonist (Kim et al. 2009, 2010). The study using donepezil (Kim et al. 2009) included two groups of patients with cognitive impairment after TBI (mean interval after injury = 5.2 months). The control group was treated only with rehabilitation ($N = 13$). The other group received rehabilitation plus donepezil medication ($N = 13$). In the donepezil-treated group, ^{18}F-FDG PET and neuropsychological test studies were carried out at treatment onset and completion. In the control group, only neuropsychological tests were performed. ^{18}F-FDG PET images were analyzed by SPM. At the beginning of the study, no significant differences in cognitive function of both groups were observed. At the end, the group given donepezil showed a significant improvement in cognitive functions compared with controls and a significant bilateral increase of cortical metabolism in the frontal, parietal, occipital, and temporal regions.

Table 43.1 FDG PET in chronic phase of traumatic brain injury

Authors	Subjects	Design/methods	Main results	Specifications
Nakayama et al. (2006)	Chronic TBI patients (higher dysfunction) (*N* = 22), minimally conscious state (*N* = 13), persistent vegetative state (*N* = 17), controls (*N* = 30)	Cross-sectional, SPM analysis	Bilateral hypometabolism pattern involving prefrontal medial region, medial frontobasal region, anterior and posterior regions of the cingulate gyrus, and thalamus	This pattern was more extensive and prominent in the group in persistent vegetative state and less in the group with higher brain dysfunction, with an intermediate level in the group with minimally conscious state
Kato et al. (2007)	Patients with clinical DAI (*N* = 32), controls (*N* = 30)	Cross-sectional, SPM, correlation analysis between regional metabolism and neuropsychological variables in the patient group	Full-scale intelligence quotient (FIQ) was found to correlate positively with metabolism in the right cingulate gyrus and the bilateral medial frontal region	
Nakashima et al. (2007)	DAI patients with neurological deficits (*N* = 12) and controls (*N* = 32)	Cross-sectional, SPM, case-by-case analysis using 3D stereotactic surface projection (SSP)	Group comparison revealed hypometabolism in the cingulate, lingual, and cuneus gyrus. Case-by-case analysis showed differences regarding the site and extension of hypometabolism in the cingulate gyrus, although hypometabolism was more frequent in the medial region of the cingulate gyrus (six patients)	
Lupi et al. (2007)	Chronic TBI (*N* = 57) and controls (*N* = 57)	Cross-sectional, visual and ROI analysis	Results showed that in most patients, there was visually increased ^{18}F-FDG uptake in the cerebellar vermis. V/C also showed a significant increase in the patients compared to controls	The time elapsed between the acute phase and the ^{18}F-FDG PET was highly variable in the patient sample (15 days–4 years)
Lupi et al. (2011)			Strong correlation between V/C ratio and the severity of TBI as determined by cognitive and performance testings. Good correlation between V/C ratio determined shortly after TBI and the clinical outcome	Findings suggest that V/C ratio may be considered an index of brain suffering

(continued)

Table 43.1 (continued)

Authors	Subjects	Design/methods	Main results	Specifications
Zhang et al. (2010)	Chronic TBI patients ($N = 81$) and controls ($N = 68$), subgroups with ($N = 35$) and without ($N = 40$) structural abnormalities	Cross-sectional, SPM analysis.	Group comparison showed extensive bilateral hypometabolism in the cerebral cortex (including the frontal and temporal lobes) and the thalamus. Cluster counting analysis showed that patients with TBI (with or without structural lesion) had a higher proportion of large clusters of hypometabolism, and they were closer to the brain edge when compared with controls	One of the most interesting findings was that the cortical–subcortical hypometabolism was similar in patients with or without structural lesion, suggesting that abnormal patterns of metabolism are similar in patients with focal or diffuse TBI
Lull et al. (2010)	Controls ($N = 10$), a group with minimally conscious or persistent vegetative state ($N = 17$), a group with posttraumatic amnesia ($N = 12$), and a group with patients emerging from posttraumatic amnesia ($N = 20$)	Cross-sectional, SPM	Hypometabolism in the thalamus was directly related to the neurological outcome	This region was the most sensitive structure when patients in different neurological states were compared, despite the small percentage of patients with structural thalamic lesions in the three groups
Garcia-Panach et al. (2011)	Same groups as Lull et al.	Cross-sectional, SPM	Significant correlation between neurological outcome and glucose metabolism in all brain regions analyzed (precuneus, frontal and temporal lobes, and thalamus); there was also a direct relationship between hypometabolism and disease severity	
Ito et al. (2016)	Patients with chronic mild/moderate traumatic brain injury ($N = 90$), with ($N = 50$) and without ($N = 40$) visible lesions on MRI	Cross-sectional, SPM	Significant decrease of metabolisms in the orbital gyrus, cingulate gyrus, and medial thalamus but increased in the parietal and occipital convexity in subjects with MRI abnormalities, but not in those without	

In the memantine study (Kim et al. 2010), a group of 17 TBI patients were evaluated (mean post-onset duration = 6.8 months). ^{18}F-FDG PET was done at the beginning and after completion of the treatment. Furthermore, a covariance analysis was performed to assess if metabolic enhancement correlated with increases in mini-mental status examination (MMSE) scores. ^{18}F-FDG PET image analysis was performed by SPM. Results showed that MMSE scores were significantly improved after memantine treatment. When ^{18}F-FDG PET data acquired before and after treatment were compared, a significant increase of metabolism in the prefrontal region and the parietal association cortex was observed. A significant correlation was also found between MMSE and metabolism in the prefrontal regions and the association parietal cortex of the left hemisphere.

Distinct mechanisms may be at play in two entities we will briefly address in the next two subsections: chronic traumatic encephalopathy and the post-concussion syndrome.

43.2.2.1 Chronic Traumatic Encephalopathy

Chronic traumatic encephalopathy is a neurodegenerative disease resulting from repetitive head injury, which involves the development of long-term neuropsychiatric sequelae. Since the neuropathological studies of Omalu et al. in American football players (Omalu et al., 2010)—which became the subject of the popular movie "Concussion"—the impact of repetitive head injury in sports and associated chronic traumatic encephalopathy has gained attention, both in research and in society. Symptoms vary according to the stage but may be related to behavior, mood, or cognition. Neuropathologically, it is characterized by deposition of hyperphosphorylated tau (p-tau) protein as neurofibrillary tangles, astrocytic tangles, and neurites in clusters around small blood vessels of the cortex, preferentially located around small vessels in the depths of sulci (McKee et al. 2016). In recent years, tau PET ligands have become available allowing in vivo identification of tauopathies. Stern and colleagues demonstrated increased Standardized Uptake Value Ratios (SUVRs) using flortaucipir PET in the former American Football League players, a population particularly prone to CTE, primarily in the bilateral superior frontal, bilateral medial temporal, and left parietal regions (Stern et al. 2019). Takahata et al. using another tau ligand, ^{11}C-PBB3, determined the "binding capacity" in patients with a history of severe TBI of repetitive head injury ($n = 30$) and controls ($n = 16$). Binding capacity was significantly increased in widespread brain regions in patients, whereas clinical symptoms (diagnosis of traumatic encephalopathy syndrome) in the patient group were related to increased binding capacity in the white matter (Takahata et al. 2019). This group also demonstrated PBB3 binding to neurofibrillary tangles in cortical gray matter by means of PBB3 fluorescence labelling and immunofluorescence of autopsied TBI brains, albeit not in the same group of patients. These results seem to confirm the potential of PET to detect tauopathy in vivo in chronic TBI patients, although it is generally noted that the tau load is significantly less when compared to Alzheimer's disease. In the context of cognitive decline after repetitive head injury, additional amyloid positivity may be demonstrated using ^{11}C-PIB scanning (Okonkwo et al. 2019).

43.2.2.2 Post-concussion Syndrome

The "post-concussion syndrome" is a complex disorder in which symptoms—such as headaches and dizziness—may persist for weeks of months after a mild traumatic brain injury. These symptoms are often present in the absence of structural brain damage, which has also been described as "complicated" mild traumatic brain injury (Lange et al. 2009). Komura and colleagues studied 89 patients who suffered a single blunt mild traumatic brain injury without structural abnormalities and persistent mental and cognitive problems (Komura et al. 2019). Reduced metabolism was reported in the bilateral prefrontal area and significantly increased around the limbic system in the patient group compared with normal controls, which is different from patterns typically implicated in DAI. Mild chronic TBI due to cerebral concussion caused by repeated blast exposure in war zones has also been evaluated using ^{18}F-FDG PET (Peskind et al. 2011). The study included a group of Iraq war veterans ($N = 12$) and a control group ($N = 12$). The patient group showed hypometabolism in the cerebellum, vermis, pons, and medial region of the temporal lobe. The patients had mild cognitive dysfunction similar to that reported for patients with cerebellar lesions.

43.2.3 PET Imaging of Specific Cellular Process in Brain Trauma

Since the mid-2000s, several papers of great interest using other PET radiotracers to study specific cellular processes in TBI pathophysiology have been published. An example of these is ^{11}C-flumazenil (FMZ), which is a marker of central-type benzodiazepine receptor (BZR). FMZ binding, i.e., coupling of BZRs with GABA-A receptors, can be used as a marker of neuronal viability. The first study using $^{15}O_2$-PET and ^{11}C-FMZ PET (the binding potential of FMZ) investigated the relation between $CMRO_2$ abnormalities and loss of neuronal integrity in symptomatic patients with chronic TBI ($N = 10$), without structural abnormalities detected by MRI (Shiga et al. 2006). The study included a control group ($N = 10$). Image evaluation was done using ROI analysis. $CMRO_2$ abnormalities were observed in all patients, while reduced uptake in ^{11}C-FMZ BP images was only found in six patients. Reduced uptake in ^{11}C-FMZ BP images was accompanied by abnormalities in $CMRO_2$ images. In 15 lesions observed in $CMRO_2$ images, no abnormalities were found in ^{11}C-FMZ BP images, suggesting that ^{11}C-FMZ PET can be useful for differentiating hypometabolism caused by selective neuronal loss from hypometabolism caused by other factors. A more recent study using ^{11}C-FMZ PET aimed at identifying regional neuronal damage occurring in chronic diffuse TBI patients with neuropsychological impairment ($N = 8$) (Kawai et al. 2010). The study included a control group ($N = 20$). 3D SSP group comparisons showed significant bilateral reductions of ^{11}C-FMZ uptake in the frontal medial gyrus, anterior cingulate gyrus, and thalamus. Case-by-case analysis also found reduced ^{11}C-FMZ uptake in these regions, although the distribution and extent were different in each case. Furthermore, FIQ and performance IQ were negatively correlated with the degree of ^{11}C-FMZ BP reduction in the right thalamus. Likewise, FIQ, verbal IQ, and performance IQ were negatively correlated with the degree of ^{11}C-FMZ BP reduction in the left frontal medial gyrus.

We consider that even though these results are promising for detection of selective neuronal loss in patients with chronic diffuse TBI, they still require validation in larger patient samples and improvement of quantification methods. A recent study was aimed at validating reference tissue kinetic modeling of ^{11}C-FMZ PET within a group of patients with TBI (Geeraerts et al. 2011). ^{11}C-FMZ PET imaging were performed on controls ($N = 16$) and patients ($N = 11$) at least 6 months after TBI. Regional non-displaceable binding potentials (BP_{ND}) were estimated from five reference tissue models and compared to BP_{ND} from arterial input models. Total distribution volume of the pons was not significantly different between controls and patients. BP_{ND} from all the reference tissue approaches significantly correlated with BP_{ND} from the plasma input models for control and patient groups. Thus this study demonstrated the validity of the pons as a reference region for calculating ^{11}C-FMZ BP in apparently normal and perilesional regions in patients with chronic TBI.

More recently, adenosine receptor imaging has been used in an effort to identify neuronal and axonal injury in patients in the chronic phase of DAI. Hayashi and colleagues used A_1 receptor (A1R) [1-methyl-^{11}C] 8-dicyclopropylmethyl-1-methyl-3-propylxanthine (MPDX) PET in ten patients in the chronic phase of DAI and reported increased BPs in the lower frontal lobe, posterior cingulate cortex, and rolandic cortex, without any apparent decreases in BP (Hayashi et al. 2018). These areas did not correlate with regions of decreased ^{11}C-FMZ binding in the same patients, suggesting that the observed alterations using MPDX PET reflect neuroprotective effects rather than neuronal loss.

Another specific cell process recently examined in chronic TBI is the activity of the cholinergic system (Östberg et al. 2011). This preliminary study was carried out in a group of patients with chronic diffuse TBI with cognitive deficit ($N = 17$) and a control group ($N = 12$). PET studies were performed with [methyl-^{11}C]*N*-methylpiperidyl-4-acetate (^{11}C-MP4A). ^{11}C-MP4A reflects acetylcholinesterase (AChE) activity. Group comparisons by SPM showed a significant bilateral reduction of AChE in several areas of the neocortex in the TBI group, more pronounced in the parietal–occipital regions. ROI analysis also showed a significant reduction of AChE in all ROIs examined, except in the medial temporal region, probably associated with the relatively small size of the sample. Since the study sample only represents a certain type of TBI, we agree with the authors that it would be interesting to study larger and more varied samples. Moreover, it would be interesting to study what percentage of cases with TBI shows cholinergic dysfunction and whether this dysfunction correlates with clinical symptoms and outcome. This methodology could also be useful to clarify differences between patients with chronic TBI who respond to treatment with AChE inhibitors and those that do not respond.

The outcome of ^{11}C-NMSP/^{18}F-FDG microPET studies aimed at evaluating the effects of neural stem cell (NSC) transplantation in a TBI model in rats was recently published (Zhang et al. 2008). ^{11}C-NMSP (^{11}C-*N*-methylspiperone) is a radioligand for the dopamine receptor subtype 2 (D_2). The combination of microPET and a

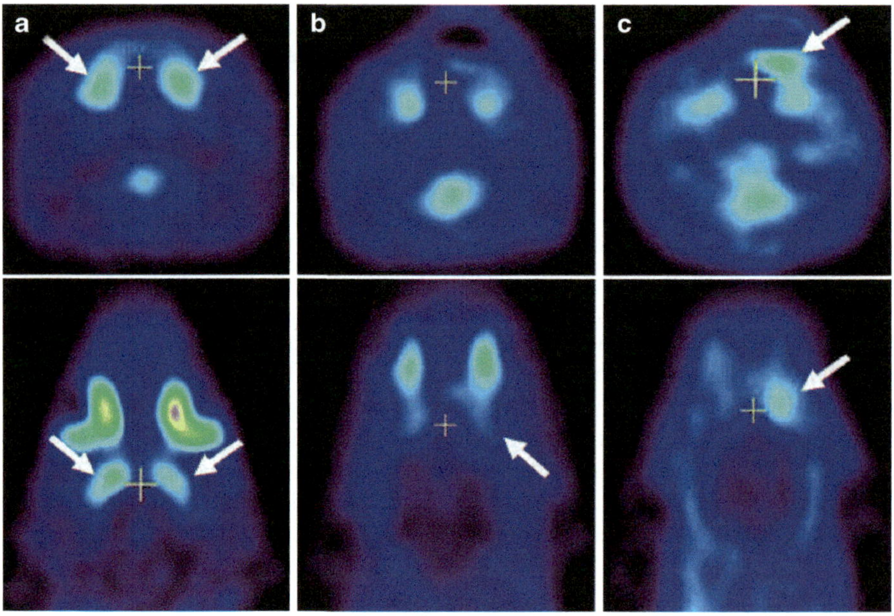

Fig. 43.1 Typical examples of ^{11}C-NMSP microPET imaging in various conditions. Coronal and axial sections of rat brain are shown. White cross markers in the coronal and axial sections indicate the same position in a scan. (**a**) Typical image of ^{11}C-NMSP microPET in normal rat brain showing high ^{11}C-NMSP accumulation in the striatum. (**b**) L/N ratio of ^{11}C-NMSP decreased after traumatic brain injury. (**c**) High accumulation of ^{11}C-NMSP indicated the existence of transplanted DRD2-positive NSCs. (From Zhang et al. (2008); with permission)

reporter gene system to track transplanted stem cells in animal experiments has allowed researchers to trace reporter gene carrying cells in vivo. The study was performed in a group of 18 rats with focal TBI in the right parietal lobe, later randomly assigned to a group that received a transplant ($N = 10$) and a control group ($N = 8$). In the former group, NSCs were transplanted in the brain lesion. ^{11}C-NMSP and ^{18}F-FDG microPET images were used to monitor changes in D_2 expression and glucose metabolism in the brain lesion before and after transplantation. Behavioral neurological function was also evaluated. Histological analysis identified viable NSCs at the transplantation site. The lesion-to-normal contralateral ratio (L/N ratio) of ^{11}C-NMSP in the brain lesion decreased from 97 to 68% after TBI, increasing to 137% 1 day after transplantation (Fig. 43.1) and later decreasing gradually. On the other hand, L/N ratio of glucose metabolism decreased to 35% in the brain lesion and then increased to 87% 2 weeks after transplantation (Fig. 43.2). The behavioral neurological function significantly improved in the transplanted group compared to the control group. Thus, this study demonstrates the feasibility of using microPET and a reporter gene system to evaluate NSC-induced D_2 expression in rat models, which could prove useful in future clinical trials of NSC transplantation therapy in TBI patients.

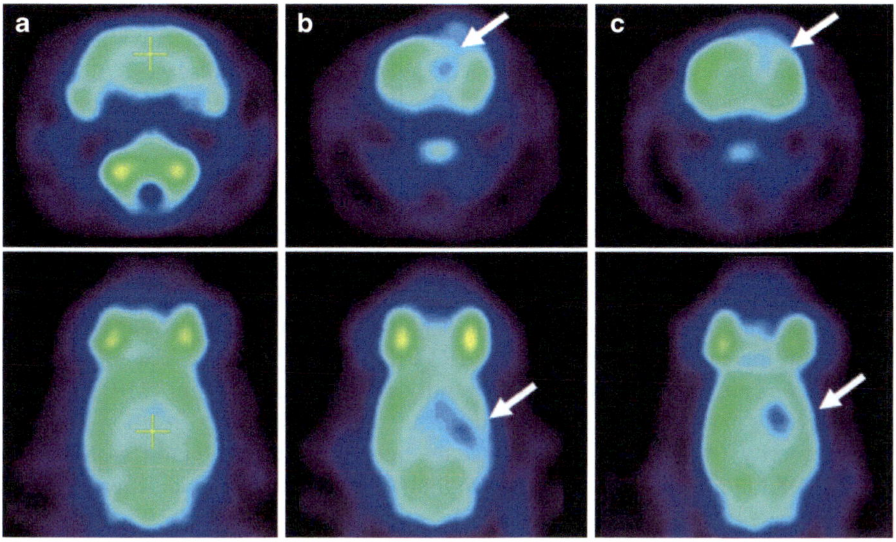

Fig. 43.2 Typical examples of ^{18}F-FDG microPET imaging in various conditions. Coronal and axial sections of rat brain are shown. (**a**) Typical image of ^{18}F-FDG microPET in normal rat brain. (**b**) As shown with *arrows*, the focal traumatic lesion appeared as a hypometabolic area in the right parietal cortex. (**c**) The regional glucose metabolism of the focal traumatic lesion recovered 14 days after NSC transplantation. (From Zhang et al. (2008); with permission)

43.2.3.1 PET Imaging of Neuroinflammation

Cellular processes that have received much attention lately are those involved in TBI neuroinflammation. Microglial, astrocyte, and neuron cells resident in the central nervous system begin to react in the acute TBI phase and eventually may be chronically activated. The role of activated microglia is to serve as the most important antigen-presenting cells and to synthesize inflammatory mediators and complement, which are crucial in the neuroinflammatory cascade after TBI. Microglia functions are very complex, since they have both neurotoxic and neuroprotective roles. In the acute phase, it may be involved in the restauration of the homeostasis in the brain. It has been hypothesized that chronic neuroinflammation may drive neurodegeneration after (repetitive) traumatic brain injury, which could be related to the release of pro-inflammatory cytokines, reactive oxygen species, nitrogen species, and excitatory neurotransmitters (Donat et al. 2017). Previous studies in TBI animal models have demonstrated that the inflammatory process may persist for at least a year, especially in the thalamus (Nagamoto-Combs et al. 2007, 2010). Human postmortem studies have also found microglial activation many years after TBI (Gentleman et al. 2004).

The neuroinflammatory response can be studied in vivo with PET using the radioligand ^{11}C-(R)-PK11195 (1-[2-chlorophenyl]-*N*-methyl-*N*-[1-methylpropyl]-3-isoquinoline carboxamide), which is a selective marker for activated microglia.

(R)-PK11195 binds to the 18 kDa translocator protein (TSPO), expressed in the mitochondria of activated microglia. ^{11}C-(R)-PK11195 PET has previously been used to study neuroinflammation in several neurodegenerative diseases.

The first studies using ^{11}C-(R)-PK11195 PET in TBI patients have been published recently (Folkersma et al. 2011; Ramlackhansingh et al. 2011). In the paper by Folkersma and coworkers, a patient group in chronic stage with moderate or severe TBI ($N = 8$) and a control group ($N = 7$) were studied. ^{11}C-(R)-PK11195 PET and MR images were acquired 6 months after TBI. ^{11}C-(R)-PK11195 BP_{ND} parametric images were generated. To generate a reference tissue input, the authors used supervised cluster analysis (Boellaard et al. 2008). Evaluation of the ^{11}C-(R)-PK11195 BP_{ND} was done in the whole brain and regionally. Group comparisons showed a significant increase of whole-brain ^{11}C-(R)-PK11195 BP_{ND} in the TBI group. This increase was not only observed in structurally affected brain regions (MRI) but also in apparently normal regions. On the other hand, there was no correlation between TBI severity (GCS) or neurological outcome (GOS) and whole-brain ^{11}C-(R)-PK11195 BP_{ND}. Although microglial activation is mostly a diffuse event in TBI, brain regions showing significant increases of ^{11}C-(R)-PK11195 BP_{ND} were the left and right frontal lobe, left and right thalamus, left parietal lobe, right temporal lobe, hippocampus and putamen, midbrain, and pons. An interesting finding was that ^{11}C-(R)-PK11195 BP_{ND} was maximal in the thalamus in six out of eight patients.

The study by Ramlackhansingh et al. (2011) investigated whether the inflammatory response persists in patients with chronic TBI and if this response was related to structural abnormalities and cognitive dysfunction. This paper included a group of patients with moderate to severe chronic TBI ($N = 10$). Five patients had focal damage visible in MR images, while the other five did not show abnormalities. ^{11}C-(R)-PK11195 PET was performed on all patients at least 11 months after TBI. Like in the previous study, ^{11}C-(R)-PK11195 BP_{ND} parametric images were generated using supervised cluster analysis. Volumetric MRI and DTI were done to evaluate focal damage and the disruption of WM. Cognitive function was also evaluated. Group comparisons showed that ^{11}C-(R)-PK11195 BP_{ND} was increased in the thalami, putamen, occipital cortices, and posterior limb of the internal capsules in the patient group compared with controls (Fig. 43.3). Unlike the study by Folkersma and coworkers, they found no increase in ^{11}C-(R)-PK11195 BP_{ND} at the original site of focal brain injury, which is probably due to the different intervals which had elapsed after TBI in both studies. In the patient sample, a positive correlation was observed between ^{11}C-(R)-PK11195 BP_{ND} in the thalamus and the degree of cognitive impairment. ^{11}C-(R)-PK11195 BP_{ND} increase was not associated with structural damage found by volumetric MRI and DTI or the time elapsed after TBI. Like in the article by Folkersma, persistent microglial activation in chronic TBI patients was confirmed especially in subcortical regions. Taking into account the long intervals after injury in the patient sample, this paper also suggests that therapeutic interventions can be beneficial even for a long time after TBI.

Over the past decades, new TSPO PET ligands have been developed with higher signal-to-noise ratios, including second- and third-generation ligands. After it

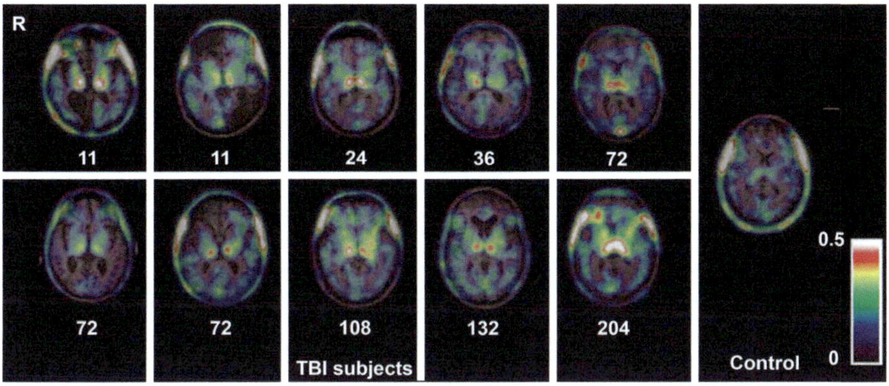

Fig. 43.3 Chronic microglial activation is present following traumatic brain injury (*TBI*). Overlay images of the transverse T1 magnetic resonance imaging at the level of the thalamus superimposed with ^{11}C-(R)-PK11195 (*PK*) images of all TBI subjects and a representative control subject. Numbers indicate time in months from the time of TBI to positron emission tomography scanning. Images illustrate the greater binding of PK in the thalami of all TBI subjects. *R* right. (From Ramlackhansingh et al. (2011); with permission)

became apparent that the binding of second-generation ligands was influenced by the rs6971 polymorphism (Ala147Thr) in the TSPO gene, efforts using third-generation ligands have shown promise to reduce this issue (Ikawa et al. 2017). Although its clinical value still has to be determined, these developments may eventually facilitate the use of TSPO PET as a biomarker after traumatic brain injury.

43.3 Single-Photon Emission Computed Tomography (SPECT)

Perfusion SPECT using ^{99m}Tc-hexamethyl-propyleneamine oxime (HMPAO) or ^{99m}Tc-ethylene cysteine dimer (ECD) has been extensively used in TBI. Reviews of this neuroimaging modality have appeared regularly in the last years (Davalos and Bennett 2002; Cihangiroglu et al. 2002; Belanger et al. 2007; Tikofsky 2010; Tong et al. 2011). These reviews coincide in pointing out that perfusion SPECT has high negative predictive value during the acute phase in mild TBI. They also agree that perfusion SPECT, like ^{18}F-FDG PET, is more sensitive than CT for identifying abnormalities in TBI during the first hours, detecting them in very early stages, when CT (or MRI) scans may still be negative. Abnormalities detected by perfusion SPECT are more extensive than those observed by structural neuroimaging. A recent study shows that the combination of structural neuroimages, such as CT, with perfusion SPECT using ^{99m}Tc-ECD is useful to determine the extent and severity of TBI lesions and tissue viability in core, edema, and perilesional tissue (Pifarré et al. 2011). Figure 43.4 shows CT and SPECT perfusion imaging of a patient with left frontal primarily brain trauma.

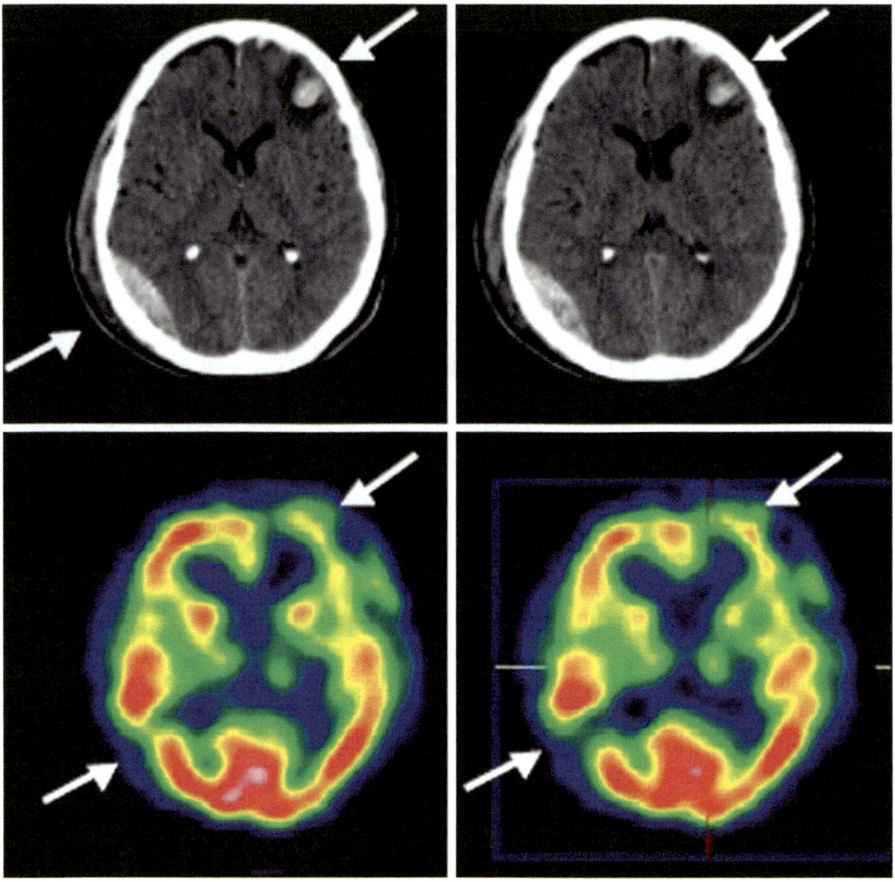

Fig. 43.4 CT and SPECT perfusion imaging of a patient with left frontal primarily brain trauma. In the hemorrhagic lesion seen on the CT in the right posterior temporal region, SPECT images show an absence of perfusion. (From Pifarré et al. (2011))

Furthermore, using SPECT, it is possible to study cell-specific processes related to TBI pathophysiology. Studies combining ^{123}I-2-β-carbomethoxy-3-β-(4-iodophenyl) tropane (β-CIT) and ^{123}I-iodobenzamide (IBZM) found nigrostriatal dysfunction in TBI patients, although the striatum was structurally relatively preserved, suggesting these studies may be useful in the evaluation of therapies directed toward reducing parkinsonian symptoms in TBI patients (Donnemiller et al. 2000). Another very recent animal study used *N′*,*N′*-diethyl-6-chloro-(4′-[^{123}I]iodophenyl) imidazo[1,2-*a*]pyridine-3-acetamide (^{123}I-CLINDE) for the in vivo monitoring of neuroinflammation by SPECT (Mattner et al. 2011). ^{123}I-CLINDE is a highly specific radioligand for TSPO. A recent perfusion SPECT activation study investigated cognitive fatigue mechanisms in patients with mild TBI (Hattori et al. 2009). In this study, it was possible to show that there is a frontocerebellar dissociation in patients with mild TBI that may explain cognitive impairment and cognitive fatigue in the chronic phase.

Technological advances in SPECT detector systems, hybrid SPECT–CT, continuous development of new gamma-emitting radioligands, and the application of modern methods of image analysis make the SPECT technique a valid alternative for the study of TBI, both for clinical practice and for research. Nevertheless, like ^{18}F-FDG PET, evidence-based imaging studies are required to demonstrate its incremental validity in TBI. The main advantage of SPECT is that it is much less costly and is still more widely available on a worldwide scale in comparison to PET.

43.4 Conclusions

In the acute TBI phase, ^{18}F-FDG PET seems to be more useful and has prognostic value in patients whose neurological state cannot be explained by structural neuroimages. However, evidence-based imaging studies are necessary to demonstrate the incremental validity of ^{18}F-FDG PET together with cost-effectiveness analysis to appropriately compare ^{18}F-FDG PET with other neuroimaging techniques. Whichever the results of these studies, ^{18}F-FDG PET and $^{15}O_2$-PET will remain very valuable tools for research of the complex and not yet fully understood pathophysiology of acute-phase TBI. In chronic TBI patients, most of the ^{18}F-FDG PET studies coincide in indicating a diffuse cortical–subcortical pattern of hypometabolism associated with cognitive impairment, even in patients without evident structural abnormalities. Preliminary studies also suggest the usefulness of ^{18}F-FDG PET for the evaluation of different therapeutic approaches for improving cognitive function in chronic TBI. In recent years, interest in studying cell-specific processes involved in TBI pathophysiology with PET is growing. Most considerably, tau PET ligands became available, which have allowed in vivo imaging of tauopathy in subjects who were exposed to (repetitive) traumatic brain injury. Another interesting application has been the imaging of markers of neuroinflammation using TSPO PET. Neuroinflammation imaging could become very attractive for detecting secondary damage after TBI, possibly with higher sensitivity than ^{18}F-FDG PET. Furthermore, it could serve in the evaluation of different therapeutic approaches, especially with the arrival of more sensitive third-generation TSPO ligands Finally, SPECT is a valid alternative for the study of TBI. However, as with PET, evidence-based imaging studies are required to demonstrate its incremental validity. SPECT is much less expensive and more widely available on a global scale.

References

Abate M, Trivedi M, Fryer TD et al (2008) Early derangements in oxygen and glucose metabolism following head injury: the ischemic penumbra and pathophysiological heterogeneity. Neurocrit Care 9:319–325

Alavi A (1989) Functional and anatomic studies of head injury. J Neuropsychiatry Clin Neurosci 1:S45–S50

Alavi A, Mirot A, Newberg A et al (1997) Fluorine-18-FDG evaluation of crossed cerebellar diaschisis in head injury. J Nucl Med 38:1717–1720

Bassett DS, Bullmore ET (2009) Human brain networks in health and disease. Curr Opin Neurol 22:340–347
Belanger HG, Vanderploeg RD, Curtiss G et al (2007) Recent neuroimaging techniques in mild traumatic brain injury. J Neuropsychiatry Clin Neurosci 19:5–20
Bergsneider M, Hovda DA, Shalmon E et al (1997) Cerebral hyperglycolysis following severe traumatic brain injury in humans: a positron emission tomography study. J Neurosurg 86:241–251
Bergsneider M, Hovda DA, Lee SM et al (2000) Dissociation of cerebral glucose metabolism and level of consciousness during the period of metabolic depression following human traumatic brain injury. J Neurotrauma 17:389–401
Bergsneider M, Hovda DA, McArthur DL et al (2001) Metabolic recovery following human traumatic brain injury based on FDG-PET: time course and relationship to neurological disability. J Head Trauma Rehabil 16:135–148
Boellaard R, Turkheimer F, Hinz R et al (2008) Performance of a modified supervised cluster algorithm for extracting reference region input function from [11C](R)-PK11195 brain PET studies. In IEEE Nucl Sci Symp Conf Rec 5400–5402
Bullock R, Chestnut RM, Clifton G et al (2007) Guidelines for the management of severe traumatic brain injury, 3rd ed. J Neurotrauma 24(Suppl 1):S26–S31
Byrnes KR, Wilson CM, Brabazon F, von Leden R, Jurgens JS, Oakes TR, Selwyn RG (2014) FDG-PET imaging in mild traumatic brain injury: a critical review. Front Neuroenerg 5:13
Cihangiroglu M, Ramsey RG, Dohrmann GJ (2002) Brain injury: analysis of imaging modalities. Neurol Res J24:7–18
Coles J, Fryer T (2004) ^{15}O PET imaging of cerebral metabolism and ischaemia following traumatic brain injury: defining the ischaemic brain volume. J Cereb Blood Flow Metab 24:191–201
Coles JP, Fryer TD, Smielewski P et al (2004a) Incidence and mechanisms of cerebral ischemia in early clinical head injury. J Cereb Blood Flow Metab 24:202–211
Coles JP, Steiner LA, Johnston AJ et al (2004b) Does induced hypertension reduce cerebral ischaemia within the traumatized human brain? Brain 127:2479–2490
Coles JP, Fryer TD, Coleman MR et al (2006) Hyperventilation following head injury: effect on ischemic burden and cerebral oxidative metabolism. Crit Care Med 35:568–578
Cunningham AS, Salvador R, Coles JP et al (2005) Physiological thresholds for irreversible tissue damage in contusional regions following traumatic brain injury. Brain 128:1931–1942
Dagal A, Lam AM (2011) Cerebral blood flow and the injured brain: how should we monitor and manipulate it? Curr Opin Anaesthesiol 24:131–137
Davalos DB, Bennett TL (2002) A review of the use of single-photon emission computerized tomography as a diagnostic tool in mild traumatic brain injury. Appl Neuropsychol 9:92–105
Diringer MN, Aiyagari V, Zazulia AR et al (2007) Effect of hyperoxia on cerebral metabolic rate for oxygen measured using positron emission tomography in patients with acute severe head injury. J Neurosurg 106:526–529
Diringer MN, Scalfani M, Zazulia A et al (2011) Effect of mannitol on cerebral blood volume in patients with head injury. Neurosurgery 70(5):1215–1219. https://doi.org/10.1227/NEU.0b013e3182417bc2
Donat CK, Scott G, Gentleman SM, Sastre M (2017) Microglial activation in traumatic brain injury. Front Aging Neurosci 9:208
Donnemiller E, Brenneis C, Wissel J et al (2000) Impaired dopaminergic neurotransmission in patients with traumatic brain injury: a SPET study using (123)I-beta-CIT and (123)I-IBZM. Eur J Nucl Med Mol Imaging 27:1410–1414
Faul M, Xu L, Wald MM et al (2010) Traumatic brain injury in the United States: Emergency Department Visits, Hospitalizations and Deaths 2002–2006. Centers for Disease Control and Prevention, National Center for Injury Prevention and Control, Atlanta. http://cdc.gov/TraumaticBrainInjury
Folkersma H, Boellaard R, Yaqub M et al (2011) Widespread and prolonged increase in (R)-(^{11})C-PK11195 binding after traumatic brain injury. J Nucl Med 52:1235–1239
Fontaine A, Azouvi P, Remy P et al (1999) Functional anatomy of neuropsychological deficits after severe traumatic brain injury. Neurology 53:1963–1968

Frey LC (2003) Epidemiology of posttraumatic epilepsy: a critical review. Epilepsia 44:11–17
Friston KJ (1994) Statistical parametric mapping. In: Thatcher RW, Hallet M, Zeffiro T, John ER, Huerta M (eds) Functional neuroimaging. Academic, New York
Garcia-Panach J, Lull N, Jose Lull J et al (2011) A voxel-based analysis of FDG-PET in traumatic brain injury: regional metabolism and relationship between the thalamus and cortical areas. J Neurotrauma 28:1707–1717
Geeraerts T, Coles JP, Aigbirhio FI et al (2011) Validation of reference tissue modelling for [(11) C]flumazenil positron emission tomography following head injury. Ann Nucl Med 25:396–405
Gentleman SM, Leclercq PD, Moyes L et al (2004) Long-term intracerebral inflammatory response after traumatic brain injury. Forensic Sci Int 146:97–104
Gupta AK, Hutchinson PJ, Fryer T et al (2002) Measurement of brain tissue oxygenation performed using positron emission tomography scanning to validate a novel monitoring method. J Neurosurg 96:263–268
Haller S, Vernooij MW, Kuijer JPA, Larsson EM, Jager HR, Barkhof F (2018) Cerebral microbleeds: imaging and clinical significance. Radiology 287(1):11–28
Hattori N, Huang SC, Wu HM et al (2003) Correlation of regional metabolic rates of glucose with Glasgow Coma Scale after traumatic brain injury. J Nucl Med 44:1709–1716
Hattori N, Huang SC, Wu HM et al (2004) Acute changes in regional cerebral ^{18}F-FDG kinetics in patients with traumatic brain injury. J Nucl Med 45:775–783
Hattori N, Swan M, Stobbe GA et al (2009) Differential SPECT activation patterns associated with PASAT performance may indicate frontocerebellar functional dissociation in chronic mild traumatic brain injury. J Nucl Med 50:1054–1061
Hayashi S, Inaji M, Nariai T, Oda K, Sakata M, Toyohara J, Ishii K, Ishiwata K, Maehara T (2018) Increased binding potential of brain adenosine A1 receptor in chronic stages of patients with diffuse axonal injury measured with [1-methyl-(11)C] 8-dicyclopropylmethyl-1-methyl-3-propylxanthine Positron Emission Tomography Imaging. J Neurotrauma 35(1):25–31
Hunter JV, Wilde EA, Tong KA et al (2012) Emerging imaging tools for use with traumatic. Brain Injury Res J Neurotrauma 29:654–671
Hutchinson PJ, Gupta AK, Fryer TF et al (2002) Correlation between cerebral blood flow, substrate delivery, and metabolism in head injury: a combined microdialysis and triple oxygen positron emission tomography study. J Cereb Blood Flow Metab 22:735–745
Hutchinson PJ, O'Connell MT, Seal A et al (2009) A combined microdialysis and FDG-PET study of glucose metabolism in head injury. Acta Neurochir 151:51–61
Ikawa M, Lohith TG, Shrestha S, Telu S, Zoghbi SS, Castellano S, Taliani S, Da Settimo F, Fujita M, Pike VW, Innis RB, Biomarkers Consortium Radioligand Project Team (2017) 11C-ER176, a radioligand for 18-kDa translocator protein, has adequate sensitivity to robustly image all three affinity genotypes in human brain. J Nucl Med 58(2):320–325
Ito K, Asano Y, Ikegame Y, Shinoda J (2016) Differences in brain metabolic impairment between chronic mild/moderate TBI patients with and without visible brain lesions based on MRI. BioMed Res Int 2016:3794029
Johnston AJ, Steiner LA, Coles JP et al (2005) Effect of cerebral perfusion pressure augmentation on regional oxygenation and metabolism after head injury. Crit Care Med 33:189–195
Kato T, Nakayama N, Yasokawa Y et al (2007) Statistical image analysis of cerebral glucose metabolism in patients with cognitive impairment following diffuse traumatic brain injury. J Neurotrauma 24:919–926
Kawai N, Nakamura T, Tamiya T et al (2008) Metabolic disturbance without brain ischemia in traumatic brain injury: a positron emission tomography study. Acta Neurochir Suppl 102:241–245
Kawai N, Maeda Y, Kudomi N et al (2010) Focal neuronal damage in patients with neuropsychological impairment after diffuse traumatic brain injury: evaluation using (11)C-flumazenil positron emission tomography with statistical image analysis. J Neurotrauma 27:2131–2138
Kim YW, Kim DY, Shin JC et al (2009) The changes of cortical metabolism associated with the clinical response to donepezil therapy in traumatic brain injury. Clin Neuropharmacol 32:63–68
Kim Y, Shin JC, Ys A (2010) Changes in cerebral glucose metabolism in patients with posttraumatic cognitive impairment after memantine therapy: a preliminary study. Ann Nucl Med 24:363–369

Komura A, Kawasaki T, Yamada Y, Uzuyama S, Asano Y, Shinoda J (2019) Cerebral glucose metabolism in patients with chronic mental and cognitive sequelae after a single blunt mild traumatic brain injury without visible brain lesions. J Neurotrauma 36(5):641–649
Kraus MF, Smith GS, Butters M et al (2005) Effects of the dopaminergic agent and NMDA receptor antagonist amantadine on cognitive function, cerebral glucose metabolism and D2 receptor availability in chronic traumatic brain injury: a study using positron emission tomography (PET). Brain Inj 19:471–479
Kubal WS (2012) Updated imaging of traumatic brain injury. Radiol Clin N Am 50:15–41
Lange RT, Iverson GL, Franzen MD (2009) Neuropsychological functioning following complicated vs. uncomplicated mild traumatic brain injury. Brain Injury 23(2):83–91
Langfitt TW, Obrist WD, Alavi A et al (1986) Computerized tomography, magnetic resonance imaging, and positron emission tomography in the study of brain trauma. J Neurosurg 64:760–767
Ley E, Park R (2010) In vivo effect of propranolol dose and timing on cerebral perfusion after traumatic brain injury. J Trauma 68:353–356
Ley EJ, Scehnet J, Park R et al (2009) The in vivo effect of propranolol on cerebral perfusion and hypoxia after traumatic brain injury. J Trauma 66:154–161
Liu YR, Cardamone L, Hogan R et al (2010) Progressive metabolic and structural cerebral perturbations after traumatic brain injury: an in vivo imaging study in the rat. J Nucl Med 51:1788–1795
Lull N, Noe E, Jose Lull J et al (2010) Voxel-based statistical analysis of thalamic glucose metabolism in traumatic brain injury: relationship with consciousness and cognition. Brain Inj 24:1098–1107
Lupi A, Bertagnoni G, Salgarello M et al (2007) Cerebellar vermis relative hypermetabolism: an almost constant PET finding in an injured brain. Clin Nucl Med 32:445–451
Lupi A, Bertagnoni G, Borghero A et al (2011) Relative hypermetabolism of vermis cerebelli in traumatic brain injured patients studied with 18FDG PET: a descriptor of brain damage and a possible predictor of outcome. Curr Radiopharm 4:167–175
Maas AI, Stocchetti N, Bullock R (2008) Moderate and severe traumatic brain injury in adults. Lancet Neurol 7:728–741
Marklund N, Sihver S, Hovda D et al (2009) Increased cerebral uptake of [18F]fluoro-deoxyglucose but not [1-14c]glucose early following traumatic brain injury in rats. J Neurotrauma 26:1281–1293
Mattner F, Bandin DL, Staykova M et al (2011) Evaluation of [(123)I]-CLINDE as a potent SPECT radiotracer to assess the degree of astroglia activation in cuprizone-induced neuroinflammation. Eur J Nucl Med Mol Imaging 38:1516–1528
McKee AC, Cantu RC, Nowinski CJ et al (2009) Chronic traumatic encephalopathy in athletes: progressive tauopathy after repetitive head injury. J Neuropathol Exp Neurol 68:709–735
McKee AC, Cairns NJ, Dickson DW, Folkerth RD, Keene CD, Litvan I, Perl DP, Stein TD, Vonsattel JP, Stewart W, Tripodis Y, Crary JF, Bieniek KF, Dams-O'Connor K, Alvarez VE, Gordon WA, TBI/CTE group (2016) The first NINDS/NIBIB consensus meeting to define neuropathological criteria for the diagnosis of chronic traumatic encephalopathy. Acta Neuropathologica 131(1):75–86
Medina LS, Blackmore CC, Applegate KE et al (2011) Principles of evidence-based imaging. In: Medina LS, Blackmore CC (eds) Evidence-based imaging: improving the quality of imaging in patient care. Springer, New York
Menon DKP, Coles JPP, Gupta AKF et al (2004) Diffusion limited oxygen delivery following head injury. Crit Care Med 32:1384–1390
Nagamoto-Combs K, Mcneal DW, Morecraft RJ et al (2007) Prolonged microgliosis in the rhesus monkey central nervous system after traumatic brain injury. J Neurotrauma 24:1719–1742
Nagamoto-Combs K, Morecraft RJ, Darling WG et al (2010) Long-term gliosis and molecular changes in the cervical spinal cord of the rhesus monkey after traumatic brain injury. J Neurotrauma 27:565–585
Nakashima T, Nakayama N, Miwa K et al (2007) Focal brain glucose hypometabolism in patients with neuropsychologic deficits after diffuse axonal injury. AJNR Am J Neuroradiol 28:236–242

Nakayama N, Okumura A, Shinoda J et al (2006) Relationship between regional cerebral metabolism and consciousness disturbance in traumatic diffuse brain injury without large focal lesions: an FDG-PET study with statistical parametric mapping analysis. J Neurol Neurosurg Psychiatry 77:856–862

Nortje J, Coles JP, Timofeev I et al (2008) Effect of hyperoxia on regional oxygenation and metabolism after severe traumatic brain injury: preliminary findings. Crit Care Med 36:273–281

O'Connell MT, Seal A, Nortje J et al (2005) Glucose metabolism in traumatic brain injury: a combined microdialysis and [(18)F]-2-fluoro-2-deoxy-D-glucose-positron emission tomography (FDG-PET) study. Acta Neurochir Suppl 95:165–168

Okonkwo DO, Puffer RC, Minhas DS, Beers SR, Edelman KL, Sharpless J, Laymon CM, Lopresti BJ, Benso S, Puccio AM, Pathak S, Ikonomovic MD, Mettenburg JM, Schneider W, Mathis CA, Mountz JM (2019) [(18)F]FDG, [(11)C]PiB, and [(18)F]AV-1451 PET imaging of neurodegeneration in two subjects with a history of repetitive trauma and cognitive decline. Front Neurol 10:831

Omalu BI, Hamilton RL, Kamboh MI, DeKosky ST, Bailes J (2010) Chronic traumatic encephalopathy (CTE) in a National Football League Player: case report and emerging medicolegal practice questions. J Forensic Nurs 6(1):40–46

Östberg A, Virta J, Rinne JO et al (2011) Cholinergic dysfunction after traumatic brain injury: preliminary findings from a PET study. Neurology 76:1046–1050

Park E, Bell JD, Baker AJ (2008) Traumatic brain injury: can the consequences be stopped? CMAJ 178:1163–1170

Peskind ER, Petrie EC, Cross DJ et al (2011) Cerebrocerebellar hypometabolism associated with repetitive blast exposure mild traumatic brain injury in 12 Iraq war Veterans with persistent post-concussive symptoms. NeuroImage 54(Suppl 1):S76–S82

Pifarré P, Cuberas G, Benejam B et al (2011) Cerebral blood flow measurement in the assessment of post-traumatic cerebral contusions. Open J Radiol 1:21–27

Ramlackhansingh AF, Brooks DJ, Greenwood RJ et al (2011) Inflammation after trauma: microglial activation and traumatic brain injury. Ann Neurol 70:374–383

Rao N, Turski PA, Polcyn RE et al (1984) F-18 positron emission computed-tomography in closed head-injury. Arch Phys Med Rehabil 65:780–785

Robertson C (2004) Mitochondrial dysfunction contributes to cell death following traumatic brain injury in adult and immature animals. J Bioenerg Biomembr 36:363–368

Shiga T, Ikoma K, Katoh C et al (2006) Loss of neuronal integrity: a cause of hypometabolism in patients with traumatic brain injury without MRI abnormality in the chronic stage. Eur J Nucl Med Mol Imaging 33:817–822

Stern RA, Adler CH, Chen K, Navitsky M, Luo J, Dodick DW, Alosco ML, Tripodis Y, Goradia DD, Martin B, Mastroeni D, Fritts NG, Jarnagin J, Devous MD, Mintun MA, Pontecorvo MJ, Shenton ME, Reiman EM (2019) Tau Positron-Emission Tomography in Former National Football League Players. N Engl J Med 380(18):1716–1725

Stryke J, Stalnacke B, Sojka P et al (2007) Traumatic brain injuries in a well-defined population: epidemiological aspects and severity. J Neurotrauma 24:1425–1436

Tagliaferri F, Compagnone C, Korsic M et al (2006) A systematic review of brain injury epidemiology in Europe. Acta Neurochir 148:255–268

Takahata K, Kimura Y, Sahara N, Koga S, Shimada H, Ichise M, Saito F, Moriguchi S, Kitamura S, Kubota M, Umeda S, Niwa F, Mizushima J, Morimoto Y, Funayama M, Tabuchi H, Bieniek KF, Kawamura K, Zhang MR, Dickson DW, Mimura M, Kato M, Suhara T, Higuchi M (2019) PET-detectable tau pathology correlates with long-term neuropsychiatric outcomes in patients with traumatic brain injury. Brain 142(10):3265–3279

Tenjin H, Ueda S, Mizukawa N et al (1990) Positron emission tomographic studies on cerebral hemodynamics in patients with cerebral contusion. Neurosurgery 26:971–979

Tikofsky RS (2010) Traumatic brain injury: SPECT and PET. In: Van Heertum RL, Tikofsky RS, Ichise M (eds) Functional cerebral SPECT and PET imaging, 4th edn. Wolters Kluwer Lippincott Williams & Wilkins, Philadelphia

Tong KA, Oyoyo UE, Holshouser BA et al (2011) Neuroimaging for traumatic brain injury. In: Medina LS, Blackmore CC (eds) Evidence-based imaging: improving the quality of imaging in patient care. Springer, New York

Vespa P, Bergsneider M, Hattori N et al (2005) Metabolic crisis without brain ischemia is common after traumatic brain injury: a combined microdialysis and positron emission tomography study. J Cereb Blood Flow Metab 25:763–774

WHO/OMS (2009) Global status report on road safety: time for action. World Health Organisation, Geneva. http://whqlibdoc.who.int/publications/2009/9789241563840_eng.pdf

Wu HM, Huang SC, Hattori N et al (2004a) Selective metabolic reduction in gray matter acutely following human traumatic brain injury. J Neurotrauma 21:149–161

Wu HM, Huang SC, Hattori N et al (2004b) Subcortical white matter metabolic chances remote from focal hemorrhagic lesions suggest diffuse injury after human traumatic brain injury. Neurosurgery 55:1306–1317

Xu Y, McArthur DL, Alger JR et al (2010) Early nonischemic oxidative metabolic dysfunction leads to chronic brain atrophy in traumatic brain injury. J Cereb Blood Flow Metab 30:883–894

Yamaki T, Yoshino E, Fujimoto M et al (1996) Chronological positron emission tomographic study of severe diffuse brain injury in the chronic stage. J Trauma 40:50–56

Zasler ND, Katz D, Zafonte RD (2007) Brain injury medicine: principles and practice. Demos Medical Publishing, New York

Zhang H, Zheng X, Yang X et al (2008) ^{11}C-NMSP/18F-FDG microPET to monitor neural stem cell transplantation in a rat model of traumatic brain injury. Eur J Nucl Med Mol Imaging 35:1699–1708

Zhang J, Mitsis EM, Chu K et al (2010) Statistical parametric mapping and cluster counting analysis of [(18)F] FDG-PET imaging in traumatic brain injury. J Neurotrauma 27:35–49

Part VIII

Other Subjects

Anaesthesia and PET of the Brain 44

Anthony Absalom and Ram Adapa

Contents

Abstract

Although drugs have been used to administer general anaesthesia for more than a century and a half, relatively little was known until recently about the molecular and cellular effects of the anaesthetic agents and the neurobiology of anaes-

A. Absalom (✉)
Department of Anesthesiology, University Medical Center Groningen, Groningen University, Groningen, The Netherlands
e-mail: a.r.absalom@umcg.nl

R. Adapa
Anaesthetic Department, Addenbrooke's Hospital, Cambridge, UK
e-mail: ra342@cam.ac.uk

R. A. J. O. Dierckx et al. (eds.), *PET and SPECT in Neurology*,
https://doi.org/10.1007/978-3-030-53168-3_44

thesia. Positron emission tomography (PET) and single-photon emission computed tomography (SPECT) studies have played a valuable role in improving this knowledge. PET studies using ^{11}C-flumazenil binding have been used to demonstrate that the molecular action of some, but not all, of the current anaesthetic agents is mediated via the $GABA_A$ receptor. Using different tracers labelled with ^{18}F, ^{11}C and ^{15}O, PET studies have shown the patterns of changes in cerebral metabolism and blood flow associated with different intravenous and volatile anaesthetic agents. Within classes of volatile agents, there are minor variations in patterns. More profound differences are found between classes of agents. Interestingly, all agents cause alterations in the blood flow and metabolism of the thalamus, providing strong support for the hypothesis that the anaesthetic agents interfere with consciousness by interfering with thalamocortical communication.

44.1 Introduction

Every day, around the world, a large number of patients receive sedative and anaesthetic agents for sedation and anaesthesia in intensive care units, in operating theatres and in other centres where diagnostic and therapeutic procedures are performed. Despite this and the fact that anaesthetic drugs have been used regularly since the 1840s, surprisingly, little is known about the state of anaesthesia, the mechanism and site of action of the anaesthetic agents and the longer-term consequences of sedation and anaesthesia. In the early 1990s, so little was known about the state of anaesthesia that Christof Koch co-wrote a serious article discussing the basic question ‘Does anaesthesia cause loss of consciousness?’ (Kulli and Koch 1991). In the decades since, significant progress has been made, thanks mostly to developments in technologies for functional imaging, such as PET, but still many fundamental questions remain unanswered! Part of the reason for slow progress is the current limited understanding of the neurobiology of consciousness.

Although anaesthesia is sometimes required for clinical PET scanning of the brain and other organs, the anaesthetic management of patients undergoing scanning will not be discussed here. Rather, this chapter will focus on the application of PET brain scanning techniques to studies of the neurobiology of anaesthesia.

44.2 Consciousness and Unconsciousness

One of the aims of anaesthesia is to induce loss of consciousness and prevent return of consciousness during a surgical procedure. Consciousness is an ethereal concept, whose nature and meaning have been debated for centuries. Today, most people believe it to be a subjective experience resulting from the electrical activity of the neurons in the brain (or more accurately the co-ordinated activity of assemblies or networks of neurons). Generally, we infer that an individual is conscious on the basis of his behaviour, his interactions with his environment and his reports of his experiences.

Medically, we define unconsciousness as an absence of wakefulness, alertness and awareness, but inferences that these are absent are usually based on the absence of behavioural responses to external stimuli. There are several circumstances when such inferences may not be true, as in patients with the 'locked-in' syndrome. In anaesthetic practice, we commonly administer doses of opioid drugs that obtund responses to stimuli (but do not necessarily by themselves prevent consciousness), and in patients presumed to be unconscious, we often administer drugs that paralyze the muscles but do not alter consciousness.

The literature contains a wide range of published incidences of the so-called problem of accidental awareness of general anaesthesia with subsequent recall of intraoperative events (AAGA). The differences arise mostly from differences in study population and methodology. The reported incidence also appears to be higher when structured postoperative interviews are used to test for explicit recall (Mashour et al. 2013; Walker et al. 2016), with incidences in large trials of the 1–2 out of every 1000 patients undergoing anaesthesia (Sandin et al. 2000; Sebel et al. 2004). A recent large UK national audit project (NAP5) indicated that the incidence of spontaneous complaints of AAGA is much lower (~1: 19,000 patients) but higher in specific patient populations and a wide range of psychological consequences (Pandit et al. 2014). The incidence of awareness during surgery without subsequent recall is not known but is likely to be much higher (Absalom and Green 2013).

44.3 Definition of Anaesthesia

Due to the combined problems of a poor understanding of consciousness and of the effects of anaesthetic drugs on the brain, anaesthesia has been very difficult to define and has largely been defined on the basis of the absence of features of consciousness. For most of the history of the practice of anaesthesia, anaesthesiologists have tended to define adequate clinical anaesthesia as a triad of 'hypnosis', analgesia and muscle relaxation. In anaesthetic jargon, anaesthetic-induced loss of consciousness is referred to as 'hypnosis' and anaesthesia-inducing drugs as 'hypnotics'. The term 'analgesia' was previously used to refer more generally to the (desired) loss of autonomic responses to painful stimuli, and muscle relaxation referred to the desire of the surgeon for a lack of patient movement and for some operations a reduction in muscle tone. Early volatile anaesthetic agents were able to suppress consciousness and, in sufficiently large doses, were able to suppress autonomic responses (tachycardia, hypertension) and reduce muscular tone. These latter effects are mediated by separate actions of the drugs on different parts of the nervous system and on the cardiovascular system and are not part of a single spectrum of effects at a single site (Prys-Roberts 1987; Kissin 1993). Thus, modern clinical practice involves administration of different 'purer' agents targeted at different elements of this triad—modest doses of hypnotic agents for suppression of consciousness, local and systemic analgesic drugs for suppression of autonomic responses and neuromuscular blocking agents for muscle relaxation or paralysis where that is required. With this approach, more attention is now focused on the cognitive aspects of anaesthesia, with anaesthesia being defined as a drug-induced reversible state of unconsciousness principally characterized by a lack of awareness of, and subsequent memory for, intraoperative events.

Thus, this chapter will focus on the use of PET technology to understand the main component of anaesthesia, 'hypnosis', and will not deal with functional imaging of pain perception and analgesia.

44.4 Why Study Anaesthesia?

In current clinical practice, many anaesthesiologists err on the side of deeper anaesthesia in the hope of avoiding the problem of anaesthetic awareness. This is not an ideal approach since all the anaesthetic agents in current use possess dose-related adverse effects, such as depression of the cardiovascular and immune systems.

Earlier studies suggested an association between excessive depth of anaesthesia (i.e. an excessive dose) and mortality within 1 and 2 years (Monk et al. 2005; Lindholm et al. 2009). A recent large randomized controlled trial however indicated that there was no difference in 1-year mortality between light general anaesthesia and deep general anaesthesia in elderly patients (Short et al. 2019).

Animal evidence suggests that in the extremes of age (i.e. in the very young and the elderly), anaesthetic agents may be neurotoxic.

There is a plethora of evidence that exposure of a wide variety of animals to the commonly used anaesthetic agents during the neonatal period results in neuronal injury and associated cognitive changes (Jevtovic-Todorovic et al. 2013). Epidemiological studies of neonatal exposure to anaesthetic agents have shown conflicting results, whereas a randomized controlled trial in human neonates showed no evidence of changes in cognitive function at 3 and 5 years after exposure (Davidson et al. 2016; McCann et al. 2019).

While there is some in vitro evidence that anaesthetic agents may promote Alzheimer's disease-type changes (Mandal and Fodale 2009; Whittington et al. 2011), so far, there is no convincing clinical evidence that anaesthetic exposure enhances neurodegenerative processes in the ageing brain.

Studies of the molecular mechanisms of action of the anaesthetic agents offer much more than simply satisfying the curiosity of anaesthesiologists. Better knowledge of the molecular mechanism may inform the development of newer agents, specifically designed to have a broader therapeutic range and fewer adverse effects.

Furthermore, studies of the mechanism of action of the anaesthetic agents may provide information about the nature of, and the mechanisms of, consciousness itself. Here, the hypnotics or sedatives used could be regarded as probes, by which investigators can interfere with different cognitive functions, to help shed light on functions such as speech processing and memory functions (Davis et al. 2007; Adapa et al. 2014; Naci et al. 2018), alertness, wakefulness, awareness and consciousness itself (Arhem et al. 2003; Lydic and Baghdoyan 2005; Hameroff 2006; Mashour 2006; Franks 2008; Alkire et al. 2008b; Brown et al. 2010; Varley et al. 2019). Once again, this knowledge has practical relevance, since a better understanding of memory function, and of the interactions among anaesthetic agents and stress on awareness and memory function, may inform methods of detecting and preventing inadvertent awareness with subsequent recall of intraoperative events.

44.5 Available Tools for Studying Anaesthesia

To fully understand anaesthesia, multiple layers and domains of knowledge are required, starting with the molecular effects (or possibly at submolecular level), explaining how these influence the function of individual neurons and how these influence the interactions or communication among networks or assemblies of other neurons, before making the jump to explain how the perturbed electrical and other activities in these assemblies or networks of neurons eventually result in impairment or absence of consciousness.

Different techniques lend themselves to study of different parts of this chain of events. Molecular biology laboratory techniques (such as identification and isolation of specific receptor types and patch-clamp techniques to measure the effects of ion fluxes in response to application of different agonists and antagonists) have been the basis for much of our improved understanding of the molecular actions of our agents. However, as will be seen below, in recent years, PET-based techniques have also been used to study receptor effects.

Cellular function is also commonly studied by molecular biology techniques and by recordings of local field potentials, usually in animals (Imas et al. 2006). PET techniques have been used very successfully to describe the indirect neurophysiological effects of anaesthetic agents such as changes in regional blood flow and metabolism secondary to changes in neuronal (electrical) activity. Occasionally, clever designs have been used to link these regional changes with specific neuronal populations.

Changes in regional neurophysiology are also detectable with functional MRI techniques, in which the scanner sequences are chosen so that regional changes in blood oxyhaemoglobin levels are detectable. This so-called BOLD or blood oxygen level-dependent signal relies on the fact that deoxyhaemoglobin is paramagnetic, whereas oxyhaemoglobin is not. When regional neuronal electrical activity increases, local blood flow and oxygen delivery increase in excess of the increase in oxygen requirements, thereby causing a reduction in the regional concentration of deoxyhaemoglobin and the MRI signal. These fMRI techniques have the benefit of superior temporal resolution compared with PET but suffer from the disadvantage of worse spatial resolution. There is also sometimes debate about the validity of fMRI techniques when anaesthetic agents are used, since, although the anaesthetic agents generally cause matched reductions in cerebral electrical activity, metabolism and flow, they can also have direct vasodilatory effects which result in oxygen delivery in excess of requirements and thus produce BOLD signal changes unrelated to changes in neuronal activity.

We assume that cognitive functions are mediated by electrical activity in networks of neurons, and so perhaps electroencephalography (EEG) can be said to be the most direct and objective measure of brain activity. It has excellent temporal resolution but only reflects cortical activity and represents the summed activity of millions of cortical pyramidal neurons in the vicinity of each electrode. Nonetheless, EEG-based monitors of anaesthetic depth have been developed and shown to assist with rational and patient-individualized titration of anaesthetic dose. These monitoring techniques suffer from the disadvantage that at best, their output correlates with the probability of consciousness but seldom gives an absolute indication of whether consciousness is present or absent. Although there are EEG patterns associated with wakefulness and also with very deep anaesthesia, there is currently no known EEG signal that can clearly detect the transition between consciousness and unconsciousness. Some early efforts have been made to integrate information obtained from electroencephalography with that from PET-based assessments of changes in regional neurophysiology (Noirhomme et al. 2009). Others have combined transcranial magnetic stimulation and EEG recording to yield insights into differences in signal transmission during wakefulness and natural sleep (Massimini et al. 2005, 2007). Finally, studies of the regional correlations in electrical activity, and in particular coherence analyses, are beginning to yield interesting insights into how anaesthetic agents might interfere with the transfer of information between regions (Lee et al. 2009).

Ultimately though, the aim of anaesthesia is to induce loss of consciousness and prevent return of consciousness during a surgical procedure. To understand how the molecular, cellular and neuronal network effects of the anaesthetic agents finally result in a change of consciousness and memory functions is possibly the most challenging step, since it remains to be explained how molecular, cellular and electrical activity generates conscious experiences at all.

In anaesthetic studies, a common aim is to correlate drug-induced regional neurophysiological changes with cognitive function changes. This can be difficult to achieve, even with the time-honoured behavioural testing techniques of cognitive neuroscience and experimental psychology. At lower, sedative doses, when some cognitive functions are still intact, behavioural and memory testing is informative. However, when the end point is loss of consciousness, observations of behaviour and memory are only partially informative. Firstly, assessment of behavioural responses usually involves application of a verbal or painful stimulus that may itself alter the state of consciousness. Secondly, the absence of behavioural responses does not always imply lack of consciousness, but may only indicate a failure of volition or motor control, and in some circumstances, movement in response to pain can occur without the presence of consciousness. Likewise, reliance on explicit memory is not always informative, since sub-sedative doses of several anaesthetic agents are associated with profound amnesia.

44.6 Early Theories of the Molecular Mechanism of Anaesthetic Action

The range of possible types of theories for the mechanism of action is from so-called unitary theories, proposing a single neuronal target, to hypotheses that propose multiple neuronal targets per drug. For most of the twentieth century, the Meyer-Overton hypothesis—a unitary theory—held sway. It was noted that the potency of the anaesthetic agents correlated with their lipid solubility, and this combined with the observation that increases in ambient pressure could reverse anaesthesia leads to the conclusion that anaesthetic effects were mediated by a non-specific physical effect on the lipid bilayer of neuronal cell membranes. It was thought that the physical presence of anaesthetic molecules within this layer caused alterations in membrane volume and fluidity, resulting in dose-dependent dysfunction of all exposed neurons.

Towards the end of the twentieth century, evidence mounted against the Meyer-Overton hypothesis. Studies showed that membrane volume changes were in fact negligible. Other evidence against a non-specific mechanism came from increasing knowledge of exceptions to the rule and biochemical experiments with known anaesthetic agents where small alterations in structure were associated with loss of anaesthetic potency. Further evidence against a simple physical mechanism came from studies showing that current flows along giant squid axons (mediated by voltage-gated Na and K channels) were insensitive to anaesthetic agents (Haydon and Urban 1983, 1986). A major breakthrough came when Franks and Lieb produced the first strong evidence that known anaesthetic agents exhibited dose-dependent effects on proteins, leading to the suggestion that anaesthetic agents acted on membrane receptors (Franks and Lieb 1984). Nonetheless, the academic community was slow to accept this, and it was only with growing evidence against non-specific membrane effects (such as the demonstration of differences in potency among optical isomers of known anaesthetic agents (Franks and Lieb 1993)) and growing evidence of specific effects at receptors (Hales and Lambert 1991; Franks and Lieb 1997) that the Meyer-Overton hypothesis was gradually rejected.

44.7 Current Theories of the Molecular Mechanism of Anaesthetic Action

Most workers in the field now agree that anaesthetic agents act to hyperpolarize neurons by either potentiating inhibitory circuits or inhibiting excitatory pathways and that they do so by specific actions at ligand-gated receptors (Franks 2008; Alkire et al. 2008b; Franks and Lieb 2004). In the case of the commonly used intravenous anaesthetic agent propofol, and for the less commonly used agents such as the barbiturates and etomidate, the chief molecular effect seems to be potentiation at the $GABA_A$ receptor. Gene knockout studies in animals suggest that the different components of the clinical effects of these agents, such as amnesia and sedation, are mediated by different $GABA_A$ receptor subtypes. In fact, sensitivity to the different anaesthetic effects may be strongly modulated by single nucleotide substitutions (Belelli et al. 1997; Mihic et al. 1997; Reynolds et al. 2003), suggesting a potential genetic basis for some of the pharmacodynamic variability seen in clinical practice. Although the $GABA_A$ receptor is posited to be the main molecular site of action, there is also evidence for effects at an array of other sites, such as at nicotinic ACh receptors and voltage-gated potassium channels, although the significance of these effects is unclear (Fig. 44.1).

Two less commonly used intravenous anaesthetic agents that have not yet been mentioned are ketamine and dexmedetomidine. Ketamine causes potent analgesia, and when used as the sole hypnotic, it causes a dissociated state (in which the patient may appear conscious but is dissociated from the environment and applied stimuli). Both effects are mediated via an antagonist effect at the NMDA glutamate receptor (Franks 2008; Alkire et al. 2008b). Dexmedetomidine also has some weaker analgesic effects and at low doses causes arousable sedation not dissimilar to a natural sleep state, with general anaesthesia occurring at much higher doses. These effects are mediated by an agonist effect at α2 adrenergic receptors, with sedative and hypnotic effects probably mediated by actions on these receptors in the locus coeruleus.

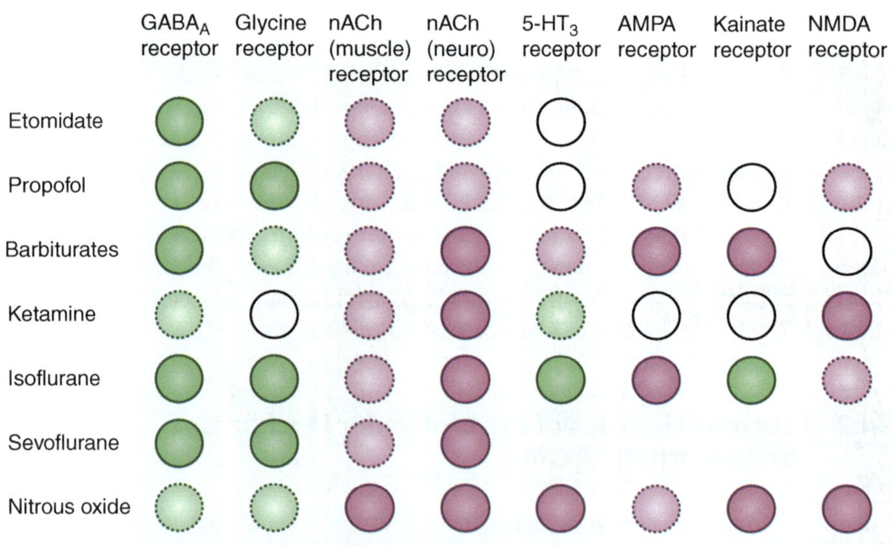

Fig. 44.1 Ligand-gated ion channels are probably the most relevant targets for general anaesthetics. A *dark green* or *pink spot* indicates significant potentiation or inhibition, respectively, of agonist actions at the receptor by the anaesthetic with an *EC50* or *IC50* that is no greater than three times higher than the EC50 for producing immobility. A *light green* or *light pink spot* indicates little potentiation or inhibition, respectively, at concentrations that were less than three times the EC50 for immobility; an *empty spot* indicates no effect at any concentration tested. (From Rudolph and Antkowiak (2004) used with permission)

For the volatile anaesthetic agents, agonist effects at the $GABA_A$ receptor appear to be important (Alkire et al. 2008b) but with binding of the agents to different binding sites than those for propofol and the barbiturates. The molecular mechanism of action of the volatile agents may also include significant potentiating effects at two-pore potassium and glycine channels and inhibitory effects at NMDA receptors (Franks 2008).

44.8 Early PET Studies of the Global and Regional Changes in Cerebral Glucose Metabolism Caused by Anaesthetic Agents

The earliest PET studies of anaesthesia were performed in rats, in which ^{18}FDG was used during propofol anaesthesia, and showed dose-dependent global reductions in cerebral glucose utilization (Ori et al. 1986; Dam et al. 1990; Cavazzuti et al. 1991). These studies led Dr Michael Alkire to perform the first PET studies of anaesthesia in humans. In that, ^{18}FDG was used before and during propofol anaesthesia, and as in the rat studies, it was found that anaesthesia caused reductions in glucose metabolism in all measured cortical and subcortical areas (Alkire et al. 1995). In this study, marked regional differences in tracer uptake were noted, with a greater suppression of cortical than subcortical activity. At this time, it was just becoming apparent that the molecular mechanism of action of propofol was mediated by the $GABA_A$ receptor. These regional differences even led Alkire and colleagues to speculate that differences in the regional distribution of $GABA_A$ receptors were responsible for the regional variations in metabolic activity.

Alkire and his group then went on to study the influence of isoflurane anaesthesia on glucose metabolism, again using the ^{18}FDG tracer (Alkire et al. 1997). Although they found a similar degree of global reduction in metabolic activity to propofol, they found less regional variability with isoflurane. They found similar reductions in cortical and subcortical activity and widespread, fairly uniform reductions in activity across all cortical and subcortical areas. This widely quoted study was taken to provide support for a non-specific, physical explanation of the mechanism of action of the anaesthetic agents.

A subsequent study with an older volatile anaesthetic agent, halothane, showed similar global reductions in metabolic activity to isoflurane and propofol (40% vs. 46% and 55%, respectively) (Alkire et al. 1999). In general, the pattern of regional metabolic effects was similar to that found with isoflurane, with the exception of the cerebellum, where metabolism was more suppressed by halothane. As with isoflurane, midbrain metabolism was more suppressed than with propofol, and here, the authors speculated that this is because the volatile anaesthetics have a strong influence on cholinergic transmission, whereas propofol does not.

Each of the above three studies involved only a small number of subjects, in whom anaesthetic dose was titrated to loss of consciousness, with concurrent EEG monitoring, using the bispectral index (BIS) monitor (Covidien, USA), a monitor of depth of anaesthesia, which gives an output of between 0 and 100, where zero indicates no brain electrical activity and 100 the completely awake state and values between 40 and 60 are taken to represent adequate anaesthesia. The authors combined the data to show that the degree of global reduction in glucose metabolism correlated strongly with the bispectral index (Alkire 1998).

Although the above findings were sometimes taken to provide evidence of a non-specific mechanism of anaesthetic activity, they also indicated differences between anaesthetic agents and regional variations in metabolic suppression, providing evidence against the theory of a single non-specific mechanism of action. In the subsequent years, the evidence against this theory continued to mount up, particularly as investigators designed more sophisticated studies, combined imaging modalities and compared the results of different drugs and modalities. PET methodology played an important role in this. Indeed, by 2005, there was sufficient evidence from studies involving PET measures of cerebral blood flow and metabolism with different anaesthetic agents for Alkire to perform a conjunction analysis. This analysis highlighted the considerable regional differences among different agents, thereby providing strong evidence for specific anaesthetic effects (Alkire and Miller 2005). Further, despite differences in molecular mechanisms and in regional neurophysiological effects, all agents with anaesthetic effects had in common a significant effect on the thalamus (see Fig. 44.2). Based on this work and on previous animal findings (Angel 1993), Alkire became a strong proponent of the 'thalamocortical switch hypothesis', the theory that thalamocortical resonant loops are essential for consciousness and that all anaesthetic agents interrupt consciousness by interrupting the thalamocortical interactions and interrupting onward transmission of ascending electrical signals (Alkire et al. 2000).

Subsequent work using PET has assessed various combinations of cerebral metabolism, blood flow, blood volume and receptor occupancy, for different drugs (sometimes in combination). To simplify the findings, they will be subdivided by drug type, starting with the intravenous agents (propofol, ketamine and the alpha2 agonists) and finishing with the inhaled agents (volatile anaesthetic agents, nitrous oxide, xenon).

44.9 PET and Propofol

The early work by Alkire et al. (1995) has already been mentioned. Although this showed global reductions in glucose metabolism, the effects of propofol on relative glucose metabolism were different for different areas (where regional metabolism as a proportion of global metabolism is considered). Thus, whereas the relative glucose metabolism decreased for most cortical areas and the thalamus, there were relative increases for the temporal lobe, hippocampus, basal ganglia, midbrain and cerebellum.

Fiset and colleagues used $H_2{}^{15}O$ PET to study changes in global and regional cerebral blood flow (rCBF) associated with mild sedation, deep sedation and unconsciousness induced by propofol (Fiset et al. 1999). Concordant with the findings of Alkire, they found dose-related decreases in global CBF. Further, they identified

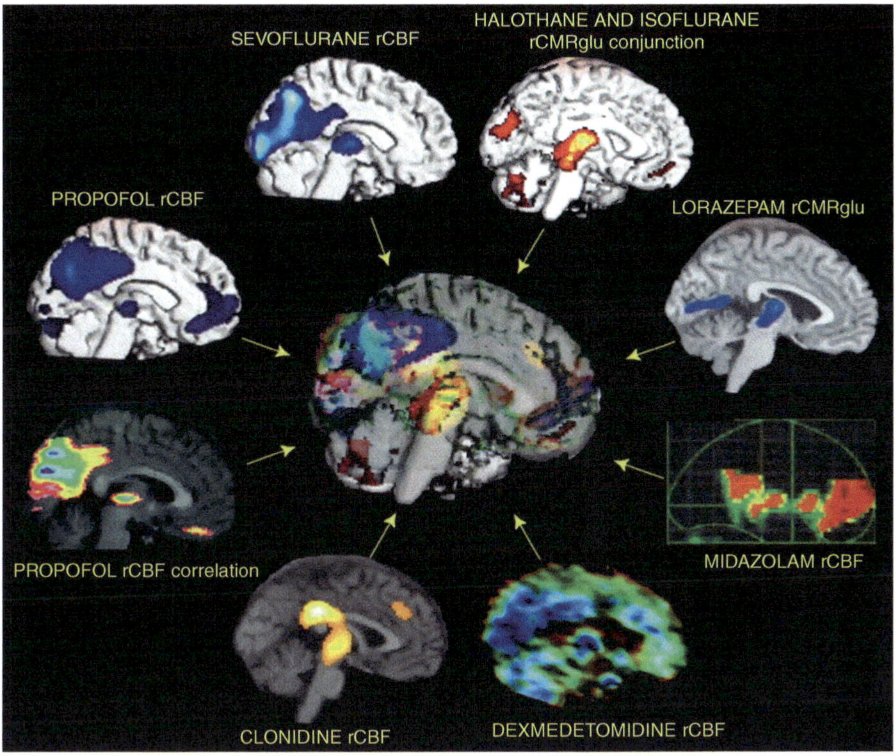

Fig. 44.2 The regional effects of anaesthetics on brain function in humans who were given various anaesthetic agents at doses that altered the level of consciousness. The data are from seven different groups of investigators and encompass the study of eight different agents. The regional effects were measured using blood-flow- or glucose-metabolism-based techniques. All images show regional decreases in activity caused by anaesthesia compared to the awake state, except the propofol correlation image, which shows increasing anaesthetic dose correlates with decreasing blood flow. The figure identifies that altered blood flow and metabolism in the thalamus are a common finding associated with anaesthetic-induced unconsciousness. (From Alkire and Miller (2005) used with permission)

evidence supporting specific molecular effects of propofol. They found that propofol preferentially decreased rCBF in brain regions involved in arousal, autonomic functions and associative functions, such as the medial thalamus, midbrain, cuneus and precuneus, posterior cingulate cortex and orbitofrontal regions. Interestingly, there were strong correlations in rCBF in the midbrain and thalamus, indicating strong functional interactions between the arousal systems of these regions.

In a more sophisticated study, this group measured CBF responses (using $H_2{}^{15}O$ PET) to vibrotactile stimulation during graded sedation and anaesthesia (Bonhomme et al. 2001). In general, this study demonstrated that propofol caused dose-dependent decreases in rCBF in the thalamus, bilateral precuneus and bilateral posterior cingulate gyri. During unconsciousness, there were widespread increases in rCBF when $PaCO_2$ was increased by 20%, which can be explained by the fact that CO_2

reactivity is preserved with propofol. In the awake state, vibrotactile stimulation produced a predicted pattern of rCBF changes—increases in relative rCBF in the left thalamus and primary somatosensory cortex (S1) and left superior frontal gyrus and bilateral secondary somatosensory (S2) cortices. Most interesting was the finding that propofol produced dose-dependent, selective regional effects on the responses to vibrotactile stimulation. At low sedative doses, the S1 responses were abolished, and at moderate sedative doses, the S2 responses were abolished (and accompanied by changes in sensory perception), whereas thalamic responses were only abolished when consciousness was lost.

Scheinin et al. in Finland used $H_2{}^{15}O$ PET to assess changes in absolute and relative CBF during graded general anaesthesia (from moderate to deep levels) with propofol and sevoflurane (Kaisti et al. 2002). Propofol caused a significant global decrease in absolute rCBF but with a ceiling effect at the lowest anaesthetic concentration studied (a target plasma concentration of 6 μg/mL, which is approximately the concentration required to suppress movement responses to pain in 50% of patients). The transition from the awake state to that at EC50 was associated with relative rCBF decreases in the thalamus, midbrain, cuneus, precuneus, posterior limbic system and parietal and frontal cortices. The lack of absolute changes in rCBF with propofol, even at 2 × EC50, suggested that flow-metabolism coupling is maintained during propofol anaesthesia. In a subsequent study by the same group, also involving propofol anaesthesia, but at a lower dose (mean measured concentration 3.7 μg/mL), similar changes in rCBF, regional oxygen metabolism and regional cerebral blood volume (assessed by $H_2{}^{15}O$, ${}^{15}O_2$ and $C_{15}O$ tracers, respectively) were found (Kaisti et al. 2003). This provided evidence of intact flow-metabolism coupling at this low dose, which suggests that low-dose propofol anaesthesia does not produce direct vasodilatory effects. Another group administered a similar level of propofol anaesthesia (targeting a BIS of 35–40) to volunteers and found similarly matched changes in flow and metabolism (in this case, metabolism was assessed with ^{18}FDG PET) (Schlunzen et al. 2012).

Most studies of the influence of propofol metabolism have assessed glucose or oxygen metabolism. One study, however, has assessed regional cerebral protein synthesis rates using the tracer L-[1-^{11}C]leucine (Bishu et al. 2009). No effect of propofol on protein synthesis was found (measured propofol concentrations were in the range 4.2–8.1 μg/mL).

The remaining studies to be discussed in this section were focused on receptor effects of propofol. Alkire and Haier performed a study in which they correlated their findings concerning regional cerebral glucose metabolism rates under propofol and isoflurane anaesthesia, with data previously published by other investigators on the regional distributions of different neurotransmitter systems (Alkire and Haier 2001). The latter data were acquired from post-mortem immunochemistry investigations (Braestrup et al. 1977; Zezula et al. 1988; Enna and Snyder 1977). They were able to show that there were significant correlations between regional reductions in glucose metabolism during propofol anaesthesia and the regional distribution of benzodiazepine binding sites (from studies using ^{3}H-diazepam which binds to both neuronal and mitochondrial benzodiazepine receptors and ^{3}H-flunitrazepam which binds only to neuronal benzodiazepine binding sites on $GABA_A$ receptors). There were also weaker correlations with the distribution of opioid binding sites but no correlations with distribution densities of adrenergic, muscarinic and serotonin binding sites.

Salmi and colleagues later showed that propofol increases ^{11}C-flumazenil binding, indicating that propofol enhances the affinity of GABA for $GABA_A$ receptors (Salmi et al. 2004). At around the same time, another group found that propofol anaesthesia was associated with a reduction in muscarinic receptor binding by the tracer [*N*-^{11}C-methyl]-benztropine (Xie et al. 2004), but this finding was difficult to interpret. Although it may have indicated binding of propofol to muscarinic receptors, it could also have been the result of a change of affinity of the receptor for benztropine or an increase in benztropine metabolism caused by propofol. Several years later, members of the same group performed an intriguing study in which they measured CBF with a $H_2{}^{15}O$ technique at baseline, after loss of consciousness with propofol and administration of the cholinesterase inhibitor, physostigmine (Xie et al. 2011). Some, but not all, volunteers regained consciousness after physostigmine administration, despite constant blood and brain concentrations of propofol. The authors found that loss of consciousness was associated with decreases in rCBF in the thalamus and precuneus and that among those that regained consciousness after physostigmine, restoration of consciousness was associated with increases in rCBF in these same structures. It is assumed that the increased ACh levels caused by physostigmine result in activation of cholinergic pathways and an increase in thalamic throughput of electrical signals sufficient to cause a return of consciousness.

Taken together, these studies indicate that propofol causes a specific pattern of changes in regional metabolic activity and CBF but with a key effect at the thalamus and that loss of consciousness is associated with interruption of thalamocortical signalling. Finally, the work from the past decade and a half supports the hypothesis that propofol acts at specific protein targets, most notably at the $GABA_A$ receptor.

44.10 PET and Ketamine

Ketamine is an older anaesthetic agent than propofol but is seldom used alone for inducing or maintaining surgical anaesthesia because of a propensity to cause troublesome psychiatric adverse effects. It remains interesting clinically and is being used with increasing frequency as an adjunct during propofol anaesthesia. Known and potential beneficial effects include improved cardiovascular stability, neuroprotection, reduced acute post-operative pain, potent antidepressant activity and attenuation of post-operative hyperalgesia and chronic pain.

Ketamine is also of scientific interest because it acts as an antagonist at the NMDA receptor and causes different neurophysiological changes to the other hypnotics. When used alone, it causes impaired consciousness but with cortical electrical activation accompanied by increases in glucose metabolism (Vollenweider et al. 1997) and rCBF. The reasons behind these effects are not clear. The drug antagonizes an excitatory pathway, but presumably, this results in activation of other excitatory pathways. Impaired consciousness is probably the result of impaired connectivity or communication between regions of the brain important for consciousness.

Långsjö and colleagues studied the effects of sub-anaesthetic doses of **racemic ketamine** on rCBF, regional oxygen metabolism ($rCMRO_2$) and regional cerebral blood volume (rCBV) using the PET tracers $H_2{}^{15}O$, ${}^{15}O_2$ and C ${}^{15}O$ (Långsjö et al. 2003). Ketamine caused global dose-dependent changes in absolute rCBF, with the biggest changes in the anterior cingulate, insula and frontal cortex (areas involved in pain processing) and also in the thalamus and putamen. As expected, mean systemic arterial pressures were increased. There were no significant changes in $rCMRO_2$, and hence, the oxygen extraction fraction was reduced. rCBV was only increased in the frontal cortex. Taken together, these findings were consistent with known behavioural and electrophysiological changes seen with ketamine sedation but did give rise to a suggestion of altered flow-metabolism coupling. The authors performed a follow-up study, this time using ^{18}FDG to assess regional changes in glucose metabolism (rCMRG) associated with sub-sedative racemic ketamine doses (at the highest dose used in the previous study) (Långsjö et al. 2004). Region of interest analyses showed global absolute increases in rCMRG but with the greatest changes in the thalamus and frontal and parietal cortex. Voxel-based analyses showed increases in relative rCMRG in frontal, temporal and parietal cortices. These changes occurred in a similar distribution and magnitude to the rCBF findings of the previous study (Långsjö et al. 2003), suggesting maintenance of flow-metabolism coupling. The authors suggested that the absence of $rCMRO_2$ changes was the result of non-oxidative glucose metabolism in response to ketamine-induced glutamate release. A recent study by Laaksonen and colleagues comparing the effects of dexmedetomidine, propofol and *S*-ketamine also identified no significant changes in rCMRG in the ketamine cohort (Laaksonen et al. 2018).

The Långsjö group also studied the effects of ***S*-ketamine** on cerebral blood flow and metabolism, using a complex study design (Långsjö et al. 2005). $H_2{}^{15}O$ and ${}^{15}O_2$ scans were performed during one session, at three moments: awake, during low-dose sub-sedative *S*-ketamine administration and during much higher dose of *S*-ketamine anaesthesia. ^{18}FDG scans were performed 3 weeks before the main study and finally also towards the end of the *S*-ketamine anaesthesia. The authors found dose-dependent increases in total CBF and in absolute rCBF in almost all regions studied. During low-dose *S*-ketamine administration, the greatest increases were in the anterior cingulate, whereas at anaesthetic doses, the largest increase (86.5%) was in the insula. At low doses, there were no significant increases in $rCMRO_2$, whereas at anaesthetic doses, $rCMRO_2$ was increased only in the frontal cortex (by 15.7%). During anaesthesia, rCMRG was only increased in the thalamus, and CBV was increased >50%. These findings show that CBF is increased in excess of metabolic needs, suggesting a disturbance of flow-metabolism coupling. While the excess flow may be perceived to be protective, these findings confirmed the long-held views of anaesthesiologists (based on the work of others using different methodologies) that ketamine is not a suitable agent for use during neurosurgery, where the increases in CBF and CBV can cause increased brain volume, increased intracranial pressure and impaired surgical access.

Finally, the same group studied the influence of sub-anaesthetic doses of ketamine on ^{11}C-flumazenil binding (Salmi et al. 2005). They showed no interference in binding, thereby confirming that ketamine has minimal effects on the $GABA_A$ receptor.

The antidepressant effect of ketamine has also been explored using PET scanning in recent years. Using [^{11}C]DASB PET in healthy volunteers, it was demonstrated that the antidepressant effect was not mediated by ketamine binding to the serotonin transporter (Spies et al. 2018). More recently, the radiotracer ^{18}F-FPEB was used to establish that ketamine leads to a downregulation of the metabotropic glutamate receptor 5 (mGluR5) (Holmes et al. 2019). These two studies highlight how PET imaging can be used to probe existing (serotonin reuptake) and novel (mGluR5) treatment targets for psychiatric disorders.

44.11 PET and Alpha2 Agonists

PET technology has only been used a few times to study the alpha2 agonists, among which clonidine and dexmedetomidine are the two agents available for clinical use. Although clonidine has been available for a long time, it has mainly been used intravenously for its antihypertensive effects. More recently, it has been used as a preoperative oral sedative premedication and perioperatively as an intravenous analgesic adjunct. Dexmedetomidine has been in use for almost 20 years in the USA. Initially, it was mostly used for ICU sedation; more recently, it has been used as a sedative during surgical procedures such as awake craniotomy. It was first registered in Europe in late 2011.

Prielipp used $H_2{}^{15}O$ scans to assess the changes in rCBF during and after low and high sedative dose infusions of dexmedetomidine. The agent caused marked reductions in global CBF and also reductions in absolute rCBF in 13 out of 14 regions of interest studied. There were no significant differences in patterns of rCBF between low and high sedative doses. Despite the rapid pharmacokinetics of dexmedetomidine, CBF remained decreased when assessed 30 min after the end of the dexmedetomidine infusion (Prielipp et al. 2002). This reduction of CBF in the absence of concomitant reduction in $CMRO_2$ raised concerns about the potential for cerebral ischaemia with dexmedetomidine. More recently however, the abovementioned comparative study by Laaksonen et al. revealed that volunteers sedated with dexmedetomidine showed the lowest rCMRG in almost all brain regions compared to other anaesthetics (Fig. 44.3).

More recent reports have studied healthy volunteers sedated with dexmedetomidine in an attempt to explore disruptions in brain functional connectivity with combined PET-fMRI studies. Unconsciousness was associated with reduced regional blood flow and CMRG in the thalamus, the default mode network (DMN) and the bilateral frontoparietal networks (FPNs) (Akeju et al. 2014). Importantly, functional connectivity within these networks was preserved, while internetwork connectivity was disrupted. As reported above, recovery from unconsciousness was associated with sustained reduction in CBF and restored DMN thalamocortical functional connectivity. Other studies have identified greater functional connectivity between the

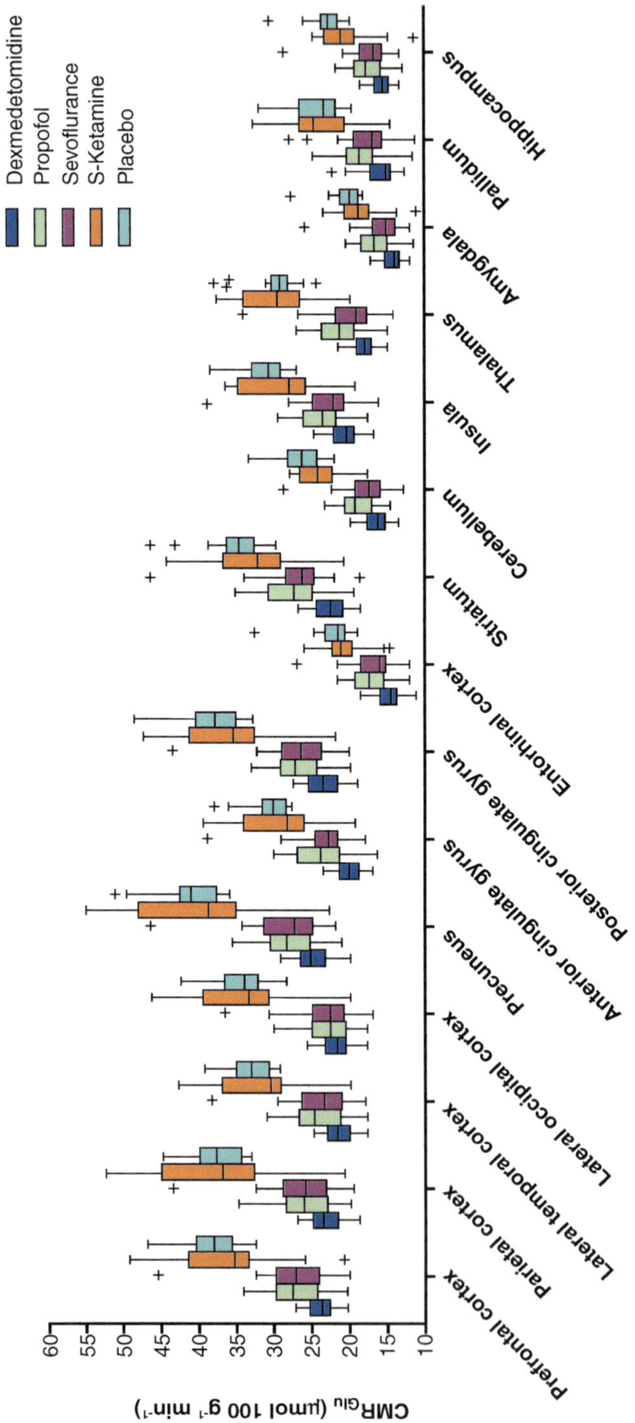

Fig. 44.3 Boxplots of regional cerebral metabolic rate of glucose (CMR_{glu}) in the 15 analyzed regions of interest (ROIs) during dexmedetomidine, propofol, sevoflurane, *S*-ketamine and placebo administration in 160 healthy subjects ($P < 0.001$ between the treatments in all ROIs). Lowest CMR_{glu} values were observed in the dexmedetomidine group. Boxes represent lower quartiles and medians and upper quartiles; whiskers represent 1.5 × interquartile ranges below and above the lower and upper quartiles, respectively. Outlying values are marked with symbols

parietal and anterior cingulate cortex upon emergence from anaesthesia, prompting suggestions of a functional network that activates with restored consciousness (Långsjö et al. 2012).

Another group studied the influence of clonidine infusions on rCBF (assessed by $H_2{}^{15}O$ PET), clinical status and EEG (Bonhomme et al. 2008). Clonidine caused rousable sedation and on the EEG spindle patterns similar to those found during non-rapid eye movement sleep. There was a negative correlation between measured plasma clonidine concentration and rCBF in a network of regions including the thalamus, prefrontal cortex, orbital and parietal association cortex, posterior cingulate cortex and precuneus. Changes in these regions are associated with natural sleep. These regions also form part of the default mode network, whose component areas show strong correlations in activity (assessed by fMRI) during the resting state, but not during task performance conditions (Mason et al. 2007; Stamatakis et al. 2010).

44.12 PET and Volatile Anaesthetic Agents

Volatile anaesthetic agents have been the subject of many PET studies. These have mainly focused on the neurophysiological changes in flow and metabolism and have shown generally concordant findings, with only minor variations between studies, possibly related to differences in dose. Minor variations were found according to drug, despite some chemical differences between the agents studied, such as structure, molecular weight, degree of halogenations and water and lipid solubility. Halothane is a halogenated hydrocarbon that is now seldom used in the First World. Isoflurane, sevoflurane and desflurane are halogenated ethers. The latter two agents are the most commonly used inhalational anaesthetic agents, although there are few PET studies involving desflurane.

The early work by Alkire, showing that isoflurane anaesthesia caused a 46% reduction in rCMRG with fairly uniform regional distribution, has already been mentioned (Alkire et al. 1997). Alkire then studied the effects of halothane on rCMRG, since this agent had been shown in earlier studies to cause less uniform rCMRG reductions (Alkire et al. 1999). Halothane anaesthesia was found to cause a 40% reduction in global rCMRG, but in keeping with the prior animal work, there were some regional differences, with the greater metabolic reductions being found in the basal forebrain, thalamus, limbic system, cerebellum and occipital cortex.

In the above studies, halothane and isoflurane were administered until an end point of loss of consciousness (the mean concentrations administered were 30% and 60% less than the concentrations required to prevent a response to a surgical incision—the so-called MAC value, a measure of potency). Kaisti studied the effects of surgical levels of sevoflurane anaesthesia—at concentrations that were 1.0, 1.5 and 2.0 multiples of the MAC value—on rCBF using $H_2{}^{15}O$ (Kaisti et al. 2002). At 1.0 MAC, sevoflurane caused global decreases in absolute rCBF (regional decreases were between 36% and 53% of baseline). Increasing doses caused a redistribution of flow, with increases in rCBF in the thalamus and cerebellum, suggesting a disturbance of flow-metabolism coupling.

In a follow-up study, using $H_2{}^{15}O$, $^{15}O_2$ and C ^{15}O to study rCBF, $rCMRO_2$ and CBV, respectively, Kaisti titrated sevoflurane and propofol anaesthesia (with and without N_2O) to a moderate depth of anaesthesia, guided by the BIS (Kaisti et al. 2003). Sevoflurane concentrations were thus lower than in the previous study—0.75 × MAC without N_2O and 0.6 MAC with 70% N_2O. Sevoflurane without N_2O reduced the total CBF but only caused rCBF decreases in some areas (the occipital cortex, cerebellum, caudate and thalamus). The most significant changes in relative rCBF were in the thalamus, cuneus, frontoparietal cortex and cerebellum. Addition of N_2O caused a global return to baseline rCBF values, with the most significant relative rCBF increases in the occipital cortex and pons. With regard to $CMRO_2$, sevoflurane caused a global reduction, with absolute decreases in $rCMRO_2$ in all areas studied. The greatest reductions in relative $rCMRO_2$ were in the thalamus, cuneus, frontoparietal cortex and cerebellum. Addition of N_2O increased $rCMRO_2$ in the parieto-occipital region and cerebellum, but not quite to baseline/awake levels. At the doses studied, sevoflurane with and without N_2O did not alter rCBV. It was associated with a tendency towards reduced oxygen extraction fraction, more marked in the presence of N_2O, indicating that metabolism was more suppressed than flow, suggesting a degree of disturbed flow-metabolism coupling.

The above findings were generally confirmed by Schlunzen et al., although some increases in rCBF were found at lower doses (Schlunzen et al. 2004). The study involved use of $H_2{}^{15}O$ to study changes in rCBF associated with sub-anaesthetic to anaesthetic doses of sevoflurane (0.2, 0.35 and 1.0 MAC multiples). At all doses, sevoflurane increased rCBF in the anterior cingulate and decreased rCBF in the cerebellum. Compared with the baseline state, 0.2 MAC sevoflurane decreased rCBF in the inferior temporal cortex and lingual gyrus. 0.35 MAC increased rCBF in the middle temporal cortex and lingual gyrus while decreasing rCBF in the thalamus. The latter finding is unsurprising given that some volunteers displayed no response to a verbal stimulus, whereas other showed only sluggish responses. Finally, compared with 0.35 MAC, 1 MAC increased rCBF in the insula and decreased rCBF in the posterior cingulated, lingual gyrus, precuneus and frontal cortex. Similar patterns of changes were found in subsequent study, using similar methodology and equipotent isoflurane doses (Schlunzen et al. 2006).

When administering anaesthesia to patients with raised intracranial pressure who require surgical excision of space-occupying lesions, anaesthesiologists often employ a degree of hyperventilation in order to reduce CBF and intracranial pressure. Schlunzen thus studied the influence of hyperventilation on rCBF in volunteers subjected to surgical levels of sevoflurane anaesthesia (1 MAC) (Schlunzen et al. 2010). A reduction of the mean $PaCO_2$ from 5.5 to 3.8 kPa reduced the total CBF by 44%. The largest reductions in rCBF were found in the thalamus, medial occipitotemporal gyrus, cerebellum, precuneus, putamen and insula. This work clearly showed that under surgical levels of sevoflurane anaesthesia, CO_2 reactivity is maintained, with stronger responses in some areas than others.

Finally, this group also studied the effects of surgical levels of sevoflurane anaesthesia (1 MAC) on $rCMRO_2$ (Schlunzen et al. 2010). Total CMRG was reduced by 56%, and absolute rCMRG was decreased in all areas studied. The most significant relative rCMRG decreases were found in the lingual gyrus, occipital lobe and thalamus.

A few studies have addressed the molecular biology of the volatile agents. Among five subjects subjected to isoflurane anaesthesia, Alkire showed that the regional distribution of changes in rCBF correlated best with ex vivo-demonstrated muscarinic acetylcholine binding density, suggesting that the molecular action of isoflurane may involve antagonism of central acetylcholine pathways (Alkire and Haier 2001). On the other hand, Salmi showed that sevoflurane increased the distribution volume of ^{11}C-flumazenil in all areas studied (except pons and white matter), suggesting the involvement of $GABA_A$ receptors in the mechanism of action of sevoflurane (Salmi et al. 2004). This was concordant with a previous study of isoflurane, which showed a dose-dependent increase in distribution volume of ^{11}C-flumazenil (Gyulai et al. 2001).

Alkire and colleagues used PET to study the effects of sevoflurane at a higher system level (Alkire et al. 2008a). In the first step, they determined that exposure to low doses of sevoflurane—0.1% and 0.2% (0.05 and 0.1 MAC, respectively)—provided a subsequent mnemonic boost for emotional arousal but not neutral stimuli, presented during the sevoflurane exposure. This mnemonic boost was absent in volunteers administered with 0.25% sevoflurane. In the second step, ^{18}FDG PET was used to assess regional changes in glucose metabolism associated with 0.25% sevoflurane. Using structural equation modelling, they demonstrated that this dose blocked emotional memory by interfering with the amygdala to hippocampal connectivity.

44.13 PET and Nitrous Oxide

Nitrous oxide used to be commonly administered concomitantly with volatile anaesthetics. Although this practice is common, it is declining in frequency as environmental concerns have resulted in some departments no longer having inbuilt nitrous oxide supplies. On its own, the gas is a weak anaesthetic (administration of a partial pressure > 1 atm is required for general anaesthesia) but a reasonably strong analgesic, thanks to the fact that the drug acts as an antagonist at the NDMA receptor.

Few studies have used PET to study the neurophysiological changes associated with administration of nitrous oxide. Reinstrup used ^{133}Xe SPECT to study CBF changes associated with inhalation of 50% N_2O (Reinstrup et al. 1994). They found global increases in CBF, which were fairly uniform during normocapnia, although it remains possible that these changes were partly the result of Xe administration. It was also unclear whether these changes were the result of direct cerebral vasodilatation or from increases in metabolism. Later, the same group used ^{18}FDG to study changes in glucose metabolism (Reinstrup et al. 2008). Inhalation of 50% nitrous oxide did not change global rCMRG, but did change the relative distribution of glucose metabolism, with 14% and 22% increases in the basal ganglia and thalamus, respectively.

In a study focused on sevoflurane and propofol, Kaisti and colleagues studied the effects of adjunct administration of 70% N_2O and found that N_2O counteracted some of the $rCMRO_2$ and rCBF reductions seen when propofol or sevoflurane was used alone (Kaisti et al. 2003). The findings all corroborated the findings of previous animal and human studies, in which other methods were used to study the cerebral blood flow and metabolic responses to N_2O.

44.14 PET and Xenon

Xenon is a rare (and expensive) noble gas and also a weak anaesthetic. Exposure to a 70% Xe will prevent purposeful movements in response to a surgical stimulus in 50% of volunteers (for comparison, the MAC of sevoflurane is 2.0%). The molecule is interesting because, like N_2O, it is also an NMDA antagonist, and it is probably for this reason that it may be neuroprotective.

PET studies of changes in rCBF have shown that in contrast to ketamine (also an NMDA antagonist), anaesthetic concentrations of Xe cause widespread decreases in rCBF, mostly marked in the cerebellum, thalamus and parietal cortex (Laitio et al. 2007). Findings for changes in rCMRG induced by Xe anaesthesia were also contrary to expectations, based on findings for N_2O and ketamine. Rex and colleagues found that Xe reduced total CMRG by 26% and decreased rCMRG in all areas studied (Rex et al. 2006). In a subsequent study, this group measured changes in rCBF associated with Xe anaesthesia, using $H_2{}^{15}O$ PET (Rex et al. 2008). Relative decreases in several cortical, subcortical and cerebellar areas were shown, with relative increases in white matter. These findings matched well with the previous pattern of findings with regard to rCBF, suggesting that flow-metabolism coupling is maintained with Xe.

Laitio and colleagues used ^{18}FDG and ^{15}O PET to study combined changes in rCMRG and rCBF associated with 67% Xe (Laitio et al. 2009). While the patterns of changes were broadly similar to those of Rex and colleagues, they found that the decreases in metabolism exceeded those of blood flow. When they calculated the rCBF/rCMRG ratio, they found that this was particularly increased in the insula, anterior and posterior cingulated and somatosensory cortex.

Although the patterns of changes in blood flow and metabolism are not too dissimilar to those found with the volatile anaesthetic agents, Xe does not influence ^{11}C-flumazenil binding, suggesting that the molecular mechanism of action of Xe does not involve an effect on the $GABA_A$ receptor (Salmi et al. 2008).

44.15 Summary and Conclusion

Early studies on the regional distribution of changes in cerebral metabolism associated with anaesthetic doses of isoflurane seemed to suggest uniform changes in keeping with a unitary hypothesis of a non-specific, physical molecular mechanism of action of the anaesthetic drugs. A limited number of studies have specifically studied the molecular mechanisms and site of action of the anaesthetic agents. In general, these studies have confirmed the findings of laboratory work using molecular biology techniques.

More recent PET studies have shown that the anaesthetic agents cause regionally specific effects on metabolism and flow and that these are probably the result of regionally specific distributions of neuronal $GABA_A$, NMDA and muscarinic ACh receptors. Most groups report global CBF and metabolic rate findings, absolute changes in rCBF and rCMRG or $rCMRO_2$ and then also changes in relative rCBF and rCMRG or $rCMRO_2$. The assumption inherent in the latter approach is that the greatest relative changes will happen in the regions where key anaesthetic effects are mediated. Different anaesthetic agents cause slightly different patterns of regional effects, but all cause an alteration in flow and/or metabolism in the thalamus. Anaesthetic-induced loss of consciousness appears to be associated with a significant reduction in blood flow and metabolism in the thalamus. While some investigators argue that this provides evidence that the thalamus is a key site of action of these agents (Alkire et al. 2000), caution is required, since these reductions in blood flow and metabolism may be the result of reduced cortical activity and thus reduced cortical input to the thalamus. EEG and electrocorticography studies suggest that the primary effect of anaesthetic agents is at the cortex, rather than at subcortical structures (Velly et al. 2007). EEG and fMRI studies provide contradictory evidence, with some suggesting that thalamocortical connectivity is maintained despite loss of consciousness (Boveroux et al. 2010; Boly et al. 2012), and others that preserved thalamocortical connectivity are a necessary prerequisite for consciousness (Barttfeld et al. 2015; Malekmohammadi et al. 2019).

Generally, the findings from PET studies of regional changes in blood flow and metabolism are in keeping with the known molecular sites of action. Xenon is one exception, since it has the same site of action as nitrous oxide and ketamine (NMDA receptor) yet has regional effects on blood flow and metabolism similar to those caused by the volatile anaesthetic agents (whose effects are mediated by action at $GABA_A$ and muscarinic Ach receptors and possibly also at K channels).

Much work remains to be done to understand how these molecular effects result in regional changes in activity and connectivity and changes in communication among distributed areas and how each of changes mediates alterations in consciousness.

References

Absalom AR, Green D (2013) NAP5: the tip of the iceberg, or all we need to know? Br J Anaesth 113(4):527–530

Adapa RM, Davis MH, Stamatakis EA, Absalom AR, Menon DK (2014) Neural correlates of successful semantic processing during propofol sedation. Hum Brain Mapp 35:2935–2949

Akeju O, Loggia ML, Catana C, Pavone KJ, Vazquez R, Rhee J et al (2014) Disruption of thalamic functional connectivity is a neural correlate of dexmedetomidine-induced unconsciousness. elife 4:e04499

Alkire MT (1998) Quantitative EEG correlations with brain glucose metabolic rate during anesthesia in volunteers. Anesthesiology 89(2):323–333

Alkire MT, Haier RJ (2001) Correlating in vivo anaesthetic effects with ex vivo receptor density data supports a GABAergic mechanism of action for propofol, but not for isoflurane. Br J Anaesth 86(5):618–626

Alkire MT, Miller J (2005) General anesthesia and the neural correlates of consciousness. Prog Brain Res 150:229–244

Alkire MT, Haier RJ, Barker SJ, Shah NK, Wu JC, Kao YJ (1995) Cerebral metabolism during propofol anesthesia in humans studied with positron emission tomography. Anesthesiology 82(2):393–403

Alkire MT, Haier RJ, Shah NK, Anderson CT (1997) Positron emission tomography study of regional cerebral metabolism in humans during isoflurane anesthesia. Anesthesiology 86(3):549–557

Alkire MT, Pomfrett CJ, Haier RJ, Gianzero MV, Chan CM, Jacobsen BP, Fallon JH (1999) Functional brain imaging during anesthesia in humans: effects of halothane on global and regional cerebral glucose metabolism. Anesthesiology 90(3):701–709

Alkire MT, Haier RJ, Fallon JH (2000) Toward a unified theory of narcosis: brain imaging evidence for a thalamocortical switch as the neurophysiologic basis of anesthetic-induced unconsciousness. Conscious Cogn 9(3):370–386

Alkire MT, Gruver R, Miller J, McReynolds JR, Hahn EL, Cahill L (2008a) Neuroimaging analysis of an anesthetic gas that blocks human emotional memory. Proc Natl Acad Sci U S A 105(5):1722–1727

Alkire MT, Hudetz AG, Tononi G (2008b) Consciousness and anesthesia. Science 322(5903):876–880

Angel A (1993) Central neuronal pathways and the process of anaesthesia. Br J Anaesth 71(1):148–163

Arhem P, Klement G, Nilsson J (2003) Mechanisms of anesthesia: towards integrating network, cellular, and molecular level modeling. Neuropsychopharmacology 28(Suppl 1):S40–S47

Barttfeld P, Bekinschtein TA, Salles A, Stamatakis EA, Adapa R, Menon DK, Sigman M (2015) Factoring the brain signatures of anesthesia concentration and level of arousal across individuals. NeuroImage Clin 9:385–391

Belelli D, Lambert JJ, Peters JA, Wafford K, Whiting PJ (1997) The interaction of the general anesthetic etomidate with the gamma-aminobutyric acid type A receptor is influenced by a single amino acid. Proc Natl Acad Sci U S A 94(20):11031–11036

Bishu S, Schmidt KC, Burlin TV, Channing MA, Horowitz L, Huang T, Liu ZH, Qin M, Vuong BK, Unterman AJ, Xia Z, Zametkin A, Herscovitch P, Quezado Z, Smith CB (2009) Propofol anesthesia does not alter regional rates of cerebral protein synthesis measured with L-[1-(11) C]leucine and PET in healthy male subjects. J Cereb Blood Flow Metab 29(5):1035–1047

Boly M, Moran R, Murphy M, Boveroux P, Bruno MA, Noirhomme Q, Ledoux D, Bonhomme V, Brichant JF, Tononi G, Laureys S, Friston K (2012) Connectivity changes underlying spectral EEG changes during propofol-induced loss of consciousness. J Neurosci 32(20):7082–7090

Bonhomme V, Fiset P, Meuret P, Backman S, Plourde G, Paus T, Bushnell MC, Evans AC (2001) Propofol anesthesia and cerebral blood flow changes elicited by vibrotactile stimulation: a positron emission tomography study. J Neurophysiol 85(3):1299–1308

Bonhomme V, Maquet P, Phillips C, Plenevaux A, Hans P, Luxen A, Lamy M, Laureys S (2008) The effect of clonidine infusion on distribution of regional cerebral blood flow in volunteers. Anesth Analg 106(3):899–909, table of contents

Boveroux P, Vanhaudenhuyse A, Bruno MA, Noirhomme Q, Lauwick S, Luxen A, Degueldre C, Plenevaux A, Schnakers C, Phillips C, Brichant JF, Bonhomme V, Maquet P, Greicius MD, Laureys S, Boly M (2010) Breakdown of within- and between-network resting state functional magnetic resonance imaging connectivity during propofol-induced loss of consciousness. Anesthesiology 113(5):1038–1053

Braestrup C, Albrechtsen R, Squires RF (1977) High densities of benzodiazepine receptors in human cortical areas. Nature 269(5630):702–704

Brown EN, Lydic R, Schiff ND (2010) General anesthesia, sleep, and coma. N Engl J Med 363(27):2638–2650, no. 1533-4406; 0028-4793

Cavazzuti M, Porro CA, Barbieri A, Galetti A (1991) Brain and spinal cord metabolic activity during propofol anaesthesia. Br J Anaesth 66(4):490–495

Dam M, Ori C, Pizzolato G, Ricchieri GL, Pellegrini A, Giron GP, Battistin L (1990) The effects of propofol anesthesia on local cerebral glucose utilization in the rat. Anesthesiology 73(3):499–505

Davidson AJ, Disma N, de Graaff JC et al (2016) Neurodevelopmental outcome at 2 years of age after general anaesthesia and awake-regional anaesthesia in infancy (GAS): an international multicentre, randomised controlled trial. Lancet 387(10015):239–250

Davis MH, Coleman MR, Absalom AR, Rodd JM, Johnsrude IS, Matta BF, Owen AM, Menon DK (2007) Dissociating speech perception and comprehension at reduced levels of awareness. Proc Natl Acad Sci U S A 104(41):16032–16037

Enna SJ, Snyder SH (1977) GABA receptor binding in frog spinal cord and brain. J Neurochem 28(4):857–860

Fiset P, Paus T, Daloze T, Plourde G, Meuret P, Bonhomme V, Hajj-Ali N, Backman SB, Evans AC (1999) Brain mechanisms of propofol-induced loss of consciousness in humans: a positron emission tomographic study. J Neurosci 19(13):5506–5513

Franks NP (2008) General anaesthesia: from molecular targets to neuronal pathways of sleep and arousal. Nat Rev Neurosci 9(5):370–386

Franks NP, Lieb WR (1984) Do general anaesthetics act by competitive binding to specific receptors? Nature 310(5978):599–601, no. 0028-0836; 0028-0836

Franks NP, Lieb WR (1993) Selective actions of volatile general anaesthetics at molecular and cellular levels. Br J Anaesth 71(1):65–76

Franks NP, Lieb WR (1997) Inhibitory synapses. Anaesthetics set their sites on ion channels. Nature 389(6649):334–335

Franks NP, Lieb WR (2004) Seeing the light: protein theories of general anesthesia. 1984. Anesthesiology 101(1):235–237

Gyulai FE, Mintun MA, Firestone LL (2001) Dose-dependent enhancement of in vivo GABA(A)-benzodiazepine receptor binding by isoflurane. Anesthesiology 95(3):585–593, no. 0003-3022; 0003-3022

Hales TG, Lambert JJ (1991) The actions of propofol on inhibitory amino acid receptors of bovine adrenomedullary chromaffin cells and rodent central neurones. Br J Pharmacol 104(3):619–628

Hameroff SR (2006) The entwined mysteries of anesthesia and consciousness: is there a common underlying mechanism? Anesthesiology 105(2):400–412

Haydon DA, Urban BW (1983) The effects of some inhalation anaesthetics on the sodium current of the squid giant axon. J Physiol 341:429–439

Haydon DA, Urban BW (1986) The actions of some general anaesthetics on the potassium current of the squid giant axon. J Physiol 373:311–327

Holmes SE, Gallezot JD, Davis MT et al (2019) Measuring the effects of ketamine on mGluR5 using [(18)F]FPEB and PET. J Cereb Blood Flow Metab. https://doi.org/10.1177/271678X19886316

Imas OA, Ropella KM, Wood JD, Hudetz AG (2006) Isoflurane disrupts anterio-posterior phase synchronization of flash-induced field potentials in the rat. Neurosci Lett 402(3):216–221

Jevtovic-Todorovic V, Absalom AR, Blomgren K, Brambrink A, Crosby G, Culley DJ et al (2013) Anaesthetic neurotoxicity and neuroplasticity: an expert group report and statement based on the BJA Salzburg Seminar. Br J Anaesth 111(2):143–151
Kaisti KK, Metsahonkala L, Teras M, Oikonen V, Aalto S, Jaaskelainen S, Hinkka S, Scheinin H (2002) Effects of surgical levels of propofol and sevoflurane anesthesia on cerebral blood flow in healthy subjects studied with positron emission tomography. Anesthesiology 96(6):1358–1370
Kaisti KK, Langsjo JW, Aalto S, Oikonen V, Sipila H, Teras M, Hinkka S, Metsahonkala L, Scheinin H (2003) Effects of sevoflurane, propofol, and adjunct nitrous oxide on regional cerebral blood flow, oxygen consumption, and blood volume in humans. Anesthesiology 99(3):603–613
Kissin I (1993) General anesthetic action: an obsolete notion? Anesth Analg 76(2):215–218
Kulli J, Koch C (1991) Does anesthesia cause loss of consciousness? Trends Neurosci 14(1):6–10
Laaksonen L, Kallioinen M, Långsjö J et al (2018) Comparative effects of dexmedetomidine, propofol, sevoflurane, and S-ketamine on regional cerebral glucose metabolism in humans: a positron emission tomography study. Br J Anaesth 121(1):281–290
Laitio RM, Kaisti KK, Långsjö JW, Aalto S, Salmi E, Maksimow A, Aantaa R, Oikonen V, Sipila H, Parkkola R, Scheinin H (2007) Effects of xenon anesthesia on cerebral blood flow in humans: a positron emission tomography study. Anesthesiology 106(6):1128–1133
Laitio RM, Långsjö JW, Aalto S, Kaisti KK, Salmi E, Maksimow A, Aantaa R, Oikonen V, Viljanen T, Parkkola R, Scheinin H (2009) The effects of xenon anesthesia on the relationship between cerebral glucose metabolism and blood flow in healthy subjects: a positron emission tomography study. Anesth Analg 108(2):593–600
Långsjö JW, Kaisti KK, Aalto S, Hinkka S, Aantaa R, Oikonen V, Sipila H, Kurki T, Silvanto M, Scheinin H (2003) Effects of subanesthetic doses of ketamine on regional cerebral blood flow, oxygen consumption, and blood volume in humans. Anesthesiology 99(3):614–623
Långsjö JW, Salmi E, Kaisti KK, Aalto S, Hinkka S, Aantaa R, Oikonen V, Viljanen T, Kurki T, Silvanto M, Scheinin H (2004) Effects of subanesthetic ketamine on regional cerebral glucose metabolism in humans. Anesthesiology 100(5):1065–1071
Långsjö JW, Maksimow A, Salmi E, Kaisti K, Aalto S, Oikonen V, Hinkka S, Aantaa R, Sipila H, Viljanen T, Parkkola R, Scheinin H (2005) S-ketamine anesthesia increases cerebral blood flow in excess of the metabolic needs in humans. Anesthesiology 103(2):258–268
Långsjö JW, Alkire MT, Kaskinoro K, Hayama H, Maksimow A, Kaisti KK, Aalto S, Aantaa R, Jääskeläinen SK, Revonsuo A, Scheinin H (2012) Returning from oblivion: imaging the neural core of consciousness. J Neurosci 32(14):4935–4943
Lee U, Kim S, Noh GJ, Choi BM, Hwang E, Mashour GA (2009) The directionality and functional organization of frontoparietal connectivity during consciousness and anesthesia in humans. Conscious Cogn 18(4):1069–1078
Lindholm ML, Traff S, Granath F, Greenwald SD, Ekbom A, Lennmarken C, Sandin RH (2009) Mortality within 2 years after surgery in relation to low intraoperative bispectral index values and preexisting malignant disease. Anesth Analg 108(2):508–512, no. 1526-7598
Lydic R, Baghdoyan HA (2005) Sleep, anesthesiology, and the neurobiology of arousal state control. Anesthesiology 103(6):1268–1295
Malekmohammadi M, Price CM, Hudson AE, DiCesare JAT, Pouratian N (2019) Propofol-induced loss of consciousness is associated with a decrease in thalamocortical connectivity in humans. Brain 142(8):2288–2302
Mandal PK, Fodale V (2009) Isoflurane and desflurane at clinically relevant concentrations induce amyloid beta-peptide oligomerization: an NMR study. Biochem Biophys Res Commun 379(3):716–720
Mashour GA (2006) Integrating the science of consciousness and anesthesia. Anesth Analg 103(4):975–982
Mashour GA, Kent C, Picton P, Ramachandran SK, Tremper KK, Turner CR, Shanks A, Avidan MS (2013) Assessment of intraoperative awareness with explicit recall: a comparison of 2 methods. Anesth Analg 116:889–891
Mason MF, Norton MI, Van Horn JD, Wegner DM, Grafton ST, Macrae CN (2007) Wandering minds: the default network and stimulus-independent thought. Science (New York, NY) 315(5810):393–395

Massimini M, Ferrarelli F, Huber R, Esser SK, Singh H, Tononi G (2005) Breakdown of cortical effective connectivity during sleep. Science 309(5744):2228–2232

Massimini M, Ferrarelli F, Esser SK, Riedner BA, Huber R, Murphy M, Peterson MJ, Tononi G (2007) Triggering sleep slow waves by transcranial magnetic stimulation. Proc Natl Acad Sci U S A 104(20):8496–8501

McCann ME, de Graaff JC, Dorris L et al (2019) Neurodevelopmental outcome at 5 years of age after general anaesthesia or awake-regional anaesthesia in infancy (GAS): an international, multicentre, randomised, controlled equivalence trial. Lancet 393(10172):664–677

Mihic SJ, Ye Q, Wick MJ, Koltchine VV, Krasowski MD, Finn SE, Mascia MP, Valenzuela CF, Hanson KK, Greenblatt EP, Harris RA, Harrison NL (1997) Sites of alcohol and volatile anaesthetic action on GABA(A) and glycine receptors. Nature 389(6649):385–389

Monk TG, Saini V, Weldon BC, Sigl JC (2005) Anesthetic management and one-year mortality after noncardiac surgery. Anesth Analg 100(1):4–10, no. 0003-2999; 0003-2999

Naci L, Haugg A, MacDonald A, Anello M, Houldin E, Naqshbandi G-LL, Arango M, Harle C, Cusack R, Owen A (2018) Functional diversity of brain networks supports consciousness and verbal intelligence. Sci Rep 8:13259

Noirhomme Q, Boly M, Bonhomme V, Boveroux P, Phillips C, Peigneux P, Soddu A, Luxen A, Moonen G, Maquet P, Laureys S (2009) Bispectral index correlates with regional cerebral blood flow during sleep in distinct cortical and subcortical structures in humans. Arch Ital Biol 147(1–2):51–57

Ori C, Dam M, Pizzolato G, Battistin L, Giron G (1986) Effects of isoflurane anesthesia on local cerebral glucose utilization in the rat. Anesthesiology 65(2):152–156

Pandit JJ, Andrade J, Bogod DG, Hitchman JM et al (2014) 5th National Audit Project (NAP5) on accidental awareness during general anaesthesia: summary of main findings and risk factors. Br J Anaesth 113(4):549–559

Prielipp RC, Wall MH, Tobin JR, Groban L, Cannon MA, Fahey FH, Gage HD, Stump DA, James RL, Bennett J, Butterworth J (2002) Dexmedetomidine-induced sedation in volunteers decreases regional and global cerebral blood flow. Anesth Analg 95(4):1052–1059, table of contents

Prys-Roberts C (1987) Anaesthesia: a practical or impractical construct? Br J Anaesth 59:1341–1345

Reinstrup P, Ryding E, Algotsson L, Berntman L, Uski T (1994) Effects of nitrous oxide on human regional cerebral blood flow and isolated pial arteries. Anesthesiology 81(2):396–402

Reinstrup P, Ryding E, Ohlsson T, Sandell A, Erlandsson K, Ljunggren K, Salford LG, Strand S, Uski T (2008) Regional cerebral metabolic rate (positron emission tomography) during inhalation of nitrous oxide 50% in humans. Br J Anaesth 100(1):66–71

Rex S, Schaefer W, Meyer PH, Rossaint R, Boy C, Setani K, Bull U, Baumert JH (2006) Positron emission tomography study of regional cerebral metabolism during general anesthesia with xenon in humans. Anesthesiology 105(5):936–943

Rex S, Meyer PT, Baumert JH, Rossaint R, Fries M, Bull U, Schaefer WM (2008) Positron emission tomography study of regional cerebral blood flow and flow-metabolism coupling during general anaesthesia with xenon in humans. Br J Anaesth 100(5):667–675

Reynolds DS, Rosahl TW, Cirone J, O'Meara GF, Haythornthwaite A, Newman RJ, Myers J, Sur C, Howell O, Rutter AR, Atack J, Macaulay AJ, Hadingham KL, Hutson PH, Belelli D, Lambert JJ, Dawson GR, McKernan R, Whiting PJ, Wafford KA (2003) Sedation and anesthesia mediated by distinct GABA(A) receptor isoforms. J Neurosci 23(24):8608–8617

Rudolph U, Antkowiak B (2004) Molecular and neuronal substrates for general anaesthetics. Nat Rev Neurosci 5(9):709–720

Salmi E, Kaisti KK, Metsahonkala L, Oikonen V, Aalto S, Nagren K, Hinkka S, Hietala J, Korpi ER, Scheinin H (2004) Sevoflurane and propofol increase 11C-flumazenil binding to gamma-aminobutyric acid A receptors in humans. Anesth Analg 99(5):1420–1426

Salmi E, Langsjo JW, Aalto S, Nagren K, Metsahonkala L, Kaisti KK, Korpi ER, Hietala J, Scheinin H (2005) Subanesthetic ketamine does not affect 11C-flumazenil binding in humans. Anesth Analg 101(3):722–725

Salmi E, Laitio RM, Aalto S, Maksimow AT, Langsjo JW, Kaisti KK, Aantaa R, Oikonen V, Metsahonkala L, Nagren K, Korpi ER, Scheinin H (2008) Xenon does not affect gamma-aminobutyric acid type A receptor binding in humans. Anesth Analg 106(1):129–134

Sandin RH, Enlund G, Samuelsson P, Lennmarken C (2000) Awareness during anaesthesia: a prospective case study. Lancet 355(9205):707–711

Schlunzen L, Vafaee MS, Cold GE, Rasmussen M, Nielsen JF, Gjedde A (2004) Effects of subanaesthetic and anaesthetic doses of sevoflurane on regional cerebral blood flow in healthy volunteers. A positron emission tomographic study. Acta Anaesthesiol Scand 48(10):1268–1276

Schlunzen L, Cold GE, Rasmussen M, Vafaee MS (2006) Effects of dose-dependent levels of isoflurane on cerebral blood flow in healthy subjects studied using positron emission tomography. Acta Anaesthesiol Scand 50(3):306–312

Schlunzen L, Vafaee MS, Juul N, Cold GE (2010) Regional cerebral blood flow responses to hyperventilation during sevoflurane anaesthesia studied with PET. Acta Anaesthesiol Scand 54(5):610–615

Schlunzen L, Juul N, Hansen KV, Cold GE (2012) Regional cerebral blood flow and glucose metabolism during propofol anaesthesia in healthy subjects studied with positron emission tomography. Acta Anaesthesiol Scand 56(2):248–255

Sebel PS, Bowdle TA, Ghoneim MM, Rampil IJ, Padilla RE, Gan TJ, Domino KB (2004) The incidence of awareness during anesthesia: a multicenter United States study. Anesth Analg 99(3):833–839

Short TG, Campbell D, Frampton C et al (2019) Anaesthetic depth and complications after major surgery: an international, randomised controlled trial. Lancet 394(10212):1907–1914

Spies M, James GM, Berroterán-Infante N, Ibeschitz H, Kranz GS, Unterholzner J, Godbersen M, Gryglewski G, Hienert M, Jungwirth J et al (2018) Assessment of ketamine binding of the serotonin transporter in humans with positron emission tomography. Int J Neuropsychopharmacol 21:145–153

Stamatakis EA, Adapa RM, Absalom AR, Menon DK (2010) Changes in resting neural connectivity during propofol sedation. PLoS One 5(12):e14224, no. 1932-6203; 1932-6203

Varley TF, Luppi A, Pappas I, Naci L, Adapa R, Owen A, Menon DK, Stamatakis EA (2019) Consciousness and brain functional complexity in propofol anaesthesia. bioRxiv: 680447

Velly LJ, Rey MF, Bruder NJ, Gouvitsos FA, Witjas T, Regis JM, Peragut JC, Gouin FM (2007) Differential dynamic of action on cortical and subcortical structures of anesthetic agents during induction of anesthesia. Anesthesiology 107(2):202–212

Vollenweider FX, Leenders KL, Oye I, Hell D, Angst J (1997) Differential psychopathology and patterns of cerebral glucose utilisation produced by (S)- and (R)-ketamine in healthy volunteers using positron emission tomography (PET). Eur Neuropsychopharmacol 7(1):25–38

Walker EM, Bell M, Cook TM, Grocott MP, Moonesinghe SR (2016) SNAP-1 investigator group. Patient reported outcome of adult perioperative anaesthesia in the United Kingdom: a cross-sectional observational study. Br J Anaesth 117:758–766

Whittington RA, Virag L, Marcouiller F et al (2011) Propofol directly increases tau phosphorylation. PLoS One 6(1):e16648

Xie G, Gunn RN, Dagher A, Daloze T, Plourde G, Backman SB, Diksic M, Fiset P (2004) PET quantification of muscarinic cholinergic receptors with [N-11C-methyl]-benztropine and application to studies of propofol-induced unconsciousness in healthy human volunteers. Synapse 51(2):91–101

Xie G, Deschamps A, Backman SB, Fiset P, Chartrand D, Dagher A, Plourde G (2011) Critical involvement of the thalamus and precuneus during restoration of consciousness with physostigmine in humans during propofol anaesthesia: a positron emission tomography study. Br J Anaesth 106(4):548–557

Zezula J, Cortes R, Probst A, Palacios JM (1988) Benzodiazepine receptor sites in the human brain: autoradiographic mapping. Neuroscience 25(3):771–795

PET Imaging in Altered States of Consciousness: Coma, Sleep, and Hypnosis

45

Estelle A. C. Bonin, Géraldine Martens, Helena Cassol, Camille Chatelle, Steven Laureys, and Aurore Thibaut

Contents

Abstract

Positron emission tomography (PET) allows studies of cerebral metabolism and blood flow and has been widely used to investigate physiological mechanisms underlying altered states of consciousness. Consciousness is characterized by two components: wakefulness and awareness. In this chapter, we review the current literature on brain metabolism during pathological loss of consciousness (vegetative/unresponsive or minimally conscious states), sleep (in healthy subjects and in patients with insomnia), and under hypnosis. By identifying brain areas specifically involved in conscious processing, these studies have contrib-

E. A. C. Bonin · G. Martens · H. Cassol · C. Chatelle · S. Laureys · A. Thibaut (✉)
Coma Science Group, GIGA-Consciousness, University of Liège, Liège, Belgium

Centre du Cerveau (C2), University Hospital of Liège, Liège, Belgium
e-mail: Estelle.Bonin@uliege.be; Geraldine.Martens@chuliege.be; hcassol@uliege.be; Steven.Laureys@uliege.be; athibaut@uliege.be

R. A. J. O. Dierckx et al. (eds.), *PET and SPECT in Neurology*,
https://doi.org/10.1007/978-3-030-53168-3_45

uted to our understanding of the underlying physiology of consciousness. The precuneal and cingulate cortices, for example, seem to be key areas for maintaining conscious awareness. FDG-PET further allowed the identification of the minimal energetic requirement for conscious awareness in this population, which corresponds to 42% of normal cortical activity. Up to now, it is the most accurate neuroimaging tool regarding the diagnosis of patients with disorders of consciousness. In the future, its use as part of multimodal assessment could improve diagnosis and prognosis in this challenging population. In sleep, a greater activity of the precuneus/posterior cingulate cortex and the frontoparietal areas during non-rapid eye movement sleep also seems to play a role in disorders such as insomnia. Other areas such as the hypothalamus, amygdala, or temporo-occipital cortex seem to play a role in different states such as rapid eye movement sleep and hypnosis. PET studies permit a better comprehension of the neural correlates of consciousness and identify the implication of specific neural areas and networks in altered states of consciousness in post-comatose patients, sleep, and induced hypnosis.

45.1 Introduction

There is at present no validated objective definition of consciousness (Noirhomme and Laureys 2011). Numerous definitions abound in the literature (Nagel et al. 1979; Searle 2000; Dehaene and Naccache 2001; Tononi 2004; Baars 2005); for a review, see Damasio and Kaspar (2009). Consciousness is a multifaceted concept described as comprising two major components: arousal and awareness (Zeman 2001). This dichotomous terminology provides a practical approach, which corresponds well to clinical settings (Posner et al. 2007). Arousal refers to the degree of wakefulness or the level of consciousness. It is clinically manifested by spontaneous eye opening (indicating wakefulness and rest cycles) and controlled mainly by the ascending reticular system in the brainstem, midbrain, and thalamus. Awareness is a term used to describe the capacity to perceive and to experience something—that is, the phenomenological experience of being (Nagel et al. 1979) or the contents of consciousness. Evidence from functional neuroimaging studies suggests that there are two anticorrelated cortical systems that mediate conscious awareness: an "extrinsic" network that encompasses lateral frontoparietal areas and has been linked with processes of external input (external awareness) and an "intrinsic" network which includes mainly medial brain areas and has been associated with internal processes (internal awareness) (Vanhaudenhuyse et al. 2011). The clinical quantification of awareness is limited to evaluating patients' motor responsiveness to commands and nonreflex behaviors, such as visual pursuit or localization to pain (Noirhomme and Laureys 2011; for a review, see Gosseries et al., 2014).

Awareness is believed to be a phenomenon emerging from cortical activity and supported by subcortical connections in particular to the thalamus. Even if awareness normally follows from arousal, the two qualities are dissociable. Hence, preserved arousal does not necessarily imply awareness (Laureys 2005). As the anatomical and physiological correlates of consciousness are complex, the interplay of arousal and awareness is incompletely understood, and a plethora of questions remain unsolved, limiting our understanding of the human consciousness.

During the last decade, researchers began to investigate brain activity in patients with disorders of consciousness (DOC) following severe brain injury. Other studies focused on hypnosis and sleep, and in conjunction, these investigations contributed to our current understanding of the minimal neural correlates of conscious awareness in both physiological and pathological states.

One way to study brain activity is by positron emission tomography (PET), measuring regional increases in cerebral blood flow (rCBF) with [^{18}F]-fluorodeoxyglucose (FDG) or using ^{15}O-labeled water (H_2O^{15}). PET imaging allows studies of regional brain functionality at rest, without the patients' active participation. The aim of this chapter is to provide an overview of the neural correlates of altered consciousness, identified by PET studies, in both physiological and pathological conditions (for summary, see Tables 45.1, 45.2, 45.3, and 45.4). We will first discuss studies on

Table 45.1 Summary of FDG-PET studies on disorders of consciousness during resting state

Authors	*N*	Diagnosis	Time since injuries	Main findings
Levy et al. (1987)	*7*	UWS	1–72	60% (53–67%) decrease in metabolism
DeVolder et al. (1990)	*7*	UWS	1–4	53% (43–65%) decrease in metabolism
Tommasino et al. (1995)	*10*	UWS	2–24	56% decrease in metabolism
Plum et al. (1998)	*3*	UWS		50% decrease in metabolism with significant regional variations
Laureys et al. (1999a)	*4*	UWS	<1–60	Frontoparietal hypometabolism and disconnections
Laureys et al. (1999b)	*1*	UWS	1	38% decrease in metabolism; recovery of consciousness = frontoparietal recovery
Rudolf et al. (1999a)	*24*	UWS	<1–6	25% decrease in metabolism (17% for acute patients (<3 months) and 33% for chronic patients (>3 months))
Schiff and Plum (1999)	*1*	UWS	240	50% decrease in metabolism with significant regional variations
Laureys et al. (2000b)	*1*	UWS	4	Recovery of consciousness = thalamocortical reconnections
Rudolf et al. (2000)	*9*	UWS	<1	Decrease in benzodiazepine receptor density in VS/UWS
Laureys et al. (2002a)	*30*	UWS	1–5	56% (37–72%) decrease in metabolism

(continued)

Table 45.1 (continued)

Authors	*N*	Diagnosis	Time since injuries	Main findings
Schiff et al. (2002)	*5*	UWS	6–240	50% (31–87%) decrease in metabolism with regional variations
Beuthien-Baumann et al. (2003)	*16*	UWS	2–12	58% decrease in metabolism; frontoparietal hypometabolism
Tengvar et al. (2004)	*1*	MCS	6	47–65% frontoparietal hypometabolism
Juengling et al. (2005)	*5*	UWS	1–48	Frontoparietal and thalamic hypometabolism
Nakayama et al. (2006)	*30*	17 UWS 13 MCS	6–60	Frontoparietal and thalamic hypometabolism in VS/UWS
				Less impaired in MCS
Majerus et al. (2009)	*36*	MCS	1–265	Hypometabolism in language-processing regions (left superior, middle and inferior temporal gyri, left inferior frontal gyrus, and the right inferior temporal gyri)
Schnakers et al. (2008)	*1*	MCS	24	Changes in the fronto-temporoparietal network and the sensorimotor area
Silva et al. (2010)	*10*	UWS	2–24	Frontoparietal hypometabolism
Lull et al. (2010)	*17*	UWS and MCS	12	Thalamus hypometabolism
Bruno et al. (2010)	*10*	UWS	3	Frontoparietal hypometabolism (VS/UWS without fixation = patients with fixation)
Phillips et al. (2011)	*13 8*	UWS LIS	<1–290	Automatic classification between VS/UWS and healthy subjects or LIS using the "relevance vector machine"
Garcia-Panach et al. (2011)	*17*	UWS and MCS	12	Cortico-thalamocortical hypometabolism correlates with less favorable outcomes
Bruno et al. (2012)	*27*	13 MCS	1–70	Left-sided metabolism MCS+ (command following) > MCS− (low level of nonreflexive behaviors)
		14 MCS+		Broca's region disconnection from language network, mesiofrontal, and cerebellar areas in MCS−
Thibaut et al. (2012)	*70*	24 UWS	<1–270	Extrinsic and intrinsic network hypometabolism in VS/UWS
Studies using resting state FDG-PET to evaluate the effects of pharmacological treatment				
Chatelle et al. (2014)	3	MCS	18 months to 7 years	Metabolism increase in bilateral dorsolateral prefrontal and mesiofrontal cortices after the administration of zolpidem
Studies using resting state FDG-PET to evaluate the effects of pharmacological treatment and as a diagnostic tool				
Stender et al. (2014)	112	UWS, MCS, LIS	<1 month to >1 year	85% of diagnosis agreement between CRS-R and FDG-PET for MCS (67% for UWS). 74% good outcome prediction

Table 45.1 (continued)

Authors	*N*	Diagnosis	Time since injuries	Main findings
Stender et al. (2015)	41	UWS, MCS, eMCS	10 days to 9 years	Regional differences between VS/UWS and MCS more pronounced in the frontoparietal cortex. In the brainstem and thalamus, metabolism declined equally in both VS/UWS and MCS
Stender et al. (2016)	131	UWS, MCS, eMCS	622–1299 days	Use of extracerebral tissue normalization. 42% of normal cortical activity = minimal energetic requirement for conscious awareness
Studies using resting state FDG-PET as part of multimodal assessment				
Soddu et al. (2016)	15	UWS, LIS	NA	High correlation between resting state fMRI total neuronal activity and PET cerebral metabolism. UWS vs. HS = decrease in lateral and medial frontoparietal networks for both techniques
Annen et al. (2016)	25	UWS, MCS, eMCS	30 days to 1.8 years	Association between functional metabolism (inferior parietal, precuneus, and frontal regions) and structural integrity of the DMN (frontal-inferior parietal, precuneus-inferior parietal, thalamo-inferior parietal, and thalamofrontal tracts)
Di Perri et al. (2016)	58	UWS, MCS, eMCS	27 months	Correlation between FDG-PET brain metabolism and fMRI connectivity. Brain metabolism increase in the thalamus, basal ganglia, and lateral frontoparietal, parieto-occipital, and temporal cortices. Correlation between brain metabolisms and CRS-R scores in the lateral frontoparietal and superior temporal regions
Bodart et al. (2017)	24	UWS, MCS, eMCS, LIS	5–1116 weeks	FDG-PET and PCI revealed preserved metabolic rates and high complexity levels in four patients who were behaviorally unresponsive.
Golkowski et al. (2017)	20	UWS, MCS	116–170 days	Glucose metabolism in the occipital lobe higher in MCS as compared to VS/UWS. FDG-PET values in the occipital cortex correlated with CRS-R on the day of measurement
Annen et al. (2018)	12	UWS, MCS	7.5–50 months	Preservation in the region of the right dorsolateral prefrontal cortex, the inferior parietal junction, and the inferior temporal gyrus in patient with signs of "covert command following"

VS/UWS vegetative state/unresponsive wakefulness syndrome, *MCS* minimally conscious state, *MCS+* patients in "MCS plus" (showing command following), *MCS−* patients in "MCS minus" (showing minimal level of behavioral interactions without command following), *LIS* locked-in syndrome, *EMCS* emergence from the minimally conscious state, *HS* healthy subject, *DMN* default mode network, *CRS-R* Coma Recovery Scale-Revised, *EEG* electroencephalogram, *fMRI* functional magnetic resonance imaging, *PCI* perturbational complexity index

Table 45.2 Summary of PET-H_2O^{15} studies in patients with disorders of consciousness during sensory stimulations

Authors	*N*	Diagnosis	Time since insult (day(s) and month(s))	Passive stimulation	Level of activation
De Jong et al. (1997)	1	UWS	2 months	Auditory (familiar voice)	High
Menon et al. (1998)	1	UWS	3 months	Visual (familiar face)	Low
Laureys et al. (2000a)	5	UWS	3–38 days	Auditory (click)	Low
Laureys et al. (2002b)	15	UWS	1 month	Pain (electrical stimulation)	Low
Schiff et al. (2002)	5	3 UWS, 2 UWS	6–300 months	Auditory (click), tactile	Low/high
Owen et al. (2002)	3	1 UWS, 2 UWS	4 months	Visual (familiar face), auditory (noise, words)	Low/high
Kassubek et al. (2003)	7	UWS	3–48 months	Pain (electrical stimulation)	High
Boly et al. (2004)	20	15 UWS, 5 MCS	1–4 months	Auditory (click)	Low/high
Laureys et al. (2004b)	1	MCS	6 months	Auditory (noise, cries, own name)	High
Owen et al. (2005)	1	UWS	4 months	Auditory (speech)	High
Giacino et al. (2006)	5	UWS	1–3 months	Visual (flash)	Low
Boly et al. (2008a)	20	15 UWS, 5 MCS	1–4 months	Pain (electrical stimulation)	Low/high
Silva et al. (2010)	5	UWS	2–22 months	Tactile	Low

UWS unresponsive wakefulness syndrome, *MCS* minimally conscious state, *LIS* locked-in syndrome

patients with disorders of consciousness, in resting state condition and during passive stimulation paradigms. We will then give an overview of sleep and hypnosis studies and discuss the clinical implications of these findings.

45.2 Disorders of Consciousness Following a Brain Injury

Following severe brain damage with loss of consciousness, patients usually evolve through different clinical stages before fully or partially recovering consciousness. Coma is defined as complete absence of arousal and awareness, with no eye opening

Table 45.3 Summary of PET studies on healthy subjects during sleep

Authors	*N*		Stage	Main findings
Maquet et al. (1990)	11	FDG	SWS	Metabolism decrease 40% (>thalami)
			REMS	Metabolism = wakefulness
Maquet et al. (1996)	7	FDG	REMS	Metabolism increase in the tegmentum, left thalamus, amygdala, ACC, and right parietal operculum
				Metabolism decrease in dorsolateral prefrontal and parietal cortices, PCC, and the precuneus
Braun et al. (1997)	37	H_2O^{15}	SWS/REMS	Metabolism decrease in centrencephalic and heteromodal association regions and increase in S1–S2
				Metabolism increase in centrencephalic and S1–S2 and decrease in the frontoparietal association cortices
Hofle et al. (1997)	11	H_2O^{15}	SWS	rCBF negatively correlates with sigma power (EEG) in the thalamus bilaterally
Maquet (1997)	11	H_2O^{15}	SWS	Metabolism decrease in the dorsal pons and mesencephalon, thalami, basal ganglia, basal forebrain/hypothalamus, orbitofrontal cortex, anterior cingulate cortex, and precuneus
Andersson et al. (1998)	19	H_2O^{15}	SWS	Metabolism decrease in the thalamus and the frontal and parietal association areas and increase in the cerebellum
Kajimura et al. (1999)	18	H_2O^{15}	SWS	Metabolism decrease in midbrain tegmentum, cerebellar vermis, basal forebrain, caudate nucleus, posterior cingulate gyrus, and neocortical regions
Nofzinger et al. (1997)	8	FDG	REMS	Metabolism increase in limbic regions and orbitofrontal, cingulate, entorhinal, and insular cortices
Peigneux et al. (2001)	12	H_2O^{15}	REMS	Correlation during REMS between the density of REMS and rCBF in the occipital and the lateral geniculate bodies of the thalamus
Nofzinger et al. (2002)	14	FDG	SWS	Metabolism decrease in frontal, parietal, temporal and occipital cortices and the thalamus
				Increases in the dorsal pontine tegmentum, hypothalamus, basal forebrain, ventral striatum, anterior cingulate cortex, and mesial temporal lobe
Dang-Vu et al. (2005)	23	H_2O^{15}	SWS	Association between rCBF in the ventromedial prefrontal regions and delta power (EEG)
Maquet et al. (2005)	207	H_2O^{15}	REMS	Metabolism decrease in frontal and parietal areas

(continued)

Table 45.3 (continued)

Authors	*N*		Stage	Main findings
Wilckens et al. (2016)	52	FDG	Wakefulness	Higher relative slow-wave activity associated with greater dorsolateral prefrontal metabolism in healthy subjects. Negative correlation between age and wake metabolism in the dorsolateral prefrontal cortex
Kay et al. (2016)	44 PI, 40 GS	FDG	Wakefulness, SWS/NREM	Insomnia associated with impaired disengagement of theleft frontoparietal and the left middle frontal cortices, the precuneus/posterior cingulate, and the fusiform/lingual gyri during NREM sleep and impaired engagement of these regions during wakefulness
Kay et al. (2019)	17 PI, 19 GS	FDG	Wakefulness, SWS/NREM	Individuals with insomnia and good sleepers showed similar relative rCMRglc responses to acute sleep restriction (lower relative rCMRglc in the left frontoparietal cortex, medial frontal cortex, posterior cingulate cortex, and thalamus)

FDG fluorodeoxyglucose, *SWS* slow-wave sleep, *REMS* rapid eye movement sleep, *NREMS* non-rapid eye movement sleep, *rCBF* regional cerebral blood flow, *ACC* anterior cingulate cortex, *S1–S2* primary and secondary sensorimotor areas, *EEG* electroencephalography, *GS* good sleeper, *PI* primary insomnia, *rCMRglc* regional cerebral metabolic rate for glucose

and only presenting reflexive behavior, in other words an "unarousable unresponsiveness" (Posner et al. 2007). When eye opening and rest-wake cycles are reestablished but the patients still only exhibit reflexive behaviors, they are said to be in a vegetative state (VS), now called unresponsive wakefulness syndrome (UWS) (The Multi-Society Task Force on PVS 1994; Laureys et al. 2010). Progression from VS/UWS usually leads to the minimally conscious state, where reproducible but fluctuating signs of consciousness are present, such as eye tracking motion or response to verbal or tactile stimuli (Giacino et al. 2002), but these patients are, by definition, unable to effectively communicate. We recently proposed a subcategorization of MCS patients based on the complexity of their behavior in two entities: "MCS −" and "MCS +." "MCS −" describes patients with minimal level of behavioral interactions without command following (e.g., visual pursuit, localization of noxious stimulation, and/or smiling/crying in contingent relationship to external stimuli). "MCS +" patients show higher-level behavioral responses such as command following (Fig. 45.1) (Bruno et al. 2012). The emergence of the MCS is characterized by the recovery of functional communication (verbal or nonverbal) or functional use of objects (Giacino et al. 2002). In rare cases, following brainstem lesions, patients can fully recover consciousness but remain totally paralyzed and aphonic, in the aptly named locked-in syndrome (Laureys et al. 2005a). These patients are able to communicate only with small eye movements (American Congress of Rehabilitation Medicine 1995). The difficulty in disentangling reflexive from voluntary responses, the fluctuation of vigilance, and the additional cognitive or sensory deficits lead to a

Table 45.4 PET studies on hypnosis, at rest, and during pain stimulation in healthy subjects

Authors	*N*	PET	Paradigm	State	Main findings
Maquet (1999)	9	H_2O^{15}	Rest	Hypnotic state	Widespread metabolism increase, mainly left sided (occipital, parietal, precentral, premotor, and ventrolateral prefrontal cortices)
Rainville et al. (1999b)	10	H_2O^{15}	Pain	Hypnotic suggestion	Increased metabolism in ACC and in the inferior frontal gyri
					Decreased metabolism in the right inferior parietal lobule, the left precuneus, and the posterior cingulate gyrus
Rainville et al. (1997)	11	H_2O^{15}	Pain	Hypnotic suggestion	Increase in ACC
Rainville et al. (1999a)	22	H_2O^{15}	Pain	Hypnotic state	Increase in ACC, insula, S1 and S2
Faymonville et al. (2000)	11	H_2O^{15}	Pain	Hypnotic state	Metabolism increase in right-sided extrastriate area and the ACC
Hofbauer et al. (2001)	10	H_2O^{15}	Pain	(a) Hypnotic state	(a) Activation of S1 and S2, ACC, and insula
				(b) Hypnotic suggestion	(b) Significant increase in pain-evoked activity within S1 and ACC
Rainville et al. (2002)	10	H_2O^{15}	Rest	Hypnotic state	Metabolism increase in the ACC, thalamus, and pontomesencephalic brainstem
					Decrease in the inferior parietal lobule, the precuneus, and the posterior temporal cortices
Faymonville et al. (2003)	19	H_2O^{15}	Pain	Hypnotic state	Increased functional connectivity between midcingulate cortex and insula, pregenual and frontal areas, pre-SMA, brainstem, thalamus, and basal ganglia
Derbyshire et al. (2004)	33	H_2O^{15}	Rest	Hypnotic suggestion	Both pain and hypnotically induced pain experience and pain stimulation induced metabolic modulations within the thalamus, ACC, insula, and prefrontal and parietal cortices
Nusbaum et al. (2011)	14	H_2O^{15}	Rest (patients with chronic low-back pain)	Hypnotic suggestion	Metabolism increase in frontotemporal area, insula, caudate, acumens, lenticular nuclei, and ACC

ACC anterior cingulate cortex, *S1–S2* primary and secondary sensorimotor cortex, *SMA* supplementary motor area

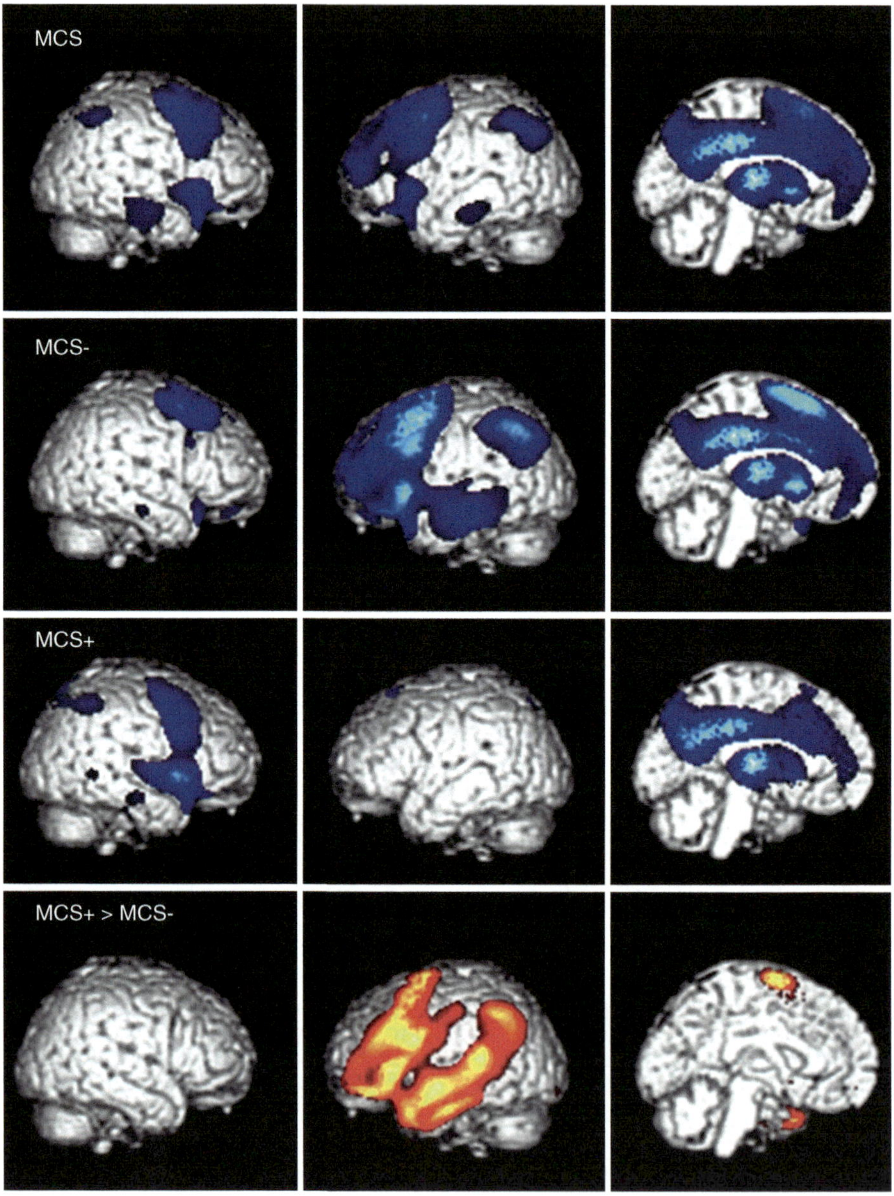

Fig. 45.1 Areas with impaired metabolism (shown in *blue*) in patients in a minimally conscious state (*MCS*), MCS− (showing nonreflex behavior), and MCS+ (showing command following). The *lowest panel* illustrates areas with higher metabolism in MCS+ as compared to MCS− (shown in *orange*). All results are shown on a 3D MRI template and thresholded at false discovery rate corrected $p < 0.05$ (from Bruno et al. (2012))

high rate of misdiagnosis between VS/UWS and MCS (Andrews et al. 1996; Childs and Mercer 1996; Schnakers et al. 2009) and locked-in syndrome (Bruno et al. 2009). The diagnosis may influence decisions about the patients' care, regarding crucial matters such as end-of-life decisions (Demertzi et al. 2011) or pain management (Demertzi et al. 2009). In this context, objective measures independent of the integrity of the motor pathways are needed to supplement behavioral assessments at the bedside. Neuroimaging provides a promising means to this end (for a review, see Schiff (2006) and Laureys and Schiff (2012)).

45.3 PET Scan and Disorders of Consciousness

45.3.1 Measuring the Brain at "Rest"

In 1987, the first FDG-PET study on VS/UWS patients showed a global decrease in brain metabolism of about 40–50% (Levy et al. 1987). These results were reproduced in several studies (DeVolder et al. 1990; Tommasino et al. 1995; Laureys et al. 1999b; Rudolf et al. 1999b; Stender et al. 2015). FDG-PET was suggested to be a good tool to complement bedside examination and reduce misdiagnosis (Schnakers et al. 2009). Indeed, regarding the diagnosis of MCS patients, FDG-PET showed 85% of good congruence with the score of the Coma Recovery Scale-Revised (i.e., CRS-R, this behavioral scale is the gold standard for the diagnosis of DOC patient) with a sensitivity to identify MCS patients of 93%. It is also a good tool to predict patient outcomes (i.e., 74% of VS/UWS and MCS patients diagnosed by FDG-PET remained respectively unconscious and conscious at follow-up) (Stender et al. 2014). Even if the diagnostic and prognostic usefulness of this technique has been shown, they still lack clear guidelines regarding the assessment of changes in brain metabolism due to the use of nonquantitative methods (i.e., visual examination). More recent studies (Table. 45.2) reported an average of 42% of global cerebral metabolism rate of glucose (CMRglc) in VS/UWS and 55% in MCS patients with more pronounced difference in the frontoparietal and precuneal cortices (Stender et al. 2015), highlighting that a minimum of 42% of global brain metabolism preservation is needed for the emergence of consciousness in post-comatose patients. In another study using an objective method to quantify FDG-PET images (i.e., by normalizing the images to extracerebral tissue and not the brainstem which could be impaired and bias the results), they confirmed that 42% of normal cortical hemispheric activity represents the minimal energetic requirement for sustained awareness (Stender et al. 2016). Moreover, in this study, all the FDG-PET images of MCS patients were normalized to their global best-hemisphere mean in order to investigate the effect of regional variation relative to resting baseline metabolism on cognitive and sensory function. The results showed an increase of this regional metabolism variation relative to resting baseline (i.e., 10–30% of increase) in response to sensory and cognitive tasks reflecting a preservation of some specific cognitive and sensory functions in MCS patients.

Regarding patients in locked-in syndrome, brain metabolism levels are closer to normal than VS/UWS patients (Levy et al. 1987). Results from studies by Laureys et al. indicated that no supratentorial cortical areas show significantly lower metabolism in acute and chronic locked-in patients when compared to age-matched healthy subjects (Laureys et al. 2003, 2004a, 2005a). However, the global brain metabolism is not directly correlated with the level of consciousness. A recovery from VS/UWS does not always imply substantial changes in global brain metabolism (Laureys et al. 1999b). Moreover, some healthy subjects show metabolic rates of glucose comparable to VS/UWS patients (Laureys 2005). Those results suggest that some brain areas are more important for the emergence of consciousness than others (Laureys et al. 1999b, 2000c, 2004a). Studies on regional brain metabolism were performed to identify areas specifically involved in loss of consciousness, comparing brain metabolism of VS/UWS and MCS patients with age-matched healthy subjects. Results highlighted a widespread impairment of the frontoparietal network, encompassing midline (i.e., anterior cingulate cortex (ACC)/mesiofrontal and posterior cingulate cortex (PCC)/precuneus) and lateral (i.e., prefrontal and posterior parietal) associative cortices being associated with a decreased level of consciousness (Laureys et al. 1999a, b; Beuthien-Baumann et al. 2003; Juengling et al. 2005; Nakayama et al. 2006; Lull et al. 2010; Silva et al. 2010; Bruno et al. 2012; Thibaut et al. 2012). Preserved areas were the midbrain and brainstem structures, known to be involved in autonomous functions such as sleep-wake cycles, thermoregulation, and respiration (Laureys et al. 2002a). Moreover, functional connectivity studies also highlighted a cortico-cortical (Laureys et al. 1999a, 2000b, 2002b) and thalamocortical (Laureys et al. 2000b) disconnection syndrome in VS/UWS patients. A recent study showed that a cortico-thalamocortical hypometabolism seems to be correlated with less favorable outcome (Garcia-Panach et al. 2011). These observations led to the hypothesis that consciousness is an emergent property of frontoparietal functional connectivity (Baars et al. 2003; Laureys 2005).

A clinical trial (Giacino et al. 2012) has shown effects of amantadine, a mixed noradrenergic and dopaminergic agonist, toward improving the speed of recovery from disorders of consciousness. A case study reported by Schnakers et al. highlighted effects on brain metabolism of the drug, in a widespread frontotemporoparietal network and the sensorimotor area (Schnakers et al. 2008). These data suggest a modulation of polymodal associative cortical metabolism and motor function by amantadine. Alongside, they underline the behavioral improvements associated with amantadine treatment (e.g., recovery of command following). Within this frontoparietal network, the precuneus seems to be a critical region (Vogt and Laureys 2005). This area is the most active in conscious resting states (Raichle and Snyder 2007) and seems to be the most widely impaired in patients with disorders of consciousness (Laureys et al. 2005b). Studies, based on the mesocircuit hypothesis (Schiff 2010), investigated the effect of zolpidem in DOC patients (Whyte and Myers 2009). Indeed, in rare cases, this non-benzodiazepine agent usually used to treat insomnia (Langtry and Benfield 1990; Sanger 2004) results in a paradoxical increase in responsiveness at bedside (Clauss and Nel 2006; Shames and Ring 2008). A case study using FDG-PET was performed in three zolpidem responders that were MCS and showed an increased metabolism in the dorsolateral prefrontal and mesiofrontal cortices following zolpidem administration (Chatelle et al. 2014). According to the mesocircuit hypothesis, zolpidem could increase thalamic activity by disinhibiting the globus pallidus interna and thereby restoring thalamocortical connectivity, preferentially with the prefrontal cortex, and, thus, induce increase in prefrontal activity. After zolpidem intake, an impaired brain metabolism was observed in the thalami and the left precuneus/posterior cingulated. These impaired brain areas did not show structural lesions, suggesting that neurologic deficits in responders are not due to brain lesions in these areas but could rather be linked to an inhibitory functional effect of the fronto-thalamic connectivity.

A study on traumatic brain-injured patients found a hypometabolism in the ACC and PCC, the medial frontobasal regions, and the thalamus. The metabolism in these regions was mostly impaired in VS/UWS patients compared to MCS. Moreover, hypometabolism was more widespread and prominent in the MCS group as compared to patients who had emerged from the MCS (Nakayama et al. 2006). Within this network, it seems possible to distinguish areas involved in external (related to external/sensory awareness) or internal consciousness (related to internal/self-awareness) (Laureys et al. 1999a; Tian et al. 2007; Boly et al. 2008b; Vanhaudenhuyse et al. 2011). These results demonstrated that both external (encompassing lateral frontoparietal cortices) and internal (midline areas) networks were impaired in VS/UWS patients, while MCS patients only had decreased metabolism in the internal network, even less affected in patients emerging from the MCS (Thibaut et al. 2012).

Cerebral PET imaging has also been employed to disentangle reflexive from nonreflexive movements. International guidelines seem to disagree whether visual fixation is compatible with the diagnosis of VS/UWS (i.e., automatic subcortical process (Royal College of Physicians 2003)) or is a sufficient sign of awareness by mandating a higher-order cortical processing (Giacino et al. 2002). It was shown that anoxic VS/UWS patients with or without visual fixation presented identical brain metabolism and cortico-cortical functional disconnections, indicating that visual fixation does not necessarily reflect awareness in anoxic patients (Bruno et al. 2010). PET scan was also used to explore other cognitive dysfunctions, such as aphasia, which could induce an underestimation of cognitive capabilities of patients with disorders of consciousness. A study by Majerus and collaborators highlights that brain metabolism in language-processing regions (left superior, middle, and inferior temporal gyri, left inferior frontal gyrus, and right inferior temporal gyri) was shown to be particularly impaired in MCS patients whatever the etiology (Majerus et al. 2009), suggesting that a significant part of this population could suffer from language disorders such as aphasia. It was further investigated whether the differences in brain metabolism supported the subcategorization of the MCS into MCS− and MCS + (Bruno et al. 2012). Patients in MCS+ showed a higher cerebral metabolism in left-sided cortical areas encompassing the language network, premotor, pre-supplementary motor, and sensorimotor cortices as compared to patients in MCS− (Fig. 45.1). FDG-PET studies also allow development of machine-learning classifiers for clinical use, by automatic assessment of the functional integrity in this frontoparietal network and calculation of a probability for a patient to be conscious or not (Phillips et al. 2011). The development of automated methods could help in the future to improve the accuracy of the diagnosis of these patients on a single-subject level.

Recently, several studies focused on the use of multimodal assessment to improve diagnostic precision in DOC patients (Table. 45.1). Indeed, transcranial magnetic stimulation combined with electroencephalography (i.e., TMS-EEG; Bodart et al. 2017) and P3-based brain-computer interface (Annen et al. 2016) showed good congruence with FDG-PET diagnosis. The combined use of FDG-PET and these techniques seems to be a reliable way to increase diagnostic accuracy in DOC patients. In the first case, TMS-EEG could be used to assess the effective connectivity of cortical neurons in patients for whom an accurate diagnosis is needed for important clinical decisions (Bodart et al. 2017). In the second case, P3-based brain-computer interface (BCI) paradigm allows the identification of patients with "covert command following" (i.e., presenting an appropriate cortical activation—measured by EEG—in response to a command, without being able to respond to command at the bedside). PET images of these patients with "covert command following" showed a higher glucose metabolism in brain regions involved in language and a good agreement with the diagnosis of MCS (Annen et al. 2018). The use of resting state functional magnetic resonance imaging (i.e., fMRI) as a complementary technique has also been investigated in several recent studies. A study comparing functional MRI neuronal activity maps and FDG-PET cerebral metabolic maps found a high correlation between these two techniques. Results suggest that resting state fMRI maps could allow the estimation of relative levels of FDG-PET metabolic activity and could be useful for clinical centers with no FDG-PET (Soddu et al. 2016). Other studies investigated the relationship between functional brain activity and structural connectivity in DOC patients by combining FDG-PET and fMRI. The results showed an association between functional metabolism (i.e., the inferior parietal, precuneus, and frontal regions) and structural integrity of the default mode network (i.e., DMN including frontal-inferior parietal, precuneus-inferior parietal, thalamo-inferior parietal, and thalamofrontal tracts) (Annen et al. 2016; Di Perri et al. 2016). Even if FDG-PET seems to have a better diagnostic precision than mental imagery fMRI, this last one could be a good complement when further investigation about preserved cognitive abilities is needed (Stender et al. 2014). A recent case series using simultaneously EEG-PET-fMRI techniques confirmed that the use of multimodal assessment could improve diagnosis and prognosis of DOC patients (Golkowski et al. 2017). Multimodal assessment could also help for the management of pharmaceutical and non-pharmacological treatment trials such as amantadine, zolpidem, and apomorphine or tDCS and DBS and to assess the effect of such therapeutic interventions on brain activity of DOC patients (Table. 45.1) (Lemaire et al. 2018; Sanz et al. 2019; Schnakers et al. 2008; for a review, see Thibaut et al., 2019).

45.3.2 Measuring the Brain During Sensory Stimulation

Since the 1990s, functional neuroimaging studies have investigated regional increases in rCBF in response to passive external stimulation (auditory, visual, or somatosensory) using ^{15}O-labeled water PET (see Table 45.3). The first studies on brain metabolism in VS/UWS patients during sensory stimulation found a residual subcortical neural activation but also gray matter region activation encompassing primary auditory (De Jong et al. 1997; Laureys et al. 2000a; Owen et al. 2002; Schiff et al. 2002; Boly et al. 2004), somatosensory (Laureys et al. 2002b; Boly et al. 2008a), or visual cortices (Menon et al. 1998; Giacino et al. 2006), depending on the stimulation. However, these studies also highlighted a functional disconnection from associative cortical areas encompassing ACC, insular, prefrontal, and posterior parietal cortices reported to be necessary for awareness (Schiff et al. 2002). These results suggest that brain processing following a stimulus is insufficient to induce a conscious integration of the stimulation in VS/UWS population (Laureys et al. 1999a, 2002b; Boly et al. 2004). In contrast, brain activation and connectivity were significantly higher in MCS than in VS/UWS patients following an auditory stimulus, suggesting that MCS patients can reach a certain level of sensory and affective perception (Boly et al. 2004). Other studies investigated the impact of an emotional auditory stimulus, such as the voice of a relative or the patients' own name. These studies demonstrated that emotional stimuli in MCS, as compared to VS/UWS, induced a higher level of activation in the internal network (i.e., ACC/mesiofrontal and PCC/precuneus) areas known to be involved in self-awareness (Laureys and Boly 2007). Modification of blood flow in response to different auditory relevant modalities, such as meaningful stories told by a relative (Bekinschtein et al. 2004) or self-referential stimuli (i.e., patients' own name) (Laureys 2004; Qin et al. 2010), also showed an activation within this network. Moreover, a linear correlation between the level of consciousness and activation of the ACC in MCS patients was identified (Qin et al. 2010). These results suggest a relative preservation of emotional perception in MCS, as compared to VS/UWS.

Differential pain sensitivity—a matter with important ethical implications—was investigated using PET imaging during nociceptive stimulation. Boly et al. reported an activation and preservation of the connectivity within the "pain matrix" in MCS patients, including ACC and insular areas, thought to be important in the affective emotional perception of pain (Kupers et al. 2005; Boly et al. 2008a). These observations should encourage physicians to systematically use analgesic treatment in MCS, even if (by definition) they cannot communicate their feelings (Demertzi et al. 2009, 2012; Schnakers et al. 2012). However, these neuroimaging data are shown at the group level and should be used with caution regarding clinical or ethical decisions at the single level.

45.4 PET Scan and Sleep

Normal sleep can be considered as a physiological state of reduction of consciousness. It is characterized by the absence of arousal and different stages of awareness—from alteration (rapid eye movement sleep, REMS) to loss of awareness (slow-wave sleep, SWS). Slow-wave activity is a part of non-rapid eye movement sleep (NREMS). During NREMS, a decrease in cerebral blood flow and glucose metabolism is observed in regions involved in cognitive, affective, and arousal system (Braun et al. 1997; Buchsbaum 2001; Nofzinger et al. 2002). A recent study in young and middle-age (i.e., range from 25 to 61 years old) healthy adults showed that greater encephalographic slow-wave activity during NREMS was related to a greater prefrontal metabolic rate during wakefulness, suggesting that neural synchrony underlying slow-wave activity leads to the restoration of waking function (Wilckens et al. 2016). In contrast, age was related to a lower semiquantitative whole-brain metabolism and superior frontal metabolism during wakefulness, but this effect was moderated by the presence of slow-wave activity. During SWS, overall brain metabolism decreases to approximately 60% of normal waking values (Maquet et al. 1997), whereas in REMS, metabolism returns to nearly normal waking values (Maquet 2000) (Table 45.4, Fig. 45.2). Further studies have investigated the related changes to regional brain metabolism and highlighted cerebral deactivations in a wide frontoparietal network encompassing the polymodal associative cortices, bilateral frontal regions, parietotemporal and posterior parietal areas, PCC,

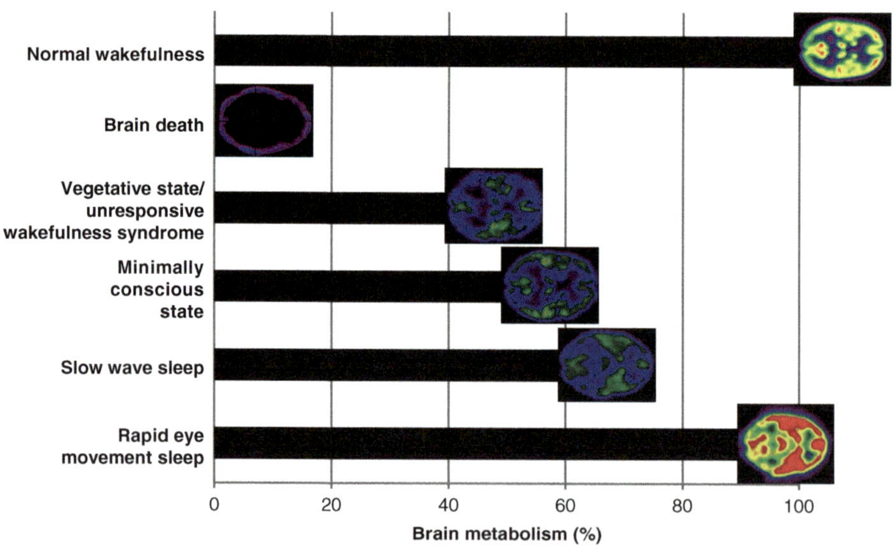

Fig. 45.2 Mean decrease in global cerebral metabolism (in percentage of normal conscious waking values) in pathological (brain death, vegetative state/unresponsive wakefulness syndrome, minimally conscious state) and physiological (sleep—slow-wave and rapid eye movement sleeps) altered states of consciousness. (Adapted from Laureys et al. (2004a) and Maquet (2000))

and mesiofrontal and precuneal cortices, while primary sensory cortices were still active (Maquet et al. 1996, 1997; Braun et al. 1997; Nofzinger et al. 2002). These frontoparietal associative cortical areas are called the "default mode network" and were shown to be mostly active in resting non-stimulated waking conditions in a functional magnetic resonance imaging study (Raichle and Mintun 2006). This network is known to be important in various functions relating to consciousness, such as attention, memory, and language (Baars et al. 2003), and its deactivation could explain the alteration of consciousness during SWS. FDG-PET studies on patients with insomnia confirmed the importance of these regions in sleep regulation. Indeed, a recent study aimed to compare regional cerebral metabolic rate of glucose in patients with insomnia and good sleepers. In good sleepers, the greater NREMS vs. wake differences were observed in the cerebellum and the prefrontal and parietal cortices. Compared to good sleepers, patients with insomnia also showed a smaller glucose metabolism difference during NREMS and wakefulness in regions involved in conscious awareness (i.e., left frontoparietal and the left middle frontal cortices, the precuneus/posterior cingulate, and the fusiform gyri). This smaller NREMS vs. wake difference could reflect a greater metabolic rate of glucose during NREMS that could explain a hyperarousal during sleep leading to insomnia (Kay et al. 2016). Another FDG-PET study investigated the impact of acute sleep deprivation on cerebral glucose metabolism during NREMS in people with insomnia and good sleepers. In good sleepers, sleep restriction leads to a decrease in whole-brain glucose metabolism during recovery of NREMS (i.e., after one night of sleep restriction) compared to baseline NREMS. In people with insomnia, no change in glucose metabolism was observed at the whole-brain level, but there was a decrease in regional glucose metabolism in the left hemisphere and the DMN (left frontoparietal cortex, right precuneus/posterior cingulate cortex, and right lingual/fusiform gyri). These results suggest that sleep deprivation, by reducing brain activity in regions involved in conscious awareness, could improve quality of sleep in people with insomnia (Kay et al. 2019). Dang-Vu et al. investigated the neural correlates of delta activity during SWS (Dang-Vu et al. 2005). The analysis characterized the cerebral correlates of delta waves (between 0 and 4 Hz; registered by electroencephalography) in areas where rCBF decreases during SWS (Maquet et al. 1997). An association was observed between rCBF in the ventromedial prefrontal regions and delta power. However, no correlation was observed with the thalamus, highlighting the importance of an extra-thalamic delta rhythm among the synchronous SWS oscillations. Therefore, rCBF could be a reflection of the cellular processes involved in cortical delta waves during SWS. These results confirm the frontal predominance of slow-wave activity during human SWS, as demonstrated by scalp electroencephalography studies (Finelli et al. 2001). On the other hand, activity in the thalamus seems to be negatively correlated with the rCBF during SWS (Hofle et al. 1997). This negative correlation may reflect the neural substrates underlying the progressive decrease in sensory awareness, motor responsiveness, and arousal that occur during SWS. Nevertheless, specific areas were found less activated, such as frontal and parietal areas encompassing the PCC, dorsolateral prefrontal and inferior parietal cortices, and precuneus (Maquet et al. 1996, Maquet et al. 2005;

Braun et al. 1997). Significant increases in rCBF were found in the pontine tegmentum, thalamus, basal forebrain, amygdala, hippocampus, and ACC (Maquet et al. 1996; Braun et al. 1997). An activation of posterior cortices (i.e., temporo-occipital areas) and a modification in connectivity in this network were also observed (Braun et al. 1998). These studies could explain the relationship between consciousness during REMS and regional patterns of brain hypometabolism in the frontal and parietal areas and the precuneus/PCC, areas known to be involved in internal and external consciousness (Laureys et al. 1999a; Boly et al. 2008b; Vanhaudenhuyse et al. 2011). Metabolic increases in regions such as the pontine tegmentum, thalamic nuclei, and limbic areas might correlate with some features of cognition, as reflected in dream reports (Maquet et al. 2005).

Functional neuroimaging has offered an increasingly refined description of brain activity across the sleep-wake cycle, from regional patterns of sleep stages to transient activations during sleep oscillations. Reports using PET demonstrated a specialized network of deactivated brain areas during SWS (i.e., the ACC, thalamus, frontal and parietal association areas) and activated/deactivated structures (i.e., decrease in frontal and parietal areas and PCC/precuneus; activation of the pontine tegmentum, thalamus, basal forebrain, amygdale, hippocampus, and ACC) during REMS.

45.5 PET Scan and Hypnosis

In 1994, hypnosis was defined as "a procedure during which a health professional or researcher suggests that a patient or subject experiences changes in sensations, perceptions, thoughts, or behavior" (The Executive Committee of the American Psychological Association – Division of Psychological Hypnosis 1994). However, this definition was criticized as being too long and presenting a theoretical limitation (i.e., concept such as "state" and "self-hypnosis" was not mentioned, and the use of hypnosis in hospital does not appear in the list of application). Eventually, hypnosis has been redefined in 2014 as "a state of consciousness involving focused attention and reduced peripheral awareness characterized by an enhanced capacity for response to suggestion" (Elkins et al. 2016). This procedure induces an altered state of awareness which could be explained by specific cortical changes (i.e., dynamic properties and neural correlates) (Maquet et al. 1999; Rainville et al. 2002; Cardeña et al. 2013). Hypnosis can be considered as an appropriate means to transiently modulate conscious cognition in healthy subjects because it does not lead to general unconsciousness (compared to pharmacological anesthesia or sleep) and does not have long-term effects on neuroplasticity (compared to meditation techniques (Holzel et al. 2008)). Even more, it is well documented to induce an altered conscious state (Oakley and Halligan 2009). The hypnotic process has three main components: absorption, dissociation, and suggestibility (Spiegel 1991). Absorption is the ability to be fully involved in a thought experiment. Dissociation can be defined as the separation of mental behavior that usually goes together (e.g., in the case of dreams where we are at the same time the actor and the observer). This condition can also cause a sensation of driving or uncontrollable feelings of discontinuity of a body part compared to others. Finally, suggestibility is the ability of the person to comply with the instructions of the professional practicing hypnosis. These processes could diminish the tendency to judge and censor, whereas hypnosis could reduce spontaneous thoughts and give the feeling of one's own response as automatic (Rainville and Price 2003; Terhune and Cardeña 2010). However, a study showed that individuals do not display a uniform response to a hypnotic induction (Terhune and Cardeña 2010).

It is important to emphasize that people under hypnosis do not lose complete control of their behavior. They are aware of their identity and their actual location, and unless amnesia is induced, they keep a souvenir of the experience during the hypnotic process. Another important thing to note is that not all individuals respond to hypnosis. There are low and highly suggestible subjects. A study conducted by Terhune and collaborators (2011) using EEG showed that highly suggestible participants reliably experienced greater state of dissociation and exhibited lower frontoparietal phase synchrony in the α-2 frequency band during hypnosis than low-suggestible participants. These findings suggest that highly suggestible individuals exhibit a disruption of the frontoparietal network that is only observable following a hypnotic induction. At the same time, the fact that cerebral responses to hypnosis are different between subjects points to the difficulty of generalizing obtained results.

Hypnosis has for many years been used, among other things, in the treatment of both somatic and psychological disorders (such as pain, gastrointestinal and dermatological diseases, depression, anxiety, stress, and addictions). In addition to its clinical application, the study of hypnosis is thought to provide leverage to investigate not only the contents of consciousness but also the neural correlates of its background states. Functional neuroimaging studies have been performed as a means of investigation of the phenomenon, mainly using PET imaging. The earliest studies found a modulation of ACC activity and highlighted changes in connectivity between ACC and prefrontal areas during hypnosis (Maquet et al. 1999; Faymonville et al. 2003, 2006) and hypnotic suggestion (Rainville et al. 1997, 1999b; Hofbauer et al. 2001). The activation in the ACC could reflect the attentional effort necessary for the subject to internally generate mental imagery, while the connectivity between ACC and prefrontal areas may indicate a modification in distributed associative processes of cognitive appraisal, attention, or memory of perceived noxious stimuli (Rainville et al. 1997, 1999a, 2002; Faymonville et al. 2000; Hofbauer et al. 2001).

Mental imagery appears to play a role in hypnosis. This notion is supported by the activation of the occipital and temporal cortices, precuneus, and other extrastriate visual areas during hypnotic state and hypnotic suggestion, which account for the altered perception of reality (Maquet 1999; Rainville et al. 1999b; Faymonville et al. 2006). This is further stressed by the fact that motor commands are processed differently than in the normal conscious state, with activity deviating toward the precuneus and extrastriate visual areas (Casale et al. 2012). After induction of a hypotonic state, an increase in rCBF was observed in the ACC, the thalami, and the mesencephalic brainstem, while brain metabolism decreased in the precuneus, the parietal lobule, and the posterior temporal cortex (Rainville et al. 2002). The hypometabolism of the precuneus during hypnosis supports the correlation between awareness and precuneal integration. The induction of a hypotonic state produced the expected increases in both mental relaxation and absorption. Regression analyses between rCBF and self-ratings confirm the hypothesized involvement of the ACC, the thalamus, and the pontomesencephalic brainstem in the generation of hypnotic states. Hypnotic relaxation further involved an increase in occipital rCBF, consistent with previous interpretation that hypnotic states are characterized by a decrease in cortical arousal and a reduction in cross-modality suppression (disinhibition). In contrast, increases in mental absorption during hypnotic state were associated with rCBF increases in a distributed network of cortical and subcortical structures described as the brain's attentional system (Rainville et al. 2002).

Because of its analgesic effects, hypnosis is increasingly used in anesthesia for several minor surgeries (such as scar correction, tooth extraction, thyroidal lobectomy, or face lifting) (Vanhaudenhuyse et al. 2008). This technique is called hypnosedation. Neuroimaging—especially PET studies—was conducted trying to understand the mechanisms underlying the anesthetic effects of hypnosis. The results showed an activation of a widespread set of cortical areas involving occipital, parietal, precentral, premotor, and ventrolateral, as well as the ACC and the prefrontal cortex during hypnotic state (Rainville et al. 1997; Faymonville et al. 2000, 2003, 2006; Hofbauer et al. 2001;). The ACC is known to be involved in interaction processes between cognitive and emotional perceptions related to changes in attentional and emotional states (Devinsky et al. 1995; Bush et al. 2000). Decrease in pain perception during hypnosedation was shown to be related to increases in connectivity between ACC and a large neural cortical and subcortical network, known to be involved in pain perception and integration (i.e., the prefrontal cortex, supplementary and premotor area, insula, striatum, thalamus, and brainstem) (Faymonville et al. 2006). These changes in connectivity between the ACC and prefrontal brain regions induced by hypnosis might reflect a change in the associative processes of judgment, attention, or memory of perceived nociceptive stimuli. In contrast with these studies, Derbyshire and collaborators used hypnosis to induce pain (Derbyshire et al. 2004). They found that both real pain-heating stimuli and hypnosis-induced pain experience modulated the activity within the thalamus, ACC, insula, and prefrontal and parietal cortices. This study showed that hypnosis is able to induce cerebral activations as real pain stimuli.

PET studies highlighted an activation of a widespread set of cortical areas involving ACC and occipital, parietal, precentral, premotor, and ventrolateral prefrontal cortices related to the hypnotic state. This pattern of activation shares some similarities with mental imagery tasks, from which it mainly differs by the relative deactivation of the precuneus. This deactivation could explain the alteration of awareness induced by hypnosis. Indeed, hypometabolism of the precuneus seems to be highly correlated with modified state of consciousness (Maquet et al. 1996, 2005; Braun et al. 1997; Laureys et al. 1999a, b; Vogt and Laureys, 2005). Nevertheless, results could be confounded, because of the differences between high- and low-suggestible individuals in terms of neuronal processes underlying hypnosis induction.

Comparing the brain activation patterns associated with the analgesic effect of hypnosis and the resting state, a reduction of affective and sensory responses to noxious stimulation was found, which is modulated by the activity in the midcingulate cortex and especially the ACC.

45.6 Conclusion

Recent advances in functional neuroimaging techniques are beginning to open the black box of altered consciousness. PET studies facilitate a better understanding of the mechanisms underlying the altered state of consciousness and highlight the involvement of specific neural areas and networks in pathologically altered states of consciousness (VS/UWS and MCS), in sleep, and under hypnosis. Results from several studies point to the importance of the precuneus and cingulate cortices in altered states of consciousness in all of these conditions. Clinically, these findings may prove important in facilitating precise differential diagnostic tools to distinguish low levels of awareness in unresponsive patient populations. Currently, FDG-PET is the most robust paraclinical technique for differential diagnosis in DOC patients. However, the use and the development of multimodal assessment could be a good complement for the examination/diagnosis and management of this sensitive population. Taken together, the frontoparietal network which is hypometabolic during SWS and mostly impaired in patients with disorders of consciousness—but not during REMS or hypnosis—could reflect the preservation of brain activity in correlation with different brain processes such as dreaming, memory consolidation (sleep), or motor imagery (hypnosis).

Acknowledgments This update is based on the work of previous authors whom we would like to thank: Johan Stender, Athena Demertzi, Claire Bernard, Roland Hustinx, and Marie-Aurélie Bruno.

References

American Congress of Rehabilitation Medicine (1995) Recommendations for use of uniform nomenclature pertinent to patients with severe alterations of consciousness. Arch Phys Med Rehabil 76:205–209

Andersson JL, Onoe H, Hetta J, Lidstrom K, Valind S, Lilja A, Sundin A, Fasth KJ, Westerberg G, Broman JE, Watanabe Y, Langstrom B (1998) Brain networks affected by synchronized sleep visualized by positron emission tomography. J Cereb Blood Flow Metab 18:701–715

Andrews K, Murphy L, Munday R, Littlewood C (1996) Misdiagnosis of the vegetative state: retrospective study in a rehabilitation unit. BMJ 313:13–16

Annen J, Heine L, Ziegler E et al (2016) Function-structure connectivity in patients with severe brain injury as measured by MRI-DWI and FDG-PET: function-structure connectivity in DOC. Hum Brain Mapp 37:3707–3720

Annen J, Blandiaux S, Lejeune N et al (2018) BCI performance and brain metabolism profile in severely brain-injured patients without response to command at bedside. Front Neurosci 12:370

Baars BJ (2005) Global workspace theory of consciousness: toward a cognitive neuroscience of human experience. Prog Brain Res 150:45–53

Baars BJ, Ramsoy TZ, Laureys S (2003) Brain, conscious experience and the observing self. Trends Neurosci 26:671–675

Bekinschtein T, Leiguarda R, Armony J, Owen A, Carpintiero S, Niklison J, Olmos L, Sigman L, Manes F (2004) Emotion processing in the minimally conscious state. J Neurol Neurosurg Psychiatry 75:788

Beuthien-Baumann B, Handrick W, Schmidt T, Burchert W, Oehme L, Kropp J, Schackert G, Pinkert J, Franke WG (2003) Persistent vegetative state: evaluation of brain metabolism and brain perfusion with PET and SPECT. Nucl Med Commun 24:643–649

Bodart O, Gosseries O, Wannez S et al (2017) Measures of metabolism and complexity in the brain of patients with disorders of consciousness. NeuroImage Clin 14:354–362

Boly M, Faymonville ME, Peigneux P, Lambermont B, Damas P, Del Fiore G, Degueldre C, Franck G, Luxen A, Lamy M, Moonen G, Maquet P, Laureys S (2004) Auditory processing in severely brain injured patients: differences between the minimally conscious state and the persistent vegetative state. Arch Neurol 61:233–238

Boly M, Faymonville ME, Schnakers C, Peigneux P, Lambermont B, Phillips C, Lancellotti P, Luxen A, Lamy M, Moonen G, Maquet P, Laureys S (2008a) Perception of pain in the minimally conscious state with PET activation: an observational study. Lancet Neurol 7:1013–1020

Boly M, Phillips C, Tshibanda L, Vanhaudenhuyse A, Schabus M, Dang-Vu TT, Moonen G, Hustinx R, Maquet P, Laureys S (2008b) Intrinsic brain activity in altered states of consciousness: how conscious is the default mode of brain function? Ann N Y Acad Sci 1129:119–129

Braun AR, Balkin TJ, Wesenten NJ, Carson RE, Varga M, Baldwin P, Selbie S, Belenky G, Herscovitch P (1997) Regional cerebral blood flow throughout the sleep-wake cycle. An H2(15)O PET study. Brain J Neurol 120(Pt 7):1173–1197

Braun AR, Balkin TJ, Wesensten NJ, Gwadry F, Carson RE, Varga M, Baldwin P, Belenky G, Herscovitch P (1998) Dissociated pattern of activity in visual cortices and their projections during human rapid eye movement sleep. Science 279:91–95

Bruno MA, Schnakers C, Damas F, Pellas F, Lutte I, Bernheim J, Majerus S, Moonen G, Goldman S, Laureys S (2009) Locked-in syndrome in children: report of five cases and review of the literature. Pediatr Neurol 41:237–246

Bruno MA, Vanhaudenhuyse A, Schnakers C, Boly M, Gosseries O, Demertzi A, Majerus S, Moonen G, Hustinx R, Laureys S (2010) Visual fixation in the vegetative state: an observational case series PET study. BMC Neurol 10:35

Bruno MA, Majerus S, Boly M, Vanhaudenhuyse A, Schnakers C, Gosseries O, Boveroux P, Kirsch M, Demertzi A, Bernard C, Hustinx R, Moonen G, Laureys S (2012) Functional neuroanatomy underlying the clinical subcategorization of minimally conscious state patients. J Neurol 259:1087–1098

Buchsbaum M (2001) Positron emission tomography with deoxyglucose-F18 imaging of sleep. Neuropsychopharmacology 25:50–56

Bush G, Luu P, Posner MI (2000) Cognitive and emotional influences in anterior cingulate cortex. Trends Cogn Sci 4:215–222

Cardeña E, Jonsson P, Terhune DB, Marcusson-Clavertz D (2013) The neurophenomenology of neutral hypnosis. Cortex 49(2):375–385

Casale AD, Ferracuti S, Rapinesi C, Serata D, Sani G, Savoja V, Kotzalidis GD, Tatarelli R, Girardi P (2012) Neurocognition under hypnosis: findings from recent functional neuroimaging studies. Int J Clin Exp Hypn 60:286–317

Chatelle C, Thibaut A, Gosseries O et al (2014) Changes in cerebral metabolism in patients with a minimally conscious state responding to zolpidem. Front Hum Neurosci 8:917

Childs NL, Mercer WN (1996) Misdiagnosing the persistent vegetative state. Misdiagnosis certainly occurs. BMJ 313:944

Clauss R, Nel W (2006) Drug induced arousal from the permanent vegetative state. NeuroRehabilitation 21(1):23–28

Damasio A, Kaspar M (2009) Consciousness: an overview of the phenomenon and of its possible neural basis. In: Laureys S, Tononi J (eds) The neurology of consciousness. Elsevier, London

Dang-Vu TT, Desseilles M, Laureys S, Degueldre C, Perrin F, Phillips C, Maquet P, Peigneux P (2005) Cerebral correlates of delta waves during non-REM sleep revisited. NeuroImage 28:14–21

De Jong B, Willemsen A, Paans A (1997) Regional cerebral blood flow changes related to affective speech presentation in persistent vegetative state. Clin Neurol Neurosurg 47:197–204

Dehaene S, Naccache L (2001) Towards a cognitive neuroscience of consciousness: basic evidence and a workspace framework. Cognition 79:1–37

Demertzi A, Schnakers C, Ledoux D, Chatelle C, Bruno MA, Vanhaudenhuyse A, Boly M, Moonen G, Laureys S (2009) Different beliefs about pain perception in the vegetative and minimally conscious states: a European survey of medical and paramedical professionals. Prog Brain Res 177:329–338

Demertzi A, Ledoux D, Bruno MA, Vanhaudenhuyse A, Gosseries O, Soddu A, Schnakers C, Moonen G, Laureys S (2011) Attitudes towards end-of-life issues in disorders of consciousness: a European survey. J Neurol 258:1058–1065

Demertzi A, Racine E, Bruno M, Ledoux D, Gosseries O, Vanhaudenhuyse A, Thonnard M, Soddu A, Moonen G, Laureys S (2012) Pain perception in disorders of consciousness: neuroscience, clinical care, and ethics in dialogue. Neuroethics 6:1–14

Derbyshire SW, Whalley MG, Stenger VA, Oakley DA (2004) Cerebral activation during hypnotically induced and imagined pain. NeuroImage 23:392–401

Devinsky O, Morrell MJ, Vogt BA (1995) Contributions of anterior cingulate cortex to behaviour. Brain 118(Pt 1):279–306

DeVolder AG, Goffinet AM, Bol A, Michel C, de Barsy T, Laterre C (1990) Brain glucose metabolism in postanoxic syndrome. Positron emission tomographic study. Arch Neurol 47:197–204

Di Perri C, Bahri MA, Amico E et al (2016) Neural correlates of consciousness in patients who have emerged from a minimally conscious state: a cross-sectional multimodal imaging study. Lancet Neurol 15:830–842

Elkins GR, Barabasz AF, Council JR, Spiegel D (2016) Advancing research and practice: the revised APA division 30 definition of hypnosis. Int J Clin Exp Hypn 63:1–9

Faymonville ME, Laureys S, Degueldre C, DelFiore G, Luxen A, Franck G, Lamy M, Maquet P (2000) Neural mechanisms of antinociceptive effects of hypnosis. Anesthesiology 92:1257–1267

Faymonville ME, Roediger L, Del Fiore G, Delgueldre C, Phillips C, Lamy M, Luxen A, Maquet P, Laureys S (2003) Increased cerebral functional connectivity underlying the antinociceptive effects of hypnosis. Brain Res Cogn Brain Res 17:255–262

Faymonville ME, Boly M, Laureys S (2006) Functional neuroanatomy of the hypnotic state. J Physiol Paris 99:463–469

Finelli LA, Borbely AA, Achermann P (2001) Functional topography of the human nonREM sleep electroencephalogram. Eur J Neurosci 13:2282–2290

Garcia-Panach J, Lull N, Lull JJ, Ferri J, Martinez C, Sopena P, Robles M, Chirivella J, Noe E (2011) A voxel-based analysis of FDG-PET in traumatic brain injury: regional metabolism and relationship between the thalamus and cortical areas. J Neurotrauma 28:1707–1717

Giacino JT, Ashwal S, Childs N, Cranford R, Jennett B, Katz DI, Kelly JP, Rosenberg JH, Whyte J, Zafonte RD, Zasler ND (2002) The minimally conscious state: definition and diagnostic criteria. Neurology 58:349–353

Giacino JT, Hirsch J, Schiff N, Laureys S (2006) Functional neuroimaging applications for assessment and rehabilitation planning in patients with disorders of consciousness. Arch Med Rehab 87:S67–S76

Giacino JT, Whyte J, Bagiella E, Kalmar K, Childs N, Khademi A, Eifert B, Long D, Katz DI, Cho S, Yablon SA, Luther M, Hammond FM, Nordenbo A, Novak P, Mercer W, Maurer-Karattup P, Sherer M (2012) Placebo-controlled trial of amantadine for severe traumatic brain injury. N Engl J Med 366:819–826

Golkowski D, Merz K, Mlynarcik C et al (2017) Simultaneous EEG–PET–fMRI measurements in disorders of consciousness: an exploratory study on diagnosis and prognosis. J Neurol 264:1986–1995

Gosseries O, Zasler ND, Laureys S (2014) Recent advances in disorders of consciousness: focus on the diagnosis. Brain Inj 28:1141–1150
Hofbauer RK, Rainville P, Duncan GH, Bushnell MC (2001) Cortical representation of the sensory dimension of pain. J Neurophys 86:402–411
Hofle N, Paus T, Reutens D, Fiset P, Gotman J, Evans AC, Jones BE (1997) Regional cerebral blood flow changes as a function of delta and spindle activity during slow wave sleep in humans. J Neurosci 17:4800–4808
Holzel BK, Ott U, Gard T, Hempel H, Weygandt M, Morgen K, Vaitl D (2008) Investigation of mindfulness meditation practitioners with voxel-based morphometry. Soc Cogn Affect Neurosci 3:55–61
Juengling FD, Kassubek J, Huppertz HJ, Krause T, Els T (2005) Separating functional and structural damage in persistent vegetative state using combined voxel-based analysis of 3-D MRI and FDG-PET. J Neurol Sci 228:179–184
Kajimura N, Uchiyama M, Takayama Y, Uchida S, Uema T, Kato M, Sekimoto M, Watanabe T, Nakajima T, Horikoshi S, Ogawa K, Nishikawa M, Hiroki M, Kudo Y, Matsuda H, Okawa M, Takahashi K (1999) Activity of midbrain reticular formation and neocortex during the progression of human non-rapid eye movement sleep. J Neurosci 19:10065–10073
Kassubek J, Juengling FD, Els T, Spreer J, Herpers M, Krause T, Moser E, Lucking CH (2003) Activation of a residual cortical network during painful stimulation in long-term postanoxic vegetative state: a 15O-H2O PET study. J Neurol Sci 212:85–91
Kay DB, Karim HT, Soehner AM et al (2016) Sleep-wake differences in relative regional cerebral metabolic rate for glucose among patients with insomnia compared with good sleepers. Sleep 39:1779–1794
Kay DB, Karim HT, Hasler BP et al (2019) Impact of acute sleep restriction on cerebral glucose metabolism during recovery non-rapid eye movement sleep among individuals with primary insomnia and good sleeper controls. Sleep Med 55:81–91
Kupers R, Faymonville ME, Laureys S (2005) The cognitive modulation of pain: hypnosis- and placebo-induced analgesia. Prog Brain Res 150:251–269
Langtry HD, Benfield P (1990) Zolpidem: a review of its pharmacodynamic and pharmacokinetic properties and therapeutic potential. Drugs 40:291–313
Laureys S (2004) Functional neuroimaging in the vegetative state. NeuroRehabilitation 19:335–341
Laureys S (2005) The neural correlate of (un)awareness: lessons from the vegetative state. Trends Cogn Sci 9:556–559
Laureys S, Boly M (2007) What is it like to be vegetative or minimally conscious? Curr Opin Neurol 20:609–613
Laureys S, Schiff ND (2012) Coma and consciousness: paradigms (re)framed by neuroimaging. NeuroImage 61:478–491
Laureys S, Goldman S, Phillips C, Van Bogaert P, Aerts J, Luxen A, Franck G, Maquet P (1999a) Impaired effective cortical connectivity in vegetative state: preliminary investigation using PET. NeuroImage 9:377–382
Laureys S, Lemaire C, Maquet P, Phillips C, Franck G (1999b) Cerebral metabolism during vegetative state and after recovery to consciousness. J Neurol Neurosurg Psychiatry 67:121
Laureys S, Faymonville ME, Degueldre C, Fiore GD, Damas P, Lambermont B, Janssens N, Aerts J, Franck G, Luxen A, Moonen G, Lamy M, Maquet P (2000a) Auditory processing in the vegetative state. Brain J Neurol 123(Pt 8):1589–1601
Laureys S, Faymonville ME, Luxen A, Lamy M, Franck G, Maquet P (2000b) Restoration of thalamocortical connectivity after recovery from persistent vegetative state. Lancet 355:1790–1791
Laureys S, Faymonville ME, Moonen G, Luxen A, Maquet P (2000c) PET scanning and neuronal loss in acute vegetative state. Lancet 355:1825–1826; author reply 1827
Laureys S, Antoine S, Boly M, Elincx S, Faymonville ME, Berre J, Sadzot B, Ferring M, De Tiege X, van Bogaert P, Hansen I, Damas P, Mavroudakis N, Lambermont B, Del Fiore G, Aerts J, Degueldre C, Phillips C, Franck G, Vincent JL, Lamy M, Luxen A, Moonen G, Goldman S, Maquet P (2002a) Brain function in the vegetative state. Acta Neurol Belg 102:177–185

Laureys S, Faymonville ME, Peigneux P, Damas P, Lambermont B, Del Fiore G, Degueldre C, Aerts J, Luxen A, Franck G, Lamy M, Moonen G, Maquet P (2002b) Cortical processing of noxious somatosensory stimuli in the persistent vegetative state. NeuroImage 17:732–741

Laureys S, Van Eeckhout P, Ferring M, Faymonville M, Mavroudakis N, Berre J, Van Bogaert P, Pellas F, Cornu P, Luxen A, Vincent J, Moonen G, Maque P, Goldman S (2003) Brain function in acute and chronic locked-in syndrome. In 9th annual meeting of the Organisation for Human Brain Mapping (OHBM), vol 19 NY, USA

Laureys S, Owen AM, Schiff ND (2004a) Brain function in coma, vegetative state, and related disorders. Lancet Neurol 3:537–546

Laureys S, Perrin F, Faymonville ME, Schnakers C, Boly M, Bartsch V, Majerus S, Moonen G, Maquet P (2004b) Cerebral processing in the minimally conscious state. Neurology 63:916–918

Laureys S, Pellas F, Van Eeckhout P, Ghorbel S, Schnakers C, Perrin F, Berre J, Faymonville ME, Pantke KH, Damas F, Lamy M, Moonen G, Goldman S (2005a) The locked-in syndrome : what is it like to be conscious but paralyzed and voiceless? Prog Brain Res 150:495–511

Laureys S, Piret S, Ledoux D (2005b) Quantifying consciousness. Lancet Neurol 4:789–790

Laureys S, Celesia GG, Cohadon F, Lavrijsen J, Leon-Carrion J, Sannita WG, Sazbon L, Schmutzhard E, von Wild KR, Zeman A, Dolce G (2010) Unresponsive wakefulness syndrome: a new name for the vegetative state or apallic syndrome. BMC Med 8:68

Lemaire J-J, Sontheimer A, Pereira B et al (2018) Deep brain stimulation in five patients with severe disorders of consciousness. Ann Clin Transl Neurol 5:1372–1384

Levy DE, Sidtis JJ, Rottenberg DA, Jarden JO, Strother SC, Dhawan V, Ginos JZ, Tramo MJ, Evans AC, Plum F (1987) Differences in cerebral blood flow and glucose utilization in vegetative versus locked-in patients. Ann Neurol 22:673–682

Lull N, Noe E, Lull JJ, Garcia-Panach J, Chirivella J, Ferri J, Lopez-Aznar D, Sopena P, Robles M (2010) Voxel-based statistical analysis of thalamic glucose metabolism in traumatic brain injury: relationship with consciousness and cognition. Brain Inj 24:1098–1107

Majerus S, Bruno MA, Schnakers C, Giacino JT, Laureys S (2009) The problem of aphasia in the assessment of consciousness in brain-damaged patients. Prog Brain Res 177:49–61

Maquet P (1997) Positron emission tomography studies of sleep and sleep disorders. J Neurol 244:S23–S28

Maquet P (1999) Brain mechanisms of sleep: contribution of neuroimaging techniques. J Psychopharmacol 13:S25–S28

Maquet P (2000) Functional neuroimaging of normal human sleep by positron emission tomography. J Sleep Res 9:207–231

Maquet P, Dive D, Salmon E, Sadzot B, Franco G, Poirrier R, von Frenckell R, Franck G (1990) Cerebral glucose utilization during sleep-wake cycle in man determined by positron emission tomography and [18F] 2-fluoro-2-deoxy-D-glucose method. Brain Res 513:136–143

Maquet P, Peters J, Aerts J, Delfiore G, Degueldre C, Luxen A, Franck G (1996) Functional neuroanatomy of human rapid-eye-movement sleep and dreaming. Nature 383:163–166

Maquet P, Degueldre C, Delfiore G, Aerts J, Peters JM, Luxen A, Franck G (1997) Functional neuroanatomy of human slow wave sleep. J Neurosci 17:2807–2812

Maquet P, Faymonville ME, Degueldre C, Delfiore G, Franck G, Luxen A, Lamy M (1999) Functional neuroanatomy of hypnotic state. Biol Psychiatry 45:327–333

Maquet P, Ruby P, Maudoux A, Albouy G, Sterpenich V, Dang-Vu T, Desseilles M, Boly M, Perrin F, Peigneux P, Laureys S (2005) Human cognition during REM sleep and the activity profile within frontal and parietal cortices: a reappraisal of functional neuroimaging data. Prog Brain Res 150:219–227

Menon DK, Owen AM, Williams EJ, Minhas PS, Allen CM, Boniface SJ, Pickard JD (1998) Cortical processing in persistent vegetative state. Wolfson Brain Imaging Centre Team. Lancet 352:200

Nagel T et al (1979) What is it like to be a bad? In: Mortal questions. Cambridge University Press, Cambridge, pp 165–180

Nakayama N, Okumura A, Shinoda J, Nakashima T, Iwama T (2006) Relationship between regional cerebral metabolism and consciousness disturbance in traumatic diffuse brain injury

without large focal lesions: an FDG-PET study with statistical parametric mapping analysis. J Neurol Neurosurg Psychiatry 77:856–862
Nofzinger EA, Mintun MA, Wiseman M, Kupfer DJ, Moore RY (1997) Forebrain activation in REM sleep: an FDG PET study. Brain Res 770:192–201
Nofzinger EA, Buysse DJ, Miewald JM, Meltzer CC, Price JC, Sembrat RC, Ombao H, Reynolds CF, Monk TH, Hall M, Kupfer DJ, Moore RY (2002) Human regional cerebral glucose metabolism during non-rapid eye movement sleep in relation to waking. Brain J Neurol 125:1105–1115
Noirhomme Q, Laureys S (2011) Altering consciousness and neuropathology. In: Winkelman E, Cardeña AM (eds) Altering consciousness: multidisciplinary perspectives, vol 2. Praeger, Santa Barbara
Nusbaum F, Redoute J, Le Bars D, Volckmann P, Simon F, Hannoun S, Ribes G, Gaucher J, Laurent B, Sappey-Marinier D (2011) Chronic low-back pain modulation is enhanced by hypnotic analgesic suggestion by recruiting an emotional network: a PET imaging study. Int J Clin Exp Hypn 59:27–44
Oakley DA, Halligan PW (2009) Hypnotic suggestion and cognitive neuroscience. Trends Cogn Sci 13:264–270
Owen AM, Menon DK, Johnsrude IS, Bor D, Scott SK, Manly T, Williams EJ, Mummery C, Pickard JD (2002) Detecting residual cognitive function in persistent vegetative state. Neurocase 8:394–403
Owen AM, Coleman MR, Menon DK, Berry EL, Johnsrude IS, Rodd JM, Davis MH, Pickard JD (2005) Using a hierarchical approach to investigate residual auditory cognition in persistent vegetative state. Prog Brain Res 150:457–471
Peigneux P, Laureys S, Delbeuck X, Maquet P (2001) Sleeping brain, learning brain. The role of sleep for memory systems. Neuroreport 12:A111–A124
Phillips CL, Bruno MA, Maquet P, Boly M, Noirhomme Q, Schnakers C, Vanhaudenhuyse A, Bonjean M, Hustinx R, Moonen G, Luxen A, Laureys S (2011) "Relevance vector machine" consciousness classifier applied to cerebral metabolism of vegetative and locked-in patients. NeuroImage 56:797–808
Plum F, Schiff N, Ribary U, Llinas R (1998) Coordinated expression in chronically unconscious persons. Philos Trans R Soc B-Biol Sci 353:1929–1933
Posner J, Saper C, Schiff N, Plum F (2007) Plum and Posner's diagnosis of stupor and coma. Oxford University Press, New York
Qin P, Di H, Liu Y, Yu S, Gong Q, Duncan N, Weng X, Laureys S, Northoff G (2010) Anterior cingulate activity and the self in disorders of consciousness. Hum Brain Mapp 31:1993–2002
Raichle ME, Mintun MA (2006) Brain work and brain imaging. Ann Rev Neurosci 29:449–476
Raichle ME, Snyder AZ (2007) A default mode of brain function: a brief history of an evolving idea. NeuroImage 37:1083–1090, discussion 1097–1089
Rainville P, Price DD (2003) Hypnosis phenomenology and the neurobiology of consciousness. Int J Clin Exp Hypn 51:105–129
Rainville P, Duncan GH, Price DD, Carrier B, Bushnell MC (1997) Pain affect encoded in human anterior cingulate but not somatosensory cortex. Science 277:968–971
Rainville P, Carrier B, Hofbauer RK, Bushnell MC, Duncan GH (1999a) Dissociation of sensory and affective dimensions of pain using hypnotic modulation. Pain 82:159–171
Rainville P, Hofbauer RK, Paus T, Duncan GH, Bushnell MC, Price DD (1999b) Cerebral mechanisms of hypnotic induction and suggestion. J Cogn Neurosci 11:110–125
Rainville P, Hofbauer RK, Bushnell MC, Duncan GH, Price DD (2002) Hypnosis modulates activity in brain structures involved in the regulation of consciousness. J Cogn Neurosci 14:887–901
Royal College of Physicians (2003) The vegetative state: guidance on diagnosis and management. Clin Med 3:249–254
Rudolf J, Ghaemi M, Haupt WF, Szelies B, Heiss WD (1999a) Cerebral glucose metabolism in acute and persistent vegetative state. J Neurosurg Anesthesiol 11:17–24
Rudolf J, Grond M, Schindler D, Heiss WD, Desnick RJ (1999b) Cerebral glucose metabolism in type I alpha-N-acetylgalactosaminidase deficiency: an infantile neuroaxonal dystrophy. J Child Neurol 14:543–547

Rudolf J, Sobesky J, Grond M, Heiss WD (2000) Identification by positron emission tomography of neuronal loss in acute vegetative state. Lancet 355:115–116
Sanger DJ (2004) The pharmacology and mechanisms of action of new generation, non-benzodiazepine hypnotic agents. CNS Drugs 18:9–15
Sanz LRD, Lejeune N, Blandiaux S et al (2019) Treating disorders of consciousness with apomorphine: protocol for a double-blind randomized controlled trial using multimodal assessments. Front Neurol 10:240
Schiff ND (2006) Multimodal neuroimaging approaches to disorders of consciousness. J Head Trauma Rehabil 21:388–397
Schiff ND (2010) Recovery of consciousness after brain injury: a mesocircuit hypothesis. Trends Neurosci 33(1):1–9
Schiff ND, Plum F (1999) Cortical function in the persistent vegetative state. Trends Cogn Sci 3:43–44
Schiff ND, Ribary U, Moreno DR, Beattie B, Kronberg E, Blasberg R, Giacino J, McCagg C, Fins JJ, Llinas R, Plum F (2002) Residual cerebral activity and behavioural fragments can remain in the persistently vegetative brain. Brain J Neurol 125:1210–1234
Schnakers C, Hustinx R, Vandewalle G, Majerus S, Moonen G, Boly M, Vanhaudenhuyse A, Laureys S (2008) Measuring the effect of amantadine in chronic anoxic minimally conscious state. J Neurol Neurosurg Psychiatry 79:225–227
Schnakers C, Vanhaudenhuyse A, Giacino J, Ventura M, Boly M, Majerus S, Moonen G, Laureys S (2009) Diagnostic accuracy of the vegetative and minimally conscious state: clinical consensus versus standardized neurobehavioral assessment. BMC Neurol 9:35
Schnakers C, Chatelle C, Demertzi A, Majerus S, Laureys S (2012) What about pain in disorders of consciousness? AAPS J 14:437–444
Searle JR (2000) Consciousness. Ann Rev Neurosci 23:557–578
Shames JL, Ring H (2008) Transient reversal of anoxic brain injury–related minimally conscious state after zolpidem administration: a case report. Arch Phys Med Rehabil 89:386–388
Silva S, Alacoque X, Fourcade O, Samii K, Marque P, Woods R, Mazziotta J, Chollet F, Loubinoux I (2010) Wakefulness and loss of awareness: brain and brainstem interaction in the vegetative state. Neurology 74:313–320
Soddu A, Gómez F, Heine L et al (2016) Correlation between resting state fMRI total neuronal activity and PET metabolism in healthy controls and patients with disorders of consciousness. Brain Behav 6(1):e00424
Spiegel D (1991) Neurophysiological correlates of hypnosis and dissociation. J Neuropsychiatr Clin Neurosci 3:440–445
Stender J, Gosseries O, Bruno M-A et al (2014) Diagnostic precision of PET imaging and functional MRI in disorders of consciousness: a clinical validation study. Lancet 384:514–522
Stender J, Kupers R, Rodell A et al (2015) Quantitative rates of brain glucose metabolism distinguish minimally conscious from vegetative state patients. J Cereb Blood Flow Metab 35:58–65
Stender J, Mortensen KN, Thibaut A et al (2016) The minimal energetic requirement of sustained awareness after brain injury. Curr Biol 26:1494–1499
Tengvar C, Johansson B, Sorensen J (2004) Frontal lobe and cingulate cortical metabolic dysfunction in acquired akinetic mutism: a PET study of the interval form of carbon monoxide poisoning. Brain Inj 18:615–625
Terhune DB, Cardeña E (2010) Differential patterns of spontaneous experiential response to a hypnotic induction: a latent profile analysis. Conscious Cogn 19:1140–1150
Terhune DB, Cardeña E, Lindgren M (2011) Differential frontal-parietal phase synchrony during hypnosis as a function of hypnotic suggestibility. Psychophysiology 48:1444–1447
The Executive Committee of the American Psychological Association – Division of Psychological Hypnosis (1994) Definition and description of hypnosis. Contemp Hypn 11:142–162
The Multi-Society Task Force on PVS (1994) Medical aspects of the persistent vegetative state (1). N Engl J Med 330:1499–1508
Thibaut A, Bruno MA, Chatelle C, Gosseries O, Vanhaudenhuyse A, Demertzi A, Schnakers C, Thonnard M, Charland-Verville V, Bernard C, Bahri MA, Phillips C, Boly M, Hustinx R,

Laureys S (2012) Metabolic activity in external and internal awareness networks in severely brain-damaged patients. J Rehab Med 44(6):487–494
Thibaut A, Schiff N, Giacino J et al (2019) Therapeutic interventions in patients with prolonged disorders of consciousness. Lancet Neurol 18:600–614
Tian L, Jiang T, Liu Y, Yu C, Wang K, Zhou Y, Song M, Li K (2007) The relationship within and between the extrinsic and intrinsic systems indicated by resting state correlational patterns of sensory cortices. NeuroImage 36:684–690
Tommasino C, Grana C, Lucignani G, Torri G, Fazio F (1995) Regional cerebral metabolism of glucose in comatose and vegetative state patients. J Neurosurg Anesthesiol 7:109–116
Tononi G (2004) An information integration theory of consciousness. BMC Neurosci 5:42
Vanhaudenhuyse A, Boveroux P, Boly M, Schnakers C, Bruno MA, Kirsch M, Demertzi A, Lamy M, Maquet P, Laureys S, Faymonville ME (2008) Hypnosis and pain perception. Rev Med Liege 63:424–428
Vanhaudenhuyse A, Demertzi A, Schabus M, Noirhomme Q, Bredart S, Boly M, Phillips C, Soddu A, Luxen A, Moonen G, Laureys S (2011) Two distinct neuronal networks mediate the awareness of environment and of self. J Cogn Neurosci 23:570–578
Vogt BA, Laureys S (2005) Posterior cingulate, precuneal and retrosplenial cortices: cytology and components of the neural network correlates of consciousness. Prog Brain Res 150:205–217
Whyte J, Myers R (2009) Incidence of clinically significant responses to zolpidem among patients with disorders of consciousness: a preliminary placebo controlled trial. Am J Phys Med Rehabil 88:410–418
Wilckens KA, Aizenstein HJ, Nofzinger EA et al (2016) The role of non-rapid eye movement slow-wave activity in prefrontal metabolism across young and middle-aged adults. J Sleep Res 25:296–306
Zeman A (2001) Consciousness. Brain J Neurol 124:1263–1289

Modulation of CNS Functions by Deep Brain Stimulation: Insights Provided by Molecular Imaging

46

Alexandre Boutet, Mehr Jain, Dave Gwun, Pablo Rusjan, Clemens Neudorfer, Gavin J. B. Elias, Jürgen Germann, Alexander Bilbily, Walter Kucharczyk, Alfonso Fasano, Gwenn S. Smith, and Andres M. Lozano

A. Boutet · W. Kucharczyk
University Health Network, Toronto, ON, Canada

Joint Department of Medical Imaging, University of Toronto, Toronto, ON, Canada
e-mail: alexandre.boutet@mail.utoronto.ca; w.kucharczyk@utoronto.ca

M. Jain · D. Gwun · C. Neudorfer · G. J. B. Elias · J. Germann
University Health Network, Toronto, ON, Canada
e-mail: mjain030@uottawa.ca

P. Rusjan
Research and Imaging Centre and Campbell Family Mental Health Research Institute at the Centre for Addiction and Mental Health, Toronto, ON, Canada
e-mail: pablo.rusjan@camhpet.ca

A. Bilbily
University Health Network, Toronto, ON, Canada

Joint Department of Medical Imaging, University of Toronto, Toronto, ON, Canada

16 Bit Inc., Toronto, ON, Canada
e-mail: alexander@16bit.ai

A. Fasano
University Health Network, Toronto, ON, Canada

Edmond J. Safra Program in Parkinson's Disease, Morton and Gloria Shulman Movement Disorders Clinic, Toronto Western Hospital, UHN, Division of Neurology, University of Toronto, Toronto, ON, Canada

Krembil Brain Institute, Toronto, ON, Canada
e-mail: alfonso.fasano@uhn.ca

G. S. Smith
Department of Psychiatry and Behavioral Sciences, John Hopkins University School of Medicine, Baltimore, MD, USA
e-mail: gsmith95@jhmi.edu

A. M. Lozano (✉)
University Health Network, Toronto, ON, Canada

Division of Neurosurgery, Toronto Western Hospital, Toronto, ON, Canada
e-mail: lozano@uhnresearch.ca

R. A. J. O. Dierckx et al. (eds.), *PET and SPECT in Neurology*,
https://doi.org/10.1007/978-3-030-53168-3_46

Contents

Abstract

Deep brain stimulation (DBS) is a neurosurgical intervention that allows probing and recalibration of dysfunctional brain circuits using electrical current delivered via implanted electrodes. While predominantly used in the treatment of Parkinson's disease and other movement disorders, DBS is increasingly being studied for its application to psychiatric diseases (e.g., major depressive disorder and obsessive-compulsive disorder) and cognitive disorders (e.g., Alzheimer's disease). Despite these growing applications of DBS, the mechanisms of action underlying DBS are poorly understood. Molecular neuroimaging modalities such as positron emission tomography (PET) and single-photon emission computed tomography (SPECT) provide a unique window into the neural changes induced by electrical stimulation; as such, they constitute invaluable research tools, with the potential to dramatically enhance both our understanding of this technology and its therapeutic impact. This chapter aims to provide an up-to-date review of insights gleaned from PET and SPECT studies in DBS patients.

Abbreviations

$[^{11}C]$dMP	$[^{11}C]$d-Threo-methylphenidate
$[^{11}C]$DTBZ	$[^{11}C]$Dihydrotetrabenazine
$[^{11}C]$NEM	$[^{11}C]$Nemonapride
$[^{11}C]$RACLO	$[^{11}C]$Raclopride

[^{123}I]FP-CIT	*N*-ω-Fluoropropyl-2β-carboxymethoxy-3β-(4-iodophenyl)tropane
[^{123}I]IBZM	[^{123}I]Iodobenzamide
[^{123}I]IMP	*N*-Isopropyl-*p*-(iodine-123)-iodoamphetamine
[^{18}F]FDG	18-Fluoro-2-deoxyglucose
[^{18}F]FDOPA	L-6-[^{18}F]Fluoro-3,4-dihydroxyphenylalanine
[^{18}F]FP	[^{18}F]Fallypride
[^{99m}Tc]ECD	^{99m}Technetium-ethylene biyldicysteinate dimer
[^{99m}Tc]HMPAO	^{99m}Technetium hexamethyl
ACC	Anterior cingulate cortex
AD	Alzheimer's disease
BOLD	Blood-oxygenation-level-dependent
CSTC	Cortico-striato-thalamo-cortical
DBS	Deep brain stimulation
fMRI	Functional magnetic resonance imaging
GPi	Globus pallidus internus
MDD	Major depressive disorder
MRI	Magnetic resonance imaging
NAcc	Nucleus accumbens
OCD	Obsessive-compulsive disorder
PCC	Posterior cingulate cortex
PD	Parkinson's disease
PDRP	Parkinson's disease-related pattern
PET	Positron emission tomography
SGC	Subgenual cingulate cortex
SMA	Supplementary motor area
SPECT	Single-photon emission computed tomography
STN	Subthalamic nucleus

46.1 Introduction

DBS is a neurosurgical procedure that involves electrical stimulation of structures deep within the brain using implanted electrodes. Since its inception in the early 1960s, the field of DBS has undergone rapid advancements, shaping how we understand and treat brain disorders today. An estimated 150,000 patients have received DBS treatment to date (Hariz 2017). While initially employed in the treatment of pain and movement disorders such as Parkinson's disease (PD), essential tremor (ET), and dystonia (DY), DBS has seen its spectrum of applications expand considerably in recent years. Today, DBS is being investigated for its therapeutic potential in psychiatric disorders such as obsessive-compulsive disorder (OCD), treatment-refractory major depressive disorder (MDD), Tourette's syndrome, and anorexia nervosa (Lozano et al. 2019). Currently ongoing clinical trials are also investigating its utility in cognitive disorders, such as Alzheimer's disease (AD), as well as

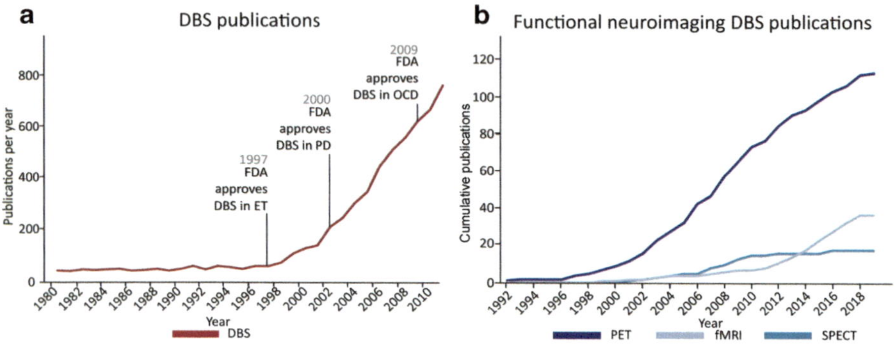

Fig. 46.1 DBS studies over time. (**a**) Cumulative number of deep brain stimulation studies published from 1980 to 2011 (modified from Neuron, 77/3, Lozano AM, Lipsman N, Probing and Regulating Dysfunctional Circuits Using Deep Brain Stimulation, 406–424, 2013, with permission from Elsevier). (**b**) Cumulative publications of positron emission tomography (PET), single-photon emission computed tomography (SPECT), and functional magnetic resonance imaging (fMRI) deep brain stimulation studies published from 1992 to 2019. Note the relative increase of PET and, more recently, fMRI studies as compared to SPECT investigations, which plateaued from 2010. *DBS* deep brain stimulation, *ET* essential tremor, *FDA* Food and Drug Administration, *fMRI* functional magnetic resonance imaging, *MRI* magnetic resonance imaging, *OCD* obsessive-compulsive disorder, *PET* positron emission tomography, *PD* Parkinson's disease, *SPECT* single-photon emission computed tomography

conditions such as morbid obesity. DBS interventions have yielded encouraging results in the treatment of chronic pain syndromes, cluster headache, and traumatic brain injury (Lozano and Lipsman 2013; Lozano et al. 2019). Due to its established and potential benefits for a broad spectrum of indications, both the number of DBS procedures conducted worldwide and the number of published DBS-related studies are rapidly increasing every year (Lozano and Lipsman 2013) (Fig. 46.1a).

DBS surgery entails the insertion of electrodes into deep brain structures through burr holes that enable access to the desired brain target. For accurate and safe electrode placement, the neurosurgeon relies on both preoperative and intraoperative imaging modalities. These typically entail multimodal, high-resolution MRI scans that allow visualization of brain structures and surrounding blood vessels (Boutet et al. 2019a). During preoperative stereotactic planning, the electrode trajectory is adjusted to accurately target the desired brain region while avoiding surrounding blood vessels and eloquent cortical areas such as the motor cortex. Following trajectory planning, electrodes are surgically implanted under local or general anesthesia. To confirm ideal electrode placement and ensure patient benefit, electrophysiological monitoring (i.e., microelectrode recordings), stimulation testing, and cranial imaging are commonly performed intraoperatively. In the final step of the surgery, an extension wire is tunneled under the skin in order to connect the electrodes to an implantable pulse generator commonly positioned in the upper chest wall (Lozano and Lipsman 2013) (Fig. 46.2a). Of note, DBS surgery is reversible; the device can be removed without long-term brain damage other than the formation of mild scar-like tissue along the implantation tracts (Erasmi et al. 2018).

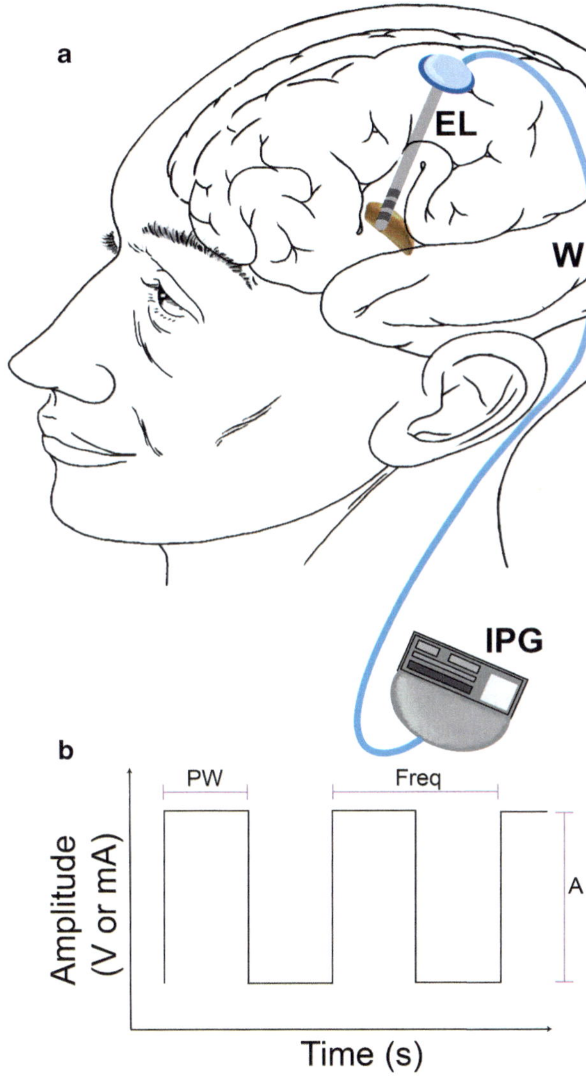

Fig. 46.2 DBS neuromodulation system. (**a**) The device consists of three components: electrode (EL), extension wire (W), and implantable pulse generator (IPG). The stimulating contacts of the electrode are placed within specific areas of the brain and receive power from the IPG that is typically placed subcutaneously in the right upper chest area. Electrode and IPG are connected via an extension wire that is tunneled under the skin. (**b**) Representation of the employed stimulation parameters during chronic DBS. Waveforms typically consist of square pulses that are applied at a predefined amplitude (A), pulse width (PW), and frequency (Freq). Parameters can be titrated individually to maximize clinical efficacy and reduce adverse effects to a minimum. V, volts; mA, milliamp; s: seconds

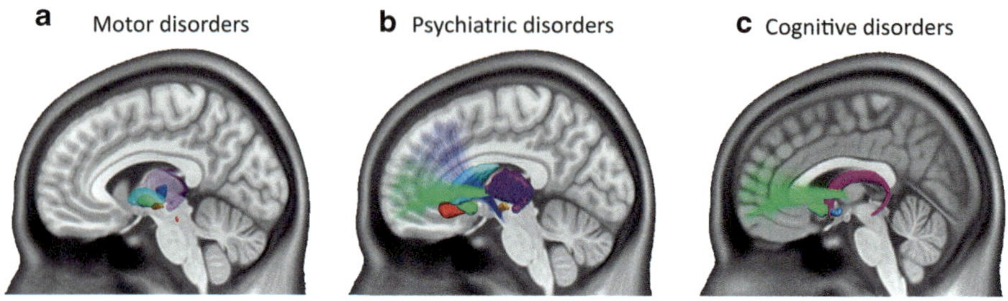

Fig. 46.3 Common DBS targets. 3D representation of brain targets overlaid on sagittal MRI (T1-weighted standard Montreal Neurological Institute brain). Apart from the caudate nucleus, only targets which have been investigated with molecular neuroimaging are displayed (Tables 46.1, 46.2, 46.3, 46.4, 46.5, 46.6, and 46.7). (**a**) Motor disorder targets: the globus pallidus externa (light blue), globus pallidus internus (green), pedunculopontine nucleus (red), subthalamic nucleus (yellow), thalamus (purple), and ventral intermediate nucleus of the thalamus (dark blue). (**b**) Psychiatric disorders targets: the caudate nucleus (light blue), middle forebrain bundle (dark blue), subgenual cingulate gyrus (red), subthalamic nucleus (yellow), thalamus (purple), and ventral capsule/ventral striatum and relevant tracts (green). (**c**) Cognitive disorder targets: the fornix (pink), nucleus basalis (blue), and ventral capsule/ventral striatum and relevant tracts (green)

To achieve maximum benefit, DBS electrodes are strategically placed within gray and white matter structures that are considered important in the pathophysiology of the respective disease. Targets are manifold and have mostly been adapted from the lesional era of neurosurgery (Miocinovic et al. 2013). In the treatment of movement disorders, established targets include the subthalamic nucleus (STN), globus pallidus internus (GPi), and ventral intermediate nucleus of the thalamus. These targets are part of a common motor circuit that processes and regulates the planning and execution of movements. In contrast, the major hubs and related white matter connections implicated—and therefore stimulated—in psychiatric diseases include structures such as the nucleus accumbens (NAcc), anterior limb of the internal capsule, anterior cingulate cortex (ACC), and medial forebrain bundle (Lozano et al. 2019). Common hubs of the major circuits targeted by DBS are shown in Fig. 46.3.

Electrical stimulation is usually not initiated immediately following electrode implantation but typically commences days to weeks after surgery, after the acute surgical effects have resolved. Local inflammatory changes of brain tissue occur surrounding the leads, which may induce temporary improvement of patients' symptoms that are unrelated to electrical stimulation (commonly referred to as "insertional effect"). Electrical stimulation is typically initiated by a physician specialized in DBS programming (Picillo et al. 2016). The stimulation parameters (i.e., voltage, frequency, and pulse width) are gradually adjusted and customized toward the patient's specific symptom constellation (Fig. 46.2b). The goal of the titration process is to maximize symptom control while reducing undesired adverse effects (e.g., speech impairment, paresthesia) that may arise from stimulation of adjacent brain structures. Stimulation programming is typically performed empirically and often involves selection of parameters on a trial-and-error basis with respect to exhibited symptoms. When adjusted properly, striking clinical improvements may be observed.

46.1.1 Electrophysiology and Functional Neuroimaging

DBS not only holds therapeutic potential for various neurological and psychiatric conditions but also offers a unique opportunity to monitor and probe neural activity in close vicinity to the chosen target structure (Lozano et al. 2018). This is accomplished, in part, through the intraoperative brain mapping techniques that are used to identify DBS target locations. Specifically, electrophysiological recordings provide insight into the dynamics of brain activity at the level of cell populations (in the case of local field potential—LFP—recordings) or individual neurons (in the case of single-unit recordings) (Rosa et al. 2013). While LFP and single-unit recordings feature a high spatial and temporal resolution, their utility is limited to confined areas in close proximity to the recording device; inferences regarding functional changes across distributed neural networks are not usually possible. To overcome these limitations, functional neuroimaging techniques such as molecular neuroimaging (e.g., positron emission tomography (PET), single-photon emission computed tomography (SPECT)), and functional magnetic resonance imaging (fMRI) have evolved that allow the study of network-level changes in response to DBS (Ko et al. 2013).

Functional neuroimaging techniques have found increasing application as research and targeting tool in DBS in recent years (Fig. 46.1b). They have provided valuable insights into how cortical and subcortical activity changes in response to different DBS paradigms (e.g., ON vs. OFF stimulation) and have gone a considerable way toward elucidating the mechanisms of DBS in movement disorders and psychiatric and neurodegenerative diseases (Ko et al. 2013). Notably, PET data have also contributed to the identification of new DBS targets for MDD and cluster headaches pinpointing key network hubs whose activity is altered in disease (May et al. 1998; Mayberg et al. 2005) (Fig. 46.4).

The selection of the appropriate functional neuroimaging modality largely depends on the experimental hypothesis and technical specifications (Friston 2009). PET and SPECT can provide information on tissue glucose consumption and cerebral blood flow and hence can be used to assess regional brain function. While these tracers measure brain activity, it is not possible to infer whether said activity is caused by the recruitment of excitatory or inhibitory neuron populations as the measurements reflect a final common pathway of brain activity (Dale and Halgren 2001; Friston 2009). As such, these methods can identify changes in neural function, but the results are not mechanistically specific. Importantly, there are established PET and SPECT radiotracers that can provide mechanistic information on specific neurotransmitter pathways (e.g., metabolism, transporters, and receptors), neuromodulators, pathological processes (e.g., inflammation), and proteins involved in neurodegenerative diseases (e.g., beta amyloid and tau proteins; Hooker and Carson 2019). Among the most commonly studied radiotracer targets of this kind are those related to monoaminergic neurotransmission (dopamine and serotonin) metabolism, receptors, and transporters. While there are several limitations of PET and SPECT imaging, mainly related to spatial and temporal resolution, these remain the only techniques available for in vivo imaging of a broad range of neurobiological mechanisms.

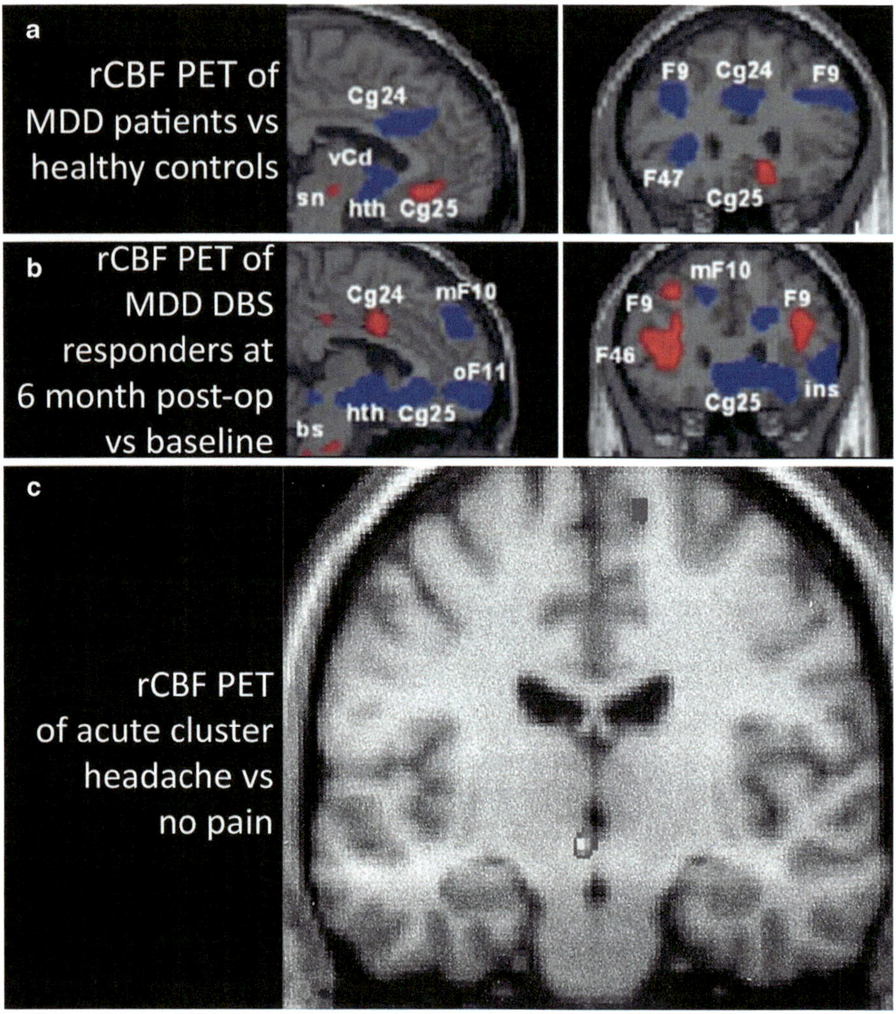

Fig. 46.4 Examples of insights from molecular neuroimaging. (**a**) In therapy-refractory major depressive disorder (MDD), PET [^{15}O]H_2O data have indicated increased blood flow within the subgenual cingulate cortex (SGC or Cg25), which has led to the investigation of this area as a potential DBS target. (**b**) Reversal of increased blood flow during SGC-DBS was associated with alleviation of depressive symptoms (**a** and **b** modified from Neuron, 45/5, Mayberg HS, Lozano AM, Voon V, McNeely HE, Seminowicz D, Hamani C, Schwalb JM, Kennedy SH, 651–660, 2005, with permission from Elsevier). (**c**) Acute episodes of headache were associated with increased hypothalamic blood flow ([^{15}O]H_2O), opening the door to hypothalamic modulation for cluster headaches (reprinted from The Lancet, 352, May A, Bahra A, Buchel C, Frackowiak RSJ, Goadsby PJ, Hypothalamic activation in cluster headache attacks, 275–278, 1998, with permission from Elsevier). *Bs* brain stem, *Cg24* anterior cingulate, *Cg 25* subgenual cingulate, *F9* dorsolateral prefrontal, *F46* prefrontal, *F47* ventrolateral prefrontal, *hth* hypothalamus, *ins* anterior insula, *mF10* medial frontal, *oF11* orbital frontal, and *vCd* ventral caudate

As neuroimaging techniques permit in vivo investigation of brain activity, PET and SPECT are often compared to magnetic resonance imaging (MRI). Compared to magnetic resonance imaging (MRI), PET and SPECT imaging technology is less widely available. The spatial (1–2 mm) and temporal resolution of MRI are superior to that of PET and SPECT imaging. The latest-generation PET scanners have reached the theoretical limit of resolution for PET (2.5 mm) (Turner and Jones 2003). The spatial resolution of PET and SPECT limits the ability to accurately quantitate radiotracer binding in small structures due to partial-volume effect that creates spillover of signal leading to less accurate signal quantification (Soret et al. 2007). MRI techniques for measuring brain function include fMRI that measures blood-oxygenation-level-dependent (BOLD) signal and arterial spin labelling that quantify blood flow, both thought to be a correlate of brain activity. MRI's signal-to-noise ratio for subcortical structures may be suboptimal, which is relevant as most DBS electrodes are placed in deep brain structures. Compared to PET, fMRI is also limited by the lack of absolute quantification (Dale and Halgren 2001; Friston 2009). In terms of participant burden, MRI involves no radiation compared to PET and SPECT. As MRI relies on strong magnetic fields and radio-frequency pulses, its application to DBS has historically been hamstrung by the risk of interference with metallic implants (Boutet et al. 2019b). Also, compared to PET and SPECT, MRI data in patients receiving DBS will be hampered to a greater extent by the metallic susceptibility artefact and associated image distortion (Fig. 46.5). Experimental designs will strongly benefit from weighting pros and cons of these modalities.

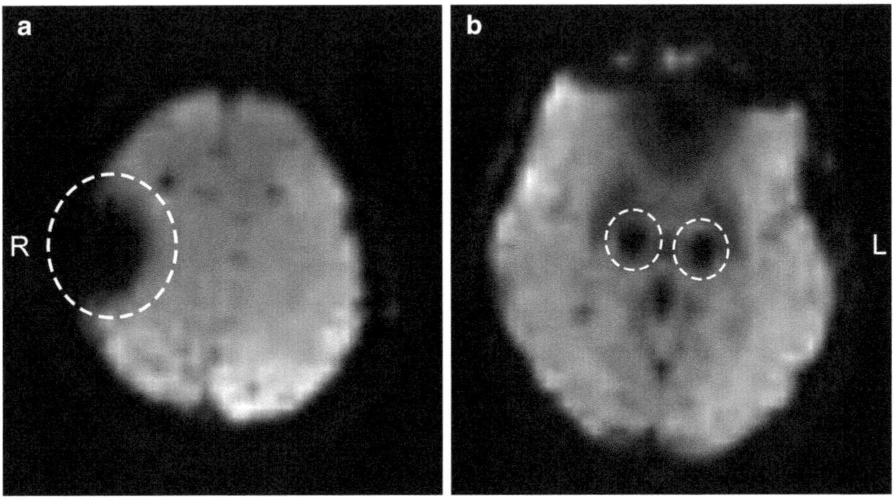

Fig. 46.5 fMRI artifacts related to the DBS device. Select axial GRE-EPI images acquired with 3 T MRI in a patient with Parkinson's disease receiving subthalamic nucleus (STN) DBS. (**a**) Artifact related to the coiled DBS extension wire under the scalp (dotted line circle). (**b**) Artifact related to the DBS leads (dotted line circle). *L* left, *R* right. *GRE-EPI* gradient recalled echo-echo planar imaging

In this chapter, we review the state-of-the-art of PET and SPECT applications in the field of DBS. First, DBS-specific experimental variables for neuroimaging studies are reviewed to guide study findings interpretation. Then, we summarize the insights gained from PET and SPECT studies in the field and provide an overview of the limitations. Finally, we provide an overview of future directions of the application of functional neuroimaging to the study of the neurobiology of DBS. Despite their potential relevance, fMRI studies were excluded as they exceed the scope of this review on molecular imaging. fMRI is briefly touched upon in Sect. 46.11.

46.2 Methods

Peer-reviewed literature pertaining to molecular neuroimaging in DBS was surveyed by searching the publicly accessible database MEDLINE. Search terms included "deep brain stimulation," "DBS," "electrical stimulation," "positron emission tomography," "PET," "PET scan," "CT PET scan," "positron emission tomography computed tomography," "single-photon emission computed tomography," "SPECT," "single-photon emission CAT scan," "single-photon emission CT scan," "single-photon emission computer assisted tomography," and "single photon emission computed radionuclide tomography." Relevant articles and reviews from other sources were included as well. We only reviewed papers published in English that involved human subjects. Data extraction from the studies is presented in the appendix and includes the following variables: study year, number of DBS patients, time of PET or SPECT after the surgery, tracer, contrast, and brain areas showing tracer increase or decrease. To remain concise, we aimed to report molecular neuroimaging findings pertaining to a single comparison (i.e., contrast representing a unique contribution) per study. In order of priority, we reported long-term changes (i.e., neuroimaging data acquired postop vs. preoperative with DBS-ON (i.e., DBS turned on) or DBS-OFF (i.e., DBS turned off)), acute changes (i.e., DBS-ON vs. DBS-OFF), and, finally, other comparisons such as OFF vs. preoperative or DBS patients vs. healthy controls.

46.3 DBS-Specific Experimental Variables

Several considerations must be kept in mind when reviewing and interpreting the results of functional neuroimaging studies involving DBS patients (Vitek et al. 2010). First, PET and SPECT findings depend on the timing between surgery and acquisition of imaging data. Indeed, inflammatory reactions as well as local swelling of brain tissue along the electrode path may confound imaging results in the immediate postoperative course. Second, changes in the medication regimen after DBS (as is done in PD patients for levodopa and dopamine agonists) and adjustment of stimulation settings prior to the imaging session (which would affect whether patients were scanned after a period of stable, optimal stimulation) have to be taken into account when investigating DBS effects. These variables may change the interpretation of the clinical and functional neuroimaging outcomes. Programming optimization is particularly problematic for psychiatric disorders for which we lack objective markers to quantify maximal symptom improvement. Third, when comparing DBS-ON and DBS-OFF, a washout period between programming and data acquisition is recommended to ensure that the prior stimulation condition does not interfere with data acquisition. Washout periods vary greatly across diseases and are determined by considerations of patient tolerability and the time course of both the re-emergence of symptoms and of the neurobiological effects. Fourth, interpretation of neuroimaging data is often complicated by the lack of information regarding electrode position. Variations in position across patients, surgeons, and institutions inevitably result in heterogeneous targeting and should ideally be assessed and accounted for to allow meaningful statements in the context of patient benefit and neuroimaging findings (Butson et al. 2007). At a single institution, the number of patients receiving DBS can be low, which results in small sample sizes unless multi-site collaboration is undertaken.

46.4 Molecular Neuroimaging Tracers

For the purpose of this chapter, PET and SPECT will be grouped under the umbrella terms "molecular neuroimaging" or "functional neuroimaging" modalities. Changes in brain activity in neural circuits upon stimulation have been the most commonly studied aspect across the DBS functional neuroimaging literature using various tracers (Fig. 46.6). In this chapter, PET (e.g., [^{18}F]FDG, [^{15}O]H_2O) and SPECT (e.g., [^{99m}Tc]ECD, [^{123}I]IMP, and [^{99m}Tc]HMPAO) tracers will be considered markers of brain "activity" or "function." However, while tracers such as [^{18}F]FDG, [^{15}O]H_2O, and [^{99m}Tc]ECD all serve to index brain function, they do so in different ways; [^{18}F]FDG, for instance, measures glucose consumption, while [^{15}O]H_2O and

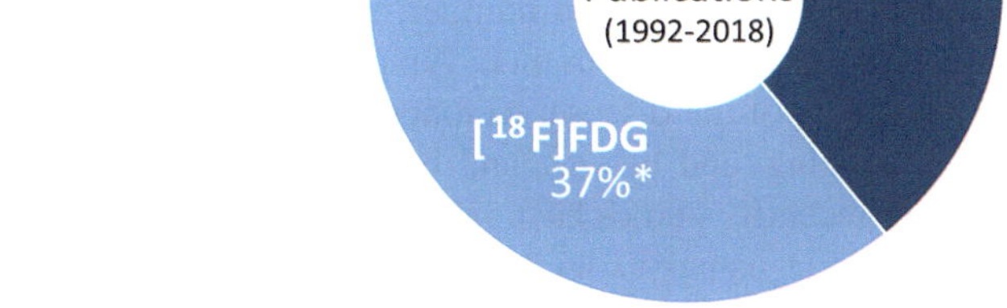

Fig. 46.6 PET and SPECT tracers commonly used in DBS studies. From 1992 to 2019, tracers used to measure brain activity (indicated by asterisk) were most commonly used. Dopaminergic tracers were also used mostly in Parkinson's disease studies

[^{99m}Tc]ECD measure cerebral blood flow. These differences should be kept in mind when comparing studies. A smaller number of PD studies have used tracers for the dopamine system, including tracers for dopamine synthesis and turnover (PET: [^{18}F]FDOPA), dopamine transporters (PET: [^{11}C]dMP; SPECT: [^{123}I]FP-CIT), vesicular monoamine transporter (PET: [^{11}C]DTBZ), and dopamine D2 receptors (PET: [^{11}C]RAC, [^{11}C]NEM, [^{18}F]FP; SPECT: [^{123}I]IBZM) (Lammertsma 2001; Shen et al. 2012).

46.5 Review of PET and SPECT Studies

The following sections provide an overview of PET and SPECT studies in DBS; studies pertaining to movement disorders, psychiatric disorders, and cognitive disorders are addressed in turn. Each section is divided into "molecular neuroimaging findings" and "contributions of molecular neuroimaging." The former summarizes the results of the literature, whereas the latter identifies insights to the field provided by these results.

46.6 Movement Disorders

Movement disorders constitute the most common indication for DBS surgery today. This is owing to the rapid and striking clinical benefits that electrical stimulation elicits in conditions such as PD, essential tremor, and dystonia (Lozano et al. 2019). The brain regions targeted in the treatment of movement disorders are subcortical motor circuit hubs that play a crucial role in the planning and execution of movement (Fig. 46.3a). Below, we will review the molecular neuroimaging findings that have provided insights into the neural substrates underlying the clinical changes that occur with DBS mainly in Parkinson's disease and, to a lesser extent, in other movement disorders.

46.6.1 Parkinson's Disease

Parkinson's disease (PD) is the second most common neurodegenerative disorder with a rapidly increasing incidence after the age of 50 (Lozano et al. 2019; Poewe et al. 2017). The disease is defined by a number of hallmark symptoms, including akinesia or bradykinesia, rigidity, and tremor. Typically, postural instability and gait issues occur in later stages of the disease. Autonomic dysfunctions including orthostatic hypotension, sweating, and bladder and bowel dysfunctions are also usually seen in late PD. More recently, studies have investigated the poorly understood non-motor manifestations of PD, namely, cognitive dysfunction (from mild executive dysfunction to distinct manifestations of dementia) and psychiatric manifestations (e.g., depression, anxiety, and psychosis) (Jankovic 2008; Rodriguez-Oroz et al. 2009).

PD is characterized by the degeneration of dopamine-rich neurons within the substantia nigra pars compacta as well as widespread accumulation of intracellular α-synuclein throughout the brain. Neurodegeneration and a-synuclein accumulation follow stages of severity known as the Braak stages: initially, the lower brain stem (including the substantia nigra compacta) undergoes pathological changes, followed by the midbrain and basal forebrain, and finally the limbic system and neocortex (Poewe et al. 2017).

The cortico-striato-thalamo-cortical (CSTC) circuit is the principal functional network for the regulation of motor activity and complex behavior in the brain. Within the circuit, information is conveyed from the cortex to major subcortical nodes such as the striatum, globus pallidus, STN, substantia nigra, and thalamus. These structures process incoming information and relay the output back to the cortex, forming a feedback loop (Albin et al. 1989; DeLong 1990) (Fig. 46.7a). For effective information processing, an equilibrium must be maintained within the circuit that readily allows adaptation to external stimuli. To this end, antagonistic regulatory subpathways have evolved within the CSTC circuit, namely, "direct," "indirect," and "hyperdirect" pathways (Fig. 46.7b). The "direct" pathway exerts inhibitory effects on the internal segment of the globus pallidus (GPi) and facilitates cortical activation via disinhibition of the thalamus. In contrast, the "indirect" pathway reduces thalamic output. This is achieved by a cascade of inhibitory and excitatory relays that promote GPi output and eventually arrest thalamic activity

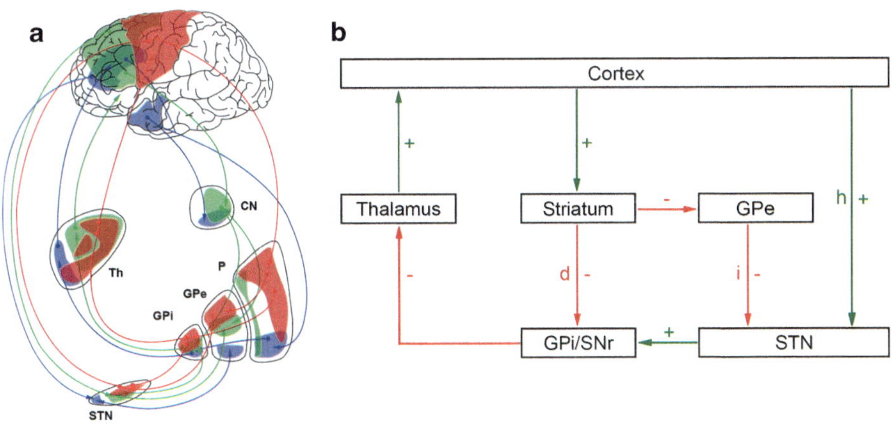

Fig. 46.7 Cortico-striato-thalamo-cortical (CSTC) circuit. (**a**) Network-wide-level representation of the CSTC circuit depicting the functional parallel reentrant loops that reside within segregated basal ganglia territories (red, sensorimotor; blue, associative; green, limbic). (**b**) Classic model of the CSTC circuit featuring direct (d) and indirect (i) and hyperdirect (h) pathway and their influence (+, excitatory; –, inhibitory) on downstream basal ganglia territories (**a** and **b** modified with permission from Springer Nature Customer Service Centre GmbH: Springer Nature, Brain Structure and Function, Neuroanatomical background and functional considerations for stereotactic interventions in the H fields of Forel, Neudorfer C, Maarouf M, 2017). *CN* caudate nucleus, *GPe* globus pallidus externa, *GPi* globus pallidus internus, *P* putamen, *SNr* substantia nigra reticulata, *STN* subthalamic nucleus, *Th* thalamus

(Chevalier and Deniau 1990; Rodriguez-Oroz et al. 2009). The "hyperdirect" pathway has only been described recently and incorporates fibers that bypass the inhibitory relay stations of the striatum and directly project to STN (Nambu et al. 2002). Functionally, the circuit is comparable to the "indirect" pathway; the projections, however, allow direct transmission of cortical input into downstream basal ganglia territories on a shorter temporal scale.

Aberrant and dysfunctional processing of information within functionally isolated loops has been associated with neurological conditions and led to the characterization of many disorders as "circuitopathies." Disruption of normal function of the basal ganglia and CSTC circuit secondary to pathological changes has been hypothesized to play a key role in PD pathophysiology (Rodriguez-Oroz et al. 2009). The classic CSTC circuit model suggests that the lack of nigrostriatal dopaminergic input secondary to neuronal loss causes aberrant processing of neural information within basal ganglia loops, leading to a disequilibrium within subpathways. Neurosurgical intervention, namely, deep brain stimulation (DBS), recalibrates dysfunctional activity by recruiting neuron populations within anatomically confined areas (Lozano and Lipsman 2013).

Molecular neuroimaging, in particular PET, has provided key insights into the functional status of the CSTC circuit in PD and other movement disorders. PET studies of cerebral glucose metabolism have defined the so-called Parkinson's disease-related pattern (PDRP) which consists of a spatial pattern of abnormal activity consistently found in PD patients (Eidelberg 2009; Ma et al. 2007). Specifically, the premotor and parieto-occipital cortical regions show relative metabolism reductions compared to the hyperactive pallidothalamic and pontine areas. In comparison to healthy controls, the expression of the PDRP is increased with disease progression and decreased with PD treatments, including levodopa and DBS. Hyperactivity of the indirect pathway causing an increase in inhibitory pallidal outflow to the thalamus and pons has, in turn, been hypothesized to underlie this pathological pattern of activity (Eidelberg 2009; Ma et al. 2007).

As mentioned, PD accounts for the largest proportion of DBS patients by far. When selected properly, the majority of PD patients highly benefit from this treatment (Okun 2012). Although multiple structures may be targeted, the STN and, to a lesser extent, GPi are most often stimulated (Fig. 46.3a). The target choice will be informed by discussion within a multidisciplinary team and dictated by the patient's unique clinical profile and needs. For example, GPi is sometimes recommended for patients with cognitive or psychiatric impairments due to the possible negative adverse effects of STN stimulation on these functions. Some symptoms such as tremor and rigidity tend to improve more than other PD manifestations including gait and speech, which may in fact worsen with stimulation. Over the years, empiric postoperative DBS programming algorithms have improved and can achieve individually optimized stimulation (Picillo et al. 2016). Immediate clinical feedback (e.g., tremor or rigidity reduction) in response to stimulation in PD patients makes DBS programming slightly easier. However, this optimization process still takes up to a year to complete. As such, clinical benefits can generally be maximized and adverse effects minimized for each patient (Lozano and Lipsman 2013; Picillo et al. 2016).

46.6.1.1 Molecular Neuroimaging Findings

Molecular neuroimaging studies have mainly focused on one of the following experimental designs to evaluate the impact of DBS on PD symptoms: (1) investigating the main effects of acute stimulation (by comparing ON and OFF stimulation conditions) or chronic stimulation (by comparing postoperative and preoperative imaging data) while the patients are at rest ("resting experiments") and (2) comparison between performance on particular tasks in ON and OFF stimulation conditions ("task experiments"). The most frequent focus of PD studies has been changes in brain function, as assessed using various PET (e.g., [^{18}F]FDG and [^{15}O]H_2O) and SPECT (e.g., [^{99m}Tc]ECD) tracers. Other PET tracers investigating dopamine metabolism ([^{11}C]NEM, [^{18}F]fallypride, [^{123}I]FP-CIT, [^{18}F]FDOPA, and [^{11}C]DTBZ) and SPECT ([^{123}I]FP-CIT and [^{123}I]IBZM) have also been used to investigate DBS mechanism of action and change in disease progression.

STN-DBS studies contrasting ON vs. OFF stimulation conditions have consistently shown changes in metabolism predominantly within major hubs of the motor circuits, although the directionality of metabolic changes is fairly heterogeneous Table 46.1. In general, STN and the neighboring thalamus show increased activity in response to STN stimulation (Asanuma et al. 2006; Garraux et al. 2011; Hershey et al. 2003; Hilker et al. 2004; 2008; Hill et al. 2013; Karimi et al. 2008; Volonte et al. 2012). Interestingly, the pallidum, which receives input from the STN, has inconsistently shown change in activity characterized by mixed directionality changes either with [^{18}F]FDG or [^{15}O]H_2O (Asanuma et al. 2006; Bradberry et al. 2012; Garraux et al. 2011; Hilker et al. 2004; 2008; Hill et al. 2013; Wang et al. 2010). Brain activity within the precentral gyrus most commonly decreases during STN-DBS, which is in line with the CSTC circuit concept (Asanuma et al. 2006; Hershey et al. 2003; Hilker et al. 2002; Trost et al. 2006). However, one study has reported increased metabolism in the motor cortex (Garraux et al. 2011). Conversely, prefrontal areas tend to preferentially show increased activity (Bradberry et al. 2012; Garraux et al. 2011; Hilker et al. 2004; Trost et al. 2006). In a few instances, the precuneus and the occipitotemporal cortex have also shown increased brain activity (Asanuma et al. 2006; Bradberry et al. 2012; Hilker et al. 2002; Trost et al. 2006). The cerebellum, an important relay of the motor network, also demonstrated mixed activity patterns with STN-DBS whether the studies were measuring metabolism or regional cerebral blood flow (rCBF) (Asanuma et al. 2006; Bradberry et al. 2012; Garraux et al. 2011; Hershey et al. 2003; Hilker et al. 2002, 2004; Nagaoka et al. 2007; Trost et al. 2006; Volonte et al. 2012; Wang et al. 2010). When investigating the effects of stimulation at the network level, resting studies have shown acute reduction (and thus normalization) of the PDRP activity with STN-DBS (Asanuma et al. 2006; Trost et al. 2006; Wang et al. 2010).

To compare across studies, we diagrammatically represented the brain areas showing changes in brain function (i.e., metabolic tracers including [^{18}F]FDG, [^{15}O]H_2O) and SPECT (e.g., [^{99m}Tc]ECD, [^{123}I]IMP, and [^{99m}Tc]HMPAO) in studies employing more conservative statistics using any method of multiple comparison corrections (e.g., family-wise error, Bonferroni, or threshold cluster corrections) (Asanuma et al. 2006; Garraux et al. 2011; Hershey et al. 2003; Hilker et al. 2004;

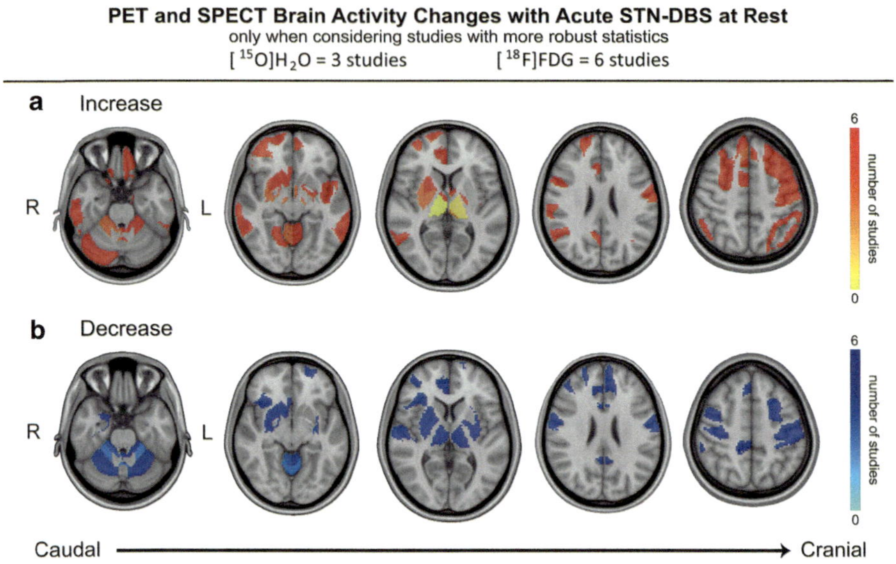

Fig. 46.8 Diagrammatic summary of activity changes with acute STN-DBS at rest. Only studies assessing acute changes with stimulation (studies with ON vs. OFF in Table 46.1) and using a form of multiple comparison correction were included to maintain robustness of reported brain regions (studies labeled with [b] in Table 46.1). First, brain regions were obtained from spatial parcellation according to published atlases (cortical, An Atlas of Intrinsic Connectivity of Homotopic Areas (Joliot et al. 2015); subcortical, Ewert et al. (2018); brain stem, Harvard Ascending Arousal Network Atlas (Edlow et al. 2012); cerebellum, Diedrichsen et al. (2009)). Then, regions were weighted according to the number of studies reporting significant changes in each region. To decide which parcellated brain areas from the atlases would be selected, we used in order of priority (1) visual representation, (2) reported coordinates, and (3) naming of areas with activation available in studies. For large activation areas, multiple parcellated brain areas were selected. Areas of brain activity changes were then overlaid on select MRI (T1-weighted Montreal Neurological Institute brain) axial images. Across studies, brain regions with an increase in activity (hot colors) are shown in (**a**), whereas brain regions with significant decrease in activity (cool colors) are shown in (**b**). Color bars represent the number of studies

Hill et al. 2013; Karimi et al. 2008; Nagaoka et al. 2007; Volonte et al. 2012; Wang et al. 2010) (Fig. 46.8).

A subset of studies have focused on *long-term changes (postop vs. preop)* associated with STN stimulation Table 46.1. The follow-up times for long-term PD studies ranged from 1 month to 20 months post operation. Interestingly, the areas demonstrating changes here differ from those linked to acute stimulation changes. Long-term changes predominantly appear to involve the frontal lobes and, to a lesser extent, the parietal and temporal lobes (Antonini et al. 2003; Cilia et al. 2009; Le Jeune et al. 2010a; Sestini et al. 2002, 2005, 2007). The direction of changes is inconsistent across studies. In contrast to ON vs. OFF stimulation studies, hubs of the motor circuit such as the STN, thalamus, GPi, and precentral gyrus seldom showed significant changes in most studies. A few studies, however, reported increased (Cilia et al. 2009; Le Jeune et al. 2010a; Peron et al. 2010; Pourfar et al. 2009; Sestini et al. 2005; Tanei et al. 2009) and decreased (Cao et al. 2017) brain activity in the cerebellum. Finally, Cao et al. (2017) reported a decrease in PDRP activity 8 months after STN-DBS surgery. When only considering more statistically stringent studies (i.e., those using any method of multiple comparison corrections), further insights into the directionality of changes in cortical areas are gleaned: the posterior parietal cortex most commonly showed increased brain activity, whereas prefrontal areas usually demonstrated decreased brain function (Antonini et al. 2003; Cao et al. 2017; Cilia et al. 2009; Le Jeune et al. 2008; 2010a; Li et al. 2006; Peron et al. 2010; Pourfar et al. 2009; Sestini et al. 2002, 2005, 2007; Smith et al. 2019; Tanei et al. 2009) (Fig. 46.9).

A subset of STN-DBS studies have investigated the functional changes associated with motor and non-motor (usually cognitive or emotional) tasks during

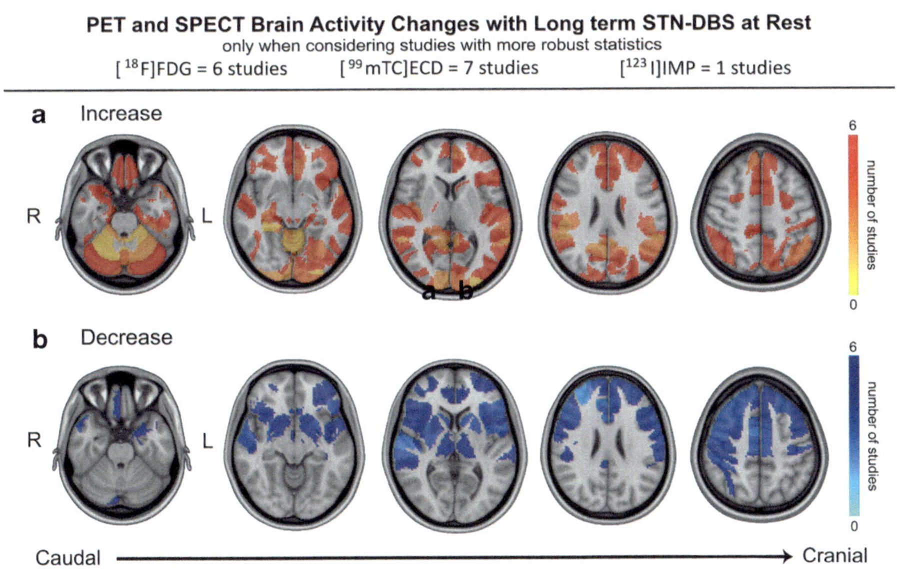

Fig. 46.9 Diagrammatic summary of activity changes with long-term STN-DBS at rest. Only studies assessing long-term changes with stimulation (studies with postop vs. preop in Table 46.1) and using a form of multiple comparison correction were included to maintain robustness of reported brain regions (studies labeled with ^{b} in Table 46.1). First, brain regions were obtained from spatial parcellation according to published atlases (cortical, An Atlas of Intrinsic Connectivity of Homotopic Areas (Joliot et al. 2015); subcortical, Ewert et al. (2018); brain stem, Harvard Ascending Arousal Network Atlas (Edlow et al. 2012); cerebellum, Diedrichsen et al. (2009)). Then, regions were weighted according to the number of studies reporting significant changes in each region. To decide which parcellated brain areas from the atlases would be selected, we used in order of priority (1) visual representation, (2) reported coordinates, and (3) naming of areas with activation available in studies. For large activation areas, multiple parcellated brain areas were selected. Areas of brain activity changes were then overlaid on select MRI (T1-weighted Montreal Neurological Institute brain) axial images. Across studies, brain regions with an increase in activity (hot colors) are shown in (**a**), whereas brain regions with significant decrease in activity (cool colors) are shown in (**b**). Color bars represent the number of studies

stimulation (Table 46.2). For the purpose of this chapter, task-based studies reported in conjunction with changes in behavior are discussed; these studies most often studied the effect of stimulation (DBS-ON vs. DBS-OFF) on tasks. Similar to resting studies, there are also inconsistencies in the results of studies using motor tasks. A likely explanation is the additional issue of variation in the motor tasks employed: motor tasks may have involved internally generated or externally cued movements as well as repetitive, random or sequential, and unilateral or bimanual movements. Modulation of motor task by STN-DBS was commonly associated with primary motor cortex and supplementary motor area (SMA) regional cerebral blood flow (rCBF) changes (Ceballos-Baumann et al. 1999; Limousin et al. 1997; Park et al. 2015; Strafella et al. 2003a). Similar to motor task studies, those using non-motor cognitive or emotional tasks provided task-specific results, with limited generalizability to other studies. In cognitive task studies (e.g., Stroop task or random number generation) investigating the effect of stimulation on cognition (i.e., interaction term), the prefrontal areas and ACC were engaged (Schroeder et al. 2002, 2003; Thobois et al. 2002, 2007; Ventre-Dominey et al. 2014). A study investigating the effect of stimulation during executive functions (spatial working memory tasks) found increased rCBF in the ACC and insula as well as decreased rCBF in the parietal lobes (Ventre-Dominey et al. 2014). Some studies also investigated the effect of motor imagery tasks. They showed rCBF changes in hubs of the motor circuit such as the precentral gyrus and SMA as well as the prefrontal cortex (Thobois et al. 2002). Specifically, Weiss et al. (2015) demonstrated that STN-DBS is associated with an increase in pedunculopontine nucleus rCBF when patients perform a gait imagination task. Interestingly, this nucleus is a DBS target for gait disturbances (Thevathasan and Moro 2019). Motor speech abilities often do not respond or respond negatively to STN-DBS (Narayana et al. 2009). A study reported decreased verbal fluency with stimulation in conjunction with decreased rCBF in the right orbitofrontal cortex, the left inferior temporal gyrus, and the left inferior frontal/insular cortex (Schroeder et al. 2003). Since a left frontotemporal network implicated in verbal fluency has been defined, this effect of STN-DBS could be related to decreased blood flow in these areas. Similarly, stuttering was worsened with STN-DBS, while the precentral gyrus, SMA, and cerebellum showed increased rCBF (Burghaus et al. 2006). Yet, a study also reported improved dysarthria in PD patients with STN stimulation causing normalization of brain activity in the motor cortex, SMA, and cerebellum (Pinto et al. 2004). These different effects of STN-DBS on various aspects of speech could be related to electrode placement, stimulation spillover on adjacent neural, and possibly related to separate circuits governing different speech facets. Various other non-motor tasks have been studied in the context of STN-DBS, such as urge to void (Herzog et al. 2006, 2008), change in pain (Dellapina et al. 2012) and smell (Cury et al. 2018; Fonoff et al. 2010), and response conflict decisions (Schroeder et al. 2002; Thobois et al. 2007) (Table 46.2). These studies usually show less engagement of the motor circuit hubs and rather changes of brain function in areas such as the thalamus, ACC, and prefrontal cortices.

A few resting studies have performed correlations with emotional changes with STN-DBS. Interestingly, worsening manic symptoms with STN-DBS have been consistently linked to increased prefrontal and ACC rCBF (Schilbach et al. 2012; Ulla et al. 2006, 2011). Worse performance in fear recognition, feeling of disgust, and worsening depression symptoms was all associated with increased (Bejjani et al. 1999) and decreased activity (Le Jeune et al. 2008; Ory et al. 2017) in the orbitofrontal cortex with STN-DBS. The STN has motor, associative, and limbic components, which explain the motor benefits and also the cognitive and emotional changes seen with DBS. These less desirable symptoms may be associated with stimulation spillover to the less desirable associative and limbic subdivisions.

As discussed, DBS electrodes may be placed in other brain targets when treating PD patients. A minority of studies have investigated PET and SPECT changes with stimulation of motor targets other than STN (Table 46.3). As with STN-DBS, GPi stimulation provides motor benefits and seems to also engage motor areas such as the motor cortex and SMA (Fukuda et al. 2001a; Valalik et al. 2009). Interestingly, one study also reported reduction (and thus normalization) of the PDRP activity with GPi-DBS (Fukuda et al. 2001b). This suggests that both STN and GPi targets provide benefits by modulating similar circuits. Additional targets are usually engaged for specific symptoms. For example, pedunculopontine nucleus (PPN) stimulation has been attempted to improve gait, while VIM stimulation is typically conducted to help patients suffering from therapy-refractory tremor (Lozano and Lipsman 2013; Lozano et al. 2019).

46.6.1.2 Studies of Dopaminergic Mechanisms

Given that degeneration of dopamine neurons within the substantia nigra is the pathophysiological hallmark of PD, investigators have used dopamine tracers to understand the role of dopamine in the mechanism of action of DBS (Poewe et al. 2017) (Tables 46.1, 46.2 and 46.3).

Dopamine tracers have been used to understand the *acute effects of STN stimulation on dopamine*. Apart from Nimura et al. (2005), most studies investigating dopamine receptor D2/3 availabilities have failed to show an acute change in striatal dopamine levels with STN stimulation whether patients were concomitantly off (Abosch et al. 2003; Arai et al. 2008; Thobois et al. 2003) or on (Strafella et al. 2003b) dopaminergic pharmacotherapy, regardless of the time duration after the stimulation was turned off. A recent study using [^{11}C]DTBZ showed a reduction in vesicular monoamine transporter 2 (VMAT2) availability which may be related to an increase of vesicular dopamine in the caudate nucleus, putamen, and some cortical and limbic regions (Smith et al. 2019). The inability of D2/3 studies to show dopamine changes with STN stimulation may be related (1) to its lack of sensitivity for detecting changes in endogenous dopamine; (2) to the slow washout of dopamine after stimulation cessation, which could last up to 12 h; and (3) to other neurotransmitters which may be involved (e.g., serotonin, gamma-aminobutyric acid (GABA), and glutamate) (Smith et al. 2019). A study comparing metabolic changes with STN-DBS and levodopa pharmacotherapy found that both treatments increased activity in SMA and decreased activity in the primary motor cortex. However, differences were seen: increased putaminal metabolism was only seen with levodopa, whereas prefrontal areas showed increased metabolism with STN-DBS

Table 46.1 STN-DBS studies in Parkinson's disease patients at rest

Studies	*n*	Postop time (month)	PD Med	Tracer	Contrast	Increase	Decrease
Hilker et al. (2002)	1	3 weeks	ON	[^{18}F]FDG	ON vs. OFF	B: MeFG, PCC, PCUN/OC, STG R: SMA, cCereb, iCereb L: PMC	B: PrG, rCereb L: Thal, hThal
Sestini et al. (2002)[a,b]	10	4.8	OFF	[^{99}mTc]ECD	ON vs. preop	B: MeFG, ACC, DLPFC, FPC; R: SFG	None
Antonini et al. (2003)[a,b]	13	6	NA	[^{99}mTc]ECD	ON (responder) vs. HC	Normalization of cortical areas	None
Hershey et al. (2003)[b]	13	2	OFF	[^{15}O]H_2O	ON vs. OFF	L: SN, RN, STN, Thal	B: SMA, PFC, MeFG R: STG, MTG, SPL, aCereb L: PrG, PoG, Cl, SFG
Hilker et al. (2003)	6	>4	OFF	[^{11}C]RACLO	ON vs. OFF	None	None
Hilker et al. (2004)[b]	8	4	NA	[^{18}F]FDG	ON vs. OFF	B: VL, STN R: DLPFC, OFC, IPL, MTG, LenN, Cereb, PCC L: ACC	L: Cereb
Haslinger et al. (2005)	6	16	OFF	[^{15}O]H_2O	Correlation between DBS frequencies (5–190 Hz) and metabolism	(Positive correlation) B: STN	(Negative correlation) B: PrG, MeFG, PMC
Hilker et al. (2005)	30	16	OFF	FDOPA	ON vs. preop	None	Unknown: CdN, Pu
Nimura et al. (2005)	3	6	ON	[^{11}C]RACLO	ON vs. preop	None	None
Sestini et al. (2005)[a–c]	10	5	OFF	[^{99}mTc]ECD	ON (5 mo) vs. ON (42 mo)	B: MeFG, SFG, aCereb, Po, SN, Thal, GPe; L: MFG, PrG, PoG	None

Asanuma et al. (2006)[b]	9	NA	ON	$[^{18}F]$FDG	ON vs. OFF	R: PCUN L: Thal, STN	B: mCereb, PrG, PoG R: Pu L: GPi, PFC (PDRP)
Li et al. (2006)[b]	5	1	OFF	$[^{18}F]$FDG	ON vs. preop	B: LG R: MFG, MidB L: PCUN, GP	B: IFG L: pHi
Trost et al. (2006)	6	6	OFF	$[^{18}F]$FDG	ON vs. OFF	Ips: PAC, PFC	Ips, contra: rPo, rMidB Ips: PrG, SMA, cerebellar vermis (PDRP)
Cilia et al. (2007)[a]	20	12	ON	$[^{99}mTc]$ECD	Correlation between verbal fluency performance and brain metabolism (stim ON)	(Positive correlation) L: DLPFC, ACC, CdN R: PMC	No negative correlation
Lokkegaard et al. (2007)[a]	35	12	ON	$[^{123}I]$FP-CIT	ON vs. preop	None	Unknown: Str
Lyoo et al. (2007)	18	2	OFF	$[^{18}F]$FDG	1. Correction between UPDRS score during DBS-ON and metabolism	(Positive correlation) unknown: SMA, ACC, PFC	(Negative correlation) none
Nagaoka et al. (2007)[b]	8	1	ON	$[^{18}F]$FDG	ON vs. OFF	R: PMC, Cereb	None
Sestini et al. (2007)[a–c]	10	5	OFF	$[^{99}mTc]$ECD	OFF vs. preop (5 months postop) OFF vs. preop (42 months postop)	L: SMA, PMC, PoG, MFG	None
Arai et al. (2008)	8	>4	OFF	$[^{18}F]$FDG, FDOPA	1. ON vs. OFF ($[^{18}F]$FDG) 2. ON vs. OFF (FDOPA)	1. Ips: Thal 2. None	1. Contra: GPi 2. None

(continued)

Table 46.1 (continued)

Studies	*n*	Postop time (month)	PD Med	Tracer	Contrast	Increase	Decrease
Campbell et al. (2008)	29	>2	OFF	[^{15}O]H_2O	ON vs. OFF	None	None
Hesse et al. (2008)[a]	18	12	OFF	[^{123}I]FP-CIT, [^{123}I]IBZM	1. ON vs. preop ([123I]FP-CIT) 2. ON vs. preop ([123I]IBZM)	1. None 2. Ips: Pu, CdN	1. None 2. None
Hilker et al. (2008)	12	6	OFF	[^{18}F]FDG	ON vs. OFF	Ips: STN Contra: GP	None
Hirano et al. (2008)	11	NA	OFF	[^{18}F]FDG, [^{15}O] H_2O	ON vs. OFF	None	None
Le Jeune et al. (2008)[b]	13	3	ON	[^{18}F]FDG	ON vs. preop	B: Cereb R: FG	B: LC, CC R SFG, PrG, MFG, STG
Karimi et al. (2008)[b]	48	>4	OFF	[^{15}O]H_2O	ON vs. OFF	B: Thal R: MidB	R: PMC
Cilia et al. (2009)[a,b]	40	12	ON	[^{99}mTc]ECD	ON vs. preop	B: OC, pHi R: Hi, PCUN, Cereb L: MTG	B: PMC, PrG, IFG, ACC, MFG R: SMA, SFG, PoG, GPe L: MeFG, Thal
Kalbe et al. (2009)	9	6	OFF	[^{18}F]FDG	ON vs. preop	None	B: vACC L: dACC
Pourfar et al. (2009)[b]	6	20	OFF	[^{18}F]FDG	OFF vs. preop	L: OC, PCUN R: SMC, pCereb, PoG	R: Pu, GP, Thal No change in PDRP expression
Tanei et al. (2009)[a,b]	7	10	ON	[^{123}I]IMP	ON vs. preop	B: CC, Cereb	B: MFG L: STG
Haegelen et al. (2010)[a]	6	3	ON	[^{18}F]FDG, HMPAO	1. ON vs. Preop ([^{18}F]FDG) 2. ON vs. Preop (HMPAO)	1. None 2. None	1. B: SFG 2. None

Le Jeune et al. (2010a)[b]	20	3	ON	$[^{18}F]FDG$	ON vs. preop	B: PCC, IFG, FG, Cereb L: MTG, pHi, MFG, OC	B: ACC, IFG, PrG, STG, PoG, MFG R: SFG, INS, MeFG L: CdN
Peron et al. (2010)[b]	13	3	ON	$[^{18}F]FDG$	ON vs. preop	B: Cereb R: IPL	B: ACC L: SFG
Wang et al. (2010)[b]	5	6	NA	$[^{18}F]FDG$	ON vs. OFF	L: MidB, Po	B: Thal, PCUN R: GPi, pCereb, SMG (PDRP)
Garraux et al. (2011)[b]	8	24	OFF	$[^{18}F]FDG$	ON vs. OFF	B: FPC, IFG, MFG, SFG, PrG, MTG, TPJ, IPL, PoG, CdN, Thal R: OFC, FO, pINS, AnG, SFG, MeFG, ACC, PPN L: TPo, STG, ITG, FuG, LG, MCC, CUN, GP, Cereb	None
Volonte et al. (2012)[b]	14	6	OFF	$[^{18}F]FDG$	ON vs. OFF	B: STN, Thal	B: Cereb
Bradberry et al. (2012)	11	24	ON	$[^{15}O]H_2O$	ON vs. OFF	B: SFG, OFC, OC, PCUN, FuG, INS, GP, Amy, Hi, Thal R: MeFG L: pCereb, IFG, PoG, Pu, MTG	B: pCereb, mCereb, PrG, SMA, MFG, PoG, SMG, Pu R: OC L: SFC, IFG, FuG, ITG, MTG, ACC
Hill et al. (2013)[b]	37	22.4	OFF	$[^{15}O]H_2O$	1. Ventral STN ON vs. ventral STN OFF 2. Dorsal STN ON vs. dorsal STN OFF	1. Ips, contra: GPi, STN, Thal 2. Ips, contra: STN, GPi	1. None 2. None

(continued)

Table 46.1 (continued)

Studies	*n*	Postop time (month)	PD Med	Tracer	Contrast	Increase	Decrease
Cao et al. (2017)[b]	8	12	OFF	[^{18}F]FDG	ON vs. preop	B: PMC, PoG, OC, SMG	B: Cereb, MFG, SFG, MeFG L: IFG, Pu (PDRP)
Smith et al. (2019)[b]	7	4–6	OFF	1. [^{11}C]DTBZ 2. [^{18}F]FDG	ON vs. preop	1. None 2. B: STG, PCUN, FG, Cereb R: pHi L: INS, IPL	1. B: PrG, Pu L: INS, STG, Amy, PCUN, IPL, CdN, Pu 2. B: CdN, STN R: Thal, Pu L: GP

Studies investigating acute (i.e., ON vs. OFF stimulation states) and long-term (i.e., postop vs. preop) effects of stimulation are listed. Clinical benefits for most patients are implicit in STN-DBS studies. *n* represents the number of patients with DBS who underwent neuroimaging. Brain areas reported to exhibit significant changes by the authors are mentioned as increase and decrease in reference to the listed contrast. However, to limit the number of abbreviations, similar areas described by different nomenclature may have been grouped under a single abbreviation with slightly less spatial specificity (e.g., middle temporal cortex was grouped under middle temporal gyrus, and thalamic subnuclei were grouped under thalamus). Most commonly, the nomenclature used to describe the areas corresponds to the terms used in the studies. *NA* not available. *PD Med* Parkinson's disease medication

[a]SPECT studies (the remainder were PET studies)

[b]This study reported a form of multiple comparison correction and was used in Figs. 46.8 and 46.9

[c]Patient overlap between these two studies

Table 46.2 Task STN-DBS studies in Parkinson's disease patients

Studies	*n*	Postop time (month)	PD Med	Tracer	Contrast	Increase	Decrease	DBS behavioral changes
Limousin et al. (1997)[a]	12	NA	OFF	$[^{15}O]H_2O$	Joystick task: effective vs. ineffective stimulation	Unknown: SMA, CC, DLPFC	None	Improvement in elbow flexion movement time
Ceballos-Baumann et al. (1999)[a]	9	>4	OFF	$[^{15}O]H_2O$	Joystick task: ON vs. OFF	Ips, contra: rSMA Ips: PMC	Ips: PrG, cSMA	Improved reaction and movement time
Strafella (2003)[a]	5	NA	OFF	$[^{15}O]H_2O$	Joystick task: Bilateral ON vs. OFF	*Contra or Ips to stimulation Ips, contra: cSMA, rSMA, GP Ips: DLPFC Contra: cACC, rACC	None	Decreased motor latency during bilateral and contralateral stimulation
Payoux et al. (2004)[a]	7	>10	OFF	$[^{15}O]H_2O$	Fist clench task: High-freq ON vs. OFF	L: STN	R: Cereb L: ACC, PrG, PoG	Improved motor symptoms (high freq)
Grafton et al. (2006)	6	4	OFF	NA	Tracking task: effective vs. ineffective stimulation	(Normalization)B: ACC R: VPMC, pCereb, IFG, SFG, CC, Pu, GP, Thal L: MeSFG, SFG, SPL, PrG, PoG, PPO	NA	Increase in extent and velocity of movement
Ballanger et al. (2009)[a]	7	47	Off	$[^{15}O]H_2O$	Go/No-Go task: ON vs. OFF	None	None	Improved motor symptoms

(continued)

Table 46.2 (continued)

Studies	*n*	Postop time (month)	PD Med	Tracer	Contrast	Increase	Decrease	DBS behavioral changes
Nozaki et al. (2013)[a]	12	32.8	OFF	[^{11}C] RACLO	Foot motion: ON vs. OFF	None	B: NAcc, CdN	Improved motor task (foot movement)
Park et al. (2015)	10		ON	[^{15}O]H_2O	1. ON: finger opposition vs. at rest 2. OFF: finger opposition vs. at rest	1. B: PrG, PoG, Cereb, CC 2. B: PrG, PoG R: SMA L: Cereb	1. Unknown: pHi 2. R: PCUN L: ITG	No difference in motor performance
Atkinson-Clement et al. (2017)	12	NA	OFF	[^{15}O]H_2O	1. Hand motion: ON vs. OFF 2. Speech production task: ON vs. OFF	1. L: PoG, IPL 2. None	1. R: Cereb L: MeFG 2. None	Improved speech and hand motion combined tasks (not in individual tasks)
Hagelweide et al. (2018)	8	NA	OFF	[^{15}O]H_2O	Serial prediction task: ON vs. OFF	R: Thal, MeOFC	None	No improvement in task
Schroeder et al. (2002)[a]	10	5	OFF	[^{15}O]H_2O	Stroop task: ON vs. OFF	L: AnG	R: ACC, Pu	Prolonged reaction time (increased Stroop effect)
Thobois et al. (2002)[a]	7	3	OFF	[^{15}O]H_2O	1. Motor imagery task: ON vs. OFF 2. Motor execution task: ON vs. OFF	1. Contra: DLPFC 2. Contra: DLPFC	1. Ips: PrG, SMA 2. Contra: SMA, PrG, IPL	Nonsignificant improvement in completion times
Schroeder et al. (2003)[a]	7	NA	NA	[^{15}O]H_2O	Fluency task: ON vs. OFF	None	R: OFC, CdN ITG, IFG, INS	Decreased verbal fluency

Burghaus et al. (2006)	1	>3	OFF	[15O]H_2O	Stuttering task: ON vs. OFF	B: ACC, Cereb R: PrG L: rSMA, BA, SMA, ACC	B: PrG, SMA, DLPFC R: WA, Cereb L: BA, aINS, ACC, rSMA	Worsening stutter (bilateral stimulation)
Geday et al. (2006)	10	NA	OFF	[15O]H_2O	1. ON: emotional faces vs. neutral visual stimuli 2. OFF: emotional situations vs. neutral visual stimuli	1. R: PFC 2. L: ACC	1. R: FuG, Pu, ITG L: INS2. R: ITG	Patients scored facial images as less pleasant
Herzog et al. (2006)[a]	11	NA	OFF	[15O]H_2O	Full bladder: ON vs. OFF	None	L: LFG	Increased urge to void volume
Thobois et al. (2007)[a]	6	>3	OFF	[15O]H_2O	Random number generation task: ON vs. OFF	R: GPi	R: ACC L: DLPFC	Decreased random number generation
Herzog et al. (2008)[a]	9	22	OFF	[15O]H_2O	Full bladder: ON vs. OFF	R: INS, Thal	None	Improved urge to void (determined by self-report scales)
Narayana et al. (2009)	1	24	NA	[15O]H_2O	1. ON: speech task vs. rest 2. OFF: speech task vs. rest	1. B: ACC, PCC, INS, Thal, BG, Cereb, pAuC/sAuC, OC R: SMA 2. B: PrG, ACC Unknown: SMA, PCC, INS, Thal, BG, Cereb, pAuC/sAuC, OC	1. L: SMA, PrG 2. None	Decrease in speech production perceptual ratings
Fonoff et al. (2010)	1	> 6	ON	[18F]FDG	Odor exposure: ON vs. OFF	B: Thal, Str, ACC, Amy, STN L: RG	None	Return of hyposmia when stimulation turned off

(continued)

Table 46.2 (continued)

Studies	*n*	Postop time (month)	PD Med	Tracer	Contrast	Increase	Decrease	DBS behavioral changes
Dellapina et al. (2012)	8	>3	OFF	[^{15}O]H_2O	Pain: ON vs. OFF	R: PoG	None	Decreased VAS and NPSI score
Ventre-Dominey et al. (2014)[a]	14	>6	OFF	[^{15}O]H_2O	1. Spatial working memory task: ON vs. OFF 2. Nonspatial working memory task: ON vs. OFF	1. R: ACC L: INS, OFC 2. R: MTG, STG	1. R: IPL, SPL, AnG L: PCUN 2 R: pHi, IPFC L: MTG	No difference in response time in all tasks
Weiss et al. (2015)[a]	10	NA	OFF	[^{15}O]H_2O	Gait imagination: ON vs. OFF	L: PPN	None	Increase in walking distance, gait velocity, and stride length
(Cury et al. (2018)	12	12	ON	[^{18}F]FDG	Smell task improvement: ON vs. OFF	R: PMC, SMA, IPL/SMG L: MidB, aCereb	None	Improved olfactory function
Mubeen et al. (2018)	7	>2	OFF	[^{15}O]H_2O	Speech task: ON vs. OFF	Unknown: Cereb Global CBF	None	CBF did not have a direct role in motor speech control

Studies investigating the effects of stimulation for a given task. For task studies, behavioral changes related to the task upon stimulation are reported, and the effect of stimulation on behavioral task (i.e., interaction term) was reported if available (i.e., ($Task_{on}$ − $Rest_{on}$) − ($Task_{off}$ − $Rest_{off}$)). *n* represents the number of patients with DBS who underwent neuroimaging. Brain areas reported to exhibit significant changes by the authors are mentioned as increase and decrease in reference to the listed contrast. However, to limit the number of abbreviations, similar areas described by different nomenclature may have been grouped under a single abbreviation with slightly less spatial specificity (e.g., middle temporal cortex was grouped under middle temporal gyrus, and thalamic subnuclei were grouped under thalamus). Most commonly, the nomenclature used to describe the areas corresponds to the terms used in the studies. Double line separates motor vs. non-motor tasks. *NA* not available. *PD Med* Parkinson's disease medication

[a]Studies reporting interaction term

Table 46.3 DBS studies in Parkinson's disease patients using other targets

Studies	DBS target	*n*	Postop time (month)	PD Med	Tracer	Contrast	Increase	Decrease	DBS behavioral changes
Deiber et al. (1993)	VIM	6	>4	NA	$[^{15}O]H_2O$	Effective stimulation: contra vs. Ips electrode	Contra: PrG, Thal	Contra: CC	NA
Fukuda et al. (2001a)	GPi	6	NA	OFF	$[^{15}O]H_2O$	Motor task: ON vs. OFF	B: SMA R: ACC L: PrG, PoG	None	Improved kinematic parameters of motor task
Fukuda et al. (2001b)	GPi	7	NA	OFF	$[^{18}F]FDG$	ON vs. OFF	Ips, contra: pCereb Ips: PMC	Ips: PDRP	NA
Nakajima et al. (2003)	GPi	6	NA	OFF	$[^{11}C]NEM$	Postop DBS or PVP vs. HC	None	Unknown: ACC	NA
Carbon and Eidelberg (2006)[a]	GPi	14	>12	NA	$[^{15}O]H_2O$ and $[^{123}I]$ FP-CIT	1. Correlation between motor learning and metabolism (PD, HC) 2. Correlation between motor learning and dopamine transporter (DAT) binding (PD)	1. B: BG, DLPFC, PMC, ACC, PL, OL L vPFC 2. L: DLPFC, vPFC	1. None 2. None	Improved motor learning and reference task performance
Valalik et al. (2009)	GPi	5	>6	ON	$[^{15}O]H_2O$	ON (joystick task) vs. OFF (rest)	R: SMA, PMC, aINS	L: PrG, PoG	Decrease in reaction time and movement time postop (DBS-ON and DBS-OFF). Reaction time: OFF > ON

(continued)

Table 46.3 (continued)

Studies	DBS target	*n*	Postop time (month)	PD Med	Tracer	Contrast	Increase	Decrease	DBS behavioral changes
Parker et al. (1992)	VIM	7	4	NA	$[^{15}O]H_2O$	Tremor: ON vs. OFF	Ips, contra: mCereb Contra: PrG, SMA, PrG, PoG, CdN,	None	NA
Wielepp et al. (2001)[a]	VIM	4	>1	NA	$[^{99}mTc]$ ECD	ON vs. HC	None	Ips, contra: PFC, ACC Ips: CdN, SMA, PrG	NA
Fukuda et al. (2004)	VIM	8	>12	OFF	$[^{15}O]H_2O$	ON vs. OFF	L: Br, Thal, OC, CUN, PCUN	R: aCereb, mCereb L: PrG, PoG	NA
Mure et al. (2011)	VIM	9	NA	OFF	$[^{18}F]FDG$	ON vs. OFF	B: CC R: aCereb L: Pu Unknown: CdN, PrG	R: PrG, PoG (PDRP)	NA
Strafella et al. (2008)	PPN	1	3	NA	$[^{15}O]H_2O$	ON vs. OFF	Ips, contra: Thal Ips: INS, Pu, Cereb	None	NA
Stefani et al. (2010)	PPN	6	>12	NA	$[^{18}F]FDG$	ON vs. OFF	B: IFG, DLPFC, OFC, ACC, SFG, IPL, SMG, SMA R: INS, STG L: vStr, SMA	R: PCC L: aCereb	NA

Davis et al. (1997)	GPi, VIM	9	>1	OFF	[^{15}O]H_2O	1. GPi: ON vs. OFF 2. VIM: ON vs. OFF	1. Ips: SMA, Pu, GPe, pHi 2. Ips: OC, DMPFC Contra: DLPFC	1. Contra: ACC 2. Ips: SAA Contra: mCereb, ACC, SMA	NA
Payoux et al. (2009)	GPi, GPe	5	>26	OFF	[^{15}O]H_2O	1. GPe ON vs. OFF (independent of motor task) 2. GPi ON vs. OFF (independent of motor task)	1. None 2. Ips: Pu	1. Ips: Cereb, PMC 2. Ips: PrG, PoG, PMC, SMA, SMA, ACC	Decreased rigidity and akinesia UPDRS scores (GPe) and decreased rigidity UPDRS score (GPi)
Velasco et al. (2015)	Raprl	5	>3	OFF	[^{18}F]FDG	ON vs. preop	Ips, contra: OFC, Cereb Unknown: Pu, SMA, Thal	None	NA
Mo et al. (2016)[a]	cZI	6	1 year	ON	[^{123}I] FP-CIT	1. PD DBS vs. PD control	None	Ips: CdN, Pu	No difference

Studies investigating the effects of stimulation at rest or during a task are listed. For rest studies, clinical benefits for most patients are implicit and no behavioral changes are reported. For task studies, behavioral changes related to the task upon stimulation are reported, and the effect of stimulation on behavioral task (i.e., interaction term) was reported if available (i.e., $(Task_{on} - Rest_{on}) - (Task_{off} - Rest_{off})$). *n* represents the number of patients with DBS who underwent neuroimaging. Brain areas reported to exhibit significant changes by the authors are mentioned as increase and decrease in reference to the listed contrast. However, to limit the number of abbreviations, similar areas described by different nomenclature may have been grouped under a single abbreviation with slightly less spatial specificity (e.g., middle temporal cortex was grouped under middle temporal gyrus, and thalamic subnuclei were grouped under thalamus). Most commonly, the nomenclature used to describe the areas corresponds to the terms used in the studies. Double lines separate DBS targets. *NA* not available. *PD Med* Parkinson's disease medication

[a]SPECT studies (the remainder were PET studies)

and decreased metabolism with levodopa (Hilker et al. 2002). These findings suggest that the dopamine system may be involved in the mechanisms of action of DBS.

Long-term dopamine changes from STN-DBS have also been studied with molecular neuroimaging. One study of the dopamine transporter failed to show a difference over time in dopaminergic function between PD patients with DBS and those treated medically (Lokkegaard et al. 2007). A second study similarly found annual rates of dopamine function decline in the caudate and putamen with STN-DBS to be comparable to other studies in PD patients treated medically (Hilker et al. 2005). However, a single D2 receptor study ([^{123}I]IBZM) reported an increase in receptor binding in the caudate nucleus and putamen with subthalamic stimulation between preop and 12 months after surgery (Hesse et al. 2008). This finding was confounded by the fact that many patients underwent changes in their dopaminergic medication regimen after surgery. The magnitude of the dopamine (or dopaminergic receptors) change over time due to DBS could be too small to detect in humans (Volkow et al. 1993). However, animal studies suggest that the dopamine increase with STN-DBS should be large enough to be detected with molecular neuroimaging (Bruet et al. 2001; Meissner et al. 2002). So far, dopaminergic molecular neuroimaging studies have not found evidence of a neuroprotective effect of STN-DBS on the dopamine system.

46.6.1.3 Contributions of Molecular Neuroimaging

PET and SPECT studies conducted in PD patients have confirmed distributed motor circuit engagement for various DBS targets. Prior literature reviews emphasized the inconsistency in the directionality of change in these areas, asserting this pattern of results supports the notion that DBS modulation is not merely inhibitory or excitatory (Boertien et al. 2011; Obeso et al. 2011). We have separated studies investigating acute (ON vs. OFF) from chronic (postop vs. preop) stimulation effects in order to disentangle these inconsistencies. Interestingly, our analysis revealed different patterns of activity changes: acute stimulation predominantly engaged primary motor hubs of the CSTC circuit, whereas chronic stimulation primarily induced changes in the frontoparietal cortex and cerebellum.

Acute changes with stimulation consistently engaged the motor hubs of the CSTC circuit including the precentral gyrus, thalamus, STN, and to a lesser extent the pallidum. In agreement with findings from PET and SPECT studies, increased brain activity of the STN and thalamus as well as pallidal activation support increased afferent inhibitory pallidothalamic tract activation (Hill et al. 2013; Volonte et al. 2012). Brain function changes in the CSTC circuit may be explained in the context of the direct and indirect pathways but may also arise from the hyperdirect pathway (Haslinger et al. 2005) (Fig. 46.7). Given the key role of the indirect pathway, the lack of consistent activity changes in the pallidum is surprising because STN and GPi modulation were demonstrated with electrophysiology upon STN stimulation (Hashimoto et al. 2003; Windels et al. 2000). Functional neuroimaging studies represent a final common pathway of neurochemical and other molecular mechanisms and may not be able to differentiate afferent and/or local inhibitory and/or excitatory synaptic activity. Combining PET and SPECT findings with electrophysiology or study employing radiotracers for GABA or glutamate would be informative.

Chronic metabolic changes with STN-DBS conform to a fairly different pattern. Instead of changes within motor CSTC hubs, diffuse changes of cortical activity were observed; specifically, decreased activity in prefrontal areas and increased activity in posterior parietal areas were shown. Contrary to acute stimulation changes, subcortical structures less commonly showed chronic changes in metabolism and displayed decreased metabolism when changes were observed. Posterior parietal increase and subcortical decrease in activity are in effect normalization of the abnormal PDRP pattern in PD patients (Asanuma et al. 2006). The decrease seen in the prefrontal areas may be a result of the STN stimulation-induced decrease in compensatory striatal hyperactivity seen in PD patients (Poston et al. 2016; Smith et al. 2019). Prefrontal decreases could also be related to the known executive impairment associated with STN-DBS (Jahanshahi et al. 2000). The posterior parietal function changes may be related to the complex interplay between the prefrontal and parietal areas as well as the caudate nucleus, which are all part of the CSTC associative loop (Alexander and Crutcher 1990). Notably, the cerebellum also commonly displayed increased activity with chronic STN-DBS. Since cerebellar lesions are known to disrupt motor planning, it is plausible that the cerebellar increases seen with long-term stimulation are a result of yet another compensatory mechanism (Manto et al. 2012).

46.6.2 Other Movement Disorders

Only a handful of studies have investigated molecular neuroimaging correlates of DBS in non-PD movement disorders; these studies most often target the motor thalamus or GPi. Table 46.4 provides a comprehensive summary of published studies in DBS for dystonia, essential tremor, and other neurodegenerative disorders. The internal segment of the globus pallidus (GPi) is the most often chosen target for DBS in dystonia (Lozano et al. 2019). As observed in PD, pallidal stimulation in dystonia patients seems to engage motor cortex and SMA (Katsakiori et al. 2009; Kefalopoulou et al. 2010; Kumar et al. 1999). Owing to the lack of studies, the overall heterogeneity of the disease etiology, and different tracers used, clear statements regarding functional changes in dystonia DBS are not possible. Indeed, dystonia studies have used [^{15}O]H_2O (Detante et al. 2004; Kumar et al. 1999; Thobois et al. 2008), [^{99}mTc]ECD (Katsakiori et al. 2009; Kefalopoulou et al. 2010), and [^{123}I]IBZM (Beukers et al. 2012). Also, they used different experimental designs such as DBS-ON vs. DBS-OFF (Katsakiori et al. 2009; Kefalopoulou et al. 2010; Thobois et al. 2008) and task-based assessments (Detante et al. 2004; Kumar et al. 1999). In essential tremor, the cerebello-thalamo-cortical tremor network is thought to be dysfunctional (Hallett 2014). Molecular neuroimaging studies have primarily reported increased rCBF in the precentral gyrus, thalamus, and cerebellum, with less involvement of diffuse cortical areas such as seen with STN-DBS (Ceballos-Baumann et al. 2001; Haslinger et al. 2003; Perlmutter et al. 2002; Reich et al. 2016).

Table 46.4 DBS studies for other movement disorders

Study	Disease	*n*	DBS target	Postop time (month)	Tracer	Contrast	Increase	Decrease
Kumar et al. (1999)[a]	Dystonia	1	GPi	12 month	$[^{15}O]$ H_2O	Joy task: ON vs. OFF	B: OC	B: DLPFC, LPMC, PrG, PoG, VLPFC, SMA, PCUN, ACC, MeTG L: STG, GP
Detante et al. (2004)	Dystonia	6	GPi	>3	$[^{15}O]$ H_2O	Execution task: ON vs. OFF	Ips: PrG, PoG, cSMA, PL Contra: mCereb	None
Thobois et al. (2008)	Tardive dystonia (depression)	5	GPi	>6	$[^{15}O]$ H_2O	ON vs. OFF	B: Cereb R: OC L: SPL	B: SMA L: PrG, ACC
Katsakiori et al. (2009)[b]	Dystonia	8	GPi, Voa	NA	$[^{99}mTc]$ ECD	ON vs. OFF	None	Unknown: PrG, SMA, ACC, DLPFC, FPC
Kefalopoulou et al. (2010)[b]	Dystonia	6	GPi, Voa	6	$[^{99}mTc]$ ECD	ON vs. OFF	None (increase seen in one patient in PrG, PMC, SMA)	Unknown: PrG, PFC
Beukers et al. (2012)[b]	Myoclonus-dystonia	3	GPi	2 years	$[^{123}I]$ IBZM	Postop vs. preop	None	None
Moro et al. (2004)[a]	HD-chorea	1	GPi	NA	$[^{15}O]$ H_2O	1. Low frequency: ON vs. OFF 2. High frequency: ON vs. OFF	1. B: SMA, ACC R: Cereb L: PrG, PoG, PMC 2. B: SMA, ACC R: Cereb L: PrG, PoG	1. None 2. None
Yianni et al. (2004)[b]	Senile chorea	1	GPi, Vop	>5	$[^{99}mTc]$ ECD	1. ON (GPi) vs. OFF 2. ON (Vop) vs. OFF	1. None 2. None	1. L: Pu, CdN, upper Br 2. L: Pu, STN, upper Br

Li et al. (2012)	Chorea-acanthocytosis	2	GPi	>1	[^{18}F] FDG	Postop vs. preop	None	None
Ceballos-Baumann et al. (2001)	ET	6	VIM	>4	[^{15}O] H_2O	Effective vs. ineffective stimulation	Ips, contra: CC Ips: PrG	Ips: IFG Contra: OC
Perlmutter et al. (2002)	ET	10	VIM	15	[^{15}O] H_2O	ON vs. OFF	Ips: Thal, SMA, PrG Contra: PPL, Cereb	None
Haslinger et al. (2003)	ET	4	VIM	9.7	[^{15}O] H_2O	1. Correlation between amplitude and blood flow 2. Correlation between frequency and blood flow	(Positive correlation) 1. B: Thal, PrG, PoG 2. B: Thal, PrG, PoG	(Negative correlation) None
Reich et al. (2016)	ET	10	Thal	23	[^{18}F] FDG	Ataxia: ON vs. OFF	B: Thal R: Cereb	None
Kefalopoulou et al. (2009)[b]	TD	1	GPi	3	[^{99}mTc] ECD	ON vs. OFF	None	Unknown: PrG, PMC, SMA
Wilcox et al. (2011)	PPFG	1	PPN	5	[^{18}F] FDG	ON vs. HC	(Normalization) B: Br, Cereb	None

Studies investigating the effects of stimulation at rest or during a task are listed. For rest studies, clinical benefits for most patients are implicit and no behavioral changes are reported. For task studies, behavioral changes related to the task upon stimulation are reported, and the effect of stimulation on behavioral task (i.e., interaction term) was reported if available (i.e., $(Task_{on} - Rest_{on}) - (Task_{off} - Rest_{off})$). *n* represents the number of patients with DBS who underwent neuroimaging. Brain areas reported to exhibit significant changes by the authors are mentioned as increase and decrease in reference to the listed contrast. However, to limit the number of abbreviations, similar areas described by different nomenclature may have been grouped under a single abbreviation with slightly less spatial specificity (e.g., middle temporal cortex was grouped under middle temporal gyrus, and thalamic subnuclei were grouped under thalamus). Most commonly, the nomenclature used to describe the areas corresponds to the terms used in the studies. Double lines separate movement disorders. *NA* not available. *PPFG* primary progressive freezing of gait, *TD* tardive dyskinesia

[a]Studies reporting interaction term

[b]SPECT studies (the remainder were PET studies)

46.7 Psychiatric Disorders

The striking clinical benefits seen in movement disorder patients have provided an impetus for applying DBS to non-motor—especially psychiatric—conditions. Neuroanatomical insights have led to the expansion of the circuit-based concept of brain function to psychiatric disease, with an emphasis on major limbic hubs and connecting white matter such as the ACC, NAcc, anterior limb of the internal capsule, subcallosal region, and medial forebrain bundle. In particular, MDD, OCD, and to a lesser extent anorexia nervosa and Tourette's syndrome have been explored as potential indications for DBS intervention (Lozano et al. 2019). The brain structures targeted in each case have been selected based on animal models, neuropathology, and functional neuroimaging studies that have characterized the neuronal circuitry associated with each disorder (Fig. 46.3b). To date, the two most common psychiatric disorders studied in the context of DBS using functional neuroimaging are MDD and OCD.

46.7.1 Major Depressive Disorder

MDD encompasses the largest cohort of psychiatric patients receiving DBS. Subgenual cingulate cortex (SGC) has been targeted in the greatest number of patients to date (Hamani et al. 2011; Mayberg et al. 2005). PET neuroimaging, particularly findings laid out in a series of seminal papers showing hypermetabolism of SGC in depression and low mood states, was instrumental in defining the SGC as a DBS target for MDD (Fig. 46.4a) (Drevets et al. 1997; Mayberg et al. 1999, 2005). Although open-label studies in general have reported meaningful clinical response in 50% of SGC-DBS patients, a recent multicenter randomized sham-controlled trial of patients who were evaluated in the first 6 months of treatment did not detect statistically significant antidepressant efficacy (Holtzheimer et al. 2017). This negative outcome may have been related to clinical features of the patient population (e.g., severe chronic depression) or heterogeneous electrode positions.

46.7.1.1 Molecular Neuroimaging Findings

Most MDD functional neuroimaging studies in DBS patients have used PET [^{18}F]FDG and [^{15}O]H_2O in the resting state to investigate brain function changes associated with stimulation (Table 46.5). The majority of these molecular neuroimaging findings were reported in conjunction with behavioral assessments, which facilitates data interpretation.

Out of eight MDD studies (Table 46.5), two studies assessed acute stimulation effects by contrasting ON and OFF stimulation states (Martin-Blanco et al. 2015; Millet et al. 2014), whereas the remaining studies investigated chronic changes, typically from 3 to 12 months after surgery (Bewernick et al. 2010; Conen et al. 2018; Fenoy et al. 2018; Lozano et al. 2008; Mayberg et al. 2005; Schlaepfer et al. 2008). Both SGC and NAcc chronic stimulation yielded changes in brain activity in the cingulate cortex, thalamus, and prefrontal cortex (Bewernick et al. 2010; Conen

Table 46.5 DBS studies for psychiatric disorders

Study	Disease	*n*	DBS target	Postop time (month)	PET tracer	Contrast	Increase	Decrease	DBS behavioral changes
Mayberg et al. (2005)[a]	MDD	3 responders	SCG	6	$[^{15}O]H_2O$	Postop vs. preop	B: PrG, AnG, DLPFC R: PAG L: CC	B: SGC, hThal, INS, SFG L OFC	Reduced HDRS-17
Lozano et al. (2008)	MDD	8 responders	SCG	>3	$[^{15}O]$ H_2O, $[^{18}F]$FDG	1. ON (FDG) vs. preop 2. ON (H_2O) vs. preop	1. Unknown: PFC, midCC, PCC 2. Unknown: PCC	1. B: MeFG, OFC, INS 2. B: OFC R: MeFG L: DLPFC Unknown: SGC	Improved HDRS-17
Schlaepfer et al. (2008)[a]	MDD	3	NAcc	1 week	$[^{18}F]$FDG	Postop vs. preop	B: NAcc, DLPFC, DMPFC, CC, Amy R: MTG, Hi, FuG, AnG L: Pu, aCereb	B: VLPFC, VMPFC R: SN, Thal, ITG, SMG L: ACC, aINS, CdN	Improved depression ratings
Bewernick et al. (2010)[a]	MDD	7	NAcc	7	$[^{18}F]$FDG	ON vs. preop	R: PrG	R: vsFS, MeFG, SGCC, PCC, dsFS L: PFC, Thal, CdN, Cereb	Improved HDRS-28, MADRS, and IDS-SR scores
Millet et al. (2014)[a]	MDD	4	NAcc	5	$[^{18}F]$FDG	ON vs. OFF	B: SFG R: ACC L: MeFG	B: Cereb R: PCC L: SFG, MeFG	Decrease in HDRS score in some patients

(continued)

Table 46.5 (continued)

Study	Disease	*n*	DBS target	Postop time (month)	PET tracer	Contrast	Increase	Decrease	DBS behavioral changes
Martin-Blanco et al. (2015)[a]	MDD	7	SCG	6	[^{18}F]FDG	ON vs. OFF	None	R: ACC, PMC, Pu	None
Conen et al. (2018)[a]	MDD	7	SCG/VAC/NAcc	>3	[^{15}O]H_2O	OFF vs. preop	R: ACC	R: MeFG L: ACC, MTG, OC, STG	Some patients remitted
Fenoy et al. (2018)[a]	MDD	6	Medial forebrain bundle	>12	[^{18}F]FDG	Postop vs. preop	None	CdN	Reduced CGI scores in all patients
Nuttin et al. (2003)[a]	OCD	3 responders	ALIC	>3	[^{18}F]FDG	ON vs. preop	B: Str, OC R: FG, MTG, STG	B: FG	Reduced Y-BOCS
Abelson et al. (2005)	OCD	3	ALIC	3 weeks	[^{18}F]FDG	ON vs. OFF	Unknown: OFC	None	Improvement in OCD and depression symptoms (Y-BOCS and HAM-D)
Rauch et al. (2006)[a]	OCD	6	VC/VS	3	[^{15}O]H_2O	ON high frequency vs. OFF	R: MeOFC, CC, Pu L: GP	None	Improved Y-BOCS
Le Jeune et al. (2010b)[a]	OCD	10	STN	6	[^{18}F]FDG	ON vs. OFF	None	L: CC, MeFG	Improved Y-BOCS
Tsai et al. (2012)	OCD	4	VC/VS	3	[^{18}F]FDG	ON vs. HC	B: VS R: SN	B: pHi L: ACC, Cereb	Improved OCD, HAM-D, and GAF scores
Figee et al. (2014)[b]	OCD	15	NAcc	12	[^{123}I] IBZM	ON vs. OFF	B: Pu	None	Improved Y-BOCS, HDRS, HARS scores

Suetens et al. (2014)[a]	OCD	16	VC/VS	68 days	[^{18}F]FDG	OFF vs. preop	R: CdN, Thal	None	Improved Y-BOCS and HAM-D
Dougherty et al. (2016)[a]	OCD	6	VC/VS	5 years	[^{15}O]H_2O	1. Ventral ON vs. OFF 2. Dorsal ON vs. OFF	1. R: dACC 2. B: GP R: Str L: Thal	None	Reduced depressive symptom severity
Goethals et al. (2008)[b]	TS	1	Thal	12	[^{99}mTc] ECD	ON vs. OFF	Ips, contra: APFC, OFC Con: DLPFC, VLPFC, LTG	None	NA
Kuhn et al. (2012)	TS	3	Thal	6 month	[^{18}F]FP	ON vs. OFF	Ips: Thal Unknown: Pu	Contra: Thal	Improved YGTSS score
Haense et al. (2016)[b]	TS	5	GPi or CM/Voi	>3	[^{99}mTc] ECD	1. GPi vs. preop 2. CM/Voi vs. preop	1. None 2. R: SMG L: PrG, PoG, MFG	1. B: MTG, Pu, Cereb R: Thal, CdN, INS, IFG, Hi L: PAL2. R: CdN, STG, MTG L: IFG	Improved YGTSS score in stimulation and sham groups
Vernaleken et al. (2009)	TS	1	STN	6 month	[^{18}F]FP	ON vs. OFF	None	B: Thal	Improved YGTSS score
Lipsman et al. (2013)	AN	6	SCG	6	[^{18}F]FDG	Postop vs. preop	R: MTG, ITG, PCUN, SMG, IPL L: PoG, CUN	B: MeFG, INS R: ACC, SGC L: CdN, Cl, mCereb	Decreased BMI
Zhang et al. (2013)	AN	4	NAcc	>3	[^{18}F]FDG	ON vs. preop	None	B: LenN, Hi, IFG	NA

(continued)

Table 46.5 (continued)

Study	Disease	*n*	DBS target	Postop time (month)	PET tracer	Contrast	Increase	Decrease	DBS behavioral changes
Heldmann et al. (2012)	AA	1	NAcc	18	$[^{15}O]H_2O$	ON vs. OFF	B: IFG, Cereb, FG R: Thal, OC, PoG, CUN L: MeGP, MTG, STG, TG, OC, FuG, OC, MFG	None	Slower and less risky choices
Giordano et al. (2016)	IED	1	VC/VS	22	$[^{18}F]FDG$	ON vs. preop	L: IFG	L: IFG, DLPFC, ITG, Un, FuG, TG, Amy	Reduced rage attacks

Studies investigating acute (i.e., ON vs. OFF stimulation states) and long-term (i.e., postop vs. preop) effects of stimulation are listed. Behavioral changes from stimulation are reported. *n* represents the number of patients with DBS who underwent neuroimaging. Brain areas reported to exhibit significant changes by the authors are mentioned as increase and decrease in reference to the listed contrast. However, to limit the number of abbreviations, similar areas described by different nomenclature may have been grouped under a single abbreviation with slightly less spatial specificity (e.g., middle temporal cortex was grouped under middle temporal gyrus, and thalamic subnuclei were grouped under thalamus). Most commonly, the nomenclature used to describe the areas corresponds to the terms used in the studies. Double lines separate psychiatric disorders. *AA* alcohol addiction, *AN* anorexia nervosa, *IED* intermittent explosive disease, *NA* not available

[a]This study reported a form of multiple comparison correction and was used in Fig. 46.10 and 46.11

[b]SPECT studies (the remainder were PET studies)

et al. 2018; Lozano et al. 2008; Mayberg et al. 2005; Schlaepfer et al. 2008). In one study ($n = 6$) that stimulated the medial forebrain bundle, significant metabolism decrease in the caudate nucleus was found when comparing ON and OFF stimulation conditions (Fenoy et al. 2018). MDD studies with stringent statistics showed a similar pattern, as well as highlighted the predominant prefrontal increase in brain function (Bewernick et al. 2010; Conen et al. 2018; Fenoy et al. 2018; Martin-Blanco et al. 2015; Mayberg et al. 2005; Millet et al. 2014; Schlaepfer et al. 2008) (Fig. 46.10).

46.7.1.2 Contributions of Molecular Neuroimaging

Functional neuroimaging studies following DBS for MDD have demonstrated that local stimulation—similar to DBS for movement disorders—exerts much of its

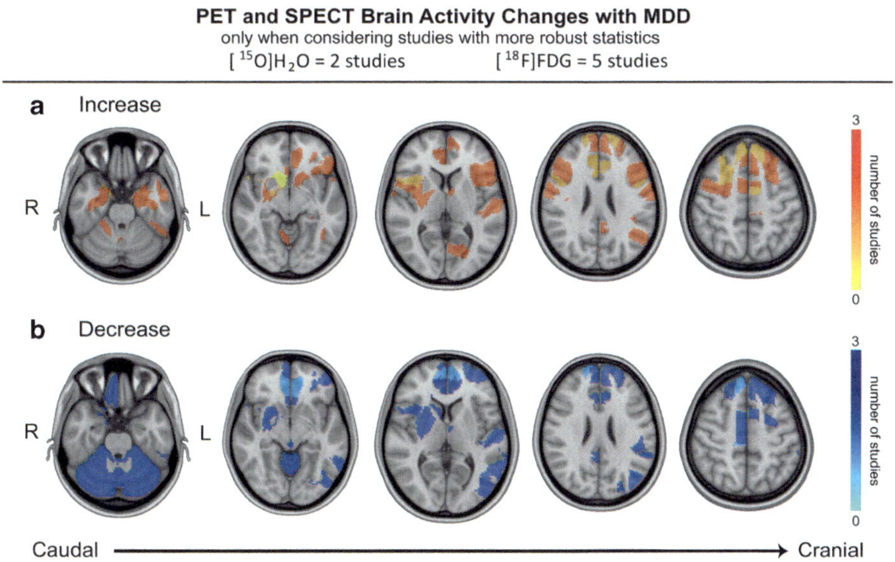

Fig. 46.10 Diagrammatic summary of activity changes in MDD. Only studies assessing either acute or long-term changes with stimulation (studies with ON vs. OFF or postop vs. preop in Table 46.5) and using a form of multiple comparison correction were included to maintain robustness of reported brain regions (studies labeled with ^{C} in Table 46.5). First, brain regions were obtained from spatial parcellation according to published atlases (cortical, An Atlas of Intrinsic Connectivity of Homotopic Areas (Joliot et al. 2015); subcortical, Ewert et al. (2018); brain stem, Harvard Ascending Arousal Network Atlas (Edlow et al. 2012); cerebellum, Diedrichsen et al. (2009)). Then, regions were weighted according to the number of studies reporting significant changes in each region. To decide which parcellated brain areas from the atlases would be selected, we used in order of priority (1) visual representation, (2) reported coordinates, and (3) naming of areas with activation available in studies. For large activation areas, multiple parcellated brain areas were selected. Areas of brain activity changes were then overlaid on select MRI (T1-weighted Montreal Neurological Institute brain) axial images. Across studies, brain regions with an increase in activity (hot colors) are shown in (**a**), whereas brain regions with significant decrease in activity (cool colors) are shown in (**b**). Color bars represent the number of studies

effect at the network level. The specificity of the engaged network is reflected by metabolic changes in a number of regions implicated in the disorders in question.

In MDD, increased SGC activity has been associated with sadness. Reduction of SGC metabolic activity is seen in response to effective pharmacological treatment with antidepressants (Mayberg et al. 2000). SGC-DBS also decreases metabolism in SGC, supporting the concept that DBS normalizes aberrant circuitry (Lozano et al. 2008; Mayberg et al. 2005). The ACC is a key player in emotional processing; its ventral aspect, the SGC, is primarily implicated in negative affect, while its dorsal section has been associated with positive emotional processing (Amodio and Frith 2006; Koski and Paus 2000; Margulies et al. 2007). Monoamine dysregulation, especially of the serotonin system, has also been implicated in MDD pathogenesis. In some studies, serotonin receptor binding (5-HT1A) is decreased in the mesiotemporal cortex in depressed patients (Savitz and Drevets 2013). In general, a visceromotor network comprising the prefrontal cortex, ACC, thalamus, caudate, and putamen demonstrates a relative hypermetabolism in the depressed state relative to the treated state (Drevets 2007; Drevets et al. 2008). Pharmacological and electroconvulsive therapy both tend to normalize metabolism in these areas (Goldapple et al. 2004; Mayberg et al. 2000; Nobler et al. 2001). Most PET and SPECT studies show that DBS for MDD also engages these aforementioned brain regions.

46.7.2 Obsessive-Compulsive Disorder

Although less commonly treated with DBS than MDD, OCD was among the first psychiatric indication to be investigated for DBS. While capsulotomy was aimed at the destruction of fronto-striatal and fronto-thalamic fibers, DBS of the anterior limb of the internal capsule was proposed as a reversible alternative (Nuttin et al. 1999). Interestingly, this target has now been refined to be more ventral (i.e., ventral striatum) and posterior (i.e., anterior commissure) than the originally defined target (Greenberg et al. 2010; Raymaekers et al. 2017). Other groups have also targeted the ventromedial associative region of the STN (Mallet et al. 2008). Most of these targets have demonstrated efficacy to some degree, although randomized, sham-controlled trials have not yet been completed. Although mostly the anterior limb of the internal capsule, thalamus, STN, and NAcc have been studied with PET and SPECT, many other brain structures including the medial forebrain bundle (Coenen et al. 2017), inferior thalamic peduncle (Lee et al. 2019), and bed nucleus of stria terminalis (Nuttin et al. 2013) have been targeted in OCD patients.

46.7.2.1 Molecular Neuroimaging Findings

Similar to MDD studies, most OCD functional neuroimaging studies in DBS patients have investigated brain activity changes associated with stimulation and provided behavioral outcomes (Table 46.5).

Increased activity in the striatum and frontal lobes was generally associated with thalamic stimulation in patients with OCD (Dougherty et al. 2016; Nuttin

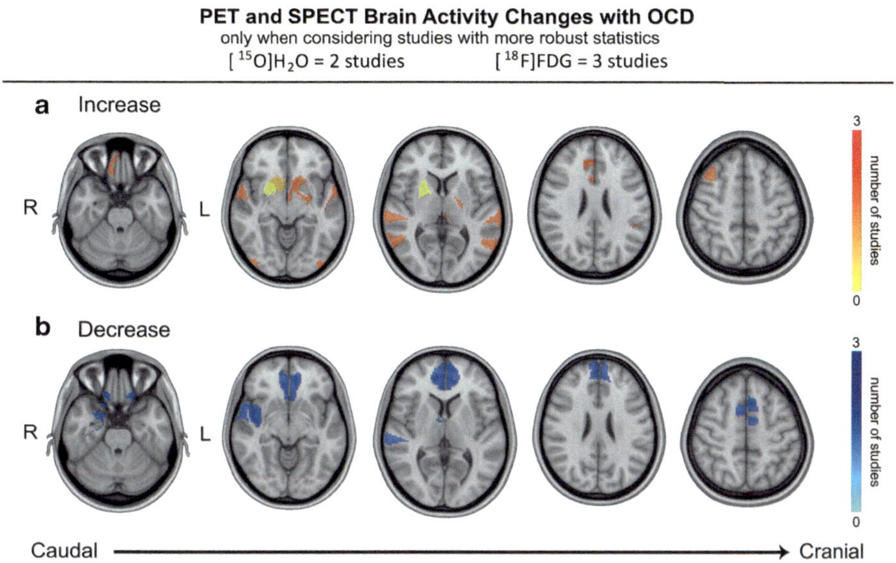

Fig. 46.11 Diagrammatic summary of activity changes with long-term OCD. Only studies assessing either acute or long-term changes with stimulation (studies with ON vs. OFF or postop vs. preop in Table 46.5) and using a form of multiple comparison correction were included to maintain robustness of reported brain regions (studies labeled with [a] in Table 46.5). First, brain regions were obtained from spatial parcellation according to published atlases (cortical, An Atlas of Intrinsic Connectivity of Homotopic Areas (Joliot et al. 2015); subcortical, Ewert et al. (2018); brain stem, Harvard Ascending Arousal Network Atlas (Edlow et al. 2012); cerebellum, Diedrichsen et al. (2009)). Then, regions were weighted according to the number of studies reporting significant changes in each region. To decide which parcellated brain areas from the atlases would be selected, we used in order of priority (1) visual representation, (2) reported coordinates, and (3) naming of areas with activation available in studies. For large activation areas, multiple parcellated brain areas were selected. Areas of brain activity changes were then overlaid on select MRI (T1-weighted Montreal Neurological Institute brain) axial images. Across studies, brain regions with an increase in activity (hot colors) are shown in (**a**), whereas brain regions with significant decrease in activity (cool colors) are shown in (**b**). Color bars represent the number of studies

et al. 2003; Suetens et al. 2014). A study with NAcc stimulation in patients with OCD found an increase in the level of striatal dopamine as well as clinical improvement with stimulation (Figee et al. 2014). Studies with robust statistics generally demonstrated frontal lobe decrease in activity, albeit less diffuse than in MDD, involving mostly the medial and basal frontal areas. These studies also showed changes in metabolism in the striatum (Dougherty et al. 2016; Le Jeune et al. 2010b; Nuttin et al. 2003; Rauch et al. 2006; Suetens et al. 2014) (Fig. 46.11). Rather than activity changes, a single study investigated striatal dopamine changes with NAcc-DBS. The authors found an increase in striatal dopamine release with acute and chronic stimulation (1 year after DBS surgery) suggested by decreased D2/3 receptor availability and increased plasma levels of homovanillic acid (Figee et al. 2014).

46.7.2.2 Contributions of Molecular Neuroimaging

Regions including the thalamus, ACC, and frontal lobes that have been implicated in OCD are also regions being modulated by DBS (Graybiel and Rauch 2000; Saxena et al. 1998; Whiteside et al. 2004). The hypermetabolic orbitofrontal cortex, which is a hallmark of OCD, is reduced with DBS (Robbins et al. 2019; Saxena et al. 1998) (Fig. 46.11).These findings support a major role for the dysfunction of the limbic circuit in OCD pathophysiology and show that DBS effectively modulates this pathway.

PET and SPECT findings in OCD (and other psychiatric disorders) support the notion that various DBS targets for psychiatric disorders represent key nodes in the same affective regulatory circuit. This concept of modulating different hubs belonging to the same circuit to achieve similar benefits was suggested in PD with STN and GPi-DBS. The more numerous and diversified DBS targets for psychiatric disorders reinforce this emerging idea. Stimulation of different brain targets for OCD seems to provide clinical benefits and modulate brain activity in similar areas such as the striatum, CC, and frontal lobes. Although different targets engaged similar areas to some degree, it is also plausible that each target provides slightly different benefits. For example, stimulation of most OCD targets seems to improve OCD symptoms as measured by commonly used scales such as Yale-Brown Obsessive-Compulsive Scale. Including other scales (e.g., Hamilton Depression Rating Scale), measuring different aspects of the disorder phenotypes (i.e., depression in OCD) may help inform the detailed benefits provided by each target. A thorough knowledge of symptom-specific networks could open the door to individualized phenotype-based DBS targeting.

46.7.3 Other Psychiatric Disorders

Findings in other psychiatric disorders including Tourette's syndrome and anorexia nervosa are summarized in Table 46.5. A study using [^{99}mTc]ECD to investigate brain function changes in Tourette's syndrome demonstrated increased activity in the superior and middle temporal gyri with either thalamic or GPi stimulation; this was associated with clinical improvements (Haense et al. 2016). Increased prefrontal activity was also noticed with thalamic stimulation inducing alternate personality state in a Tourette's syndrome patient (Goethals et al. 2008). Increased thalamic dopaminergic transmission was suggested in two studies due to decrease D2/3 receptor availability (Kuhn et al. 2012; Vernaleken et al. 2009). Interestingly, thalamic stimulation was used in one study, whereas STN stimulation was used in the second study. Both anorexia nervosa PET [^{18}F]FDG studies showed that DBS normalizes the activity in disease-implicated areas: SGC-DBS was shown to reverse the abnormalities seen in the anterior cingulate, insula, and parietal lobe (Lipsman et al. 2013), whereas hypermetabolism in the frontal lobe, hippocampus, and lentiform nucleus was decreased after NAcc-DBS (Zhang et al. 2013).

46.8 Cognitive Disorders

46.8.1 Alzheimer's Disease

Alzheimer's disease (AD) is the most common neurodegenerative disease and has a significant socioeconomic burden (Scheltens et al. 2016). Our understanding of its genetics and neuropathological hallmarks has improved in recent years. Furthermore, neuroimaging findings have identified the topography of dysfunctional brain areas in AD as well as characterize abnormalities which may eventually be used as biomarkers (Femminella et al. 2018). Although the structures of the memory circuits are affected most severely, pathological changes such as brain atrophy and change in brain metabolism can be seen globally in AD. Despite these advances, the therapeutic options remain limited. Pharmacotherapies augmenting acetylcholine availability are the mainstay of treatment. Additional experimental therapies aiming at reversing neuropathological abnormalities including amyloid plaques and tau protein accumulation are subject to extensive preclinical and clinical investigations (Graham et al. 2017).

Therapeutic modulation of the limbic and memory circuits has been a recent focus of DBS studies. Several targets have been investigated in humans including the fornix, entorhinal cortex, and nucleus basalis of Meynert (NBM) (Kuhn et al. 2015; Lozano et al. 2016) (Fig. 46.3c). The majority of studies have involved the fornix and have consistently shown sustained cortical metabolic activity in AD patients (Laxton et al. 2010; Lozano et al. 2016). The one randomized, double-blind study targeting the fornix (the main hippocampal inflow and outflow tract) identified an interaction between patient age and treatment outcomes, suggesting that older patients may be more likely to benefit from this treatment (Lozano et al. 2016). As with other DBS indications, AD patient selection (including such variables as age and severity of pathology) will likely be of paramount importance for optimizing treatment outcomes.

46.8.1.1 Molecular Neuroimaging Findings

Functional neuroimaging studies in AD DBS have used PET [18F]FDG to investigate the biological underpinnings of electrical stimulation in patients in the resting state (Table 46.6). Fornix stimulation increased metabolism mainly in the parietal and temporal lobes. Mesial temporal lobe structures such as the hippocampus also demonstrated increased metabolic activity (Fontaine et al. 2013; Lozano et al. 2016). Areas of the default mode network including the posterior cingulate cortex and precuneus also showed increased activity (Laxton et al. 2010; Smith et al. 2012). Importantly, the increase in metabolism was correlated with less decline in cognitive function. Also, increased functional connectivity in cortical-limbic networks was observed. A correlation between the nucleus basalis metabolism and cognitive scores was found when that structure was stimulated; no other significant change in metabolic activity was reported (Kuhn et al. 2015). Given that few studies listed in Table 46.6 used a form of multiple comparison correction, no diagrammatic representation was generated for cognitive disorders. To date, no molecular imaging human studies assessed the effects of stimulation on amyloid plaques or tau proteins.

Table 46.6 DBS studies for cognitive disorders

Study	Disease	*n*	DBS target	Postop time (month)	Tracer	Contrast	Increase	Decrease	DBS behavioral changes
Scharre et al. (2018)	AD	3	VC/VS	>4 weeks	[^{18}F] FDG	ON vs. OFF	Unknown: OFC, VMPFC, DLPFC	None	Activation only seen in responders (2/3 patients)
Laxton et al. (2010)[a]	AD	6	Fornix	>1	[^{18}F] FDG	ON vs. preop	B: PrG, PoG, STG, PCUN, IPL, mCereb R: PrG, LG L: MTG, PCC, Cl, Cereb	R: IFG L: ACC, MFG	Worsening of ADAS-cog score over 12 months
Smith et al. (2012)	AD	6	Fornix	>1	[^{18}F] FDG	Correlation between ADAS-cog score and metabolism	(Positive correlation) B: PrG, OC, Pu, Thal, cuneus R: PoG	(Negative correlation) B: ACC, SFG, MeFG, STG, PCUN, PCC, mCereb R: IFG, INS, IPL, SMG L: MTG, FuG	Worsening of ADAS-cog score
Fontaine et al. (2013)	AD	1	Fornix	6	[^{18}F] FDG	ON vs. preop	B: MeTG	None	Husband reported improvement in daily functioning, behavior, and mood
Kuhn et al. (2015)	AD	4	Nucleus basalis	12	[^{18}F] FDG	Correlation between ADAS-cog and MMSE score and metabolism	(Positive correlation) R: NuB	None	Nonsignificant worsening of ADAS-cog score after 12 months

Lozano et al. (2016)[a]	AD	42	Fornix	6	[^{18}F] FDG	1. ON (6 months postop) vs. OFF 2. ON (12 months postop) vs. OFF	1. Unknown: PrG, PoG, TAC, Hi, PAC, OC, Cereb 2. None	1. None 2. None	No difference in ADAS-cog 13 and CDR-SB sores

Studies investigating acute (i.e., ON vs. OFF stimulation states) and long-term (i.e., postop vs. preop) effects of stimulation are listed. Behavioral changes from stimulation are reported. *n* represents the number of patients with DBS who underwent neuroimaging. Brain areas reported to exhibit significant changes by the authors are mentioned as increase and decrease in reference to the listed contrast. However, to limit the number of abbreviations, similar areas described by different nomenclature may have been grouped under a single abbreviation with slightly less spatial specificity (e.g., middle temporal cortex was grouped under middle temporal gyrus, and thalamic subnuclei were grouped under thalamus). Most commonly, the nomenclature used to describe the areas corresponds to the terms used in the studies. *NA* not available

46.8.1.2 Contributions of Molecular Neuroimaging

Insights provided by PET [^{18}F]FDG have been instrumental in identifying the functional neuroanatomical changes associated with AD and monitoring the effects of DBS as a treatment for AD. Neuroimaging findings have consistently demonstrated a pattern of functional and morphometric change in patients with AD involving primarily the parietal and temporal lobes. These changes include temporal-parietal hypometabolism, decreased functional connectivity, and atrophy (Ferreira and Busatto 2011; Frisoni et al. 2010). PET findings associated with DBS of the hippocampal outflow tract (i.e., the fornix) demonstrated network-wide metabolic effects including persistent (1 year after DBS surgery) increased metabolism in the parietal and temporal lobes as well as in the mesial temporal lobe structures which are crucial components of the memory circuit (Laxton et al. 2010; Lozano et al. 2016; Smith et al. 2012). These PET findings confirm network engagement and target specificity. Interestingly, fornix-DBS also seems to increase default mode network (DMN) activity, which is known to be dysfunctional in AD patients (Greicius et al. 2004; Sperling et al. 2009). Similar to psychiatric disorders, molecular neuroimaging was able to substantiate stimulation-induced metabolic changes within the faulty circuits that seem to be of relevance in AD DBS (viz., the memory circuit). Understanding DBS mechanism of action with selective radiotracers (e.g., beta-amyloid, tau, muscarinic, or nicotinic receptors) may also inform the development of more effective treatments. Furthermore, identifying pattern of metabolic changes in AD may help refine patient selection and serve as predictors of response (Smith et al. 2012).

As beta-amyloid plaque and tau protein accumulation are neuropathological hallmarks of AD and radiotracers for these proteins are available, studies could be performed to determine whether DBS decreases or stabilizes their accumulation over time. Preclinical studies have shown the neurobiological effects of DBS on temporal lobe structures and AD pathology. Chronic entorhinal cortex stimulation in a mouse model of AD decreased beta-amyloid plaque and tau protein accumulation in the hippocampus and prefrontal cortex (Mann et al. 2018). Further, rodent studies reported rapid modulation of neurotrophic factors and markers of synaptic plasticity in the hippocampus with fornix-DBS (Gondard et al. 2015).

46.9 Other DBS Indications

Since DBS has shown therapeutic modulation of specific circuits hypothesized to underlie neurobiological disorders, it is being investigated for multiple other disorders. Indications include chronic pain, traumatic brain injury, and headache. Notably, hypothalamic DBS for cluster headache provides significant improvement in headache frequency, and the selection of the target was informed by PET studies that identify areas of increased hypothalamic metabolism during induced headaches (May et al. 1998) (Fig. 46.4c). For these less common indications and targets, the sample sizes are usually small and heterogeneous. Table 46.7 summarizes the molecular neuroimaging studies for these indications.

Table 46.7 DBS studies for other disorders

Study	Disease	n	DBS target	Postop time (month)	PET tracer	Contrast	Increase	Decrease	DBS behavioral changes
Duncan et al. (1998)	Pain	5	Thal	>36	$[^{15}O]H_2O$	ON vs. preop	Ips: aINS, Thal, LenN, IC	None	Satisfactory pain relief following DBS
Davis et al. (2000)	Pain	5	Thal	>4	$[^{15}O]H_2O$	ON vs. OFF	Ips: GP, IC Contra: ACC	Ips, contra: IPL Ips: OC, ITG, PrG Contra: sAuC, OC, Cereb	None
Kupers et al. (2000)	Pain	1	Thal	NA	$[^{15}O]H_2O$	ON vs. OFF	R: VMPFC L: Amy, aINS	None	Complete reduction of pain following DBS
Pereira et al. (2007)	Pain	3	VPL, PVG	5	HMPAO	1. VPL-ON vs. VPL-OFF 2. PVG-ON vs. PVG-OFF 3. VPL, PVG-ON vs. PVG-OFF	1. Ips, contra: PVG, Thal Contra: OC 2. Ips, contra: PVG, Thal Ips: INS, LenN Contra: LTG, anterior subcortical area 3. Ips, contra: PVG, Thal, OC	1. Ips, contra: LenN, PTC Ips: LTG, OC, SPL, OFC Contra: PrG, PoG 2. Ips, contra: PrG, PoG, Po, MidB, Thal Ips: LenN Contra: LTG, PVG, anterior subcortical area, DFG 3. Ips, contra: LTG, PVG Ips: SPL, LTG, INS Contra: anterior subcortical area, PTC, OC, ACC	Reduced pain

(continued)

Table 46.7 (continued)

Study	Disease	*n*	DBS target	Postop time (month)	PET tracer	Contrast	Increase	Decrease	DBS behavioral changes
Sims-Williams et al. (2017)	Pain	5	PAG	7	[^{11}C]DPN, [^{15}O]H_2O	1. ON vs. OFF [^{11}C] DPN 2. ON vs. OFF [^{15}O] H_2O	1. None 2. None	1. PAG 2. None	None
Rezai et al. (2016)	TBI	4	NAcc	2 years	[^{18}F]FDG	Correlation between cognitive score and brain metabolism	None	(Negative correlation) B: MeFG, aINS, NAcc R: Thal L: OFC, MFG, IFG, ACC, ITG	Negative correlation between cognitive score and brain metabolism
Lemaire et al. (2018)	TBI	5	mPal	5	[^{18}F]FDG	ON vs. preop	Unknown: DMN	None	Increased internally oriented cortex activation following low-frequency DBS
May et al. (2006)	HA	10	hThal	>2 years	[^{15}O]H_2O	ON vs. OFF	Contra: aINS Ips: hThal, Thal, primary PoG, PCUN, ACC, TN Unknown: ITG, PCC, aINS, mCereb, MTG	Ips, contra: ITG Unknown: SFG, MTG, PCC	Improved headache frequency

Studies investigating acute (i.e., ON vs. OFF stimulation states) and long-term (i.e., postop vs. preop) effects of stimulation are listed. Behavioral changes from stimulation are reported. *n* represents the number of patients with DBS who underwent neuroimaging. Brain areas reported to exhibit significant changes by the authors are mentioned as increase and decrease in reference to the listed contrast. However, to limit the number of abbreviations, similar areas described by different nomenclature may have been grouped under a single abbreviation with slightly less spatial specificity (e.g., middle temporal cortex was grouped under middle temporal gyrus, and thalamic subnuclei were grouped under thalamus). Most commonly, the nomenclature used to describe the areas corresponds to the terms used in the studies. Double lines separate the disorders. *HA* headache, *NA* not available. *TBI* traumatic brain injury

46.10 Limitations

The DBS literature has several limitations. Patient demographics, etiology, disease duration, and dominant disease phenotype vary considerably across studies. Moreover, selection of appropriate patient candidates is particularly challenging in psychiatric disorders as there is a lack of consensus on the definition of treatment resistance in many conditions. Patient selection is also challenging in AD in which the optimal target population is still being established. Also, the medication status varies across studies, which is particularly relevant in PD studies given the striking clinical improvements after dopaminergic medication intake and the dose reductions observed after DBS surgery. Most studies involving PD patients include an OFF-medication period of 12 h before neuroimaging data acquisition. However, it is also plausible that chronic pharmacotherapy has long-lasting influences on brain responses. Cross-study comparisons of imaging findings are thus hampered by considerable differences between study populations and the limited number and small sample size of studies conducted to date.

Data regarding electrode position and the circuitry being stimulated is not typically reported and represents an important limitation when interpreting DBS clinical and neuroimaging studies. This data is of paramount importance as targets are often in close proximity to other eloquent structures that might account for symptom improvements. For example, SGC (an MDD target) is surrounded by many white matter bundles including the forceps minor and uncinate fasciculus (Riva-Posse et al. 2018). A detailed description of electrode position is particularly pertinent in psychiatric conditions because—unlike in the case of movement disorder DBS—intraoperative electrophysiological monitoring (i.e., microelectrode recordings) is not generally conducted during psychiatric DBS surgery. Detailed position of the active contact (and DBS settings) will provide a detailed understanding of the neural structures being stimulated (Boutet et al. 2019a).

Another issue is the insufficient details regarding the stimulation programming. Optimization of stimulation parameters in psychiatric DBS is particularly challenging owing to the lack of objective biomarkers to verify patient response and the delayed onset of response which may take several weeks or months (Lozano and Lipsman 2013). Programming algorithms and whether or not patients are deemed optimized based on established scales should be included in publications. In fact, the limited successes in clinical trials for psychiatric disorders have been partly attributed to suboptimal programming. In psychiatric and cognitive disorders, the outcomes are more complex, and approaches are being developed to determine sensitive outcome measures (Kucewicz et al. 2018). While optimization status is seldom reported in PD studies, presumably because most patients benefit from the treatment, the programming process can also take months to achieve optimal symptom control. There may be variability in symptom control between patients, all of which should thus be reported in detail (Picillo et al. 2016). In addition, the lack of comparisons between effective and ineffective stimulation is a limitation. Indeed, it becomes difficult to differentiate areas with artifactual metabolic changes that are not clinically relevant from those providing clinical benefits.

Neuroimaging data in response to stimulation would be highly informative if multiple clinical outcomes were reported to untangle the meaning of the pattern of changes seen. Indeed, the common sole assessment of motor changes in PD studies is problematic since STN stimulation is known to have widespread connections and effects. Similarly, psychiatric and cognitive disorders are known to have multiple comorbidities that should be taken into account into clinical outcomes. In other words, neuroimaging findings may not be entirely attributable to a single measured behavioral change. Including multidimensional clinical outcomes (e.g., motor, mood, cognition assessments) would help with data interpretation.

Finally, there is a specific caveat when interpreting functional neuroimaging data for PD and movement disorders in general. DBS leads to a change in clinical state (e.g., decreased rigidity or tremor), introducing a possible confound for signal interpretation. It is therefore difficult to differentiate whether the observed brain response was a direct DBS-driven effect rather than a consequence of clinical improvement due to the stimulation itself.

46.11 Future Directions

As emphasized throughout this chapter, DBS studies are associated with experimental variables that should be taken into consideration when reporting the results (e.g., medication status, electrode location, programming optimization status). Guidelines to standardize data in DBS publications have been published (Vitek et al. 2010). Similarly, we also recommend a minimal set of required data specific to DBS studies including neuroimaging, which are necessary to facilitate the interpretation and comparison of results across DBS studies (Fig. 46.12).

Fig. 46.12 Guidelines for data reporting in DBS neuroimaging studies. Standardized data reporting in DBS neuroimaging studies should be followed to improve experimental design, data interpretation, and comparison across studies

<u>Standardized data to report in DBS studies</u>

Patients

- Medication status at time of scan
- Disease duration
- DBS system status (i.e., externalized or internalized)

Stimulation

- Electrode and contact locations (e.g., coordinates)
- Stimulation parameters (i.e., volume of tissue activated)
- Stimulation programming status (i.e., optimization status, measure of behavior changes)

Functional neuroimaging

- Time between DBS surgery and functional neuroimaging acquisition
- Washout period between imaging acquisitions

Most DBS patient samples from a single institution are unlikely to be sufficient to permit recruitment of an ideal and homogeneous patient cohort. Experiments are thus usually associated with numerous limitations related to sample size that constrain their generalizability. As the number of patients with DBS grows and as large-scale clinical trials are increasingly incorporating functional neuroimaging, the enabled larger sample size should enhance data analysis and interpretation. Also, multidimensional outcome assessments and novel network analysis methods (e.g., scaled subprofile modeling and partial least squares) should also be entertained to improve our ability to detect results and improve reproducibility across studies (Krishnan et al. 2011; Spetsieris and Eidelberg 2011). Furthermore, methodological guidelines have been developed (e.g., the Alzheimer's Disease Neuroimaging Initiative) to standardize imaging acquisition and to combine data for analysis across institutions.

Reporting precise electrode location will inform the slight variation of neural substrates being stimulated across patients. Commercially available and open-source software offer a method pipeline to accurately locate electrodes on CT or MRI (Horn et al. 2019). Importantly, recent neuroimaging advances have also enabled comparison of stimulation across patients: (1) precise transformation of patients' brain into standardized brain space (i.e., nonlinear normalization to Montreal Neurological Institute brain template), (2) DBS electrode localization, and (3) estimation of the volume of tissue activated (VTA) (Ewert et al. 2019; Horn et al. 2019; McIntyre et al. 2004) (Fig. 46.13). Easy-to-use imaging analysis

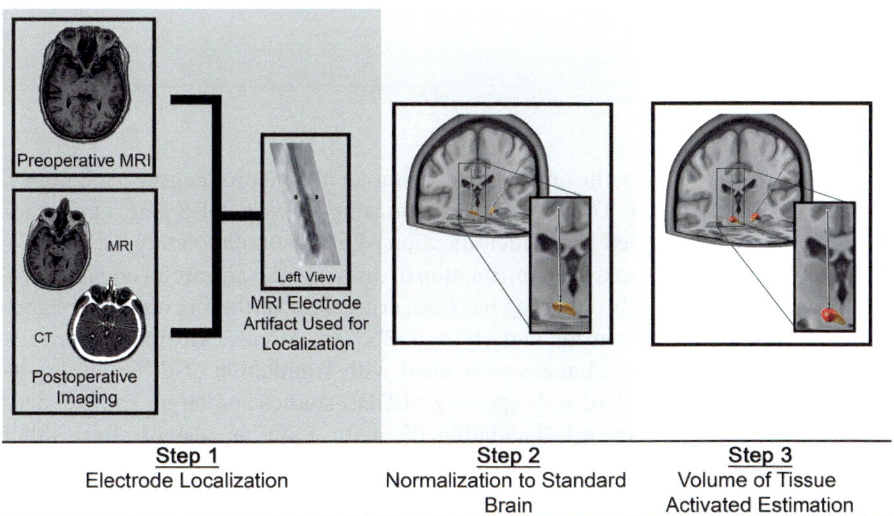

Fig. 46.13 Pipeline for electrode localization. Step 1: The electrodes are localized on postoperative imaging using the metallic artifact. Step 2: To enable group analysis, electrode positions are transformed into standardized brain space (Montreal Neurological Institute brain) using preoperative imaging (i.e., normalization). The subthalamic nucleus is shown in shaded orange. Step 3: Volume of tissue activated (shaded red) is computed based on the programming settings

pipelines have been developed to streamline this process. The variations in stimulated neural substrates across patients can be taken into account by incorporating electrode positions or alternatively distance to a target as covariates may improve the analysis. Alternatively, recent studies tend to compute VTA, thought to be a more accurate measure to compare differences of stimulation across patients.

In summary, the majority of functional neuroimaging studies have focused on PET glucose metabolism studies as an outcome. One of the main advantages of PET and SPECT is the experimental versatility that is afforded by the wide range of tracers available. Future MDD or anorexia studies investigating network-level serotonin changes (e.g., 5-HTR tracers) upon stimulation would further inform DBS mechanism of action as well as pathophysiology.

Owing to technological advancements in neuroimaging and DBS hardware, many challenges of performing MRI in patients with neurostimulators have been partially overcome. Recent studies, however, have demonstrated the feasibility of safe 3 T MRI (and fMRI) using a high-resolution body-transmit coil—the contemporary gold standard for clinical and research MRI—in patients receiving DBS, under specific conditions (Boutet et al. 2019b, c; Hancu et al. 2019). These studies potentially open the door to PET-MRI imaging in DBS patients. It should be noted that, due to the intense radio-frequency pulses required, arterial spin labelling cannot be performed safely in patients with DBS (Boutet et al. 2019b). While PET and SPECT have the major advantages of assessing specific molecules, fMRI may investigate changes in brain circuitry with a superior spatial-temporal resolution. As new fMRI studies are emerging, it will be interesting to compare BOLD changes with PET/SPECT findings; this new data should further inform DBS mechanism of action.

46.12 Conclusion

This chapter emphasizes the importance of molecular neuroimaging techniques, namely, PET and SPECT. The symbiotic relationship between DBS and neuroimaging research has to date led to the identification of new stimulation targets, the validation of current targets, and the confirmation of disease-relevant circuit engagement. In this way, functional neuroimaging has been critical for furthering our understanding of the network mechanisms underlying DBS. In particular, distinct patterns of metabolic and blood flow changes associated with stimulation of different targets can be appreciated. Standardized reporting of DBS studies and larger sample sizes would go a long way toward elucidating them. In addition, insights from other emerging neuroimaging modalities such as fMRI can and should be integrated in order to further our understanding and interpretation of PET and SPECT data. Continued functional neuroimaging research will likely contribute to improved patient selection and surgical targeting as well as to the identification of biomarkers of treatment efficacy.

Conflicts of Interest Dr. Bilbily is the co-founder and CEO of 16 Bit Inc. Dr. Fasano reports grants, personal fees, and nonfinancial support from AbbVie; grants, personal fees, and nonfinancial support from Medtronic; grants and personal fees from Boston Scientific; personal fees from Sunovion; personal fees from Chiesi Farmaceutici, personal fees from UCB; and grants and personal fees from Ipsen, outside the submitted work. Dr. Lozano serves as a consultant for Medtronic, Abbott, Boston Scientific, and Functional Neuromodulation, during the conduct of the study, and reports grants from GE Healthcare, outside the submitted work. Other authors report no conflict of interest.

Funding: This chapter was supported by the RR Tasker Chair in Functional Neurosurgery at University Health Network and a Tier 1 Canada Research Chair in Neuroscience and the German Research Foundation (Deutsche Forschungsgemeinschaft, DFG NE 2276/1-1) (C.N.). The corresponding author confirms that he had full access to all the data in the study and had final responsibility for the decision to submit for publication.

Appendix

Abbreviations Used in Tables

a	Anterior
Amy	Amygdala
AnG	Angular gyrus
BA	Broca's area
BG	Basal ganglia
Br	Brain stem
c	Caudal
CC	Cingulate cortex
CdN	Caudate nucleus
Cereb	Cerebellum
Cl	Claustrum
CUN	Cuneus
d	Dorsal
DMN	Default mode network
FG	Frontal gyrus
FO	Frontal operculum
FPC	Frontopolar cortex
FS	Frontal sulcus
FuG	Fusiform gyrus
GP	Globus pallidus
GPe	Globus pallidus externus
GPi	Globus pallidus internus
Hi	Hippocampus
hThal	Hypothalamus
i	Inferior
IC	Internal capsule
INS	Insula
l	Lateral
LC	Limbic cortex

LenN	Lentiform nucleus
LG	Lingual gyrus
m	Middle
me	Medial
MidB	Midbrain
NAcc	Nucleus accumbens
NuB	Nucleus basalis
OC	Occipital cortex
OFC	Orbitofrontal cortex
p	Posterior
PAC	Parietal association cortex
PAG	Periaqueductal gray
PAL	Pallidum
pAuC/sAuC	Primary/secondary auditory cortex
PCUN	Precuneus
PFC	Prefrontal cortex
pHi	Parahippocampus
PL	Parietal lobe
PMC	Premotor cortex
Po	Pons
PoG	Postcentral gyrus
PPN	Pedunculopontine nucleus
PPO	Postcentral parietal operculum
PrG	Precentral gyrus
PTC	Parietotemporal cortex
Pu	Putamen
PVG	Periventricular gray
r	Rostral
RC	Retrosplenial cortex
RN	Red nucleus
s	Superior
SAA	Sensory association area
SG	Subgenual
SMA	Supplementary motor cortex
SMG	Supramarginal gyrus
SN	Substantia nigra
Str	Striatum
TAC	Temporal association cortex
TG	Temporal gyrus
Thal	Thalamus (includes all parts of the thalamus)
TN	Trigeminal nucleus
TPJ	Temporoparietal junction
TPo	Temporal pole
Un	Uncus
v	Ventral
WA	Wernicke's area

References

Abelson JL et al (2005) Deep brain stimulation for refractory obsessive-compulsive disorder. Biol Psychiatry 57:510–516. https://doi.org/10.1016/j.biopsych.2004.11.042

Abosch A et al (2003) Stimulation of the subthalamic nucleus in Parkinson's disease does not produce striatal dopamine release. Neurosurgery 53:1095–1102. , discussion 1095–1102. https://doi.org/10.1227/01.neu.0000088662.69419.1b

Albin RL, Young AB, Penney JB (1989) The functional anatomy of basal ganglia disorders. Trends Neurosci 12:366–375

Alexander GE, Crutcher MD (1990) Functional architecture of basal ganglia circuits: neural substrates of parallel processing. Trends Neurosci 13:266–271

Amodio DM, Frith CD (2006) Meeting of minds: the medial frontal cortex and social cognition. Nat Rev Neurosci 7:268–277. https://doi.org/10.1038/nrn1884

Antonini A et al (2003) Brain flow changes before and after deep brain stimulation of the subthalamic nucleus in Parkinson's disease. Neurol Sci 24:151–152. https://doi.org/10.1007/s10072-003-0104-4

Arai N et al (2008) Mechanisms of unilateral STN-DBS in patients with Parkinson's disease: a PET study. J Neurol 255:1236–1243. https://doi.org/10.1007/s00415-008-0906-7

Asanuma K et al (2006) Network modulation in the treatment of Parkinson's disease. Brain 129:2667–2678. https://doi.org/10.1093/brain/awl162

Atkinson-Clement C et al (2017) Subthalamic nucleus stimulation effects on single and combined task performance in Parkinson's disease patients: a PET study. Brain Imaging Behav 11:1139–1153. https://doi.org/10.1007/s11682-016-9588-4

Ballanger B et al (2009) Stimulation of the subthalamic nucleus and impulsivity: release your horses. Ann Neurol 66:817–824. https://doi.org/10.1002/ana.21795

Bejjani BP et al (1999) Transient acute depression induced by high-frequency deep-brain stimulation. N Engl J Med 340:1476–1480. https://doi.org/10.1056/NEJM199905133401905

Beukers RJ, Contarino MF, Speelman JD, Schuurman PR, Booij J, Tijssen MA (2012) Deep brain stimulation of the pallidum is effective and might stabilize striatal D(2) receptor binding in myoclonus-dystonia. Front Neurol 3:22. https://doi.org/10.3389/fneur.2012.00022

Bewernick BH et al (2010) Nucleus accumbens deep brain stimulation decreases ratings of depression and anxiety in treatment-resistant depression. Biol Psychiatry 67:110–116. https://doi.org/10.1016/j.biopsych.2009.09.013

Boertien T et al (2011) Functional imaging of subthalamic nucleus deep brain stimulation in Parkinson's disease. Mov Disord 26:1835–1843. https://doi.org/10.1002/mds.23788

Boutet A et al (2019a) Neuroimaging technological advancements for targeting in functional neurosurgery. Curr Neurol Neurosci Rep 19:42. https://doi.org/10.1007/s11910-019-0961-8

Boutet A et al (2019b) 3-Tesla MRI of deep brain stimulation patients: safety assessment of coils and pulse sequences. J Neurosurg 32(2):586–594. https://doi.org/10.3171/2018.11.JNS181338

Boutet A et al (2019c) Functional MRI safety and artifacts during deep brain stimulation: experience in 102 patients. Radiology 293(1):174–183. https://doi.org/10.1148/radiol.2019190546

Bradberry TJ et al (2012) Common and unique responses to dopamine agonist therapy and deep brain stimulation in Parkinson's disease: an H(2)(15)O PET study. Brain Stimul 5:605–615. https://doi.org/10.1016/j.brs.2011.09.002

Bruet N, Windels F, Bertrand A, Feuerstein C, Poupard A, Savasta M (2001) High frequency stimulation of the subthalamic nucleus increases the extracellular contents of striatal dopamine in normal and partially dopaminergic denervated rats. J Neuropathol Exp Neurol 60:15–24. https://doi.org/10.1093/jnen/60.1.15

Burghaus L et al (2006) Deep brain stimulation of the subthalamic nucleus reversibly deteriorates stuttering in advanced Parkinson's disease. J Neural Transm (Vienna) 113:625–631. https://doi.org/10.1007/s00702-005-0341-1

Butson CR, Cooper SE, Henderson JM, CC MI (2007) Patient-specific analysis of the volume of tissue activated during deep brain stimulation. Neuroimage 34:661–670. https://doi.org/10.1016/j.neuroimage.2006.09.034

Campbell MC et al (2008) Neural correlates of STN DBS-induced cognitive variability in Parkinson disease. Neuropsychologia 46:3162–3169. https://doi.org/10.1016/j.neuropsychologia.2008.07.012

Cao C et al (2017) Modified fluorodeoxyglucose metabolism in motor circuitry by subthalamic deep brain stimulation. Stereotact Funct Neurosurg 95:93–101. https://doi.org/10.1159/000455930

Carbon M, Eidelberg D (2006) Functional imaging of sequence learning in Parkinson's disease. J Neurol Sci 248:72–77. https://doi.org/10.1016/j.jns.2006.05.005

Ceballos-Baumann AO et al (1999) A positron emission tomographic study of subthalamic nucleus stimulation in Parkinson disease: enhanced movement-related activity of motor-association cortex and decreased motor cortex resting activity. Arch Neurol 56:997–1003. https://doi.org/10.1001/archneur.56.8.997

Ceballos-Baumann AO et al (2001) Thalamic stimulation for essential tremor activates motor and deactivates vestibular cortex. Neurology 56:1347–1354. https://doi.org/10.1212/wnl.56.10.1347

Chevalier G, Deniau JM (1990) Disinhibition as a basic process in the expression of striatal functions. Trends Neurosci 13:277–280

Cilia R et al (2007) Brain networks underlining verbal fluency decline during STN-DBS in Parkinson's disease: an ECD-SPECT study parkinsonism. Relat Disord 13:290–294. https://doi.org/10.1016/j.parkreldis.2006.11.011

Cilia R et al (2009) Clinical and cerebral activity changes induced by subthalamic nucleus stimulation in advanced Parkinson's disease: a prospective case-control study. Clin Neurol Neurosurg 111:140–146. https://doi.org/10.1016/j.clineuro.2008.09.018

Coenen VA et al (2017) The medial forebrain bundle as a target for deep brain stimulation for obsessive-compulsive disorder. CNS Spectr 22:282–289. https://doi.org/10.1017/S1092852916000286

Conen S, Matthews JC, Patel NK, Anton-Rodriguez J, Talbot PS (2018) Acute and chronic changes in brain activity with deep brain stimulation for refractory depression. J Psychopharmacol 32:430–440. https://doi.org/10.1177/0269881117742668

Cury RG et al (2018) Effects of subthalamic stimulation on olfactory function in Parkinson disease. World Neurosurg 114:e559–e564. https://doi.org/10.1016/j.wneu.2018.03.033

Dale AM, Halgren E (2001) Spatiotemporal mapping of brain activity by integration of multiple imaging modalities. Curr Opin Neurobiol 11:202–208

Davis KD, Taub E, Houle S, Lang AE, Dostrovsky JO, Tasker RR, Lozano AM (1997) Globus pallidus stimulation activates the cortical motor system during alleviation of parkinsonian symptoms. Nat Med 3:671–674

Davis KD, Taub E, Duffner F, Lozano AM, Tasker RR, Houle S, Dostrovsky JO (2000) Activation of the anterior cingulate cortex by thalamic stimulation in patients with chronic pain: a positron emission tomography study. J Neurosurg 92:64–69. https://doi.org/10.3171/jns.2000.92.1.0064

Deiber MP et al (1993) Thalamic stimulation and suppression of parkinsonian tremor. Evidence of a cerebellar deactivation using positron emission tomography. Brain 116(Pt 1):267–279. https://doi.org/10.1093/brain/116.1.267

Dellapina E et al (2012) Effect of subthalamic deep brain stimulation on pain in Parkinson's disease. Pain 153:2267–2273. https://doi.org/10.1016/j.pain.2012.07.026

DeLong MR (1990) Primate models of movement disorders of basal ganglia origin. Trends Neurosci 13:281–285

Detante O et al (2004) Globus pallidus internus stimulation in primary generalized dystonia: a H215O PET study. Brain 127:1899–1908. https://doi.org/10.1093/brain/awh213

Diedrichsen J, Balsters JH, Flavell J, Cussans E, Ramnani N (2009) A probabilistic MR atlas of the human cerebellum. Neuroimage 46:39–46. https://doi.org/10.1016/j.neuroimage.2009.01.045

Dougherty DD et al (2016) Acute deep brain stimulation changes in regional cerebral blood flow in obsessive-compulsive disorder. J Neurosurg 125:1087–1093. https://doi.org/10.3171/2015.9.JNS151387

Drevets WC (2007) Orbitofrontal cortex function and structure in depression. Ann N Y Acad Sci 1121:499–527. https://doi.org/10.1196/annals.1401.029

Drevets WC, Price JL, Simpson JR Jr, Todd RD, Reich T, Vannier M, Raichle ME (1997) Subgenual prefrontal cortex abnormalities in mood disorders. Nature 386:824–827. https://doi.org/10.1038/386824a0
Drevets WC, Price JL, Furey ML (2008) Brain structural and functional abnormalities in mood disorders: implications for neurocircuitry models of depression. Brain Struct Funct 213:93–118. https://doi.org/10.1007/s00429-008-0189-x
Duncan GH, Kupers RC, Marchand S, Villemure JG, Gybels JM, Bushnell MC (1998) Stimulation of human thalamus for pain relief: possible modulatory circuits revealed by positron emission tomography. J Neurophysiol 80:3326–3330. https://doi.org/10.1152/jn.1998.80.6.3326
Edlow BL et al (2012) Neuroanatomic connectivity of the human ascending arousal system critical to consciousness and its disorders. J Neuropathol Exp Neurol 71:531–546. https://doi.org/10.1097/NEN.0b013e3182588293
Eidelberg D (2009) Metabolic brain networks in neurodegenerative disorders: a functional imaging approach. Trends Neurosci 32:548–557. https://doi.org/10.1016/j.tins.2009.06.003
Erasmi R, Granert O, Zorenkov D, Falk D, Wodarg F, Deuschl G, Witt K (2018) White matter changes along the electrode lead in patients treated with deep brain stimulation. Front Neurol 9:983. https://doi.org/10.3389/fneur.2018.00983
Ewert S et al (2018) Toward defining deep brain stimulation targets in MNI space: a subcortical atlas based on multimodal MRI, histology and structural connectivity. Neuroimage 170:271–282. https://doi.org/10.1016/j.neuroimage.2017.05.015
Ewert S, Horn A, Finkel F, Li N, Kuhn AA, Herrington TM (2019) Optimization and comparative evaluation of nonlinear deformation algorithms for atlas-based segmentation of DBS target nuclei. Neuroimage 184:586–598. https://doi.org/10.1016/j.neuroimage.2018.09.061
Femminella GD, Thayanandan T, Calsolaro V, Komici K, Rengo G, Corbi G, Ferrara N (2018) Imaging and molecular mechanisms of Alzheimer's disease: a review. Int J Mol Sci 19(12):3702. https://doi.org/10.3390/ijms19123702
Fenoy AJ et al (2018) A longitudinal study on deep brain stimulation of the medial forebrain bundle for treatment-resistant depression. Transl Psychiatry 8:111. https://doi.org/10.1038/s41398-018-0160-4
Ferreira LK, Busatto GF (2011) Neuroimaging in Alzheimer's disease: current role in clinical practice and potential future applications. Clinics (Sao Paulo) 66(Suppl 1):19–24. https://doi.org/10.1590/s1807-59322011001300003
Figee M et al (2014) Deep brain stimulation induces striatal dopamine release in obsessive-compulsive disorder. Biol Psychiatry 75:647–652. https://doi.org/10.1016/j.biopsych.2013.06.021
Fonoff ET et al (2010) Pet findings in reversible improvement of olfactory dysfunction after STN stimulation in a Parkinson's disease patient. Mov Disord 25:2466–2468. https://doi.org/10.1002/mds.23253
Fontaine D, Deudon A, Lemaire JJ, Razzouk M, Viau P, Darcourt J, Robert P (2013) Symptomatic treatment of memory decline in Alzheimer's disease by deep brain stimulation: a feasibility study. J Alzheimers Dis 34:315–323. https://doi.org/10.3233/JAD-121579
Frisoni GB, Fox NC, Jack CR Jr, Scheltens P, Thompson PM (2010) The clinical use of structural MRI in Alzheimer disease. Nat Rev Neurol 6:67–77. https://doi.org/10.1038/nrneurol.2009.215
Friston KJ (2009) Modalities, modes, and models in functional neuroimaging. Science 326:399–403. https://doi.org/10.1126/science.1174521
Fukuda M et al (2001a) Functional correlates of pallidal stimulation for Parkinson's disease. Ann Neurol 49:155–164
Fukuda M et al (2001b) Networks mediating the clinical effects of pallidal brain stimulation for Parkinson's disease: a PET study of resting-state glucose metabolism. Brain 124:1601–1609. https://doi.org/10.1093/brain/124.8.1601
Fukuda M et al (2004) Thalamic stimulation for parkinsonian tremor: correlation between regional cerebral blood flow and physiological tremor characteristics. Neuroimage 21:608–615. https://doi.org/10.1016/j.neuroimage.2003.09.068

Garraux G, Bahri MA, Lemaire C, Degueldre C, Salmon E, Kaschten B (2011) Brain energization in response to deep brain stimulation of subthalamic nuclei in Parkinson's disease. J Cereb Blood Flow Metab 31:1612–1622. https://doi.org/10.1038/jcbfm.2011.41

Geday J, Ostergaard K, Gjedde A (2006) Stimulation of subthalamic nucleus inhibits emotional activation of fusiform gyrus. Neuroimage 33:706–714. https://doi.org/10.1016/j.neuroimage.2006.06.056

Giordano F et al (2016) Deep brain stimulation of the anterior limb of the internal capsule may be efficacious for explosive aggressive behaviour. Stereotact Funct Neurosurg 94:371–378. https://doi.org/10.1159/000449171

Goethals I, Jacobs F, Van der Linden C, Caemaert J, Audenaert K (2008) Brain activation associated with deep brain stimulation causing dissociation in a patient with Tourette's syndrome. J Trauma Dissociation 9:543–549

Goldapple K, Segal Z, Garson C, Lau M, Bieling P, Kennedy S, Mayberg H (2004) Modulation of cortical-limbic pathways in major depression: treatment-specific effects of cognitive behavior therapy. Arch Gen Psychiatry 61:34–41. https://doi.org/10.1001/archpsyc.61.1.34

Gondard E, Chau HN, Mann A, Tierney TS, Hamani C, Kalia SK, Lozano AM (2015) Rapid modulation of protein expression in the rat hippocampus following deep brain stimulation of the fornix. Brain Stimul 8:1058–1064. https://doi.org/10.1016/j.brs.2015.07.044

Grafton ST, Turner RS, Desmurget M, Bakay R, Delong M, Vitek J, Crutcher M (2006) Normalizing motor-related brain activity: subthalamic nucleus stimulation in Parkinson disease. Neurology 66:1192–1199. https://doi.org/10.1212/01.wnl.0000214237.58321.c3

Graham WV, Bonito-Oliva A, Sakmar TP (2017) Update on Alzheimer's disease therapy and prevention strategies. Annu Rev Med 68:413–430. https://doi.org/10.1146/annurev-med-042915-103753

Graybiel AM, Rauch SL (2000) Toward a neurobiology of obsessive-compulsive disorder. Neuron 28:343–347

Greenberg BD et al (2010) Deep brain stimulation of the ventral internal capsule/ventral striatum for obsessive-compulsive disorder: worldwide experience. Mol Psychiatry 15:64–79. https://doi.org/10.1038/mp.2008.55

Greicius MD, Srivastava G, Reiss AL, Menon V (2004) Default-mode network activity distinguishes Alzheimer's disease from healthy aging: evidence from functional MRI. Proc Natl Acad Sci U S A 101:4637–4642. https://doi.org/10.1073/pnas.0308627101

Haegelen C et al (2010) SPECT and PET analysis of subthalamic stimulation in Parkinson's disease: analysis using a manual segmentation. J Neurol 257:375–382. https://doi.org/10.1007/s00415-009-5327-8

Haense C et al (2016) Effect of deep brain stimulation on regional cerebral blood flow in patients with medically refractory tourette syndrome. Front Psychiatry 7:118. https://doi.org/10.3389/fpsyt.2016.00118

Hagelweide K, Schonberger AR, Kracht LW, Grundler TOJ, Fink GR, Schubotz RI (2018) Motor cognition in patients treated with subthalamic nucleus deep brain stimulation: limits of compensatory overactivity in Parkinson's disease. Neuropsychologia 117:491–499. https://doi.org/10.1016/j.neuropsychologia.2018.07.007

Hallett M (2014) Tremor: pathophysiology parkinsonism. Relat Disord 20(Suppl 1):S118–S122. https://doi.org/10.1016/S1353-8020(13)70029-4

Hamani C, Mayberg H, Stone S, Laxton A, Haber S, Lozano AM (2011) The subcallosal cingulate gyrus in the context of major depression. Biol Psychiatry 69:301–308. https://doi.org/10.1016/j.biopsych.2010.09.034

Hancu I et al (2019) On the (non-)equivalency of monopolar and bipolar settings for deep brain stimulation fMRI studies of Parkinson's disease patients. J Magn Reson Imaging 49:1736–1749. https://doi.org/10.1002/jmri.26321

Hariz M (2017) My 25 stimulating years with DBS in Parkinson's disease. J Parkinsons dis 7:S35–S43. https://doi.org/10.3233/JPD-179007

Hashimoto T, Elder CM, Okun MS, Patrick SK, Vitek JL (2003) Stimulation of the subthalamic nucleus changes the firing pattern of pallidal neurons. J Neurosci 23:1916–1923

Haslinger B et al (2003) Differential modulation of subcortical target and cortex during deep brain stimulation. NeuroImage 18:517–524

Haslinger B, Kalteis K, Boecker H, Alesch F, Ceballos-Baumann AO (2005) Frequency-correlated decreases of motor cortex activity associated with subthalamic nucleus stimulation in Parkinson's disease. Neuroimage 28:598–606. https://doi.org/10.1016/j.neuroimage.2005.06.034

Heldmann M et al (2012) Deep brain stimulation of nucleus accumbens region in alcoholism affects reward processing. PLoS One 7:e36572. https://doi.org/10.1371/journal.pone.0036572

Hershey T et al (2003) Cortical and subcortical blood flow effects of subthalamic nucleus stimulation in PD. Neurology 61:816–821. https://doi.org/10.1212/01.wnl.0000083991.81859.73

Herzog J et al (2006) Subthalamic stimulation modulates cortical control of urinary bladder in Parkinson's disease. Brain 129:3366–3375. https://doi.org/10.1093/brain/awl302

Herzog J et al (2008) Improved sensory gating of urinary bladder afferents in Parkinson's disease following subthalamic stimulation. Brain 131:132–145. https://doi.org/10.1093/brain/awm254

Hesse S et al (2008) Effects of subthalamic nucleus stimulation on striatal dopaminergic transmission in patients with Parkinson's disease within one-year follow-up. J Neurol 255:1059–1066. https://doi.org/10.1007/s00415-008-0849-z

Hilker R, Voges J, Thiel A, Ghaemi M, Herholz K, Sturm V, Heiss WD (2002) Deep brain stimulation of the subthalamic nucleus versus levodopa challenge in Parkinson's disease: measuring the on- and off-conditions with FDG-PET. J Neural Transm (Vienna) 109:1257–1264. https://doi.org/10.1007/s00702-002-0696-5

Hilker R et al (2003) Deep brain stimulation of the subthalamic nucleus does not increase the striatal dopamine concentration in parkinsonian humans. Mov Disord 18:41–48. https://doi.org/10.1002/mds.10297

Hilker R et al (2004) Subthalamic nucleus stimulation restores glucose metabolism in associative and limbic cortices and in cerebellum: evidence from a FDG-PET study in advanced Parkinson's disease. J Cereb Blood Flow Metab 24:7–16. https://doi.org/10.1097/01.WCB.0000092831.44769.09

Hilker R et al (2005) Disease progression continues in patients with advanced Parkinson's disease and effective subthalamic nucleus stimulation. J Neurol Neurosurg Psychiatry 76:1217–1221. https://doi.org/10.1136/jnnp.2004.057893

Hilker R et al (2008) STN-DBS activates the target area in Parkinson disease: an FDG-PET study. Neurology 71:708–713. https://doi.org/10.1212/01.wnl.0000312380.01852.77

Hill KK et al (2013) Cerebral blood flow responses to dorsal and ventral STN DBS correlate with gait and balance responses in Parkinson's disease. Exp Neurol 241:105–112. https://doi.org/10.1016/j.expneurol.2012.12.003

Hirano S et al (2008) Dissociation of metabolic and neurovascular responses to levodopa in the treatment of Parkinson's disease. J Neurosci 28:4201–4209. https://doi.org/10.1523/JNEUROSCI.0582-08.2008

Holtzheimer PE et al (2017) Subcallosal cingulate deep brain stimulation for treatment-resistant depression: a multisite, randomised, sham-controlled trial. Lancet Psychiatry 4:839–849. https://doi.org/10.1016/S2215-0366(17)30371-1

Hooker JM, Carson RE (2019) Human positron emission tomography neuroimaging. Annu Rev Biomed Eng 21:551–581. https://doi.org/10.1146/annurev-bioeng-062117-121056

Horn A et al (2019) Lead-DBS v2: towards a comprehensive pipeline for deep brain stimulation imaging. Neuroimage 184:293–316. https://doi.org/10.1016/j.neuroimage.2018.08.068

Jahanshahi M et al (2000) The impact of deep brain stimulation on executive function in Parkinson's disease. Brain 123(Pt 6):1142–1154. https://doi.org/10.1093/brain/123.6.1142

Jankovic J (2008) Parkinson's disease: clinical features and diagnosis. J Neurol Neurosurg Psychiatry 79:368–376. https://doi.org/10.1136/jnnp.2007.131045

Joliot M et al (2015) AICHA: an atlas of intrinsic connectivity of homotopic areas. J Neurosci Methods 254:46–59. https://doi.org/10.1016/j.jneumeth.2015.07.013

Kalbe E et al (2009) Frontal FDG-PET activity correlates with cognitive outcome after STN-DBS in Parkinson disease. Neurology 72:42–49. https://doi.org/10.1212/01.wnl.0000338536.31388.f0

Karimi M et al (2008) Subthalamic nucleus stimulation-induced regional blood flow responses correlate with improvement of motor signs in Parkinson disease. Brain 131:2710–2719. https://doi.org/10.1093/brain/awn179

Katsakiori PF et al (2009) Deep brain stimulation for secondary dystonia: results in 8 patients. Acta Neurochir (Wien) 151:473–478.; ; discussion 478. https://doi.org/10.1007/s00701-009-0281-x

Kefalopoulou Z, Paschali A, Markaki E, Vassilakos P, Ellul J, Constantoyannis C (2009) A double-blind study on a patient with tardive dyskinesia treated with pallidal deep brain stimulation. Acta Neurol Scand 119:269–273. https://doi.org/10.1111/j.1600-0404.2008.01115.x

Kefalopoulou Z, Paschali A, Markaki E, Ellul J, Chroni E, Vassilakos P, Constantoyannis C (2010) Regional cerebral blood flow changes induced by deep brain stimulation in secondary dystonia. Acta Neurochir (Wien) 152:1007–1014. https://doi.org/10.1007/s00701-010-0612-y

Ko JH, Tang CC, Eidelberg D (2013) Brain stimulation and functional imaging with fMRI and PET. Handb Clin Neurol 116:77–95. https://doi.org/10.1016/B978-0-444-53497-2.00008-5

Koski L, Paus T (2000) Functional connectivity of the anterior cingulate cortex within the human frontal lobe: a brain-mapping meta-analysis. Exp Brain Res 133:55–65. https://doi.org/10.1007/s002210000400

Krishnan A, Williams LJ, McIntosh AR, Abdi H (2011) Partial Least Squares (PLS) methods for neuroimaging: a tutorial and review. Neuroimage 56:455–475. https://doi.org/10.1016/j.neuroimage.2010.07.034

Kucewicz MT et al (2018) Evidence for verbal memory enhancement with electrical brain stimulation in the lateral temporal cortex. Brain 141:971–978. https://doi.org/10.1093/brain/awx373

Kuhn J et al (2012) In vivo evidence of deep brain stimulation-induced dopaminergic modulation in Tourette's syndrome. Biol Psychiatry 71:e11–e13. https://doi.org/10.1016/j.biopsych.2011.09.035

Kuhn J et al (2015) Deep brain stimulation of the nucleus basalis of Meynert in Alzheimer's dementia. Mol Psychiatry 20:353–360. https://doi.org/10.1038/mp.2014.32

Kumar R, Dagher A, Hutchison WD, Lang AE, Lozano AM (1999) Globus pallidus deep brain stimulation for generalized dystonia: clinical and PET investigation. Neurology 53:871–874. https://doi.org/10.1212/wnl.53.4.871

Kupers RC, Gybels JM, Gjedde A (2000) Positron emission tomography study of a chronic pain patient successfully treated with somatosensory thalamic stimulation. Pain 87:295–302

Lammertsma AA (2001) PET/SPECT: functional imaging beyond flow. Vision Res 41:1277–1281. https://doi.org/10.1016/s0042-6989(00)00262-5

Laxton AW et al (2010) A phase I trial of deep brain stimulation of memory circuits in Alzheimer's disease. Ann Neurol 68:521–534. https://doi.org/10.1002/ana.22089

Le Jeune F et al (2008) Subthalamic nucleus stimulation affects orbitofrontal cortex in facial emotion recognition: a PET study. Brain 131:1599–1608. https://doi.org/10.1093/brain/awn084

Le Jeune F et al (2010a) Subthalamic nucleus stimulation affects limbic and associative circuits: a PET study. Eur J Nucl Med Mol Imaging 37:1512–1520. https://doi.org/10.1007/s00259-010-1436-y

Le Jeune F et al (2010b) Decrease of prefrontal metabolism after subthalamic stimulation in obsessive-compulsive disorder: a positron emission tomography study. Biol Psychiatry 68:1016–1022. https://doi.org/10.1016/j.biopsych.2010.06.033

Lee DJ et al (2019) Inferior thalamic peduncle deep brain stimulation for treatment-refractory obsessive-compulsive disorder: a phase 1 pilot trial. Brain Stimul 12:344–352. https://doi.org/10.1016/j.brs.2018.11.012

Lemaire JJ et al (2018) Deep brain stimulation in five patients with severe disorders of consciousness. Ann Clin Transl Neurol 5:1372–1384. https://doi.org/10.1002/acn3.648

Li D, Zuo C, Guan Y, Zhao Y, Shen J, Zan S, Sun B (2006) FDG-PET study of the bilateral subthalamic nucleus stimulation effects on the regional cerebral metabolism in advanced Parkinson disease. Acta Neurochir Suppl 99:51–54

Li P et al (2012) Deep brain stimulation of the globus pallidus internal improves symptoms of chorea-acanthocytosis. Neurol Sci 33:269–274. https://doi.org/10.1007/s10072-011-0741-y

Limousin P, Greene J, Pollak P, Rothwell J, Benabid AL, Frackowiak R (1997) Changes in cerebral activity pattern due to subthalamic nucleus or internal pallidum stimulation in Parkinson's disease. Ann Neurol 42:283–291. https://doi.org/10.1002/ana.410420303

Lipsman N et al (2013) Subcallosal cingulate deep brain stimulation for treatment-refractory anorexia nervosa: a phase 1 pilot trial. Lancet 381:1361–1370. https://doi.org/10.1016/S0140-6736(12)62188-6

Lokkegaard A et al (2007) Dopamine transporter imaging and the effects of deep brain stimulation in patients with Parkinson's disease. Eur J Nucl Med Mol Imaging 34:508–516. https://doi.org/10.1007/s00259-006-0257-5

Lozano AM, Lipsman N (2013) Probing and regulating dysfunctional circuits using deep brain stimulation. Neuron 77:406–424. https://doi.org/10.1016/j.neuron.2013.01.020

Lozano AM, Mayberg HS, Giacobbe P, Hamani C, Craddock RC, Kennedy SH (2008) Subcallosal cingulate gyrus deep brain stimulation for treatment-resistant depression. Biol Psychiatry 64:461–467. https://doi.org/10.1016/j.biopsych.2008.05.034

Lozano AM et al (2016) A phase II study of fornix deep brain stimulation in mild Alzheimer's disease. J Alzheimers Dis 54:777–787. https://doi.org/10.3233/JAD-160017

Lozano CS, Ranjan M, Boutet A, Xu DS, Kucharczyk W, Fasano A, Lozano AM (2018) Imaging alone versus microelectrode recording-guided targeting of the STN in patients with Parkinson's disease. J Neurosurg:1–6. https://doi.org/10.3171/2018.2.JNS172186

Lozano AM et al (2019) Deep brain stimulation: current challenges and future directions. Nat Rev Neurol 15(Suppl 1):1. https://doi.org/10.1038/s41582-018-0128-2

Lyoo CH, Aalto S, Rinne JO, Lee KO, Oh SH, Chang JW, Lee MS (2007) Different cerebral cortical areas influence the effect of subthalamic nucleus stimulation on parkinsonian motor deficits and freezing of gait. Mov Disord 22:2176–2182. https://doi.org/10.1002/mds.21609

Ma Y, Tang C, Spetsieris PG, Dhawan V, Eidelberg D (2007) Abnormal metabolic network activity in Parkinson's disease: test-retest reproducibility. J Cereb Blood Flow Metab 27:597–605. https://doi.org/10.1038/sj.jcbfm.9600358

Mallet L et al (2008) Subthalamic nucleus stimulation in severe obsessive-compulsive disorder. N Engl J Med 359:2121–2134. https://doi.org/10.1056/NEJMoa0708514

Mann A et al (2018) Chronic deep brain stimulation in an Alzheimer's disease mouse model enhances memory and reduces pathological hallmarks. Brain Stimul 11:435–444. https://doi.org/10.1016/j.brs.2017.11.012

Manto M et al (2012) Consensus paper: roles of the cerebellum in motor control--the diversity of ideas on cerebellar involvement in movement. Cerebellum 11:457–487. https://doi.org/10.1007/s12311-011-0331-9

Margulies DS, Kelly AM, Uddin LQ, Biswal BB, Castellanos FX, Milham MP (2007) Mapping the functional connectivity of anterior cingulate cortex. Neuroimage 37:579–588. https://doi.org/10.1016/j.neuroimage.2007.05.019

Martin-Blanco A et al (2015) Immediate cerebral metabolic changes induced by discontinuation of deep brain stimulation of subcallosal cingulate gyrus in treatment-resistant depression. J Affect Disord 173:159–162. https://doi.org/10.1016/j.jad.2014.10.035

May A, Bahra A, Buchel C, Frackowiak RS, Goadsby PJ (1998) Hypothalamic activation in cluster headache attacks. Lancet 352:275–278. https://doi.org/10.1016/S0140-6736(98)02470-2

May A, Leone M, Boecker H, Sprenger T, Juergens T, Bussone G, Tolle TR (2006) Hypothalamic deep brain stimulation in positron emission tomography. J Neurosci 26:3589–3593. https://doi.org/10.1523/JNEUROSCI.4609-05.2006

Mayberg HS et al (1999) Reciprocal limbic-cortical function and negative mood: converging PET findings in depression and normal sadness. Am J Psychiatry 156:675–682. https://doi.org/10.1176/ajp.156.5.675

Mayberg HS, Brannan SK, Tekell JL, Silva JA, Mahurin RK, McGinnis S, Jerabek PA (2000) Regional metabolic effects of fluoxetine in major depression: serial changes and relationship to clinical response. Biol Psychiatry 48:830–843

Mayberg HS et al (2005) Deep brain stimulation for treatment-resistant depression. Neuron 45:651–660. https://doi.org/10.1016/j.neuron.2005.02.014

McIntyre CC, Grill WM, Sherman DL, Thakor NV (2004) Cellular effects of deep brain stimulation: model-based analysis of activation and inhibition. J Neurophysiol 91:1457–1469. https://doi.org/10.1152/jn.00989.2003

Meissner W, Harnack D, Paul G, Reum T, Sohr R, Morgenstern R, Kupsch A (2002) Deep brain stimulation of subthalamic neurons increases striatal dopamine metabolism and induces contralateral circling in freely moving 6-hydroxydopamine-lesioned rats. Neurosci Lett 328:105–108. https://doi.org/10.1016/s0304-3940(02)00463-9

Millet B et al (2014) Limbic versus cognitive target for deep brain stimulation in treatment-resistant depression: accumbens more promising than caudate. Eur Neuropsychopharmacol 24:1229–1239. https://doi.org/10.1016/j.euroneuro.2014.05.006

Miocinovic S, Somayajula S, Chitnis S, Vitek JL (2013) History, applications, and mechanisms of deep brain stimulation. JAMA Neurol 70:163–171. https://doi.org/10.1001/2013.jamaneurol.45

Mo SJ, Linder J, Blomstedt P, Granasen G, Forsgren L, Hariz M (2016) Long-term dopamine transporter imaging in Parkinson's disease treated with zona incerta stimulation. Nucl Med Commun 37:499–508. https://doi.org/10.1097/MNM.0000000000000469

Moro E et al (2004) Bilateral globus pallidus stimulation for Huntington's disease. Ann Neurol 56:290–294. https://doi.org/10.1002/ana.20183

Mubeen AM, Ardekani B, Tagliati M, Alterman R, Dhawan V, Eidelberg D, Sidtis JJ (2018) Global and multi-focal changes in cerebral blood flow during subthalamic nucleus stimulation in Parkinson's disease. J Cereb Blood Flow Metab 38:697–705. https://doi.org/10.1177/0271678X17705042

Mure H et al (2011) Parkinson's disease tremor-related metabolic network: characterization, progression, and treatment effects. Neuroimage 54:1244–1253. https://doi.org/10.1016/j.neuroimage.2010.09.028

Nagaoka T, Katayama Y, Kano T, Kobayashi K, Oshima H, Fukaya C, Yamamoto T (2007) Changes in glucose metabolism in cerebral cortex and cerebellum correlate with tremor and rigidity control by subthalamic nucleus stimulation in Parkinson's disease: a positron emission tomography study. Neuromodulation 10:206–215. https://doi.org/10.1111/j.1525-1403.2007.00110.x

Nakajima T, Nimura T, Yamaguchi K, Ando T, Itoh M, Yoshimoto T, Shirane R (2003) The impact of stereotactic pallidal surgery on the dopamine D2 receptor in Parkinson disease: a positron emission tomography study. J Neurosurg 98:57–63. https://doi.org/10.3171/jns.2003.98.1.0057

Nambu A, Tokuno H, Takada M (2002) Functional significance of the cortico-subthalamo-pallidal 'hyperdirect' pathway. Neurosci Res 43:111–117

Narayana S et al (2009) A noninvasive imaging approach to understanding speech changes following deep brain stimulation in Parkinson's disease. Am J Speech Lang Pathol 18:146–161. https://doi.org/10.1044/1058-0360(2008/08-0004)

Nimura T et al (2005) Attenuation of fluctuating striatal synaptic dopamine levels in patients with Parkinson disease in response to subthalamic nucleus stimulation: a positron emission tomography study. J Neurosurg 103:968–973. https://doi.org/10.3171/jns.2005.103.6.0968

Nobler MS, Oquendo MA, Kegeles LS, Malone KM, Campbell CC, Sackeim HA, Mann JJ (2001) Decreased regional brain metabolism after ECT. Am J Psychiatry 158:305–308. https://doi.org/10.1176/appi.ajp.158.2.305

Nozaki T et al (2013) Effect of subthalamic nucleus stimulation during exercise on the mesolimbocortical dopaminergic region in Parkinson's disease: a positron emission tomography study. J Cereb Blood Flow Metab 33:415–421. https://doi.org/10.1038/jcbfm.2012.183

Nuttin B, Cosyns P, Demeulemeester H, Gybels J, Meyerson B (1999) Electrical stimulation in anterior limbs of internal capsules in patients with obsessive-compulsive disorder. Lancet 354:1526. https://doi.org/10.1016/S0140-6736(99)02376-4

Nuttin BJ et al (2003) Long-term electrical capsular stimulation in patients with obsessive-compulsive disorder. Neurosurgery 52:1263–1272.; ; discussion 1272-1264. https://doi.org/10.1227/01.neu.0000064565.49299.9a

Nuttin B et al (2013) Targeting bed nucleus of the stria terminalis for severe obsessive-compulsive disorder: more unexpected lead placement in obsessive-compulsive disorder than in surgery for movement disorders. World Neurosurg 80:S30 e11–S30 e36. https://doi.org/10.1016/j.wneu.2012.12.029

Obeso I, Ray NJ, Antonelli F, Cho SS, Strafella AP (2011) Combining functional imaging with brain stimulation in Parkinson's disease. Int Rev Psychiatry 23:467–475. https://doi.org/10.3109/09540261.2011.621414

Okun MS (2012) Deep-brain stimulation for Parkinson's disease. N Engl J Med 367:1529–1538. https://doi.org/10.1056/NEJMct1208070

Ory S et al (2017) Pre-frontal-insular-cerebellar modifications correlate with disgust feeling blunting after subthalamic stimulation: a positron emission tomography study in Parkinson's disease. J Neuropsychol 11:378–395. https://doi.org/10.1111/jnp.12094

Park HJ et al (2015) A network analysis of (1)(5)O-H(2)O PET reveals deep brain stimulation effects on brain network of Parkinson's disease. Yonsei Med J 56:726–736. https://doi.org/10.3349/ymj.2015.56.3.726

Parker F, Tzourio N, Blond S, Petit H, Mazoyer B (1992) Evidence for a common network of brain structures involved in parkinsonian tremor and voluntary repetitive movement. Brain Res 584:11–17. https://doi.org/10.1016/0006-8993(92)90872-7

Payoux P et al (2004) Subthalamic nucleus stimulation reduces abnormal motor cortical overactivity in Parkinson disease. Arch Neurol 61:1307–1313. https://doi.org/10.1001/archneur.61.8.1307

Payoux P et al (2009) Contrasting changes in cortical activation induced by acute high-frequency stimulation within the globus pallidus in Parkinson's disease. J Cereb Blood Flow Metab 29:235–243. https://doi.org/10.1038/jcbfm.2008.107

Pereira EA, Green AL, Bradley KM, Soper N, Moir L, Stein JF, Aziz TZ (2007) Regional cerebral perfusion differences between periventricular grey, thalamic and dual target deep brain stimulation for chronic neuropathic pain. Stereotact Funct Neurosurg 85:175–183. https://doi.org/10.1159/000101296

Perlmutter JS et al (2002) Blood flow responses to deep brain stimulation of thalamus. Neurology 58:1388–1394. https://doi.org/10.1212/wnl.58.9.1388

Peron J et al (2010) Subthalamic nucleus stimulation affects theory of mind network: a PET study in Parkinson's disease. PLoS One 5:e9919. https://doi.org/10.1371/journal.pone.0009919

Picillo M, Lozano AM, Kou N, Puppi Munhoz R, Fasano A (2016) Programming deep brain stimulation for Parkinson's disease: the Toronto Western Hospital Algorithms. Brain Stimul 9:425–437. https://doi.org/10.1016/j.brs.2016.02.004

Pinto S et al (2004) Subthalamic nucleus stimulation and dysarthria in Parkinson's disease: a PET study. Brain 127:602–615. https://doi.org/10.1093/brain/awh074

Poewe W et al (2017) Parkinson disease. Nat Rev Dis Primers 3:17013. https://doi.org/10.1038/nrdp.2017.13

Poston KL et al (2016) Compensatory neural mechanisms in cognitively unimpaired Parkinson disease. Ann Neurol 79:448–463. https://doi.org/10.1002/ana.24585

Pourfar M, Tang C, Lin T, Dhawan V, Kaplitt MG, Eidelberg D (2009) Assessing the microlesion effect of subthalamic deep brain stimulation surgery with FDG PET. J Neurosurg 110:1278–1282. https://doi.org/10.3171/2008.12.JNS08991

Rauch SL et al (2006) A functional neuroimaging investigation of deep brain stimulation in patients with obsessive-compulsive disorder. J Neurosurg 104:558–565. https://doi.org/10.3171/jns.2006.104.4.558

Raymaekers S, Vansteelandt K, Luyten L, Bervoets C, Demyttenaere K, Gabriels L, Nuttin B (2017) Long-term electrical stimulation of bed nucleus of stria terminalis for obsessive-compulsive disorder. Mol Psychiatry 22:931–934. https://doi.org/10.1038/mp.2016.124

Reich MM et al (2016) Progressive gait ataxia following deep brain stimulation for essential tremor: adverse effect or lack of efficacy? Brain 139:2948–2956. https://doi.org/10.1093/brain/aww223

Rezai AR et al (2016) Improved function after deep brain stimulation for chronic, severe traumatic brain injury. Neurosurgery 79:204–211. https://doi.org/10.1227/NEU.0000000000001190

Riva-Posse P et al (2018) A connectomic approach for subcallosal cingulate deep brain stimulation surgery: prospective targeting in treatment-resistant depression. Mol Psychiatry 23:843–849. https://doi.org/10.1038/mp.2017.59

Robbins TW, Vaghi MM, Banca P (2019) Obsessive-compulsive disorder: puzzles and prospects. Neuron 102:27–47. https://doi.org/10.1016/j.neuron.2019.01.046

Rodriguez-Oroz MC, Jahanshahi M, Krack P, Litvan I, Macias R, Bezard E, Obeso JA (2009) Initial clinical manifestations of Parkinson's disease: features and pathophysiological mechanisms. Lancet Neurol 8:1128–1139. https://doi.org/10.1016/S1474-4422(09)70293-5

Rosa M, Marceglia S, Barbieri S, Priori A (2013) Local field potential and deep brain stimulation (DBS). In: Jaeger D, Jung R (eds) Encyclopedia of computational neuroscience. Springer, New York, pp 1–20. https://doi.org/10.1007/978-1-4614-7320-6_547-1

Savitz JB, Drevets WC (2013) Neuroreceptor imaging in depression. Neurobiol Dis 52:49–65. https://doi.org/10.1016/j.nbd.2012.06.001

Saxena S, Brody AL, Schwartz JM, Baxter LR (1998) Neuroimaging and frontal-subcortical circuitry in obsessive-compulsive disorder. Br J Psychiatry Suppl:26–37

Scharre DW et al (2018) Deep brain stimulation of frontal lobe networks to treat Alzheimer's disease. J Alzheimers Dis 62:621–633. https://doi.org/10.3233/JAD-170082

Scheltens P, Blennow K, Breteler MM, de Strooper B, Frisoni GB, Salloway S, Van der Flier WM (2016) Alzheimer's disease. Lancet 388:505–517. https://doi.org/10.1016/S0140-6736(15)01124-1

Schilbach L, Weiss PH, Kuhn J, Timmermann L, Klosterkotter J, Huff W (2012) Pharmacological treatment of deep brain stimulation-induced hypomania leads to clinical remission while preserving motor benefits. Neurocase 18:152–159. https://doi.org/10.1080/13554794.2011.568502

Schlaepfer TE et al (2008) Deep brain stimulation to reward circuitry alleviates anhedonia in refractory major depression. Neuropsychopharmacology 33:368–377. https://doi.org/10.1038/sj.npp.1301408

Schroeder U et al (2002) Subthalamic nucleus stimulation affects striato-anterior cingulate cortex circuit in a response conflict task: a PET study. Brain 125:1995–2004. https://doi.org/10.1093/brain/awf199

Schroeder U et al (2003) Subthalamic nucleus stimulation affects a frontotemporal network: a PET study. Ann Neurol 54:445–450. https://doi.org/10.1002/ana.10683

Sestini S, Scotto di Luzio A, Ammannati F, De Cristofaro MT, Passeri A, Martini S, Pupi A (2002) Changes in regional cerebral blood flow caused by deep-brain stimulation of the subthalamic nucleus in Parkinson's disease. J Nucl Med 43:725–732

Sestini S, Ramat S, Formiconi AR, Ammannati F, Sorbi S, Pupi A (2005) Brain networks underlying the clinical effects of long-term subthalamic stimulation for Parkinson's disease: a 4-year follow-up study with rCBF SPECT. J Nucl Med 46:1444–1454

Sestini S, Pupi A, Ammannati F, Silvia R, Sorbi S, Castagnoli A (2007) Are there adaptive changes in the human brain of patients with Parkinson's disease treated with long-term deep brain stimulation of the subthalamic nucleus? A 4-year follow-up study with regional cerebral blood flow SPECT. Eur J Nucl Med Mol Imaging 34:1646–1657. https://doi.org/10.1007/s00259-007-0428-z

Shen LH, Liao MH, Tseng YC (2012) Recent advances in imaging of dopaminergic neurons for evaluation of neuropsychiatric disorders. J Biomed Biotechnol 2012:259349. https://doi.org/10.1155/2012/259349

Sims-Williams H, Matthews JC, Talbot PS, Love-Jones S, Brooks JC, Patel NK, Pickering AE (2017) Deep brain stimulation of the periaqueductal gray releases endogenous opioids in humans. Neuroimage 146:833–842. https://doi.org/10.1016/j.neuroimage.2016.08.038

Smith GS, Laxton AW, Tang-Wai DF, McAndrews MP, Diaconescu AO, Workman CI, Lozano AM (2012) Increased cerebral metabolism after 1 year of deep brain stimulation in Alzheimer disease. Arch Neurol 69:1141–1148. https://doi.org/10.1001/archneurol.2012.590

Smith GS et al (2019) Effect of STN DBS on vesicular monoamine transporter 2 and glucose metabolism in Parkinson's disease. Parkinsonism Relat Disord 64:235–241. https://doi.org/10.1016/j.parkreldis.2019.04.006

Soret M, Bacharach SL, Buvat I (2007) Partial-volume effect in PET tumor imaging. J Nucl Med 48:932–945. https://doi.org/10.2967/jnumed.106.035774

Sperling RA et al (2009) Amyloid deposition is associated with impaired default network function in older persons without dementia. Neuron 63:178–188. https://doi.org/10.1016/j.neuron.2009.07.003

Spetsieris PG, Eidelberg D (2011) Scaled subprofile modeling of resting state imaging data in Parkinson's disease: methodological issues. Neuroimage 54:2899–2914. https://doi.org/10.1016/j.neuroimage.2010.10.025

Stefani A, Pierantozzi M, Ceravolo R, Brusa L, Galati S, Stanzione P (2010) Deep brain stimulation of pedunculopontine tegmental nucleus (PPTg) promotes cognitive and metabolic changes: a target-specific effect or response to a low-frequency pattern of stimulation? Clin EEG Neurosci 41:82–86. https://doi.org/10.1177/155005941004100207

Strafella AP, Dagher A, Sadikot AF (2003a) Cerebral blood flow changes induced by subthalamic stimulation in Parkinson's disease. Neurology 60:1039–1042. https://doi.org/10.1212/01.wnl.0000052691.48076.92

Strafella AP, Sadikot AF, Dagher A (2003b) Subthalamic deep brain stimulation does not induce striatal dopamine release in Parkinson's disease. Neuroreport 14:1287–1289. https://doi.org/10.1097/00001756-200307010-00020

Strafella AP, Lozano AM, Ballanger B, Poon YY, Lang AE, Moro E (2008) rCBF changes associated with PPN stimulation in a patient with Parkinson's disease: a PET study. Mov Disord 23:1051–1054. https://doi.org/10.1002/mds.22055

Suetens K, Nuttin B, Gabriels L, Van Laere K (2014) Differences in metabolic network modulation between capsulotomy and deep-brain stimulation for refractory obsessive-compulsive disorder. J Nucl Med 55:951–959. https://doi.org/10.2967/jnumed.113.126409

Tanei T, Kajita Y, Nihashi T, Kaneoke Y, Takebayashi S, Nakatsubo D, Wakabayashi T (2009) Changes in regional blood flow induced by unilateral subthalamic nucleus stimulation in patients with Parkinson's disease. Neurol Med Chir (Tokyo) 49:507–513. https://doi.org/10.2176/nmc.49.507

Thevathasan W, Moro E (2019) What is the therapeutic mechanism of pedunculopontine nucleus stimulation in Parkinson's disease? Neurobiol Dis 128:67–74. https://doi.org/10.1016/j.nbd.2018.06.014

Thobois S et al (2002) Effects of subthalamic nucleus stimulation on actual and imagined movement in Parkinson's disease: a PET study. J Neurol 249:1689–1698. https://doi.org/10.1007/s00415-002-0906-y

Thobois S et al (2003) Chronic subthalamic nucleus stimulation and striatal D2 dopamine receptors in Parkinson's disease--a [(11)C]-raclopride PET study. J Neurol 250:1219–1223. https://doi.org/10.1007/s00415-003-0188-z

Thobois S, Hotton GR, Pinto S, Wilkinson L, Limousin-Dowsey P, Brooks DJ, Jahanshahi M (2007) STN stimulation alters pallidal-frontal coupling during response selection under competition. J Cereb Blood Flow Metab 27:1173–1184. https://doi.org/10.1038/sj.jcbfm.9600425

Thobois S et al (2008) Globus pallidus stimulation reduces frontal hyperactivity in tardive dystonia. J Cereb Blood Flow Metab 28:1127–1138. https://doi.org/10.1038/sj.jcbfm.9600610

Trost M et al (2006) Network modulation by the subthalamic nucleus in the treatment of Parkinson's disease. Neuroimage 31:301–307. https://doi.org/10.1016/j.neuroimage.2005.12.024

Tsai HC, Chang CH, Pan JI, Hsieh HJ, Tsai ST, Hung HY, Chen SY (2012) Pilot study of deep brain stimulation in refractory obsessive-compulsive disorder ethnic Chinese patients. Psychiatry Clin Neurosci 66:303–312. https://doi.org/10.1111/j.1440-1819.2012.02352.x

Turner R, Jones T (2003) Techniques for imaging neuroscience. Br Med Bull 65:3–20. https://doi.org/10.1093/bmb/65.1.3

Ulla M et al (2006) Manic behaviour induced by deep-brain stimulation in Parkinson's disease: evidence of substantia nigra implication? J Neurol Neurosurg Psychiatry 77:1363–1366. https://doi.org/10.1136/jnnp.2006.096628

Ulla M et al (2011) Contact dependent reproducible hypomania induced by deep brain stimulation in Parkinson's disease: clinical, anatomical and functional imaging study. J Neurol Neurosurg Psychiatry 82:607–614. https://doi.org/10.1136/jnnp.2009.199323

Valalik I, Emri M, Lengyel Z, Mikecz P, Tron L, Csokay A, Marian T (2009) Pallidal deep brain stimulation and L-dopa effect on PET motor activation in advanced Parkinson's disease. J Neuroimaging 19:253–258. https://doi.org/10.1111/j.1552-6569.2008.00304.x

Velasco F et al (2015) Metabolic changes induced by electrical stimulation of prelemniscal radiations for the treatment of Parkinson disease. Stereotact Funct Neurosurg 93:333–341. https://doi.org/10.1159/000438997

Ventre-Dominey J, Bourret S, Mollion H, Broussolle E, Dominey PF (2014) Dissociable dorsal and ventral frontostriatal working memory circuits: evidence from subthalamic stimulation in Parkinson's disease. Hum Brain Mapp 35:552–566. https://doi.org/10.1002/hbm.22205

Vernaleken I et al (2009) Bithalamical deep brain stimulation in tourette syndrome is associated with reduction in dopaminergic transmission. Biol Psychiatry 66:e15–e17. https://doi.org/10.1016/j.biopsych.2009.06.025

Vitek JL et al (2010) Standard guidelines for publication of deep brain stimulation studies in Parkinson's disease (Guide4DBS-PD). Mov Disord 25:1530–1537. https://doi.org/10.1002/mds.23151

Volkow ND et al (1993) Reproducibility of repeated measures of carbon-11-raclopride binding in the human brain. J Nucl Med 34:609–613

Volonte MA et al (2012) Changes in brain glucose metabolism in subthalamic nucleus deep brain stimulation for advanced Parkinson's disease. Parkinsonism Relat Disord 18:770–774. https://doi.org/10.1016/j.parkreldis.2012.03.016

Wang J, Ma Y, Huang Z, Sun B, Guan Y, Zuo C (2010) Modulation of metabolic brain function by bilateral subthalamic nucleus stimulation in the treatment of Parkinson's disease. J Neurol 257:72–78. https://doi.org/10.1007/s00415-009-5267-3

Weiss PH et al (2015) Subthalamic nucleus stimulation improves parkinsonian gait via brainstem locomotor centers. Mov Disord 30:1121–1125. https://doi.org/10.1002/mds.26229

Whiteside SP, Port JD, Abramowitz JS (2004) A meta-analysis of functional neuroimaging in obsessive-compulsive disorder. Psychiatry Res 132:69–79. https://doi.org/10.1016/j.pscychresns.2004.07.001

Wielepp JP, Burgunder JM, Pohle T, Ritter EP, Kinser JA, Krauss JK (2001) Deactivation of thalamocortical activity is responsible for suppression of parkinsonian tremor by thalamic stimulation: a 99mTc-ECD SPECT study. Clin Neurol Neurosurg 103:228–231

Wilcox RA, Cole MH, Wong D, Coyne T, Silburn P, Kerr G (2011) Pedunculopontine nucleus deep brain stimulation produces sustained improvement in primary progressive freezing of gait. J Neurol Neurosurg Psychiatry 82:1256–1259. https://doi.org/10.1136/jnnp.2010.213462

Windels F, Bruet N, Poupard A, Urbain N, Chouvet G, Feuerstein C, Savasta M (2000) Effects of high frequency stimulation of subthalamic nucleus on extracellular glutamate and GABA in substantia nigra and globus pallidus in the normal rat. Eur J Neurosci 12:4141–4146

Yianni J et al (2004) Senile chorea treated by deep brain stimulation: a clinical, neurophysiological and functional imaging study. Mov Disord 19:597–602. https://doi.org/10.1002/mds.10716

Zhang HW, Li DY, Zhao J, Guan YH, Sun BM, Zuo CT (2013) Metabolic imaging of deep brain stimulation in anorexia nervosa: a 18F-FDG PET/CT study. Clin Nucl Med 38:943–948. https://doi.org/10.1097/RLU.0000000000000261

Radionuclide Imaging Studies in Pediatric Neurology

47

Ajay Kumar, Csaba Juhasz, and Harry T. Chugani

Contents

Abstract

Functional imaging modalities, such as positron emission tomography (PET) and single-photon emission computed tomography (SPECT), can noninvasively provide very useful qualitative (visual) and quantitative information about a variety of physiological and biological processes in the brain, which may be altered during disease conditions. The use of these techniques not only can shed light upon the underlying pathology but also can provide biomarkers to aid in the

A. Kumar (✉) · C. Juhasz
Departments of Pediatrics and Neurology, PET Center, Children's Hospital of Michigan, Detroit Medical Center, Wayne State University School of Medicine, Detroit, MI, USA
e-mail: ajaykumar@med.wayne.edu

H. T. Chugani
Department of Neurology, NYU School of Medicine, New York, NY, USA

R. A. J. O. Dierckx et al. (eds.), *PET and SPECT in Neurology*,
https://doi.org/10.1007/978-3-030-53168-3_47

diagnosis, localization, follow-up, treatment development, and/or treatment response evaluation and prognostication in various diseases. PET and SPECT have been used clinically in the evaluation of medically refractory epilepsy to select candidates for surgical intervention, especially when structural imaging (CT, MRI, etc.) is normal or discordant with other localizing information. In addition, functional neuroimaging can assist evaluation of some specific epileptic syndromes, such as tuberous sclerosis, to identify noninvasively the epileptic tuber, as well as conditions like infantile spasms or Lennox-Gastaut syndrome, to reveal a focal region for surgical resection in otherwise cryptogenic cases. Similarly, these techniques are instrumental to investigate the underlying basis for various neurocognitive and behavioral abnormalities in children, where other imaging modalities are often normal or reveal only subtle and nonspecific changes. Even when structural imaging is abnormal, PET and SPECT abnormalities may precede or extend beyond the structural changes, which can have immense therapeutic and prognostic implications.

47.1 Introduction

Functional imaging modalities, such as positron emission tomography (PET) and single-photon emission computed tomography (SPECT), can provide noninvasively qualitative (visual) and quantitative information about a variety of physiological and biological processes in the brain. These techniques not only allow in vivo visualization of these processes but also have revolutionized our understanding of various brain functions and etiopathogenesis of several neurological disorders. PET and SPECT imaging techniques use gamma ray emission from the *nuclear* disintegration of radioisotopes or radiolabeled molecules to study the perfusion or function of an organ. With both methods, a very small amount of a selected radiotracer is injected into the patient. The radiotracer is selected on the basis of the desired purpose, i.e., which organs and what functions are of interest. Once inside the body, these radiotracers become distributed in a specific way depending upon the nature of the radiotracer and the function of the targeted organs. The gamma rays emitted by the radiotracers are detected externally with the help of detectors, and an image of the spatial distribution of these radiotracers is generated. Theoretically, any organ or its function can be studied, provided appropriate and suitable radiotracers are available. The reason for applying PET and SPECT in neurology is based on the fact that the metabolism (particularly of glucose), neurochemical production/distribution, receptor density/expression, or cerebral blood flow may be altered in various neurological disorders, and these events can be visualized or quantified using PET or SPECT. Therefore, the use of these techniques not only can shed some light upon the underlying pathology but also can help in the diagnosis, localization, follow-up, treatment development, and/or treatment response evaluation and prognostication, once these pathologies are known/established. In this chapter, we will discuss the role and application of PET and SPECT in various pediatric neurological disorders.

47.2 Epileptic Disorders

Presently, neither PET nor SPECT is used in the primary diagnosis or evaluation of recent-onset epilepsy; however, they play a very unique and important role in certain specific situations, such as in the evaluation of medically refractory cases for epilepsy surgery, particularly when structural imaging (CT, MRI, etc.) is normal, or in the evaluation of some specific epileptic syndromes, such as tuberous sclerosis. As of now, neither PET nor SPECT can identify precisely the epileptogenic zone to be resected; however, they can help in the general identification of these regions, including functional deficit zone, and quite often can provide some information related to the observed neurocognitive and behavioral abnormalities.

PET in pediatric epilepsy is performed using 2-deoxy-2(^{18}F)-fluoro-D-glucose (FDG), which shows hypometabolism or decreased glucose consumption in the epileptic cortex in the interictal state. The hypometabolism can result from a variety of mechanisms, including neuronal loss, diaschisis, or reduction in synaptic density. It appears that cortical hypometabolism may be associated with duration, frequency, and severity of the seizures, as focal hypometabolism is found in only one-fifth of children with new-onset epilepsy compared to 80–85% of adults with intractable seizures (Gaillard et al. 2002). Persistent or increased seizure frequency may lead to enlargement of the hypometabolic area, whereas seizure control may be associated with decrease in the size of hypometabolic cortex or even its resolution, as demonstrated by longitudinal PET studies (Benedek et al. 2006). The time interval between PET acquisition and the most recent seizure also may affect the extent and severity of the cortical abnormality, with shorter duration leading to larger extent or severity of the hypometabolism on FDG PET scan (Bouvard et al. 2005). Pure ictal PET is rarely possible, as seizures usually last for a few seconds to minutes, whereas FDG PET shows cumulative FDG uptake over a period of 30–45 min; thus, the metabolic pattern usually reflects a summation of interictal, ictal, and postictal metabolic changes and is difficult to interpret in patients who had coincidental seizure(s) during the tracer uptake period. While a rare finding, interictal PET **hypermetabolism** does occur and may help identify epileptogenic zones with careful analysis (Schur et al. 2018).

FDG PET usually shows larger areas of hypometabolism compared to the abnormality shown on MRI (if there is one), and ictal or intracranial subdural EEG-determined epileptogenic region. An early study from our group compared the exact locations of objectively defined cortical hypometabolic regions on PET to ictal and interictal epileptiform abnormalities from subdural EEG recordings (Juhasz et al. 2000a). We found that the overlap between hypometabolic areas and seizure-onset electrodes was only partial, with seizure onset extending beyond the hypometabolic cortex, while glucose metabolic abnormalities incorporated non-epileptogenic regions also. This observation was subsequently confirmed in other studies (Alkonyi et al. 2009; Jeong et al. 2017; Tomás et al. 2019). Therefore, FDG PET abnormalities cannot be solely relied upon to determine the surgical margin; however, they can help in lateralization or *general* localization of the epileptic focus, which can facilitate surgical planning and subsequent placement of intracranial electrodes, particularly in cases of normal MRI and non-localizing scalp EEG. Various co-registration and objective analytic methods, such as statistical parametric mapping (SPM), a voxel-based whole-brain analysis, or SPM extent analysis with asymmetry index, can be quite helpful in these cases (Van Bogaert et al. 2000; Kim et al. 2006; Akman et al. 2010; Kumar et al. 2010).

It has been shown that the sensitivity of FDG PET can be increased by co-registration of PET images with structural MRI, particularly in patients with cortical dysplasia (Lerner et al. 2009). Co-registration can lead to detection of mild type I cortical dysplasia in up to 98% of the cases and can add useful localizing value in one-third of patients with non-concordant EEG and MRI findings (Salamon et al. 2008). FDG PET has a clear advantage over MRI in detecting mild malformations of cortical development, which can be missed in about 2/3 of the cases (Kim et al. 2011). Use of higher-strength MRI (3 T) images co-registered with FDG PET can further increase the detection of focal abnormalities (Ding et al. 2018). A recent study showed the utility of quantitative PET processing in combination with morphometric analysis to automatically and objectively identify epileptogenic abnormalities in the cohort of MRI-negative epilepsy patients (Lin et al. 2018). It demonstrated that the complete resection of MRI/PET-positive regions was associated with seizure-free outcome, and this effect was more robust in the extratemporal subgroup as compared to those with temporal lobe epilepsy. Another study found that hypometabolism confined to the epileptogenic zone as defined by EEG and MRI is associated with a favorable postoperative outcome in both temporal lobe and extratemporal lobe epilepsy patients (Tomás et al. 2019).

Sometimes, hypometabolism can be quite extensive and may even extend into the contralateral hemisphere, perhaps depending upon the type, location, duration, and severity of the seizure and maturity of the brain (Kumar et al. 2010). Long-standing severe seizures, particularly in the immature pediatric brain, may show extensive areas of hypometabolism, likely involving seizure propagation pathways, or the seizure effect on connected brain regions. FDG PET is particularly useful in the evaluation of the functional status of the rest of the brain when an epileptogenic lesion is considered for surgical resection, as postsurgical neurocognitive outcome will also depend upon the integrity of the remaining (unresected) cortex. This is particularly important in children, because brain plasticity following resection is more likely to involve functionally intact regions.

Several other PET tracers, such as ^{11}C-flumazenil (FMZ) and ^{11}C-alpha-methyl-L-tryptophan (AMT), used for the evaluation of gamma-aminobutyric acid type A ($GABA_A$) receptors and serotonin/kynurenine metabolism, respectively, have also been investigated in epilepsy and have been found to be useful in certain situations. FMZ PET may be clinically useful in cases of temporal lobe epilepsy (Ryvlin et al. 1998), particularly in identifying medial temporal lobe involvement (Henry et al. 1993; Koepp et al. 1996). AMT PET is very useful in patients with tuberous sclerosis and certain types of epileptogenic cortical malformations (Chugani et al. 1998a, b; Asano et al. 2000; Fedi et al. 2003; Chugani et al. 2011, 2013a, b). These applications are discussed in further detail below. Several other PET tracers, such as radioligands for opiate, histamine, NMDA, acetylcholine, dopamine, and other neuro-receptors, have been investigated in epilepsy. PET imaging using these tracers shows either increased (^{11}C-carfentanyl (μ-opioid receptor agonist), ^{11}C-methylnaltrindole (δ-opioid receptor antagonist), ^{18}F-cyclofoxy (μ-, κ-opioid receptor antagonist), ^{11}C-doxepin (H1 receptor antagonist), and ^{11}C-L-deprenyl (MAO-B inhibitor)) or decreased (^{11}C-diprenorphine (μ-, δ-, κ-opioid receptor antagonist), ^{11}C/^{18}F-FCWAY ($5HT_{1A}$ receptor antagonist), ^{18}F-MPPF ($5HT_{1A}$ receptor antagonist), ^{18}F-altanserin ($5HT_{2A}$ receptor antagonist), ^{11}C-(S)-[*N-methyl*]-ketamine (NMDA receptor antagonist), ^{11}C-NMBP ($_{m}$Ach receptor antagonist), and ^{123}I-iododexetimide ($_{m}$Ach receptor antagonist)) binding in the presumed epileptogenic region. However, only a limited number of studies are available regarding these tracers, and the clinical role and additional value of these tracers in epilepsy evaluation are yet to be established.

For epilepsy evaluation, SPECT is usually performed using ^{99m}Tc-labeled ethylcysteinate dimer (ECD) or hexamethylpropylene amine oxime (HMPAO) and demonstrates increased or decreased cerebral perfusion in the epileptic cortex when performed in the ictal or interictal state, respectively. During the ictal phase, blood flow in the epileptic region can increase up to 300%, which can be seen as an area of hyperperfusion on *ictal* SPECT (Hougaard et al. 1976). *Interictal* SPECT shows hypoperfusion or normal perfusion in the epileptogenic region; however, hypoperfusion may be very mild and sometimes difficult to distinguish from the surrounding normal brain on visual examination. The main role of interictal SPECT at present is to assist in the evaluation of ictal SPECT, visually or quantitatively, using statistical parametric mapping (SPM) or subtraction ictal SPECT co-registered to MRI (SISCOM), by providing a baseline blood flow image. Use of these registration techniques can increase the sensitivity and specificity of ictal SPECT. Studies have shown that SPM can increase the sensitivity of SPECT (and also PET) scan over visual analysis (Lee et al. 2000; Bruggemann et al. 2004; Tae et al. 2005). However, lack of age-matched controls can make its use difficult, particularly in children less than 6 years of age (Muzik et al. 2000a). SISCOM, on the other hand, appears to be very useful in children. The probability of localizing an ictal-onset zone is reported to be higher with SISCOM, compared to ictal EEG and MRI (O'Brien et al. 1998, 1999). Use of SISCOM can help in the detection of subtle MRI changes, initially reported as normal (Chiron et al. 1999a; Lawson et al. 2000). Recent pediatric studies demonstrated the complementary value of SISCOM, especially in localizing extratemporal foci (Kim et al. 2009). Outcome studies have also shown that the area of the resected SISCOM abnormality is associated with the surgical result; the larger the area of resected SISCOM abnormality, the better the outcome (O'Brien et al. 1998, 1999, 2000; von Oertzen et al. 2011). Simultaneous use of FDG PET and iomazenil SPECT may be particularly useful in patients with non-lesional epilepsy in identifying the seizure focus and predicting a seizure-free outcome (Fujimoto et al. 2018). The major limitation of SPECT in children is difficulty in acquiring a good ictal study because children may have very frequent and short-lasting seizures (such as infantile spasms or myoclonic epilepsy) so the ictal phase is missed. Another limitation is the poor spatial resolution (10–15 mm) of SPECT, compared to FDG PET (about 5–6 mm), which becomes even more crucial in small pediatric brains. Overall, the performance of ictal SPECT versus FDG PET has been variable, depending on the patient population and study design (Sturm et al. 2000; Kim et al. 2001; Seo et al. 2011; Jalota et al. 2016).

47.2.1 Epilepsy

47.2.1.1 Temporal Lobe Epilepsy

As stated above, FDG PET does not have much role in temporal lobe epilepsy evaluation if MRI is positive and concordant with localization suggested by EEG and seizure semiology. However, MRI is negative in a large number of patients, particularly in the pediatric population. Many times, the EEG can be noncontributory, generalized, or bilateral, depending upon various factors, such as seizure duration, seizure severity, or location of a seizure focus close to the midline (Lamusuo et al. 2001). PET can play an important role in these conditions, particularly considering that almost a quarter of epileptic patients become refractory and may have normal MRI and sometimes equivocal EEG (Fig. 47.1). FDG PET can help to identify the epileptic temporal lobe in almost half of the patients with noncontributory EEG (Theodore et al. 1997). It can be particularly helpful in cases with dual pathology

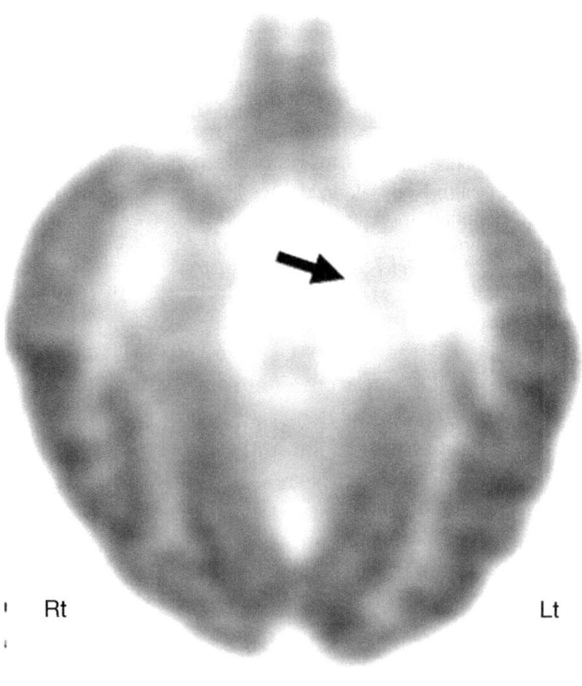

Fig. 47.1 Axial 2-deoxy-2(^{18}F)-fluoro-D-glucose PET scan in a child with intractable temporal lobe epilepsy and normal MRI. EEG changes were occasionally bilateral or equivocal. PET scan showed hypometabolism in the left medial temporal region (*arrow*) and increased the confidence for epilepsy surgery. The child underwent surgery, which showed mild sclerotic changes in the medial temporal lobe on histopathology, and is seizure-free after the surgery

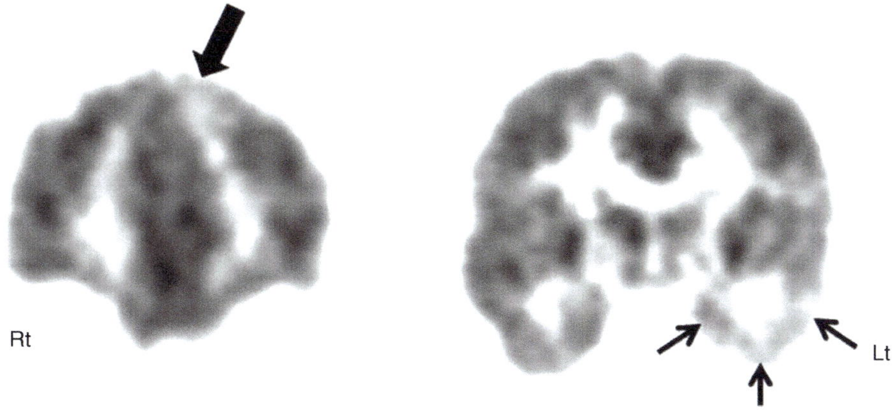

Fig. 47.2 2-Deoxy-2(^{18}F)-fluoro-D-glucose PET in a child with dual pathology. Coronal PET showing an area of decreased glucose metabolism in the left medial frontal cortex (*thick arrow*), in addition to hypometabolic left temporal lobe (*small thin arrows*) in a child with intractable temporal lobe epilepsy and bilateral epileptiform discharges on EEG. The child underwent epilepsy surgery with simultaneous resection of the left medial frontal cortex and hippocampus and is seizure-free

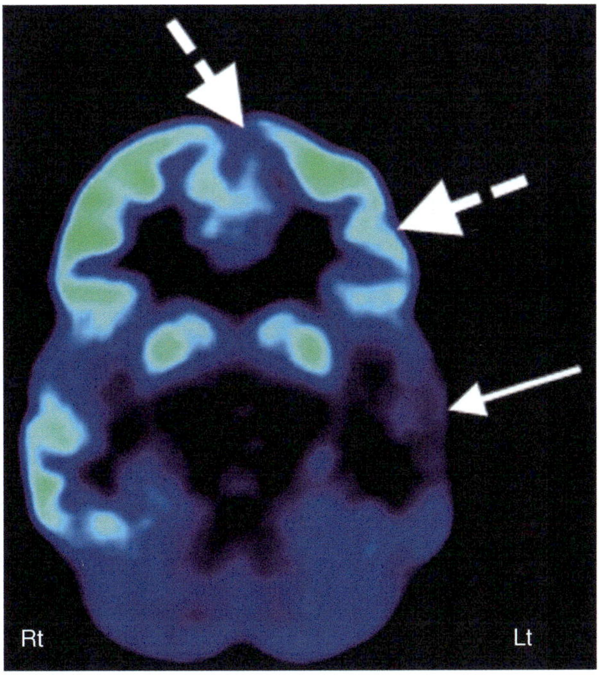

Fig. 47.3 2-Deoxy-2(^{18}F)-fluoro-D-glucose PET scan in a case of suspected secondary epileptic focus. A child with long-standing temporal lobe epilepsy (primary seizure focus) developed a change in seizure semiology with independent epileptiform discharges from frontal regions. PET scan showed severe hypometabolism of the left temporal lobe (*arrow*) along with reduced glucose metabolism in the left inferior frontal lobe (*broken arrows*), suggesting a possible secondary epileptic focus presumably due to persistent kindling through the uncinate fasciculus

(Fig. 47.2) or secondary epileptic foci (Fig. 47.3). The overall sensitivity of FDG PET in identifying the epileptic temporal lobe is in the range of 85–90% (Swartz et al. 1989; Gaillard et al. 1995; Knowlton et al. 1997; Ryvlin et al. 1998). Importantly, FDG PET can provide additional information about the epileptic focus in many patients, affecting ultimate surgical decision-making in 50–70% of patients (Ollenberger et al. 2005; Uijl et al. 2007), with it alone being the basis of surgical decision in almost 17% of patients (Uijl et al. 2007). FDG PET also has prognostic value, as unilateral PET hypometabolism appears to predict a good surgical outcome, even in patients with negative MRI or equivocal EEG (Willmann et al. 2007). An odds ratio of 7.1 has been reported for FDG PET in predicting a seizure-free outcome (Knowlton et al. 2008). It has been recently proposed that the difference in metabolic patterns, depending on the lateralization of medial temporal lobe epilepsy, may represent distinct epileptic networks in patients with right versus left medial temporal lobe epilepsy and can guide preoperative counseling and surgical planning (Cahill et al. 2019).

Another PET tracer, FMZ, has been investigated by quite a few centers. FMZ binds to the $GABA_A$ receptors, the main binding sites of the inhibitory neurotransmitter γ-aminobutyric acid (GABA). Since neurons in the normal hippocampus and amygdala have strong $GABA_A$ receptor expression, FMZ PET has been found to be particularly useful in detecting medial temporal lobe epileptic foci, which often show decreased FMZ binding, and may sometimes delineate abnormalities, either not seen or appearing subtle on FDG PET (Fig. 47.4). FMZ PET can also show decreased $GABA_A$ receptor binding in the epileptogenic neocortex, and the extent of abnormality is usually less than that seen on FDG PET scan (Henry et al. 1993; Savic et al. 1993; Szelies et al. 1996; Ryvlin et al. 1998). FMZ PET is almost 100% sensitive in cases of hippocampal sclerosis and can reveal contralateral abnormality

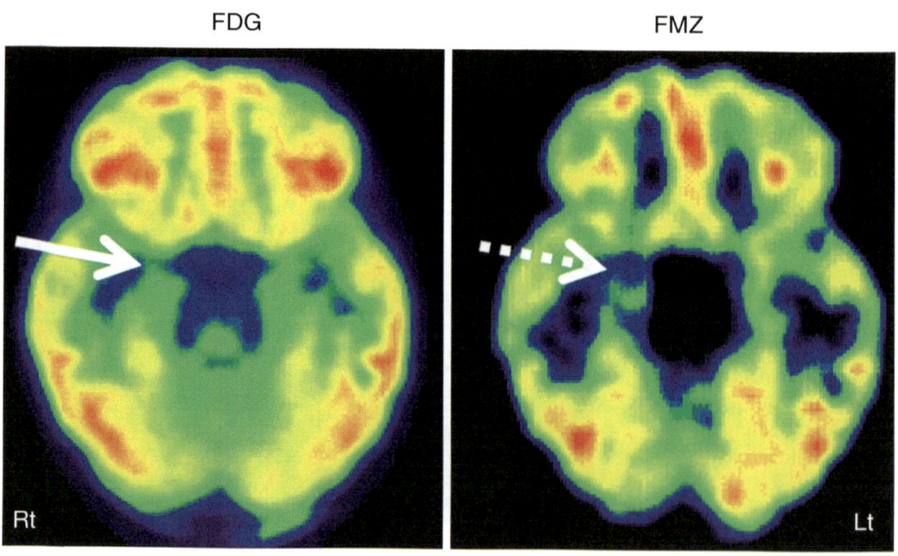

Fig. 47.4 ^{11}C-Flumazenil PET (*right image*) showing better delineation of right hippocampal abnormality (*broken arrow*) in a child with medial temporal lobe epilepsy, compared to 2-deoxy-2(^{18}F)-fluoro-D-glucose PET (*left image*) which showed only subtle changes (*solid arrow*) in this region

in almost one-third of patients with apparently unilateral hippocampal sclerosis on MRI (Henry et al. 1993; Koepp et al. 1996). FMZ PET can sometimes show increased FMZ binding in cases of cortical developmental malformations (Koepp et al. 1997) or microdysgenesis in the white matter (Hammers et al. 2002). Still, clinical use of FMZ PET in temporal lobe epilepsy is not established. Increasing availability of novel, ^{18}F-labeled (thus, longer half-life) flumazenil tracers may facilitate further exploration of this technique as a clinical tool.

Several other PET tracers have been tested in temporal lobe epilepsy for receptor imaging with variable results. AMT PET has been reported to be somewhat useful in identifying the epileptic foci in patients with temporal lobe epilepsy and normal hippocampal volume, but not in those with hippocampal sclerosis (Natsume et al. 2003); however, the added clinical value in individual cases remains uncertain. Studies of opiate receptor PET imaging have reported both increased (Frost et al. 1988; Madar et al. 1997) and normal (Mayberg et al. 1991; Theodore et al. 1992) receptor density in patients with temporal lobe epilepsy. Similarly, the level of monoamine oxidase B has been found to be both high (Kumlien et al. 1992) and low (Kumlien et al. 2001) in temporal lobe epilepsy. While significantly reduced dopamine receptor binding has been reported in the epileptogenic temporal lobe (Werhahn et al. 2006), no binding alterations were found in PET studies using ^{11}C-verapamil, a P-glycoprotein substrate (Langer et al. 2007). Patients with temporal lobe epilepsy have also been shown to have reduced NMDA receptor binding (Kumlien et al. 1999) but increased ^{11}C-doxepine uptake (Iinuma et al. 1993) in the epileptogenic temporal cortex. Recently, evidence of inflammatory changes was found in the hippocampus, parahippocampal gyrus, amygdala, and fusiform gyrus, ipsilateral to the epileptic focus in patients with temporal lobe epilepsy who underwent PET scanning with the translocator protein (TSPO) tracer ^{11}C-PBR28 (Hirvonen et al. 2012). A subsequent study also using ^{11}C-PBR28 found increased binding in temporal lobe regions both ipsilateral and contralateral to the epileptic focus, suggesting that inflammation may be an important pathophysiological mechanism in temporal lobe epilepsy (Gershen et al. 2015). In patients with neocortical epilepsy, ^{11}C-PBR28 PET revealed both focal and more distributed inflammation, as well as significant variability, thus limiting its role in clinical application (Dickstein et al. 2019).

Although limited SPECT data exist in the pediatric epilepsy population, it has been reported to be consistent with other noninvasive presurgical examinations in up to 95% of patients (O'Brien et al. 1998; Chiron et al. 1999a; Vera et al. 1999; Lawson et al. 2000; Kaminska et al. 2003; Lee et al. 2005; Kurian et al. 2007). Interictal SPECT has very low sensitivity (less than 50%) in the detection of epileptogenic regions in temporal lobe epilepsy, with false-positive or false-negative findings in 20–75% of cases. In contrast, ictal SPECT can correctly localize the epileptic foci in 70–90% of cases with unilateral temporal lobe epilepsy (Fig. 47.5) (Rowe et al. 1991; Harvey et al. 1993; Lee et al. 2005; Benifla et al. 2006). Various registration techniques, such as SPM or subtraction ictal SPECT co-registered to MRI (SISCOM), can further increase the sensitivity and specificity of ictal SPECT but require two separate SPECT studies including interictal and ictal scans. In children,

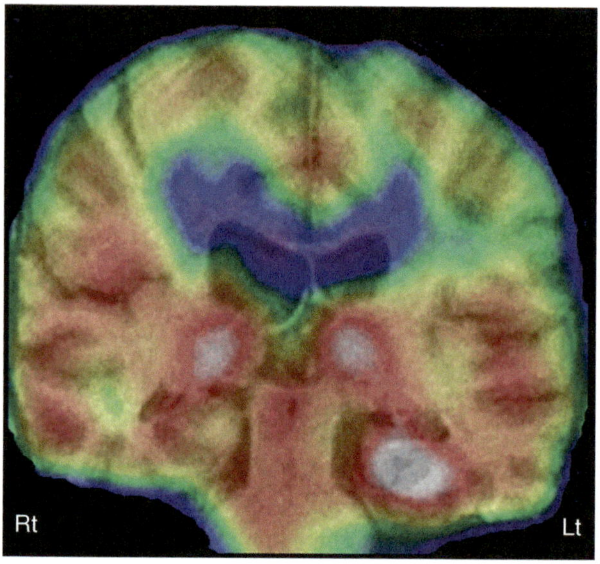

Fig. 47.5 Ictal ^{99m}Tc-ethyl cysteinate dimer SPECT (coronal view, co-registered onto the corresponding MRI slice) in a child with temporal lobe epilepsy showing increased perfusion in the left hippocampus, suggesting an epileptic focus. Also noted is increased perfusion in bilateral thalami, which can be seen during the ictal phase

SISCOM has been reported to be helpful in identifying the epileptogenic region in up to 95% of cases (Chiron et al. 1999b). In comparison to intracranial EEG findings, ictal ECD SPECT was found to correctly localize the seizure-onset zone in 80% of children with intractable epilepsy (Kaminska et al. 2003). In addition, in the majority of children with favorable outcome following resective epilepsy surgery, the surgical margin coincided with the SPECT focus. Postictal SPECT is also more sensitive (70–90%) than interictal SPECT, and its accuracy also can improve further with the use of SISCOM (Rowe et al. 1989; O'Brien et al. 1999). SISCOM can be particularly useful in cases of dysembryoplastic neuroepithelial tumor (DNET), which is often located in the temporal lobe and most prevalent in the pediatric population. SISCOM can demonstrate some additional dysplastic cortical areas around the DNET, and removal of these areas is essential for better surgical outcome. The use of SISCOM can increase the focus detection rate up to 93%, compared to 74% without it (Chiron et al. 1999b; Vera et al. 1999; Valenti et al. 2002). More rigorous studies in 113 children show less favorable results, with overall sensitivity of 64.8% and specificity of 40.7% in identifying the epileptogenic region (Aungaroon et al. 2018). Recently, a new approach PET interictal subtracted ictal SPECT co-registered with MRI (PISCOM) has been explored, and preliminary studies suggest promising results, but more data are required (Perissinotti et al. 2018).

47.2.1.2 Extratemporal Lobe Epilepsy

FDG PET plays a relatively more important role in extratemporal lobe epilepsy in children, compared to adults, due to its higher incidence in children with a large majority having noncontributory MRI (Wyllie et al. 1998). Normal MRI is perhaps due to the higher incidence of subtle cortical dysplasia in children compared to the adults, as these lesions are often difficult to detect on MRI. Here, FDG PET can play

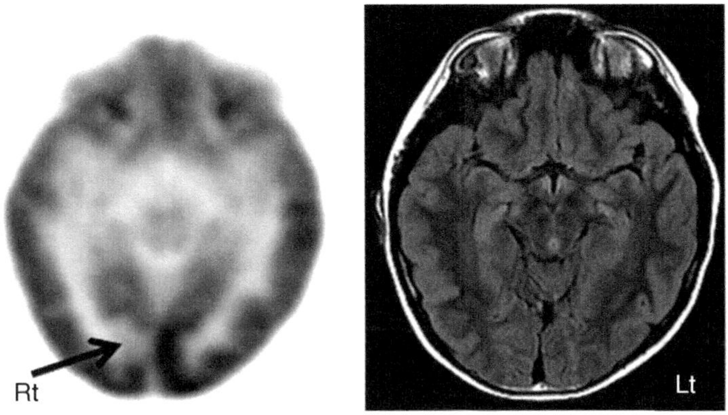

Fig. 47.6 2-Deoxy-2(^{18}F)-fluoro-D-glucose PET (*left image*) in a child with intractable epilepsy, normal fluid-attenuated inversion recovery (FLAIR) MRI (*right image*), and bilateral synchrony on EEG showed a very focal area of hypometabolism (*arrow*), which is strongly suspected to be cortical dysplasia

a valuable role, as the dysplastic cortex is usually hypometabolic (Fig. 47.6). Even when MRI is positive, it does not provide the full extent of the dysplasia, which is more obvious on FDG PET scan. FDG PET can also sometimes reveal additional epileptic foci, which can have a huge impact on surgical planning. Although a variable sensitivity of 45–92% has been reported for FDG PET in extratemporal lobe epilepsy, usually, it is less sensitive than in temporal lobe epilepsy (Henry et al. 1991; Swartz et al. 1995; da Silva et al. 1997; Kim et al. 2002; Honbolygo et al. 2006; Patil et al. 2007). The wide range of sensitivity is likely due to the variable patient populations studied and the lack of standardized analytic techniques across studies. Presurgical evaluation by co-registration of FDG PET and MRI could improve the identification of the epileptogenic focus and may further guide the surgical decision-making and improve the outcome of the refractory extratemporal lobe epilepsy with normal MRI (Ding et al. 2018). It seems that the combination of morphometric analysis, magnetoencephalography (MEG), and subtraction ictal SPECT co-registered to MRI (SISCOM) can be further useful, with morphometric analysis providing the highest yield of unique information when other tests are negative or non-localizing (Wang et al. 2019).

FMZ PET has a sensitivity of 60–100% for detecting the epileptogenic cortex in extratemporal epilepsy (Savic et al. 1995; Ryvlin et al. 1998; Muzik et al. 2000b), although most studies included a highly biased surgical population. FMZ PET abnormalities tend to be smaller than the area of FDG hypometabolism and sometimes may show better concordance with intracranial EEG findings (Arnold et al. 2000; Juhasz et al. 2000b; Szelies et al. 2002) (Fig. 47.7). FMZ PET can reveal abnormality even in patients with normal MRI (Muzik et al. 2000a; Koepp and Woermann 2005), and the complete surgical resection of FMZ abnormality has been found to be associated with good seizure outcome (Muzik et al. 2000b; Juhasz et al. 2001). The use of SPM can further increase the usefulness of FMZ PET, providing objective detection

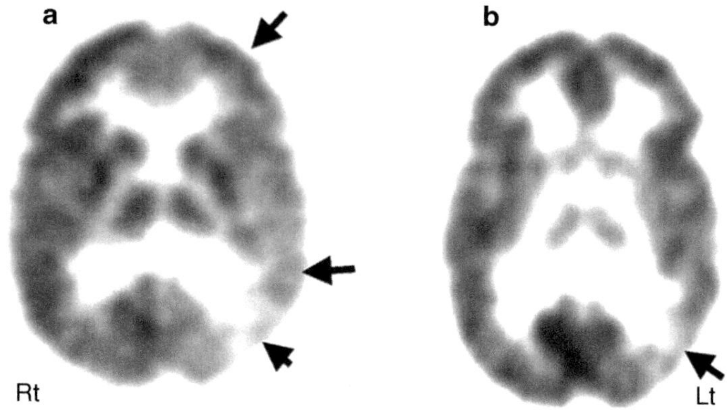

Fig. 47.7 ^{11}C-flumazenil PET (**b**) showing much smaller area of reduced flumazenil binding (*arrow*) compared to the extensive area of reduced glucose uptake in 2-deoxy-2(^{18}F)-fluoro-D-glucose PET scan (**a**) in the left temporal and frontal lobe, which was more consistent with predominantly posterior quadrant epileptiform activity on EEG

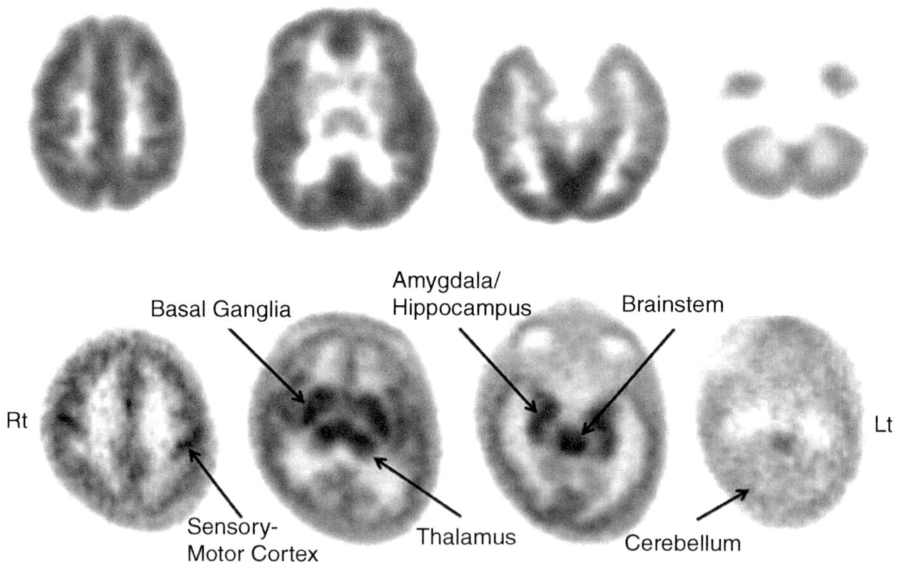

Fig. 47.8 ^{11}C-Flumazenil PET scan in an adult (upper row) and newborn (lower row) showing different pattern of FMZ-receptor binding in the newborn compared to the adult. In the newborn, highest receptor binding is seen in the amygdala-hippocampus, sensory-motor cortex, thalamus, brain stem, and basal ganglia, in that order; whereas the cerebellum and most of the cerebral cortex show relatively low binding, receptor binding is higher in the cortex compared to the basal ganglia and thalamus in normal adults

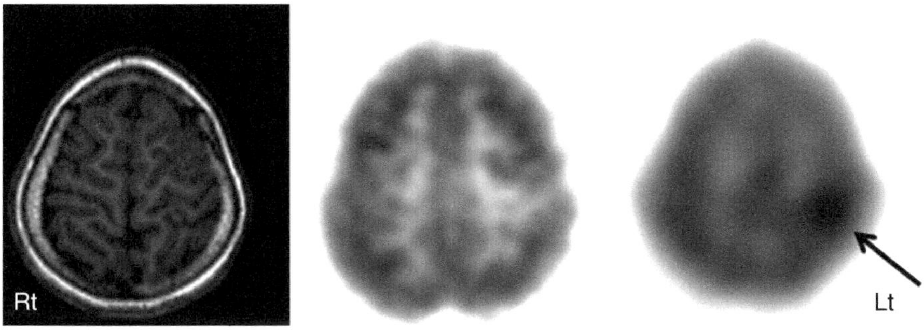

Fig. 47.9 T1-weighted MRI (*left image*), 2-deoxy-2(^{18}F)-fluoro-D-glucose (*middle image*), and ^{11}C-alpha-methyl tryptophan PET scan (*right image*) in a child with intractable epilepsy and a left frontal epileptic focus on the EEG. Whereas MRI was normal and 2-deoxy-2(^{18}F)-fluoro-D-glucose PET showed only mild hypometabolism in the left frontal region, ^{11}C-alpha-methyl tryptophan PET scan showed a focal area of increased tracer uptake interictally in this region (*arrow*). Postsurgical histopathology revealed focal cortical dysplasia

of cortical $GABA_A$ receptor abnormalities in those with or without normal MRI (Richardson et al. 1998, 2001). It should be emphasized that interpretation of FMZ PET images in very young children must take into account the normal developmental patterns seen at this age (Chugani et al. 2013a, b; Chugani 2018) (Fig. 47.8).

Another PET tracer, AMT, a ^{11}C-labeled tryptophan tracer, appears to have an important role in tuberous sclerosis (see below) and some role in selected cases, particularly in patients with cortical dysplasia and normal MRI and mild FDG changes (Juhasz et al. 2003; Wakamoto et al. 2008; Kumar et al. 2011). In these cases, AMT PET sometimes shows increased tracer uptake, particularly in patients with cortical dysplasia type IIB, who usually have very good surgical outcome (Chugani et al. 2011) (Fig. 47.9). This is an important development as it demonstrates, for the first time, that an in vivo imaging technique appears to be able to predict pathologic subtype and thus may provide presurgical prognostic information. Although the *specificity* of AMT PET is very high for detecting the seizure-onset lobe in both lesional (97%) and non-lesional neocortical epilepsies (up to 100%), its *sensitivity* is much lower (47% in lesional vs. 29% in non-lesional cases) (Wakamoto et al. 2008).

There have been a few studies which have evaluated various other brain receptors in extratemporal epilepsy. Lower opiate receptor availability was reported in the left parietal-temporal-occipital cortex in patients with reading epilepsy (Koepp et al. 1998). While reduced dopamine receptor binding in the right putamen was reported in autosomal dominant nocturnal frontal lobe epilepsy (Fedi et al. 2008), another group of investigators found increased tracer binding to nicotinic acetylcholine receptors in the midbrain, pons, and cerebellum and reduced binding in the dorsolateral prefrontal cortex in this condition (Picard et al. 2006).

Obtaining useful SPECT in pediatric extratemporal epilepsy is often difficult, as seizures are usually of short duration and propagate rapidly (such as infantile spasms

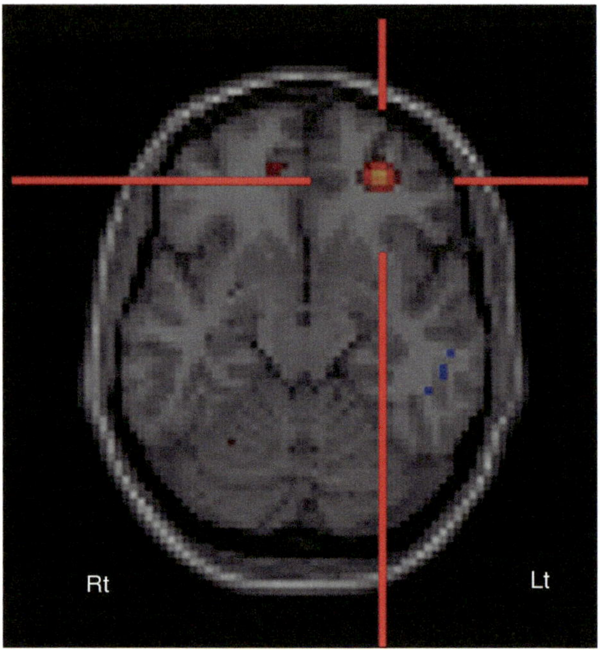

Fig. 47.10 Subtraction ictal SPECT co-registered to MRI (SISCOM) image in a patient with intractable epilepsy, normal MRI, and non-localizing surface EEG. SISCOM revealed a focal area of hyperperfusion in the left inferior frontal cortex (*red cross*)

or myoclonic epilepsy), thus making it difficult to acquire an ictal SPECT study. Postictal scans also appear less helpful because, unlike in temporal lobe epilepsy, seizure-induced perfusion changes do not always extend into the postictal phase. However, a success rate of 70% has been reported for ictal HMPAO SPECT in localizing epileptic foci (Hwang et al. 2001), and under certain conditions, it can be very useful, particularly in children with non-localizing EEG (Marks et al. 1992). Again, the use of SISCOM can further increase its localizing value (O'Brien et al. 1998; Vera et al. 1999) (Fig. 47.10). In two studies, ictal SPECT and SISCOM were found to be more sensitive than FDG PET in the detection of epileptic foci (Sturm et al. 2000; Seo et al. 2011). However, in another study of occipital lobe epilepsy, ictal HMPAO SPECT was found to be less sensitive than FDG PET (Kim et al. 2001). The use of SISCOM appears to increase the diagnostic yield in extratemporal lobe epilepsy also and correlates better with postsurgical outcome (O'Brien et al. 2000; Knowlton et al. 2008). Nevertheless, a multimodal imaging approach may provide the most benefit in children with non-lesional epilepsy (Seo et al. 2011).

47.2.2 Pediatric Epilepsy Syndromes

47.2.2.1 Infantile Spasms or West Syndrome

PET can play an important role in the evaluation of patients with infantile spasms, particularly those diagnosed with cryptogenic infantile spasms (Chugani et al. 1990, 1993). For example, uni- or multifocal cortical metabolic abnormalities were found

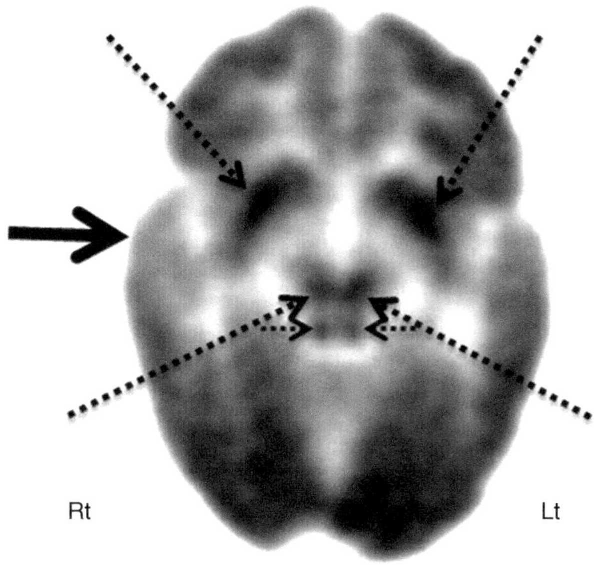

Fig. 47.11 2-Deoxy-2 (^{18}F)-fluoro-D-glucose PET showed focal hypometabolism in the right temporal cortex (*solid arrow*) in a child with infantile spasms and normal MRI. This child may be considered for focal cortical resection for possible seizure control and cognitive improvement. Also noted is hypermetabolism in the bilateral basal ganglia and brain stem nuclei (*dotted arrows*), likely implicating their role in spasm generation

in 95% of children with an initial diagnosis of cryptogenic infantile spasms (Chugani and Conti 1996). Four different patterns of FDG hypometabolism were observed: unifocal in 20%, multifocal in 65%, diffuse in 5%, and bitemporal hypometabolism in 10% of children (Chugani and Conti 1996). Out of these, the patients with unifocal lesion can be considered for epilepsy surgery if they have uncontrolled spasms with the majority of EEG changes corresponding to the PET-defined lesion, as the surgical removal of focal brain lesion leads not only to cessation of the spasms but also to improved neurocognitive outcome (Fig. 47.11) (Branch and Dyken 1979; Mimaki et al. 1983; Palm et al. 1988; Ruggieri et al. 1989; Uthman et al. 1991; Chugani et al. 1993, Chugani et al. 2015; Asarnow et al. 1997; Jonas et al. 2005; Yum et al. 2011). Occasionally, patients with a multifocal pattern can also be considered for palliative surgery, with improved quality of life but guarded developmental outcome, if the majority of seizures originate from one region (Chugani et al. 2010; Ilyas et al. 2014). The diffuse metabolic pattern is likely associated with underlying metabolic, genetic, or neurodegenerative pathology, and these patients are unlikely to be surgical candidates. Interestingly, children with bitemporal hypometabolism show a distinct clinical phenotype characterized by severe developmental delay, particularly in the language domain, and autism or pervasive developmental disorder (Chugani et al. 1996). These children are unlikely to become surgical candidates. Longitudinal studies have shown that the PET abnormalities are not always static, but may evolve as the brain matures (Sakaguchi et al. 2018).

FDG PET can also shed some light on the possible pathomechanism of epileptic spasms. For example, these patients may show a focal cortical hypometabolism along with prominent glucose metabolism in the lenticular nuclei and brain stem, suggesting complex cortical-subcortical interactions (Fig. 47.11) (Chugani et al. 1992). Basal ganglia and brain stem involvement likely suggests their role in the secondary generalization of focal cortical discharges, resulting in spasms. It appears that the spasms result primarily from focal or diffuse cortical abnormalities interacting with the brain stem and lenticular nuclei and that this type of generalization accounts for the bilateral motor involvement and relative symmetry of the majority of spasms even in the presence of a discrete focal lesion (Chugani et al. 1992). Ictal and interictal brain SPECT can also provide some interesting clues regarding the probable origin and propagation of electrical events responsible for spasms. Interictal SPECT studies have shown perfusion abnormalities, ranging from cortical hypoperfusion (Chiron et al. 1993; Miyazaki et al. 1994; Hwang et al. 1996; Sztriha et al. 1997; Haginoya et al. 1998, 2001) to cortical hyperperfusion (Chiron et al. 1993). Ictal SPECT has shown areas of cortical hyperperfusion with occasional hyperperfusion of the subcortical structures (Haginoya et al. 1998, 2001), consistent with FDG PET findings. Recent studies, using a combination of interictal and ictal SPECT, found ictal *hyper*perfusion of a cortical lesion and basal ganglia, supporting the notion that secondary generalization from a cortical focus may account for the spasms (Mori et al. 2007; Kakisaka et al. 2009). The finding of localized cortical perfusion defects in some children with West syndrome confirms that focal cortical lesions play an important role in its development (Haginoya et al. 2000). Interestingly, in infants, hyperperfusion has been found interictally in the area of cortical dysgenesis and appears to be specific for this young population (Hwang et al. 1996; Haginoya et al. 2000). These findings corroborate the notion that infantile spasms result from complex cortical-subcortical interaction with age and brain maturity playing an important role. Rapid involvement of the basal ganglia and brain stem likely results in the secondary generalization of a seemingly partial seizure, arising from a focal cortical lesion (Chugani et al. 1992). What leads to this interaction is yet to be elucidated.

47.2.2.2 Tuberous Sclerosis

Tuberous sclerosis complex (TSC) is an autosomal dominant neurocutaneous disorder characterized by multiple cortical tubers, caused by inactivating mutations in the TSC genes. Epilepsy is the main manifestation of this condition, with a prevalence of 80–90% (Osborne et al. 1991), becoming refractory to medical treatment in 50–80% of cases, as early as 2 years of age (Evans et al. 2012). As intractable seizures have a detrimental effect on neurocognitive development, these patients often benefit from epilepsy surgery (Perot et al. 1966). However, many times it is difficult to localize the epileptic focus, due to multifocal EEG changes and multiplicity of cortical tubers, even though a single tuber may be epileptogenic. In these cases, PET can play a valuable role by noninvasively lateralizing and localizing the epileptic focus *interictally* and rendering these patients surgical candidates. FDG PET can show the tubers (Asano et al. 2000, 2005; Ohta et al. 2001; Karenfort et al. 2002; Chandra et al. 2006; Weiner et al. 2006; Moshel et al. 2010; Wu et al. 2010; Carlson et al. 2011); however, it cannot identify the epileptogenic one, as all tubers appear hypometabolic (Fig. 47.12). AMT PET has been reported to be very useful in this condition, as it shows increased tracer uptake in epileptogenic tubers only (Fig. 47.12) (Chugani et al. 1998a, 2013a, b; Asano et al. 2000; Fedi et al. 2003;

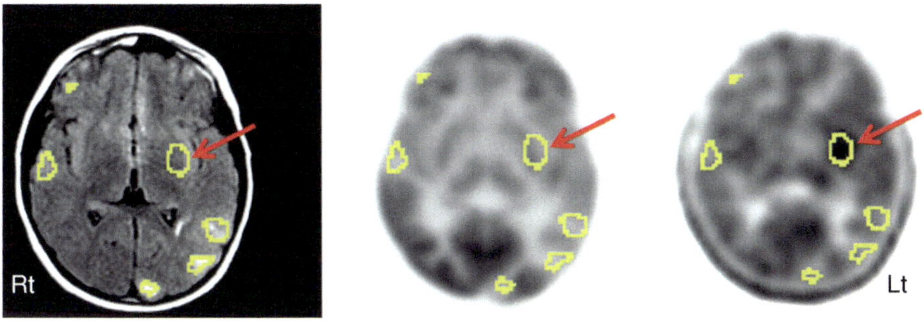

Fig. 47.12 FLAIR MRI (*left image*), 2-deoxy-2(^{18}F)-fluoro-D-glucose (*middle image*), and ^{11}C-alpha-methyl tryptophan PET (*right image*) scan in a patient with multiple tubers (*encircled* with "region of interests"), intractable seizures, and non-localizing scalp EEG. While 2-deoxy-2(^{18}F)-fluoro-D-glucose PET showed hypometabolism in all the tubers and overlying cortices, interictal ^{11}C-alpha-methyl tryptophan PET scan revealed increased alpha-methyl tryptophan uptake in an insular tuber (*arrow*)

Rubí et al. 2013), sometimes at one of its edges only with some involvement of the adjacent apparently normal cortex; such cortical regions usually turn out to be dysplastic on histopathological examination (Kagawa et al. 2005). The increased AMT uptake appears to be due to the activation of the kynurenine pathway, leading to the production of quinolinic acid, a proconvulsant, in the tuber and dysplastic cortex (Chugani et al. 1998a). AMT PET with quantitative evaluation of lesional uptake levels can identify epileptogenic tuber(s) in almost two-thirds of children with tuberous sclerosis and intractable epilepsy and is almost 100% specific (Chugani et al. 1998a; Asano et al. 2000; Fedi et al. 2003). Tubers with at least 10% increase of AMT uptake appear to be invariably epileptogenic, and a cutoff threshold of 1.02 for AMT uptake ratio provides 83% accuracy for detecting tubers that need to be resected to achieve a seizure-free outcome (Asano et al. 2000; Kagawa et al. 2005). The high specificity of increased AMT uptake is also suggested by the good correlation between resections of epileptogenic tubers, showing increased AMT uptake and seizure outcome (Kagawa et al. 2005). However, its sensitivity is suboptimal, likely depending upon the underlying pathology and method of data analysis. It appears that MRI-based quantitative assessment can increase the sensitivity of AMT PET to 79% from 44% with visual assessment (Juhasz et al. 2002). This may be related to the fact that non-epileptic tubers show decreased AMT uptake and the epileptogenic ones with relatively increased AMT uptake but still close to the surrounding normal cortex, and therefore, these increases might appear subtle and be missed on visual analysis. SPECT can also play an important role in identifying epileptic tubers, by showing them hyperperfused during ictal phase (Koh et al. 1999; Romanelli et al. 2002; Weiner et al. 2006; Moshel et al. 2010; Aboian et al. 2011; Carlson et al. 2011). A good correlation has been reported between ictal SPECT and ictal scalp EEG (Koh et al. 1999; Mori et al. 2007). SISCOM further increases the usefulness of SPECT in identifying the epileptogenic zone and in guiding the location and extent of epilepsy surgery in children with tuberous sclerosis complex and multifocal abnormalities (Aboian et al. 2011). Complete resection of the SISCOM hyperperfusion abnormality was found to be associated with seizure freedom. SPECT, using ^{123}I-iomazenil, has been used to evaluate benzodiazepine receptor status in patients with tuberous sclerosis (Kuki et al. 2008, 2012; Mori et al. 2012). GABA receptor binding was found to be decreased in cortical tubers (Mori et al. 2012), suggesting that decreased neuronal inhibition might have a role in epileptogenesis in this condition.

47.2.2.3 Lennox-Gastaut Syndrome

FDG PET can help in the metabolic characterization of the brain in *Lennox-Gastaut syndrome*, a triad of multiple seizure types including tonic seizures, developmental delay, and 1–2.5 Hz generalized "slow" spike-and-wave EEG pattern, which may have implication for prognosis, as well as treatment planning (Gur et al. 1982; Chugani et al. 1987b; Iinuma et al. 1987; Theodore et al. 1987; Miyauchi et al. 1988; Ferrie et al. 1996; You et al. 2007; Zhai et al. 2010; Hur et al. 2011). These patients may show four metabolic patterns on FDG PET scan: unilateral focal hypometabolism, unilateral diffuse hypometabolism, bilateral diffuse hypometabolism, and normal patterns (Chugani et al. 1987b). Interictal SPECT usually shows multiple areas of hypoperfusion (Heiskala et al. 1993). Patients with unilateral focal pattern may be occasionally considered for cortical resection provided there is good concordance between PET and ictal EEG findings (You et al. 2007; Hur et al. 2011).

47.2.2.4 Sturge-Weber Syndrome

In children with *Sturge-Weber syndrome* (*SWS*), FDG PET reveals hypometabolism in the involved cortex and usually identifies additional areas of abnormal cortex extending beyond the abnormality seen on MRI (Chugani et al. 1989; Juhasz et al. 2007). However, affected infants may show a paradoxical pattern of *increased* glucose metabolism interictally in the cortex underlying the leptomeningeal angioma; as the disease progresses, the hypermetabolic area becomes hypometabolic (Fig. 47.13) (Chugani et al. 1989). The presence of early cortical hypermetabolism on PET may be an imaging marker of subsequent severe epilepsy, requiring surgery (Alkonyi et al. 2011). In some young patients, serial FDG PET scans show rapidly progressing and severe hypometabolism in the affected area, probably because of rapid demise of the brain tissue associated with the angioma: these patients will have improvement in seizure status and paradoxical preservation of cognitive function and therefore may not require surgical intervention (Behen et al. 2011). Early and rapid progression in unilateral cases of SWS leads to early and more efficient reorganization in the contralateral cortex. On the other hand, persistent mild hypometabolism of the lesion may indicate ongoing functional disturbance, and these patients may show persistent seizures and developmental arrest (Lee et al. 2001b; Behen et al. 2011). These are the patients who require surgical intervention for seizure control and possible cognitive improvement by promoting effective reorganization in the contralateral hemisphere while brain plasticity is still at a maximum during development. In SWS, detrimental metabolic changes mostly occur before 3–4 years of age (Juhasz et al. 2007), coinciding with a sharp increase in

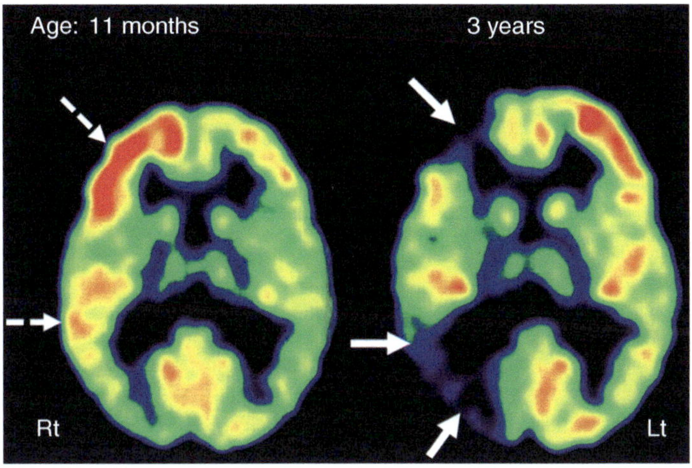

Fig. 47.13 Serial 2-deoxy-2(^{18}F)-fluoro-D-glucose PET scan showing progression of glucose metabolic abnormalities in the affected right hemisphere (MRI showed extensive leptomeningeal enhancement on that side) in a child with Sturge-Weber syndrome. PET scan at 11 months of age showed a transient increase of metabolism, most prominent in the frontal lobe and mild in the temporal cortex (*dashed arrows*). Repeat PET at 3 years of age showed severe hypometabolism in the right frontal and temporal cortices (*solid arrows*)

developmentally regulated cerebral metabolic demand (Chugani et al. 1987a). Progressive hypometabolism is associated with high seizure frequency in these children. However, metabolic abnormalities may remain limited or even partially recover later in some children with well-controlled seizures. Metabolic recovery accompanied by neurological improvement suggests a critical window for therapeutic intervention in children with unilateral SWS (Juhasz et al. 2007). FDG PET can also be used to assess for cognitive function and regional functional reorganization (Bosnyák et al. 2016; Kim et al. 2018).

Perfusion SPECT, using xenon-133, showed hyperperfusion in the lesion even before seizure onset (Pinton et al. 1997), analogous to the transient hypermetabolism seen on PET (Chugani et al. 1989; Juhasz et al. 2007). After 1 year of age, these areas typically show hypoperfusion, as revealed by another xenon-133 SPECT study (Chiron et al. 1989). In a single case report on a patient with failed functional hemispherectomy, ictal ECD SPECT showed hyperperfusion in the residual lesion with falsely lateralized EEG; further surgery resulted in seizure freedom (Bilgin et al. 2008). In recent years, SPECT studies have been largely replaced by perfusion MRI, which can be performed in conjunction with conventional clinical MRI and provide quantitative maps of blood volume and blood flow in children with Sturge-Weber syndrome (Alkonyi et al. 2012).

47.2.2.5 Hemimegalencephaly

Hemimegalencephaly is a severe congenital malformation of hemispheric development with a unilateral enlarged and defectively developed hemisphere and

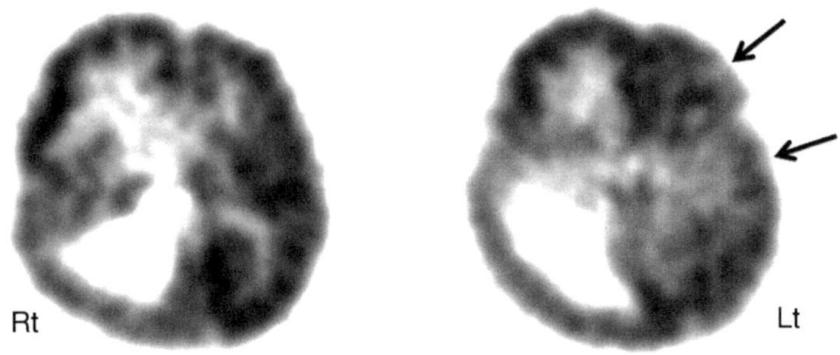

Fig. 47.14 2-Deoxy-2(^{18}F)-fluoro-D-glucose PET scan in a child with right hemimegalencephaly showing an enlarged right hemisphere with increased glucose metabolism in the right frontal lobe because of epileptic activity during the radiotracer uptake period. Also noted are mildly hypometabolic areas in the frontal and temporal regions of the left hemisphere (*arrows*), indicating functional impairment of this hemisphere, which appeared to be normal on MRI. Although right hemispherectomy resulted in seizure freedom, the child remained developmentally delayed because of an abnormal left hemisphere

intractable seizures. PET and SPECT usually show variable appearance in the involved hemisphere: hypo- and/or hypermetabolism on the FDG PET and hypo- and/or hyperperfusion on HMPAO or ECD SPECT, depending upon the seizure status at the time of scanning. Early hemisphere disconnection in these children may lead to seizure control and improved cognitive development, provided the other hemisphere is normal. Therefore, the main role of PET or SPECT is the evaluation of the apparently normal hemisphere (Fig. 47.14). In children with hemimegalencephaly, FDG PET often shows additional less pronounced abnormalities in the opposite hemisphere, which probably accounts for the suboptimal cognitive outcome even with complete seizure control after surgical removal of the profoundly abnormal hemisphere (Rintahaka et al. 1993). Thus, FDG PET can be useful in such cases to assess the functional integrity of the contralateral hemisphere prior to hemispherectomy and help predict cognitive outcome.

47.2.2.6 Rasmussen's Encephalitis and Epilepsy of Suspected Inflammatory Origin

FDG PET can show both hyper- or hypometabolism in cases of Rasmussen's encephalitis, depending upon the seizure status during the scan (Tien et al. 1992; Fiorella et al. 2001; Lee et al. 2001a). It can particularly help in the unequivocal identification of the affected cerebral hemisphere in patients whose MR imaging findings are subtle or distributed bilaterally (Fiorella et al. 2001). FDG PET can further help in guiding the site of biopsy when indicated, thus assisting in earlier diagnosis. Interictal hypometabolism expands over time and usually precedes the anatomical changes, thus further helping in clarifying the equivocal cases or assessing the functional impairment and its evolution (Lee et al. 2001a). Perfusion SPECT also shows hyper- or hypometabolism of the affected cortex, depending upon the seizure status during the tracer injection, and can guide the histopathological evaluation or surgical planning (Yacubian et al. 1997; Burneo et al. 2006). It appears that benzodiazepine SPECT and FDG PET can detect the ictal-onset area efficiently even in the absence of MRI abnormalities (Kuki et al. 2018).

Neuroinflammation is the underlying cause for intractable epilepsy in Rasmussen's encephalitis, as well as some other epileptic conditions. Neuroinflammation is mediated by activated microglia, which secrete a number of proinflammatory molecules such as cytokines, chemokines, and neurotoxins, free radicals, nitric oxide, proteinases, eicosanoids, and excitotoxins, which may play a role in epileptogenesis. Although the exact mechanisms are unclear, it appears that the inflammatory mediators act by increasing glutamatergic neurotransmission, decreasing GABA-mediated currents and inducing neovascularization, and damaging the blood-brain barrier. Detection of microglia is not possible with current radiological methods or biochemical techniques; however, they can be imaged with PET tracers binding to the activated microglia. ^{11}C-PK11195 is the most commonly used radioligand which binds specifically to the translocator protein receptors, predominantly expressed by the activated microglia in cases of neuroinflammation, thus making the in vivo detection of neuroinflammation possible (Banati et al. 1999). PET scanning using ^{11}C-PK11195 can help in the early diagnosis of Rasmussen's syndrome or other inflammatory conditions with intractable seizures, where CT and MRI are often normal for several months after the

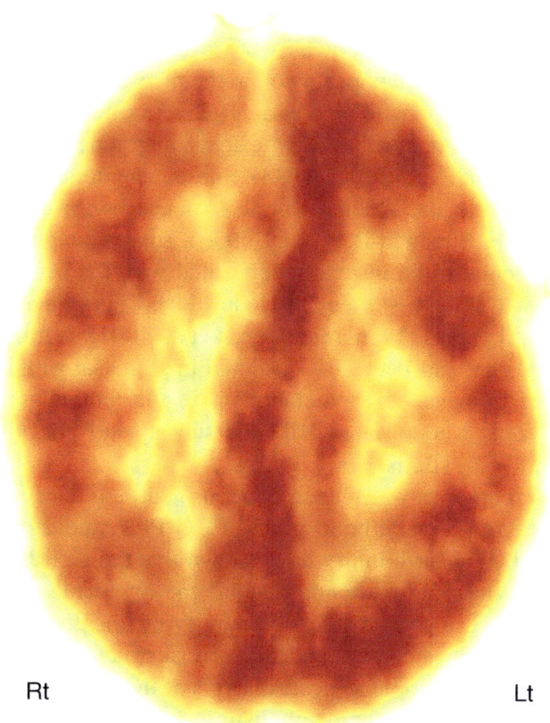

Fig. 47.15 ^{11}C-PK11195 PET scan showing increased radiotracer binding in the left hemisphere, indicating neuroinflammation mediated by activated microglia, in a child with Rasmussen's encephalitis

clinical manifestation of the disease (Fig. 47.15). Localization of the most affected brain regions may also provide a guide in deciding the site of brain biopsy in order to avoid sampling errors and can help in the surgical removal of that region (Kumar et al. 2008).

Autoimmune encephalitis is increasingly being recognized as an important cause of intractable epilepsy in adults and children, and a number of antibodies targeting brain proteins have been identified (reviewed in Spatola and Dalmau 2017). Depending upon the specific antibody, different brain regions may be involved, but in general, FDG PET shows hypermetabolism in the acute stages and hypometabolism in the chronic stages (Guerin et al. 2019). Further studies with PET and SPECT using radioligands targeting microglia (neuroinflammation) in autoimmune encephalitis will be potentially useful clinically, but a major obstacle in performing such studies is the rapid availability of the tracer in the acute setting when anti-inflammatory treatment cannot be withheld ethically.

47.3 Other Neurological Disorders

47.3.1 Perinatal Hypoxic Ischemic Brain Injury and Cerebral Palsy

PET scanning of cerebral glucose metabolism can be helpful to assess severity of brain damage in infants with hypoxic ischemic encephalopathy (HIE) and brain injury. Early FDG PET studies found areas of hypometabolism, extending beyond the affected regions shown by CT scan (Doyle et al. 1983). Cerebral perfusion PET showed relative hypoperfusion in the parasagittal regions in full-term neonates with perinatal asphyxia (Volpe et al. 1985). In preterm infants with intraventricular and intracerebral hemorrhage, large areas of hypoperfusion were reported in the affected hemisphere (Volpe et al. 1983). Subsequent studies suggested that persistently low cerebral glucose metabolism is associated with delayed development in children with HIE (Suhonen-Polvi et al. 1993). Total brain glucose metabolic rates (CMRglc) were found to be inversely correlated with the severity of HIE: neonates with the lowest CMRglc subsequently developed permanent neurological symptoms and cerebral palsy (Thorngren-Jerneck et al. 2001). A transient increase of glucose metabolic rates has been also observed in the basal ganglia in the neonatal period, followed by severe hypometabolism in the lenticular nuclei and thalami, in some newborns who suffered HIE and subsequently developed dystonic cerebral palsy (Fig. 47.16) (Batista et al. 2007).

Cerebral palsy is a heterogeneous neurological condition that sometimes may be related to perinatal brain injury. FDG PET studies of these children with cerebral palsy due to birth injury have shown that the distribution of metabolic impairment almost invariably extends beyond the apparent anatomical involvement seen on MRI. PET also can help in identifying the location and severity of functional involvement of cortical and subcortical structures in the major subtypes of cerebral palsy in the chronic stages. Analysis of these different subtypes demonstrated focal areas of cortical hypometabolism in spastic diplegic patients, without any obvious

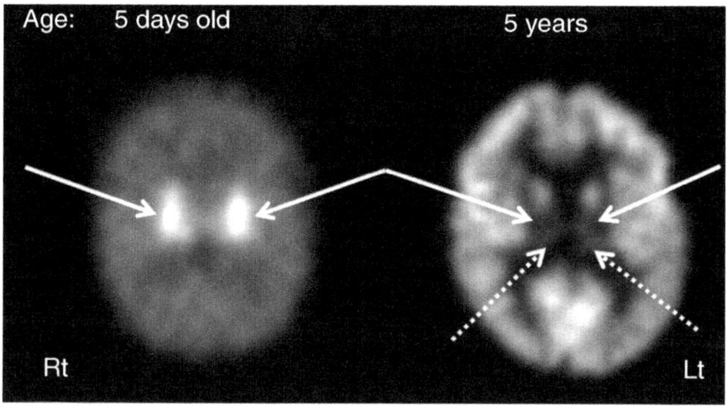

Fig. 47.16 2-Deoxy-2(^{18}F)-fluoro-D-glucose PET scans of a child who suffered hypoxic ischemic encephalopathy at birth and later developed dystonic/choreoathetoid cerebral palsy. The *left image* from the newborn period showed intense hypermetabolism in the basal ganglia (*solid arrows*). The *right image* at 5 years of age showed severe hypometabolism in the lenticular nuclei (*solid arrows*) and thalami (*dotted arrows*). Note the relative preservation of metabolism in the cerebral cortex

cortical lesion on structural imaging; in contrast, a relatively normal pattern of cortical metabolism is seen in some children with choreoathetoid cerebral palsy, who often show hypometabolism in the thalamus and lenticular nuclei (Kerrigan et al. 1991). Relative sparing of the cerebral cortex is consistent with the clinical observation that many of these children have good cognitive function despite suffering from severe motor impairment. Use of FMZ PET has demonstrated increased GABA receptor binding in the bilateral motor and visual cortex and decreased binding in the brain stem, suggesting a role of abnormal GABA mechanisms in poor motor control (Lee et al. 2007). In addition, recent studies with a rabbit model of intrauterine brain injury suggested that PET imaging of activated microglia in newborns, using ^{11}C-PK11195, can detect neuroinflammatory changes in the white matter that later develops severe structural damage causing symptoms of cerebral palsy (Kannan et al. 2007).

47.3.2 Autism

Functional neuroimaging in autism is currently a clinical research tool and has been utilized to identify neuroanatomic substrates involved in various symptoms associated with the disease. In early studies with PET scanning, increased glucose metabolic rates were reported in multiple brain regions in autistic adults, but no common regional abnormality could be identified (Rumsey et al. 1985). In a subsequent study involving 18 autistic children, neither the rates nor the regional distribution of brain glucose metabolism was different from those in control subjects (De Volder et al. 1987). Similarly, no significant abnormality in regional cerebral blood flow, oxygen consumption, and metabolism was reported in six adult autistic subjects (Herold et al. 1988). However, another study found some reversed (left > right) asymmetry of glucose metabolism in the anterior rectal gyrus (Siegel et al. 1992). A combined MRI and PET study in high-functioning autistic patients reported volume loss and associated hypometabolism in the anterior and posterior cingulate (Haznedar et al. 1997, 2000). Perfusion PET studies using radiolabeled water found hypoperfusion in the right dentate nucleus and left frontal cortex during verbal auditory and expressive language tasks (Muller et al. 1998) and hypoperfusion of the superior temporal cortex during acoustic stimulation and the cerebellum during nonverbal auditory perception task (Muller et al. 1999). Subsequently, lower glucose metabolism was reported in the medial frontal cortex and cingulate (Hazlett et al. 2004) and in the ventral caudate, putamen, and thalamus (Haznedar et al. 2006) during verbal memory task in autistic subjects.

Simultaneously with glucose PET studies, several SPECT studies attempted to find global or focal cerebral perfusion abnormalities in autistic subjects in the 1990s; most early studies were small, and the results were mixed. One study found no regional perfusion abnormalities in 21 autistic children on xenon-133 SPECT (Zilbovicius et al. 1992). Another smaller HMPAO SPECT study found global hypoperfusion as well as regions with hypoperfusion, including the right lateral temporal lobe and frontal lobes in four autistic adults (George et al. 1992). In a subsequent longitudinal study, the same group reported frontal hypoperfusion in autistic children at ages 3–4 years, which disappeared by the ages of 6–7 years, suggesting a delayed frontal maturation in childhood autism. Yet another HMPAO SPECT study showed decreased blood flow in the temporoparietal region in six autistic patients between 9 and 21 years of age, without any apparent clinical correlation (Mountz et al. 1995). A relatively larger ECD SPECT study, including 23 children with infantile autism compared to 26 non-autistic controls (matched for age and IQ), reported decreased regional blood flow in the bilateral insula, superior temporal gyri, and left prefrontal cortices and found several clinico-imaging correlations (Ohnishi et al. 2000). First, altered perfusion in the medial prefrontal cortex and anterior cingulate gyrus was associated with impairments in communication and social interaction (related to deficits in the theory of mind), and second, altered perfusion in the right medial temporal lobe was related to the obsessive desire for sameness. Thus, these findings pointed to specific locations of brain dysfunction underlying abnormal behavioral patterns in autistic patients. More recent studies have utilized objective analytic approaches such as SPM to identify abnormal cerebral blood flow patterns in autism. One such study, using ECD SPECT, also reported both global reductions and an increased right-left perfusion asymmetry in 11 autistic children, as compared to age-matched healthy children; the asymmetries were particularly prominent in the temporoparietal areas associated with language and comprehension of music and sound (Burroni et al. 2008). Another study, using a similar approach in 23 children with autistic spectrum disorder (mostly boys), found bilateral frontal, temporal, and basal ganglia hypoperfusion in autistic children (Yang et al. 2011). Interestingly, there were greater asymmetries in children with Asperger syndrome than autism, suggesting different neurobiological mechanisms. Recently, cerebral hypoperfusion using functional neuroimaging in autism subjects has been reviewed (Bjørklund et al. 2018).

PET imaging with various radiotracers allows the study of global and regional cerebral abnormalities of specific neurotransmitter systems and their potential roles in the pathophysiology of autism. These studies have been designed based on previous work demonstrating alterations in neurotransmitters, hormones, and their metabolites in the blood, cerebrospinal fluid (CSF), and urine of autistic patients. In a PET study using [^{18}F]-labeled fluorodopa (F-DOPA, a precursor of dopamine, accumulated in dopaminergic terminals) in 14 medication-free autistic children, decreased dopaminergic activity was found only in the anterior medial prefrontal cortex in the autistic group, suggesting that decreased dopaminergic function in the prefrontal cortex may contribute to the cognitive impairment seen in autism (Ernst et al. 1997). A subsequent study of 20 adults with autism also demonstrated increased dopamine transporter binding in the orbitofrontal cortex, and these abnormalities were inversely correlated with serotonin transporter binding, suggesting a potential interplay between the dopaminergic and serotonergic systems in affected brain regions (Nakamura et al. 2010).

Abnormalities of the serotonergic system have been long implicated in the pathophysiology of autism. Tryptophan depletion, leading to decreased serotonin levels, resulted in an exacerbation of symptoms in autistic subjects (McDougle et al. 1996b). Conversely, serotonin reuptake inhibitors may result in the improvement of compulsive symptoms, repetitive movements, and social difficulties in autistic adults (Cook et al. 1992; Gordon et al. 1993; McDougle et al. 1996a). Chugani et al. (1997) used AMT PET scanning to study children with autism and their healthy non-autistic siblings. AMT PET demonstrated robust AMT uptake asymmetries in the frontal cortex, thalamus, and cerebellum in seven autistic boys (Fig. 47.17); however, this pattern was not seen in one autistic girl and in four of the five siblings. Specifically, decreased AMT accumulation was seen in the left frontal cortex and

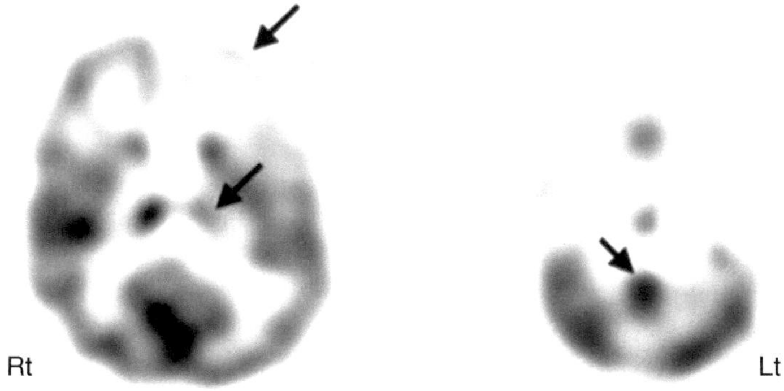

Fig. 47.17 ^{11}C-Alpha-methyl tryptophan PET showing asymmetric alpha-methyl tryptophan uptake in the frontal cortex, thalamus, and dentate nucleus of the cerebellum in a boy with autism spectrum disorder, with decreased uptake in the ipsilateral frontal cortex and thalamus and with increased uptake in the contralateral dentate nucleus (*arrows*), suggesting the involvement of dentato-thalamo-cortical pathway in autism

thalamus in five of seven autistic boys, while elevated AMT accumulation was present in the right cerebellum, in the dentate nucleus. The same children showed a normal pattern of brain glucose metabolism and normal MRI on visual evaluation, supporting that the observed novel focal cerebral abnormalities on AMT PET were specific for serotonergic abnormalities. In a subsequent larger study, Chugani et al. (1999) also reported global brain values for serotonin synthesis capacity of 54 children: 30 healthy seizure-free autistic children (24 males, 2–15 years), eight healthy non-autistic siblings (six males, 2–14 years), and 16 epileptic children without autism (nine males, 3 months–13 years). Non-autistic children showed a nonlinear change in global serotonin synthesis capacity: their values reached >200% of adult values until the age of about 5 years and then gradually declined toward adult values. In autistic children, a different developmental pattern was found: serotonin synthesis capacity increased gradually between the ages of 2 and 15 years to values 1.5 times of the adult normal values. The data indicated a period of relatively high brain serotonin synthesis capacity during childhood and that the normal developmental process is disrupted in autistic children. These results prompted further larger-scale imaging studies of the serotonergic system of the developing brain in autism. When data of a larger group (n = 117) of autistic children were analyzed, additional focal patterns were recognized, including right cortical and left cortical decreases and a subgroup with no abnormal asymmetry (Chandana et al. 2005). Children with left cortical AMT uptake decreases showed a higher prevalence of severe language impairment, whereas right cortical decreases were associated with left and mixed handedness. These studies, altogether, suggested that both global and focal asymmetric development in the serotonergic system may be implicated in abnormal "wiring" of neural circuits related to hemispheric specialization. Therefore, restoration of serotonin levels pharmacologically in a critical age window may alter developmental trajectory and improve symptoms of autistic children. Indeed, molecular imaging using various radiotracers may provide important biomarkers and pave the way for new therapeutic interventions (Hwang et al. 2017).

47.3.3 Developmental Dyslexia

Dyslexia is a specific learning disability that manifests primarily with difficulty in written language, particularly with reading and spelling. Various PET studies have shown the predominant involvement of bilateral posterior temporal and parietal cortices. Initial cerebral blood flow studies, using Xe-133, found increased left more than right asymmetry and reduced anterior to posterior difference (Rumsey et al. 1987), as well as hypoperfusion in the left superior temporal region with hyperperfusion in the more posterior temporoparietal region (Flowers et al. 1991). Subsequently, PET studies using ^{15}O-labeled water in dyslexic subjects showed a failure to activate the left temporoparietal cortex during a rhyme detection task and reduced activation/unusual deactivation in the mid- and posterior temporal cortex bilaterally and also in inferior parietal cortex, predominantly on the left side (Rumsey et al. 1992, 1997). Other PET studies showed less activation in the right superior temporal and right postcentral gyri and left cerebellum (McCrory et al. 2000) or in the right cerebellar cortex and left cingulate gyrus (Nicolson et al. 1999). Functional disconnection of the left angular gyrus from other parts of the reading network has also been reported in adults with persistent developmental dyslexia (Horwitz et al. 1998). A recent ^{15}O PET study of the learning of phoneme categorization found a less strongly left-lateralized activation involving the superior temporal, inferior parietal, and inferior lateral frontal cortex during the speech mode (Dufor et al. 2007). Frontal and parietal subparts of these left-sided regions were found to be significantly less activated in the dyslexic subjects. However, larger activations in the right frontal cortex for both speech and acoustic modes compared to the rest and an unexpected large deactivation in the medial occipital cortex for the acoustic mode were noted in the dyslexic subjects. Subsequently, the same group found activity enhancement in left premotor cortex, likely related to the persistence of motor coding for allophonic representations of speech (Dufor et al. 2009).

FDG PET studies have shown diminished asymmetry in glucose metabolism in prefrontal and lingual (inferior) regions of the occipital lobe during reading in dyslexic subjects, indicating that brain regions are activated differently in this disorder (Gross-Glenn et al. 1991). Another FDG PET study showed significantly higher absolute and relative brain metabolism along an anterior-posterior gradient, including the medial temporal lobe, in dyslexic subjects, during an auditory syllable discrimination task, suggesting more effortful processing in dyslexia (Hagman et al. 1992). Perfusion SPECT has also shown hypoperfusion in areas involved in the reading and writing processes, predominantly in the temporal lobe (Kaneko et al. 1998; Arduini et al. 2006; Sauer et al. 2006).

47.3.4 Landau-Kleffner Syndrome

Landau-Kleffner syndrome (LKS) is characterized by the sudden or gradual development of aphasia in children who had previously developed typically with normal language until disease onset. While many of the affected children have clinical seizures, some may have only electrographic seizures. FDG PET usually shows bilateral temporal lobe involvement, in the form of hyper- or hypometabolism depending upon the electrographic status of this region, particularly of the superior and medial part (Maquet et al. 1990; Rintahaka et al. 1995; da Silva et al. 1997; Honbolygo et al. 2006; Shiraishi et al. 2007). During the phase of aphasia, frequent epileptiform spiking is seen in these regions, associated with glucose hypermetabolism on FDG PET, which becomes quiescent during remission, manifested as hypometabolism on FDG PET scan. FDG PET can also show the possible involvement of temporal lobes in the generation of continuous spike waves during slow-wave sleep (Maquet et al. 1990, 1995; Rintahaka et al. 1995). FDG PET can be further useful to monitor dynamic changes of glucose metabolism in the temporal lobe during episodes of aphasia and remission, where it shows hyper- and hypometabolism, likely related to presence or absence of continuous spiking on scalp EEG, respectively, during these periods (Fig. 47.18) (Luat et al. 2006). Using ^{15}O-labeled water PET, posterior

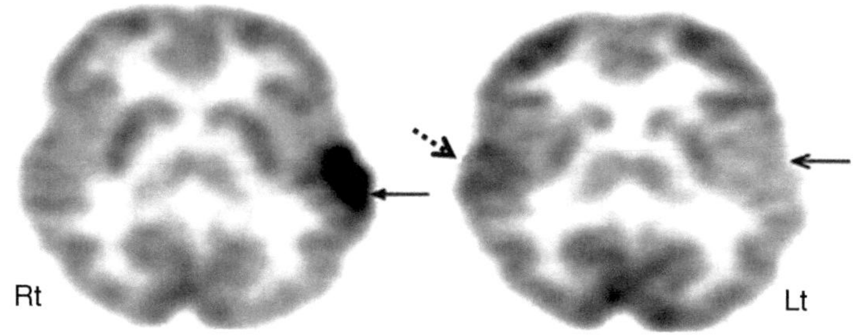

Fig. 47.18 2-Deoxy-2(^{18}F)-fluoro-D-glucose PET scan in a child with Landau-Kleffner syndrome showing marked hypermetabolism in the left temporal region (*arrow*) during the peak of his aphasic episode. EEG, performed during PET scan, showed frequent spike-and-wave activity from this region. A repeat PET scan during his remission state showed hypometabolism in the same region (*arrow*). Interestingly, a mildly increased glucose metabolism is noted in the second PET scan on the other side (right superior temporal cortex—*broken arrow*), which corresponded to some spike-and-wave discharges from this region

superior temporal gyri were found to have decreased perfusion/activation, long after remission was achieved in patients with LKS, and residual impairment in verbal short-term memory, suggesting an important role played by the temporal lobe in this condition (Majerus et al. 2003). FMZ PET revealed a deficit in benzodiazepine receptor binding at the tip of the left temporal lobe in a child affected by LKS, suggesting that the tip of the left temporal lobe might play an important role in the pathogenesis of this disease (Shiraishi et al. 2007). SPECT studies have also shown variable perfusion abnormalities, predominantly in uni- or bilateral temporal lobes, ranging from hypo- to hyperperfusion, likely related to the timing of the SPECT (Hu et al. 1989; O'Tuama et al. 1992; Guerreiro et al. 1996; Harbord et al. 1999; Sayit et al. 1999; Sinclair and Snyder 2005; Shiraishi et al. 2007).

47.3.5 Tourette Syndrome

Tourette syndrome is an inherited neuropsychiatric disorder with onset in childhood and is characterized by the presence of multiple motor tics and at least one vocal tic for more than 1 year. Initial studies using FDG PET, in a limited number of children with Tourette syndrome, failed to show any consistent glucose metabolic abnormalities. Decreased metabolic rates were reported in various regions, including paralimbic and ventral prefrontal cortices (Braun et al. 1993). Decreases were also observed in subcortical regions, including the ventral striatum (nucleus accumbens/ventromedial caudate) and in the midbrain. These changes were more robust and occurred with greater frequency in the left hemisphere and were associated with bilateral increases in metabolic activity of the supplementary motor, lateral premotor, and Rolandic cortices. Subsequently, cerebral perfusion PET studies were used for the investigation of neuronal circuits involved in tic generation. An ^{15}O PET cerebral blood flow study showed widely distributed tic-associated activation in the medial and lateral premotor cortices, anterior cingulate cortex, dorsolateral rostral prefrontal cortex, inferior parietal cortex, putamen, and caudate, as well as the primary motor cortex, Broca's area, superior temporal gyrus, insula, and claustrum (Stern et al. 2000). Another ^{15}O PET study showed robust activation of the cerebellum, insula, thalamus, and putamen during tic release (Lerner et al. 2007). Based on these studies, it can be postulated that aberrant activity in the interrelated sensorimotor, language, executive, and paralimbic circuits may account for the initiation and execution of diverse motor and vocal behaviors in Tourette syndrome.

Imaging studies of dopaminergic transmission sought to determine the potential contribution of abnormalities in the dopaminergic system to the pathophysiology of Tourette syndrome. Several aspects of dopaminergic abnormalities have been studied, including striatal dopamine transporter levels, which were elevated (Krause et al. 2002); presynaptic DOPA decarboxylase activity (Ernst et al. 1999); and D2 receptor availability, which was found to be decreased (Gilbert et al. 2006). These abnormalities again could be detected in widespread cortical and subcortical regions (e.g., the orbitofrontal cortex, primary motor cortex, anterior cingulate gyrus, mediodorsal nucleus of thalamus, and hippocampus), suggesting abnormalities in brain networks important for motivation and reward, sensory gating, movement, and attention. Another study also demonstrated increased dopamine release in the striatum, particularly the putamen, of Tourette patients (Singer et al. 2002; Wong et al. 2008). A recent meta-analysis of 16 PET and SPECT studies in Tourette subjects showed trends but no significant findings in dopaminergic alterations. While the studies supported the general notion of dopamine mechanism involvement in the pathophysiology of Tourette syndrome, the lack of significant findings was attributed to the heterogeneity of this disorder (Hienert et al. 2018). Imaging data using AMT PET appear to support the role of abnormal serotonergic neurotransmission in the pathophysiology of Tourette syndrome and some of its comorbid conditions, such as ADHD and OCD (Behen et al. 2007). Increased serotonin receptor binding was found not only in regions closely related to subcortical regions in patients with Tourette syndrome but also in most other brain regions (Haugbol et al. 2007). Decreased AMT uptake in bilateral dorsolateral prefrontal cortical and bilaterally increased uptake in the thalamus with bilateral increased ratio of AMT uptake in subcortical structures to dorsolateral prefrontal cortex was reported in Tourette syndrome children (Behen et al. 2007). However, thalamic and basal ganglia asymmetry in AMT uptake is also frequently found in these children (Fig. 47.19). Recent studies have suggested that alterations in the serotonergic system in Tourette syndrome may be related to comorbid obsessive-compulsive disorder rather than the primary cause of the disease (Müller-Vahl et al. 2019).

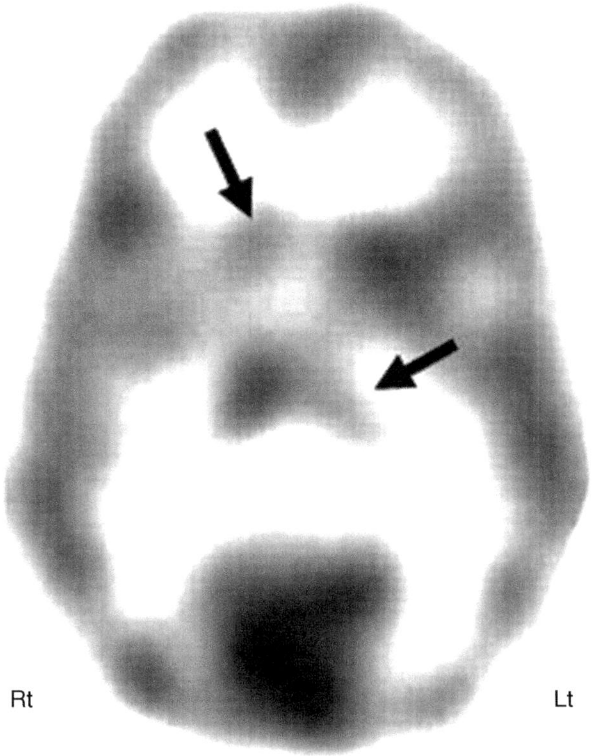

Fig. 47.19 A unique pattern of abnormality seen on ^{11}C-alpha-methyl tryptophan PET scan in a child with Tourette syndrome, with decreased alpha-methyl tryptophan uptake in the basal ganglia and contralateral thalamus (*arrows*)

47.3.6 Neuronal Ceroid Lipofuscinosis or Spielmeyer-Vogt (or Batten) Disease

The neuronal ceroid lipofuscinoses are a group of autosomal recessive neurodegenerative disorders, resulting from excessive accumulation of lipopigments (lipofuscin) in the tissue. The disorder is generally characterized by seizures, developmental regression, and progressive visual impairment. MRI can show nonspecific cortical and cerebellar atrophy and T2 hyperintensities of the white matter (D'Incerti 2000). On PET imaging, children with the juvenile form (CLN-3) or Spielmeyer-Vogt (or Batten) disease show decreased glucose metabolism in the calcarine cortex early in the course of the disease, while children with late infantile neuronal ceroid lipofuscinosis (CLN-2, Jansky-Bielschowsky disease with curvilinear inclusions) show rapid degeneration with generalized cortical and subcortical hypometabolism (De Volder et al. 1990; Iannetti et al. 1994; Philippart et al. 1994, 1997; Philippart and Chugani 1995). As the juvenile form of the disease progresses, a rostral spread of glucose hypometabolism to other cortical areas is observed (Philippart et al. 1994). Therefore, FDG PET can play a role in the early diagnosis, follow-up, and monitoring of the disease progression. PET studies have also shown reduced dopamine D1 receptors in both the caudate and putamen in juvenile neuronal ceroid lipofuscinosis (Ruottinen et al. 1997; Rinne et al. 2002).

An exhaustive review of PET imaging in the many rare neurodegenerative disorders of childhood is beyond the scope of this chapter. Suffice it to say that a recent review of the topic found adequate evidence to indicate that glucose metabolism PET scans are clinically useful in children with neurodegenerative disorders. In addition, PET imaging provides biomarkers which will be important as treatments become available for these rare disorders (Chugani 2019).

47.4 Multimodal Imaging with Simultaneous PET-MR

Both MRI and PET are powerful imaging tools used to study structure and function in pediatric neurological disorders, yet they offer complementary imaging perspectives. The simultaneous use of these tools in a single setting with recently available PET-MR scanners offers many research and clinical advantages. This new technology is a significant advancement to biomedical research because it allows simultaneously acquired noninvasive and quantitative comparisons of anatomical, functional, and metabolic tissue measures. Indeed, the fundamental advantages of simultaneous acquisition of PET and MR data reach far beyond simple co-registration of PET and MR image volumes. Important issues for children include automated motion correction for PET dynamic studies using MR navigator sequences; both structural and functional image acquisition at the same time requiring only one sedation (if necessary); image-derived arterial input function, thus eliminating the need for arterial blood sampling for quantitative modeling; and lower radioactivity exposure as the need for a transmission CT for attenuation correction used by current PET/CT technology is eliminated.

When using the PET-MR, scanning time is dictated more by MRI acquisition (approximately 40 min depending on desired sequences) than PET (approximately 10 min). We have taken advantage of this, particularly in children, by reducing the FDG dose by more than 50% and increasing PET acquisition time

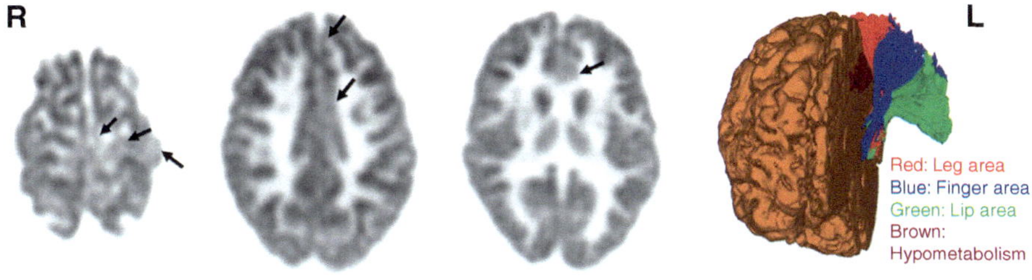

Fig. 47.20 FDG PET in a 14-year-old girl with uncontrolled seizures for 8 years, beginning with right leg shaking, nonlateralized EEG, and normal MRI, showing hypometabolism in the left motor cortex, extending into left anteromedial frontal cortex (*arrows*). The diffusion tensor analysis showing superimposition of hypometabolic region upon corticospinal tract

to equal that required for the MRI. In epilepsy surgery patients, we routinely include diffusion tensor imaging (DTI) in order to study the location of motor or language fibers in relation to the PET and MRI abnormalities (Fig. 47.20) in order to minimize damage to these vital regions during resection. PET-MR is also rapidly becoming an important research tool in the study of epilepsy by allowing a powerful approach to study anatomical-functional relationships or dual functional relationships, e.g., MR spectroscopy or functional MRI in relation to PET molecular imaging.

References

Aboian MS, Wong-Kisiel LC, Rank M, Wetjen NM, Wirrell EC, Witte RJ (2011) SISCOM in children with tuberous sclerosis complex-related epilepsy. Pediatr Neurol 45:83–88

Akman CI, Ichise M, Olsavsky A, Tikofsky RS, Van Heertum RL, Gilliam F (2010) Epilepsy duration impacts on brain glucose metabolism in temporal lobe epilepsy: results of voxel-based mapping. Epilepsy Behav 17:373–380

Alkonyi B, Juhasz C, Muzik O, Asano E, Saporta A, Shah A, Chugani HT (2009) Quantitative brain surface mapping of an electrophysiologic/metabolic mismatch in human neocortical epilepsy. Epilepsy Res 87:77–87

Alkonyi B, Chugani HT, Juhasz C (2011) Transient focal cortical increase of interictal glucose metabolism in Sturge-Weber syndrome: implications for epileptogenesis. Epilepsia 52:1265–1272

Alkonyi B, Miao Y, Wu J, Cai Z, Hu J, Chugani HT, Juhasz C (2012) A perfusion-metabolic mismatch in Sturge-Weber syndrome: a multimodality imaging study. Brain Dev 34:553–562

Arduini RG, Capellini SA, Ciasca SM (2006) Comparative study of the neuropsychological and neuroimaging evaluations in children with dyslexia. Arq Neuropsiquiatr 64:369–375

Arnold S, Berthele A, Drzezga A, Tolle TR, Weis S, Werhahn KJ, Henkel A, Yousry TA, Winkler PA, Bartenstein P, Noachtar S (2000) Reduction of benzodiazepine receptor binding is related to the seizure onset zone in extratemporal focal cortical dysplasia. Epilepsia 41:818–824

Asano E, Chugani DC, Muzik O, Shen C, Juhasz C, Janisse J, Ager J, Canady A, Shah JR, Shah AK, Watson C, Chugani HT (2000) Multimodality imaging for improved detection of epileptogenic foci in tuberous sclerosis complex. Neurology 54:1976–1984

Asano E, Juhasz C, Shah A, Muzik O, Chugani DC, Shah J, Sood S, Chugani HT (2005) Origin and propagation of epileptic spasms delineated on electrocorticography. Epilepsia 46:1086–1097

Asarnow RF, LoPresti C, Guthrie D, Elliott T, Cynn V, Shields WD, Shewmon DA, Sankar R, Peacock WJ (1997) Developmental outcomes in children receiving resection surgery for medically intractable infantile spasms. Dev Med Child Neurol 39:430–440

Aungaroon G, Trout A, Radhakrishnan R, Horn PS, Arya R, Tenney JR, Arthur TM, Holland KD, Mangano FT, Leach JL, Rozhkov L, Greiner HM (2018) Impact of radiotracer injection latency and seizure duration on subtraction ictal SPECT co-registered to MRI (SISCOM) performance in children. Clin Neurophysiol 129(9):1842–1848

Banati RB, Goerres GW, Myers R, Gunn RN, Turkheimer FE, Kreutzberg GW, Brooks DJ, Jones T, Duncan JS (1999) [11C](R)-PK11195 positron emission tomography imaging of activated microglia in vivo in Rasmussen's encephalitis. Neurology 53:2199–2203

Batista CE, Chugani HT, Juhasz C, Behen ME, Shankaran S (2007) Transient hypermetabolism of the basal ganglia following perinatal hypoxia. Pediatr Neurol 36:330–333

Behen M, Chugani HT, Juhasz C, Helder E, Ho A, Maqbool M, Rothermel RD, Perry J, Muzik O (2007) Abnormal brain tryptophan metabolism and clinical correlates in Tourette syndrome. Mov Disord 22:2256–2262

Behen ME, Juhasz C, Wolfe-Christensen C, Guy W, Halverson S, Rothermel R, Janisse J, Chugani HT (2011) Brain damage and IQ in unilateral Sturge-Weber syndrome: support for a "fresh start" hypothesis. Epilepsy Behav 22:352–357

Benedek K, Juhasz C, Chugani DC, Muzik O, Chugani HT (2006) Longitudinal changes in cortical glucose hypometabolism in children with intractable epilepsy. J Child Neurol 21:26–31

Benifla M, Otsubo H, Ochi A, Weiss SK, Donner EJ, Shroff M, Chuang S, Hawkins C, Drake JM, Elliott I, Smith ML, Snead OC III, Rutka JT (2006) Temporal lobe surgery for intractable epilepsy in children: an analysis of outcomes in 126 children. Neurosurgery 59:1203–1213; discussion 1213–1214

Bilgin O, Vollmar C, Peraud A, la Fougere C, Beleza P, Noachtar S (2008) Ictal SPECT in Sturge-Weber syndrome. Epilepsy Res 78:240–243

Bjørklund G, Kern JK, Urbina MA, Saad K, El-Houfey AA, Geier DA, Chirumbolo S, Geier MR, Mehta JA, Aaseth J (2018) Cerebral hypoperfusion in autism spectrum disorder. Acta Neurobiol Exp (Wars) 78(1):21–29

Bosnyák E, Behen ME, Guy WC, Asano E, Chugani HT, Juhasz C (2016) Predictors of cognitive functions in children with Sturge-Weber syndrome: a longitudinal study. Pediatr Neurol 61:38–45

Bouvard S, Costes N, Bonnefoi F, Lavenne F, Mauguiere F, Delforge J, Ryvlin P (2005) Seizure-related short-term plasticity of benzodiazepine receptors in partial epilepsy: a [11C]flumazenil-PET study. Brain 128:1330–1343

Branch CE, Dyken PR (1979) Choroid plexus papilloma and infantile spasms. Ann Neurol 5:302–304

Braun AR, Stoetter B, Randolph C, Hsiao JK, Vladar K, Gernert J, Carson RE, Herscovitch P, Chase TN (1993) The functional neuroanatomy of Tourette's syndrome: an FDG-PET study. I Regional changes in cerebral glucose metabolism differentiating patients and controls. Neuropsychopharmacology 9:277–291

Bruggemann JM, Som SS, Lawson JA, Haindl W, Cunningham AM, Bye AM (2004) Application of statistical parametric mapping to SPET in the assessment of intractable childhood epilepsy. Eur J Nucl Med Mol Imaging 31:369–377

Burneo JG, Hamilton M, Vezina W, Parrent A (2006) Utility of Ictal SPECT in the presurgical evaluation of Rasmussen's encephalitis. Can J Neurol Sci 33:107–110

Burroni L, Orsi A, Monti L, Hayek Y, Rocchi R, Vattimo AG (2008) Regional cerebral blood flow in childhood autism: a SPET study with SPM evaluation. Nucl Med Commun 29:150–156

Cahill V, Sinclair B, Malpas CB, McIntosh AM, Chen Z, Vivash LE, O'Shea MF, Wilson SJ, Desmond PM, Berlangieri SU, Hicks RJ, Rowe CC, Morokoff AP, King JA, Fabinyi GC, Kaye AH, Kwan P, Berkovic SF, O'Brien TJ (2019) Metabolic patterns and seizure outcomes following anterior temporal lobectomy. Ann Neurol 85(2):241–250

Carlson C, Teutonico F, Elliott RE, Moshel YA, LaJoie J, Miles D, Devinsky O, Weiner HL (2011) Bilateral invasive electroencephalography in patients with tuberous sclerosis complex: a path to surgery? J Neurosurg Pediatr 7:421–430

Chandana SR, Behen ME, Juhasz C, Muzik O, Rothermel RD, Mangner TJ, Chakraborty PK, Chugani HT, Chugani DC (2005) Significance of abnormalities in developmental trajectory and asymmetry of cortical serotonin synthesis in autism. Int J Dev Neurosci 23:171–182

Chandra PS, Salamon N, Huang J, Wu JY, Koh S, Vinters HV, Mathern GW (2006) FDG-PET/MRI coregistration and diffusion-tensor imaging distinguish epileptogenic tubers and cortex in patients with tuberous sclerosis complex: a preliminary report. Epilepsia 47:1543–1549

Chiron C, Raynaud C, Tzourio N, Diebler C, Dulac O, Zilbovicius M, Syrota A (1989) Regional cerebral blood flow by SPECT imaging in Sturge-Weber disease: an aid for diagnosis. J Neurol Neurosurg Psychiatry 52:1402–1409

Chiron C, Dulac O, Bulteau C, Nuttin C, Depas G, Raynaud C, Syrota A (1993) Study of regional cerebral blood flow in West syndrome. Epilepsia 34:707–715

Chiron C, Vera P, Kaminska A, Hollo A, Cieuta C, Ville D, Dulac O (1999a) Single-photon emission computed tomography: ictal perfusion in childhood epilepsies. Brain Dev 21:444–446

Chiron C, Vera P, Kaminska A, Cieuta C, Hollo A, Ville D, Gardin I, Stievenart JL, Dulac O (1999b) Ictal SPECT in the epileptic child. Contribution of subtraction interictal images and superposition of with MRI. Rev Neurol (Paris) 155:477–481
Chugani HT (2018) Imaging brain metabolism in the newborn. J Child Neurol 33(13):851–860
Chugani HT (2019) Positron Emission Tomography in Pediatric Neurodegenerative Disorders. Pediatr Neurol 100:12–25
Chugani HT, Conti JR (1996) Etiologic classification of infantile spasms in 140 cases: role of positron emission tomography. J Child Neurol 11:44–48
Chugani HT, Phelps ME, Mazziotta JC (1987a) Positron emission tomography study of human brain functional development. Ann Neurol 22:487–497
Chugani HT, Mazziotta JC, Engel J Jr, Phelps ME (1987b) The Lennox-Gastaut syndrome: metabolic subtypes determined by 2-deoxy-2[18F]fluoro-D-glucose positron emission tomography. Ann Neurol 21:4–13
Chugani HT, Mazziotta JC, Phelps ME (1989) Sturge-Weber syndrome: a study of cerebral glucose utilization with positron emission tomography. J Pediatr 114:244–253
Chugani HT, Shields WD, Shewmon DA, Olson DM, Phelps ME, Peacock WJ (1990) Infantile spasms: I. PET identifies focal cortical dysgenesis in cryptogenic cases for surgical treatment. Ann Neurol 27:406–413
Chugani HT, Shewmon DA, Sankar R, Chen BC, Phelps ME (1992) Infantile spasms: II. Lenticular nuclei and brain stem activation on positron emission tomography. Ann Neurol 31:212–219
Chugani HT, Shewmon DA, Shields WD, Sankar R, Comair Y, Vinters HV, Peacock WJ (1993) Surgery for intractable infantile spasms: neuroimaging perspectives. Epilepsia 34:764–771
Chugani HT, Da Silva E, Chugani DC (1996) Infantile spasms: III. Prognostic implications of bitemporal hypometabolism on positron emission tomography. Ann Neurol 39:643–649
Chugani DC, Muzik O, Rothermel R, Behen M, Chakraborty P, Mangner T, da Silva EA, Chugani HT (1997) Altered serotonin synthesis in the dentatothalamocortical pathway in autistic boys. Ann Neurol 42:666–669
Chugani DC, Muzik O, Chakraborty P, Mangner T, Chugani HT (1998a) Human brain serotonin synthesis capacity measured in vivo with alpha-[C-11]methyl-L-tryptophan. Synapse 28:33–43
Chugani DC, Chugani HT, Muzik O, Shah JR, Shah AK, Canady A, Mangner TJ, Chakraborty PK (1998b) Imaging epileptogenic tubers in children with tuberous sclerosis complex using alpha-[11C]methyl-L-tryptophan positron emission tomography. Ann Neurol 44:858–866
Chugani DC, Muzik O, Behen M, Rothermel R, Janisse JJ, Lee J, Chugani HT (1999) Developmental changes in brain serotonin synthesis capacity in autistic and nonautistic children. Ann Neurol 45:287–295
Chugani HT, Asano E, Sood S (2010) Infantile spasms: who are the ideal surgical candidates? Epilepsia 51(Suppl 1):94–96
Chugani HT, Kumar A, Kupsky W, Asano E, Sood S, Juhasz C (2011) Clinical and histopathologic correlates of (11) C-alpha-methyl-L-tryptophan (AMT) PET abnormalities in children with intractable epilepsy. Epilepsia 52(9):1692–1698
Chugani HT, Kumar A, Muzik O (2013a) GABA(A) receptor imaging with positron emission tomography in the human newborn: a unique binding pattern. Pediatr Neurol 48(6):459–462
Chugani HT, Luat AF, Kumar A, Govindan R, Pawlik K, Asano E (2013b) α-[11C]-Methyl-L-tryptophan-PET in 191 patients with tuberous sclerosis complex. Neurology 81:674–680
Chugani HT, Ilyas M, Kumar A, Juhász C, Kupsky WJ, Sood S, Asano E (2015) Surgical treatment for refractory epileptic spasms: The Detroit series. Epilepsia 56(12):1941–1949
Cook EH Jr, Rowlett R, Jaselskis C, Leventhal BL (1992) Fluoxetine treatment of children and adults with autistic disorder and mental retardation. J Am Acad Child Adolesc Psychiatry 31:739–745
D'Incerti L (2000) MRI in neuronal ceroid lipofuscinosis. Neurol Sci 21:S71–S73
da Silva EA, Chugani DC, Muzik O, Chugani HT (1997) Identification of frontal lobe epileptic foci in children using positron emission tomography. Epilepsia 38:1198–1208
De Volder A, Bol A, Michel C, Congneau M, Goffinet AM (1987) Brain glucose metabolism in children with the autistic syndrome: positron tomography analysis. Brain Dev 9:581–587

De Volder AG, Cirelli S, de Barsy T, Brucher JM, Bol A, Michel C, Goffinet AM (1990) Neuronal ceroid-lipofuscinosis: preferential metabolic alterations in thalamus and posterior association cortex demonstrated by PET. J Neurol Neurosurg Psychiatry 53:1063–1067

Dickstein LP, Liow JS, Austermuehle A, Zoghbi S, Inati SK, Zaghloul K, Zanotti-Fregonara P, Theodore WH (2019) Neuroinflammation in neocortical epilepsy measured by PET imaging of translocator protein. Epilepsia 60(6):1248–1254

Ding Y, Zhu Y, Jiang B, Zhou Y, Jin B, Hou H (2018) 18F-FDG PET and high-resolution MRI co-registration for pre-surgical evaluation of patients with conventional MRI-negative refractory extra-temporal lobe epilepsy. Eur J Nucl Med Mol Imaging 45:1567–1572

Doyle LW, Nahmias C, Firnau G, Kenyon DB, Garnett ES, Sinclair JC (1983) Regional cerebral glucose metabolism of newborn infants measured by positron emission tomography. Dev Med Child Neurol 25:143–151

Dufor O, Serniclaes W, Sprenger-Charolles L, Demonet JF (2007) Top-down processes during auditory phoneme categorization in dyslexia: a PET study. NeuroImage 34:1692–1707

Dufor O, Serniclaes W, Sprenger-Charolles L, Demonet JF (2009) Left premotor cortex and allophonic speech perception in dyslexia: a PET study. NeuroImage 46:241–248

Ernst M, Zametkin AJ, Matochik JA, Pascualvaca D, Cohen RM (1997) Low medial prefrontal dopaminergic activity in autistic children. Lancet 350:638

Ernst M, Zametkin AJ, Jons PH, Matochik JA, Pascualvaca D, Cohen RM (1999) High presynaptic dopaminergic activity in children with Tourette's disorder. J Am Acad Child Adolesc Psychiatry 38:86–94

Evans LT, Morse R, Roberts DW (2012) Epilepsy surgery in tuberous sclerosis: a review. Neurosurg Focus 32:E5

Fedi M, Reutens DC, Andermann F, Okazawa H, Boling W, White C, Dubeau F, Nakai A, Gross DW, Andermann E, Diksic M (2003) alpha-[11C]-Methyl-L-tryptophan PET identifies the epileptogenic tuber and correlates with interictal spike frequency. Epilepsy Res 52:203–213

Fedi M, Berkovic SF, Scheffer IE, O'Keefe G, Marini C, Mulligan R, Gong S, Tochon-Danguy H, Reutens DC (2008) Reduced striatal D1 receptor binding in autosomal dominant nocturnal frontal lobe epilepsy. Neurology 71:795–798

Ferrie CD, Maisey M, Cox T, Polkey C, Barrington SF, Panayiotopoulos CP, Robinson RO (1996) Focal abnormalities detected by 18FDG PET in epileptic encephalopathies. Arch Dis Child 75:102–107

Fiorella DJ, Provenzale JM, Coleman RE, Crain BJ, Al-Sugair AA (2001) (18)F-fluorodeoxyglucose positron emission tomography and MR imaging findings in Rasmussen encephalitis. AJNR Am J Neuroradiol 22:1291–1299

Flowers DL, Wood FB, Naylor CE (1991) Regional cerebral blood flow correlates of language processes in reading disability. Arch Neurol 48:637–643

Frost JJ, Mayberg HS, Fisher RS, Douglass KH, Dannals RF, Links JM, Wilson AA, Ravert HT, Rosenbaum AE, Snyder SH et al (1988) Mu-opiate receptors measured by positron emission tomography are increased in temporal lobe epilepsy. Ann Neurol 23:231–237

Fujimoto A, Okanishi T, Kanai S, Sato K, Itamura S, Baba S, Nishimura M, Masui T, Enoki H (2018) Double match of (18)F-fluorodeoxyglucose-PET and iomazenil-SPECT improves outcomes of focus resection surgery. Acta Neurochir 160(9):1875–1882

Gaillard WD, Bhatia S, Bookheimer SY, Fazilat S, Sato S, Theodore WH (1995) FDG-PET and volumetric MRI in the evaluation of patients with partial epilepsy. Neurology 45:123–126

Gaillard WD, Kopylev L, Weinstein S, Conry J, Pearl PL, Spanaki MV, Fazilat S, Venzina LG, Dubovsky E, Theodore WH (2002) Low incidence of abnormal (18)FDG-PET in children with new-onset partial epilepsy: a prospective study. Neurology 58:717–722

George MS, Costa DC, Kouris K, Ring HA, Ell PJ (1992) Cerebral blood flow abnormalities in adults with infantile autism. J Nerv Ment Dis 180:413–417

Gershen LD, Zanotti-Fregonara P, Dustin IH, Liow JS, Hirvonen J, Kreisl WC, Jenko KJ, Inati SK, Fujita M, Morse CL, Brouwer C, Hong JS, Pike VW, Zoghbi SS, Innis RB, Theodore WH (2015) Neuroinflammation in temporal lobe epilepsy measured using positron emission tomographic imaging of translocator protein. JAMA Neurol 72(8):882–888

Gilbert DL, Christian BT, Gelfand MJ, Shi B, Mantil J, Sallee FR (2006) Altered mesolimbocortical and thalamic dopamine in Tourette syndrome. Neurology 67:1695–1697

Gordon CT, State RC, Nelson JE, Hamburger SD, Rapoport JL (1993) A double-blind comparison of clomipramine, desipramine, and placebo in the treatment of autistic disorder. Arch Gen Psychiatry 50:441–447

Gross-Glenn K, Duara R, Barker WW, Loewenstein D, Chang JY, Yoshii F, Apicella AM, Pascal S, Boothe T, Sevush S et al (1991) Positron emission tomographic studies during serial word-reading by normal and dyslexic adults. J Clin Exp Neuropsychol 13:531–544

Guerin J, Watson RE, Carr CM, Liebo GB, Kotsenas AL (2019) Autoimmune epilepsy: findings on MRI and FDG-PET. Br J Radiol 92(1093):20170869

Guerreiro MM, Camargo EE, Kato M, Menezes Netto JR, Silva EA, Scotoni AE, Silveira DC, Guerreiro CA (1996) Brain single photon emission computed tomography imaging in Landau-Kleffner syndrome. Epilepsia 37:60–67

Gur RC, Sussman NM, Alavi A, Gur RE, Rosen AD, O'Connor M, Goldberg HI, Greenberg JH, Reivich M (1982) Positron emission tomography in two cases of childhood epileptic encephalopathy (Lennox-Gastaut syndrome). Neurology 32:1191–1194

Haginoya K, Kon K, Takayanagi M, Yoshihara Y, Kato R, Tanaka S, Yokoyama H, Munakata M, Nagai M, Maruoka S, Yamazaki T, Abe Y, Iinuma K (1998) Heterogeneity of ictal SPECT findings in nine cases of West syndrome. Epilepsia 39(Suppl 5):26–29

Haginoya K, Kon K, Yokoyama H, Tanaka S, Kato R, Munakata M, Yagi T, Takayanagi M, Yoshihara Y, Nagai M, Yamazaki T, Maruoka S, Iinuma K (2000) The perfusion defect seen with SPECT in West syndrome is not correlated with seizure prognosis or developmental outcome. Brain Dev 22:16–23

Haginoya K, Munakata M, Yokoyama H, Kato R, Tanaka S, Hirose M, Ishitobi M, Kon K, Yoshihara Y, Takayanagi M, Yamazaki T, Iinuma K (2001) Mechanism of tonic spasms in West syndrome viewed from ictal SPECT findings. Brain Dev 23:496–501

Hagman JO, Wood F, Buchsbaum MS, Tallal P, Flowers L, Katz W (1992) Cerebral brain metabolism in adult dyslexic subjects assessed with positron emission tomography during performance of an auditory task. Arch Neurol 49:734–739

Hammers A, Koepp MJ, Hurlemann R, Thom M, Richardson MP, Brooks DJ, Duncan JS (2002) Abnormalities of grey and white matter [11C]flumazenil binding in temporal lobe epilepsy with normal MRI. Brain 125:2257–2271

Harbord MG, Singh R, Morony S (1999) SPECT abnormalities in Landau-Kleffner syndrome. J Clin Neurosci 6:9–16

Harvey AS, Bowe JM, Hopkins IJ, Shield LK, Cook DJ, Berkovic SF (1993) Ictal 99mTc-HMPAO single photon emission computed tomography in children with temporal lobe epilepsy. Epilepsia 34:869–877

Haugbol S, Pinborg LH, Regeur L, Hansen ES, Bolwig TG, Nielsen FA, Svarer C, Skovgaard LT, Knudsen GM (2007) Cerebral 5-HT2A receptor binding is increased in patients with Tourette's syndrome. Int J Neuropsychopharmacol 10:245–252

Hazlett EA, Buchsbaum MS, Hsieh P, Haznedar MM, Platholi J, LiCalzi EM, Cartwright C, Hollander E (2004) Regional glucose metabolism within cortical Brodmann areas in healthy individuals and autistic patients. Neuropsychobiology 49:115–125

Haznedar MM, Buchsbaum MS, Metzger M, Solimando A, Spiegel-Cohen J, Hollander E (1997) Anterior cingulate gyrus volume and glucose metabolism in autistic disorder. Am J Psychiatry 154:1047–1050

Haznedar MM, Buchsbaum MS, Wei TC, Hof PR, Cartwright C, Bienstock CA, Hollander E (2000) Limbic circuitry in patients with autism spectrum disorders studied with positron emission tomography and magnetic resonance imaging. Am J Psychiatry 157:1994–2001

Haznedar MM, Buchsbaum MS, Hazlett EA, LiCalzi EM, Cartwright C, Hollander E (2006) Volumetric analysis and three-dimensional glucose metabolic mapping of the striatum and thalamus in patients with autism spectrum disorders. Am J Psychiatry 163:1252–1263

Heiskala H, Launes J, Pihko H, Nikkinen P, Santavuori P (1993) Brain perfusion SPECT in children with frequent fits. Brain Dev 15:214–218

Henry TR, Sutherling WW, Engel J Jr, Risinger MW, Levesque MF, Mazziotta JC, Phelps ME (1991) Interictal cerebral metabolism in partial epilepsies of neocortical origin. Epilepsy Res 10:174–182
Henry TR, Frey KA, Sackellares JC, Gilman S, Koeppe RA, Brunberg JA, Ross DA, Berent S, Young AB, Kuhl DE (1993) In vivo cerebral metabolism and central benzodiazepine-receptor binding in temporal lobe epilepsy. Neurology 43:1998–2006
Herold S, Frackowiak RS, Le Couteur A, Rutter M, Howlin P (1988) Cerebral blood flow and metabolism of oxygen and glucose in young autistic adults. Psychol Med 18:823–831
Hienert M, Gryglewski G, Stamenkovic M, Kasper S, Lanzenberger R (2018) Striatal dopaminergic alterations in Tourette's syndrome: a meta-analysis based on 16 PET and SPECT neuroimaging studies. Transl Psychiatry 8(1):143
Hirvonen J, Kreisl WC, Fujita M, Dustin I, Khan O, Appel S, Zhang Y, Morse C, Pike VW, Innis RB, Theodore WH (2012) Increased in vivo expression of an inflammatory marker in temporal lobe epilepsy. J Nucl Med 53:234–240
Honbolygo F, Csepe V, Fekeshazy A, Emri M, Marian T, Sarkozy G, Kalmanchey R (2006) Converging evidences on language impairment in Landau-Kleffner Syndrome revealed by behavioral and brain activity measures: a case study. Clin Neurophysiol 117:295–305
Horwitz B, Rumsey JM, Donohue BC (1998) Functional connectivity of the angular gyrus in normal reading and dyslexia. Proc Natl Acad Sci U S A 95:8939–8944
Hougaard K, Oikawa T, Sveinsdottir E, Skinoj E, Ingvar DH, Lassen NA (1976) Regional cerebral blood flow in focal cortical epilepsy. Arch Neurol 33:527–535
Hu SX, Wu XR, Lin C, Hao SY (1989) Landau-Kleffner syndrome with unilateral EEG abnormalities–two cases from Beijing, China. Brain Dev 11:420–422
Hur YJ, Kang HC, Kim DS, Choi SR, Kim HD, Lee JS (2011) Uncovered primary seizure foci in Lennox-Gastaut syndrome after corpus callosotomy. Brain Dev 33:672–677
Hwang PA, Otsubo H, Koo BK, Gilday DL, Chuang SH, Jay V, Hoffman HJ (1996) Infantile spasms: cerebral blood flow abnormalities correlate with EEG, neuroimaging, and pathologic findings. Pediatr Neurol 14:220–225
Hwang SI, Kim JH, Park SW, Han MH, Yu IK, Lee SH, Lee DS, Lee SK, Chung CK, Chang KH (2001) Comparative analysis of MR imaging, positron emission tomography, and ictal single-photon emission CT in patients with neocortical epilepsy. AJNR Am J Neuroradiol 22:937–946
Hwang BJ, Mohamed MA, Brašić JR (2017) Molecular imaging of autism spectrum disorder. Int Rev Psychiatry 29(6):530–554
Iannetti P, Messa C, Spalice A, Lucignani G, Fazio F (1994) Positron emission tomography in neuronal ceroid lipofuscinosis (Jansky-Bielschowsky disease): a case report. Brain Dev 16:459–462
Iinuma K, Yanai K, Yanagisawa T, Fueki N, Tada K, Ito M, Matsuzawa T, Ido T (1987) Cerebral glucose metabolism in five patients with Lennox-Gastaut syndrome. Pediatr Neurol 3:12–18
Iinuma K, Yokoyama H, Otsuki T, Yanai K, Watanabe T, Ido T, Itoh M (1993) Histamine H1 receptors in complex partial seizures. Lancet 341:238
Ilyas M, Sivaswamy L, Asano E, Sood S, Zidan M, Chugani H (2014) Seizure control following palliative resective surgery for intractable epilepsy-a pilot study. Pediatr Neurol 51(3):330–335
Jalota A, Rossi MA, Pylypyuk V, Stein M, Stoub T, Balabanov A (2016) Resecting critical nodes from an epileptogenic circuit in refractory focal-onset epilepsy patients using subtraction ictal SPECT coregistered to MRI. J Neurosurg 125:1565–1576
Jeong JW, Asano E, Pilli V, Nakai Y, Chugani HT, Juhasz C (2017) Objective 3D surface evaluation of intracranial electrophysiologic correlates of cerebral glucose metabolic abnormalities in children with focal epilepsy. Hum Brain Mapp 38:3098–3112
Jonas R, Asarnow RF, LoPresti C, Yudovin S, Koh S, Wu JY, Sankar R, Shields WD, Vinters HV, Mathern GW (2005) Surgery for symptomatic infant-onset epileptic encephalopathy with and without infantile spasms. Neurology 64:746–750
Juhasz C, Chugani DC, Muzik O, Watson C, Shah J, Shah A, Chugani HT (2000a) Is epileptogenic cortex truly hypometabolic on interictal positron emission tomography? Ann Neurol 48:88–96

Juhasz C, Chugani DC, Muzik O, Watson C, Shah J, Shah A, Chugani HT (2000b) Electroclinical correlates of flumazenil and fluorodeoxyglucose PET abnormalities in lesional epilepsy. Neurology 55:825–835

Juhasz C, Chugani DC, Muzik O, Shah A, Shah J, Watson C, Canady A, Chugani HT (2001) Relationship of flumazenil and glucose PET abnormalities to neocortical epilepsy surgery outcome. Neurology 56:1650–1658

Juhasz C, Chugani DC, Asano E, Shah A, Shah J, Muzik O, Sood S, Chugani HT (2002) Alpha[11C]methyl-L-tryptophan positron emission tomography scanning in 176 patients with intractable epilepsy. Ann Neurol 52:S118. (abstract)

Juhasz C, Chugani DC, Muzik O, Shah A, Asano E, Mangner TJ, Chakraborty PK, Sood S, Chugani HT (2003) Alpha-methyl-L-tryptophan PET detects epileptogenic cortex in children with intractable epilepsy. Neurology 60:960–968

Juhasz C, Batista CE, Chugani DC, Muzik O, Chugani HT (2007) Evolution of cortical metabolic abnormalities and their clinical correlates in Sturge-Weber syndrome. Eur J Paediatr Neurol 11:277–284

Kagawa K, Chugani DC, Asano E, Juhasz C, Muzik O, Shah A, Shah J, Sood S, Kupsky WJ, Mangner TJ, Chakraborty PK, Chugani HT (2005) Epilepsy surgery outcome in children with tuberous sclerosis complex evaluated with alpha-[11C]methyl-L-tryptophan positron emission tomography (PET). J Child Neurol 20:429–438

Kakisaka Y, Haginoya K, Ishitobi M, Togashi N, Kitamura T, Wakusawa K, Sato I, Hino-Fukuyo N, Uematsu M, Munakata M, Yokoyama H, Iinuma K, Kaneta T, Higano S, Tsuchiya S (2009) Utility of subtraction ictal SPECT images in detecting focal leading activity and understanding the pathophysiology of spasms in patients with West syndrome. Epilepsy Res 83:177–183

Kaminska A, Chiron C, Ville D, Dellatolas G, Hollo A, Cieuta C, Jalin C, Delalande O, Fohlen M, Vera P, Soufflet C, Dulac O (2003) Ictal SPECT in children with epilepsy: comparison with intracranial EEG and relation to postsurgical outcome. Brain 126:248–260

Kaneko M, Uno A, Kaga M, Matsuda H, Inagaki M, Haruhara N (1998) Cognitive neuropsychological and regional cerebral blood flow study of a developmentally dyslexic Japanese child. J Child Neurol 13:457–461

Kannan S, Saadani-Makki F, Muzik O, Chakraborty P, Mangner TJ, Janisse J, Romero R, Chugani DC (2007) Microglial activation in perinatal rabbit brain induced by intrauterine inflammation: detection with 11C-(R)-PK11195 and small-animal PET. J Nucl Med 48:946–954

Karenfort M, Kruse B, Freitag H, Pannek H, Tuxhorn I (2002) Epilepsy surgery outcome in children with focal epilepsy due to tuberous sclerosis complex. Neuropediatrics 33:255–261

Kerrigan JF, Chugani HT, Phelps ME (1991) Regional cerebral glucose metabolism in clinical subtypes of cerebral palsy. Pediatr Neurol 7:415–425

Kim SK, Lee DS, Lee SK, Kim YK, Kang KW, Chung CK, Chung JK, Lee MC (2001) Diagnostic performance of [18F]FDG-PET and ictal [99mTc]-HMPAO SPECT in occipital lobe epilepsy. Epilepsia 42:1531–1540

Kim YK, Lee DS, Lee SK, Chung CK, Chung JK, Lee MC (2002) (18)F-FDG PET in localization of frontal lobe epilepsy: comparison of visual and SPM analysis. J Nucl Med 43:1167–1174

Kim MA, Heo K, Choo MK, Cho JH, Park SC, Lee JD, Yun M, Park HJ, Lee BI (2006) Relationship between bilateral temporal hypometabolism and EEG findings for mesial temporal lobe epilepsy: analysis of 18F-FDG PET using SPM. Seizure 15:56–63

Kim JT, Bai SJ, Choi KO, Lee YJ, Park HJ, Kim DS, Kim HD, Lee JS (2009) Comparison of various imaging modalities in localization of epileptogenic lesion using epilepsy surgery outcome in pediatric patients. Seizure 18:504–510

Kim YH, Kang HC, Kim DS, Kim SH, Shim KW, Kim HD (2011) Neuroimaging in identifying focal cortical dysplasia and prognostic factors in pediatric and adolescent epilepsy surgery. Epilepsia 52:722–727

Kim JA, Jeong JW, Behen ME, Pilli VK, Luat A, Chugani HT, Juhasz C (2018) Metabolic correlates of cognitive function in children with unilateral Sturge-Weber syndrome: evidence for regional functional reorganization and crowding. Hum Brain Mapp 39(4):1596–1606

Knowlton RC, Laxer KD, Ende G, Hawkins RA, Wong ST, Matson GB, Rowley HA, Fein G, Weiner MW (1997) Presurgical multimodality neuroimaging in electroencephalographic lateralized temporal lobe epilepsy. Ann Neurol 42:829–837
Knowlton RC, Elgavish RA, Bartolucci A, Ojha B, Limdi N, Blount J, Burneo JG, Ver Hoef L, Paige L, Faught E, Kankirawatana P, Riley K, Kuzniecky R (2008) Functional imaging: II. Prediction of epilepsy surgery outcome. Ann Neurol 64:35–41
Koepp MJ, Woermann FG (2005) Imaging structure and function in refractory focal epilepsy. Lancet Neurol 4:42–53
Koepp MJ, Richardson MP, Brooks DJ, Poline JB, Van Paesschen W, Friston KJ, Duncan JS (1996) Cerebral benzodiazepine receptors in hippocampal sclerosis. An objective in vivo analysis. Brain 119(Pt 5):1677–1687
Koepp MJ, Labbe C, Richardson MP, Brooks DJ, Van Paesschen W, Cunningham VJ, Duncan JS (1997) Regional hippocampal [11C]flumazenil PET in temporal lobe epilepsy with unilateral and bilateral hippocampal sclerosis. Brain 120(Pt 10):1865–1876
Koepp MJ, Richardson MP, Brooks DJ, Duncan JS (1998) Focal cortical release of endogenous opioids during reading-induced seizures. Lancet 352:952–955
Koh S, Jayakar P, Resnick T, Alvarez L, Liit RE, Duchowny M (1999) The localizing value of ictal SPECT in children with tuberous sclerosis complex and refractory partial epilepsy. Epileptic Disord 1:41–46
Krause KH, Dresel S, Krause J, Kung HF, Tatsch K, Lochmuller H (2002) Elevated striatal dopamine transporter in a drug naive patient with Tourette syndrome and attention deficit//hyperactivity disorder: positive effect of methylphenidate. J Neurol 249:1116–1118
Kuki I, Kawawaki H, Oba S, Okazaki S, Ikeda H, Tomiwa K (2008) 123I iomazenil SPECT and identification of the epileptogenic tubers in patients with tuberous sclerosis. No To Hattatsu 40:54–56
Kuki I, Kawawaki H, Okazaki S, Inoue T, Nukui M, Tomiwa K, Amou K, Togawa M, Shiomi M (2012) Usefulness of 123I-iomazenil SPECT in pediatric patients with neurological disease. No To Hattatsu 44:5–12
Kuki I, Matsuda K, Kubota Y, Fukuyama T, Takahashi Y, Inoue Y, Shintaku H (2018) Functional neuroimaging in Rasmussen syndrome. Epilepsy Res 140:120–127
Kumar A, Chugani HT, Luat A, Asano E, Sood S (2008) Epilepsy surgery in a case of encephalitis: use of 11C-PK11195 positron emission tomography. Pediatr Neurol 38:439–442
Kumar A, Juhasz C, Asano E, Sood S, Muzik O, Chugani HT (2010) Objective detection of epileptic foci by 18F-FDG PET in children undergoing epilepsy surgery. J Nucl Med 51:1901–1907
Kumar A, Asano E, Chugani HT (2011) alpha-[(1)(1)C]-methyl-L-tryptophan PET for tracer localization of epileptogenic brain regions: clinical studies. Biomark Med 5:577–584
Kumlien E, Hilton-Brown P, Spannare B, Gillberg PG (1992) In vitro quantitative autoradiography of [3H]-L-deprenyl and [3H]-PK 11195 binding sites in human epileptic hippocampus. Epilepsia 33:610–617
Kumlien E, Hartvig P, Valind S, Oye I, Tedroff J, Langstrom B (1999) NMDA-receptor activity visualized with (S)-[N-methyl-11C]ketamine and positron emission tomography in patients with medial temporal lobe epilepsy. Epilepsia 40:30–37
Kumlien E, Nilsson A, Hagberg G, Langstrom B, Bergstrom M (2001) PET with 11C-deuterium-deprenyl and 18F-FDG in focal epilepsy. Acta Neurol Scand 103:360–366
Kurian M, Spinelli L, Delavelle J, Willi JP, Velazquez M, Chaves V, Habre W, Meagher-Villemure K, Roulet E, Villeneuve JG, Seeck M (2007) Multimodality imaging for focus localization in pediatric pharmacoresistant epilepsy. Epileptic Disord 9:20–31
Lamusuo S, Jutila L, Ylinen A, Kalviainen R, Mervaala E, Haaparanta M, Jaaskelainen S, Partanen K, Vapalahti M, Rinne J (2001) [18F]FDG-PET reveals temporal hypometabolism in patients with temporal lobe epilepsy even when quantitative MRI and histopathological analysis show only mild hippocampal damage. Arch Neurol 58:933–939
Langer O, Bauer M, Hammers A, Karch R, Pataraia E, Koepp MJ, Abrahim A, Luurtsema G, Brunner M, Sunder-Plassmann R, Zimprich F, Joukhadar C, Gentzsch S, Dudczak R, Kletter

K, Muller M, Baumgartner C (2007) Pharmacoresistance in epilepsy: a pilot PET study with the P-glycoprotein substrate R-[(11)C]verapamil. Epilepsia 48:1774–1784

Lawson JA, O'Brien TJ, Bleasel AF, Haindl W, Vogrin S, Cook MJ, Bye AM (2000) Evaluation of SPECT in the assessment and treatment of intractable childhood epilepsy. Neurology 55:1391–1393

Lee JD, Kim HJ, Lee BI, Kim OJ, Jeon TJ, Kim MJ (2000) Evaluation of ictal brain SPET using statistical parametric mapping in temporal lobe epilepsy. Eur J Nucl Med 27:1658–1665

Lee JS, Juhasz C, Kaddurah AK, Chugani HT (2001a) Patterns of cerebral glucose metabolism in early and late stages of Rasmussen's syndrome. J Child Neurol 16:798–805

Lee JS, Asano E, Muzik O, Chugani DC, Juhasz C, Pfund Z, Philip S, Behen M, Chugani HT (2001b) Sturge-Weber syndrome: correlation between clinical course and FDG PET findings. Neurology 57:189–195

Lee JJ, Kang WJ, Lee DS, Lee JS, Hwang H, Kim KJ, Hwang YS, Chung JK, Lee MC (2005) Diagnostic performance of 18F-FDG PET and ictal 99mTc-HMPAO SPET in pediatric temporal lobe epilepsy: quantitative analysis by statistical parametric mapping, statistical probabilistic anatomical map, and subtraction ictal SPET. Seizure 14:213–220

Lee JD, Park HJ, Park ES, Kim DG, Rha DW, Kim EY, Kim DI, Kim JJ, Yun M, Ryu YH, Lee J, Jeong JM, Lee DS, Lee MC, Park CI (2007) Assessment of regional GABA(A) receptor binding using 18F-fluoroflumazenil positron emission tomography in spastic type cerebral palsy. NeuroImage 34:19–25

Lerner A, Bagic A, Boudreau EA, Hanakawa T, Pagan F, Mari Z, Bara-Jimenez W, Aksu M, Garraux G, Simmons JM, Sato S, Murphy DL, Hallett M (2007) Neuroimaging of neuronal circuits involved in tic generation in patients with Tourette syndrome. Neurology 68:1979–1987

Lerner JT, Salamon N, Hauptman JS, Velasco TR, Hemb M, Wu JY (2009) Assessment and surgical outcomes for mild type I and severe type II cortical dysplasia: a critical review and the UCLA experience. Epilepsia 50:1310–1335

Lin Y, Fang YD, Wu G, Jones SE, Prayson RA, Moosa ANV (2018) Quantitative positron emission tomography-guided magnetic resonance imaging postprocessing in magnetic resonance imaging-negative epilepsies. Epilepsia 59:1583–1594

Luat AF, Chugani HT, Asano E, Juhasz C, Trock G, Rothermel R (2006) Episodic receptive aphasia in a child with Landau-Kleffner Syndrome: PET correlates. Brain Dev 28:592–596

Madar I, Lesser RP, Krauss G, Zubieta JK, Lever JR, Kinter CM, Ravert HT, Musachio JL, Mathews WB, Dannals RF, Frost JJ (1997) Imaging of delta- and mu-opioid receptors in temporal lobe epilepsy by positron emission tomography. Ann Neurol 41:358–367

Majerus S, Laureys S, Collette F, Del Fiore G, Degueldre C, Luxen A, Van der Linden M, Maquet P, Metz-Lutz MN (2003) Phonological short-term memory networks following recovery from Landau and Kleffner syndrome. Hum Brain Mapp 19:133–144

Maquet P, Hirsch E, Dive D, Salmon E, Marescaux C, Franck G (1990) Cerebral glucose utilization during sleep in Landau-Kleffner syndrome: a PET study. Epilepsia 31:778–783

Maquet P, Hirsch E, Metz-Lutz MN, Motte J, Dive D, Marescaux C, Franck G (1995) Regional cerebral glucose metabolism in children with deterioration of one or more cognitive functions and continuous spike-and-wave discharges during sleep. Brain 118(Pt 6):1497–1520

Marks DA, Katz A, Hoffer P, Spencer SS (1992) Localization of extratemporal epileptic foci during ictal single photon emission computed tomography. Ann Neurol 31:250–255

Mayberg HS, Sadzot B, Meltzer CC, Fisher RS, Lesser RP, Dannals RF, Lever JR, Wilson AA, Ravert HT, Wagner HN Jr et al (1991) Quantification of mu and non-mu opiate receptors in temporal lobe epilepsy using positron emission tomography. Ann Neurol 30:3–11

McCrory E, Frith U, Brunswick N, Price C (2000) Abnormal functional activation during a simple word repetition task: a PET study of adult dyslexics. J Cogn Neurosci 12:753–762

McDougle CJ, Naylor ST, Cohen DJ, Volkmar FR, Heninger GR, Price LH (1996a) A double-blind, placebo-controlled study of fluvoxamine in adults with autistic disorder. Arch Gen Psychiatry 53:1001–1008

McDougle CJ, Naylor ST, Cohen DJ, Aghajanian GK, Heninger GR, Price LH (1996b) Effects of tryptophan depletion in drug-free adults with autistic disorder. Arch Gen Psychiatry 53:993–1000

Mimaki T, Ono J, Yabuuchi H (1983) Temporal lobe astrocytoma with infantile spasms. Ann Neurol 14:695–696

Miyauchi T, Nomura Y, Ohno S, Kishimoto H, Matsushita M (1988) Positron emission tomography in three cases of Lennox-Gastaut syndrome. Jpn J Psychiatry Neurol 42:795–804

Miyazaki M, Hashimoto T, Fujii E, Tayama M, Kuroda Y (1994) Infantile spasms: localized cerebral lesions on SPECT. Epilepsia 35:988–992

Mori K, Toda Y, Hashimoto T, Miyazaki M, Saijo T, Ito H, Fujii E, Yamaue T, Kuroda Y (2007) Patients with West syndrome whose ictal SPECT showed focal cortical hyperperfusion. Brain Dev 29:202–209

Mori K, Mori T, Toda Y, Fujii E, Miyazaki M, Harada M, Kagami S (2012) Decreased benzodiazepine receptor and increased GABA level in cortical tubers in tuberous sclerosis complex. Brain Dev 34:478–486

Moshel YA, Elliott R, Teutonico F, Sellin J, Carlson C, Devinsky O, Weiner HL (2010) Do tubers contain function? Resection of epileptogenic foci in perirolandic cortex in children with tuberous sclerosis complex. Epilepsia 51:1242–1251

Mountz JM, Tolbert LC, Lill DW, Katholi CR, Liu HG (1995) Functional deficits in autistic disorder: characterization by technetium-99m-HMPAO and SPECT. J Nucl Med 36:1156–1162

Muller RA, Chugani DC, Behen ME, Rothermel RD, Muzik O, Chakraborty PK, Chugani HT (1998) Impairment of dentato-thalamo-cortical pathway in autistic men: language activation data from positron emission tomography. Neurosci Lett 245:1–4

Muller RA, Behen ME, Rothermel RD, Chugani DC, Muzik O, Mangner TJ, Chugani HT (1999) Brain mapping of language and auditory perception in high-functioning autistic adults: a PET study. J Autism Dev Disord 29:19–31

Müller-Vahl KR, Szejko N, Wilke F, Jakubovski E, Geworski L, Bengel F, Berding G (2019) Serotonin transporter binding is increased in Tourette syndrome with obsessive compulsive disorder. Sci Rep 9(1):972

Muzik O, Chugani DC, Juhasz C, Shen C, Chugani HT (2000a) Statistical parametric mapping: assessment of application in children. NeuroImage 12:538–549

Muzik O, da Silva EA, Juhasz C, Chugani DC, Shah J, Nagy F, Canady A, von Stockhausen HM, Herholz K, Gates J, Frost M, Ritter F, Watson C, Chugani HT (2000b) Intracranial EEG versus flumazenil and glucose PET in children with extratemporal lobe epilepsy. Neurology 54:171–179

Nakamura K, Sekine Y, Ouchi Y, Tsujii M, Yoshikawa E, Futatsubashi M, Tsuchiya KJ, Sugihara G, Iwata Y, Suzuki K, Matsuzaki H, Suda S, Sugiyama T, Takei N, Mori N (2010) Brain serotonin and dopamine transporter bindings in adults with high-functioning autism. Arch Gen Psychiatry 67:59–68

Natsume J, Kumakura Y, Bernasconi N, Soucy JP, Nakai A, Rosa P, Fedi M, Dubeau F, Andermann F, Lisbona R, Bernasconi A, Diksic M (2003) Alpha-[11C] methyl-L-tryptophan and glucose metabolism in patients with temporal lobe epilepsy. Neurology 60:756–761

Nicolson RI, Fawcett AJ, Berry EL, Jenkins IH, Dean P, Brooks DJ (1999) Association of abnormal cerebellar activation with motor learning difficulties in dyslexic adults. Lancet 353:1662–1667

O'Brien TJ, So EL, Mullan BP, Hauser MF, Brinkmann BH, Bohnen NI, Hanson D, Cascino GD, Jack CR Jr, Sharbrough FW (1998) Subtraction ictal SPECT co-registered to MRI improves clinical usefulness of SPECT in localizing the surgical seizure focus. Neurology 50:445–454

O'Brien TJ, So EL, Mullan BP, Hauser MF, Brinkmann BH, Jack CR Jr, Cascino GD, Meyer FB, Sharbrough FW (1999) Subtraction SPECT co-registered to MRI improves postictal SPECT localization of seizure foci. Neurology 52:137–146

O'Brien TJ, So EL, Mullan BP, Cascino GD, Hauser MF, Brinkmann BH, Sharbrough FW, Meyer FB (2000) Subtraction peri-ictal SPECT is predictive of extratemporal epilepsy surgery outcome. Neurology 55:1668–1677

O'Tuama LA, Urion DK, Janicek MJ, Treves ST, Bjornson B, Moriarty JM (1992) Regional cerebral perfusion in Landau-Kleffner syndrome and related childhood aphasias. J Nucl Med 33:1758–1765

Ohnishi T, Matsuda H, Hashimoto T, Kunihiro T, Nishikawa M, Uema T, Sasaki M (2000) Abnormal regional cerebral blood flow in childhood autism. Brain 123(Pt 9):1838–1844

Ohta Y, Nariai T, Akimoto H, Shimohira M, Sugimoto J, Ohno K, Senda M, Hirakawa K (2001) Tuberous sclerosis: epileptogenicity and multimodal presurgical evaluations. Childs Nerv Syst 17:313–319

Ollenberger GP, Byrne AJ, Berlangieri SU, Rowe CC, Pathmaraj K, Reutens DC, Berkovic SF, Scheffer IE, Scott AM (2005) Assessment of the role of FDG PET in the diagnosis and management of children with refractory epilepsy. Eur J Nucl Med Mol Imaging 32:1311–1316

Osborne JP, Fryer A, Webb D (1991) Epidemiology of tuberous sclerosis. Ann N Y Acad Sci 615:125–127

Palm DG, Brandt M, Korinthenberg R (1988) West syndrome and Lennox-Gastaut syndrome in children with porencephalic cysts: long-term follow-up after neurosurgical treatment. In: Niedermeyer E, Degen R (eds) The Lennox-Gastaut syndrome. Alan R. Liss, New York, pp 419–426

Patil S, Biassoni L, Borgwardt L (2007) Nuclear medicine in pediatric neurology and neurosurgery: epilepsy and brain tumors. Semin Nucl Med 37:357–381

Perissinotti A, Niñerola-Baizán A, Rubí S, Carreño M, Marti-Fuster B, Aparicio J, Mayoral M, Donaire A, Sanchez-Izquierdo N, Bargalló N, Rumiá J, Boget T, Pons F, Lomeña F, Ros D, Pavía J, Setoain X (2018) PISCOM: a new procedure for epilepsy combining ictal SPECT and interictal PET. Eur J Nucl Med Mol Imaging 45(13):2358–2367

Perot P, Weir B, Rasmussen T (1966) Tuberous sclerosis. Surgical therapy for seizures. Arch Neurol 15:498–506

Philippart M, Chugani B (1995) Neuronal ceroid-lipofuscinosis: late infantile form or juvenile form? Brain Dev 17:225

Philippart M, Messa C, Chugani HT (1994) Spielmeyer-Vogt (Batten, Spielmeyer-Sjogren) disease. Distinctive patterns of cerebral glucose utilization. Brain 117(Pt 5):1085–1092

Philippart M, da Silva E, Chugani HT (1997) The value of positron emission tomography in the diagnosis and monitoring of late infantile and juvenile lipopigment storage disorders (so-called Batten or neuronal ceroid lipofuscinoses). Neuropediatrics 28:74–76

Picard F, Bruel D, Servent D, Saba W, Fruchart-Gaillard C, Schollhorn-Peyronneau MA, Roumenov D, Brodtkorb E, Zuberi S, Gambardella A, Steinborn B, Hufnagel A, Valette H, Bottlaender M (2006) Alteration of the in vivo nicotinic receptor density in ADNFLE patients: a PET study. Brain 129:2047–2060

Pinton F, Chiron C, Enjolras O, Motte J, Syrota A, Dulac O (1997) Early single photon emission computed tomography in Sturge-Weber syndrome. J Neurol Neurosurg Psychiatry 63:616–621

Richardson MP, Koepp MJ, Brooks DJ, Duncan JS (1998) 11C-flumazenil PET in neocortical epilepsy. Neurology 51:485–492

Richardson MP, Hammers A, Brooks DJ, Duncan JS (2001) Benzodiazepine-GABA(A) receptor binding is very low in dysembryoplastic neuroepithelial tumor: a PET study. Epilepsia 42:1327–1334

Rinne JO, Ruottinen HM, Nagren K, Aberg LE, Santavuori P (2002) Positron emission tomography shows reduced striatal dopamine D1 but not D2 receptors in juvenile neuronal ceroid lipofuscinosis. Neuropediatrics 33:138–141

Rintahaka PJ, Chugani HT, Messa C, Phelps ME (1993) Hemimegalencephaly: evaluation with positron emission tomography. Pediatr Neurol 9:21–28

Rintahaka PJ, Chugani HT, Sankar R (1995) Landau-Kleffner syndrome with continuous spikes and waves during slow-wave sleep. J Child Neurol 10:127–133

Romanelli P, Najjar S, Weiner HL, Devinsky O (2002) Epilepsy surgery in tuberous sclerosis: multistage procedures with bilateral or multilobar foci. J Child Neurol 17:689–692

Rowe CC, Berkovic SF, Austin M, McKay WJ, Bladin PF (1989) Postictal SPET in epilepsy. Lancet 1:389–390

Rowe CC, Berkovic SF, Austin MC, McKay WJ, Bladin PF (1991) Patterns of postictal cerebral blood flow in temporal lobe epilepsy: qualitative and quantitative analysis. Neurology 41:1096–1103

Rubí S, Costes N, Heckemann RA, Bouvard S, Hammers A, Martí Fuster B, Ostrowsky K, Montavont A, Jung J, Setoain X, Catenoix H, Hino K, Liger F, Le Bars D, Ryvlin P (2013) Positron emission tomography with α-[11C]methyl-L-tryptophan in tuberous sclerosis complex-related epilepsy. Epilepsia 54(12):2143–2150

Ruggieri V, Caraballo R, Fejerman N (1989) Intracranial tumors and West syndrome. Pediatr Neurol 5:327–329

Rumsey JM, Duara R, Grady C, Rapoport JL, Margolin RA, Rapoport SI, Cutler NR (1985) Brain metabolism in autism. Resting cerebral glucose utilization rates as measured with positron emission tomography. Arch Gen Psychiatry 42:448–455

Rumsey JM, Berman KF, Denckla MB, Hamburger SD, Kruesi MJ, Weinberger DR (1987) Regional cerebral blood flow in severe developmental dyslexia. Arch Neurol 44:1144–1150

Rumsey JM, Andreason P, Zametkin AJ, Aquino T, King AC, Hamburger SD, Pikus A, Rapoport JL, Cohen RM (1992) Failure to activate the left temporoparietal cortex in dyslexia. An oxygen 15 positron emission tomographic study. Arch Neurol 49:527–534

Rumsey JM, Nace K, Donohue B, Wise D, Maisog JM, Andreason P (1997) A positron emission tomographic study of impaired word recognition and phonological processing in dyslexic men. Arch Neurol 54:562–573

Ruottinen HM, Rinne JO, Haaparanta M, Solin O, Bergman J, Oikonen VJ, Jarvela I, Santavuori P (1997) [18F]fluorodopa PET shows striatal dopaminergic dysfunction in juvenile neuronal ceroid lipofuscinosis. J Neurol Neurosurg Psychiatry 62:622–625

Ryvlin P, Bouvard S, Le Bars D, De Lamerie G, Gregoire MC, Kahane P, Froment JC, Mauguiere F (1998) Clinical utility of flumazenil-PET versus [18F]fluorodeoxyglucose-PET and MRI in refractory partial epilepsy. A prospective study in 100 patients. Brain 121(Pt 11):2067–2081

Sakaguchi Y, Kidokoro H, Ogawa C, Okai Y, Ito Y, Yamamoto H, Ohno A, Nakata T, Tsuji T, Nakane T, Kawai H, Kato K, Naganawa S, Natsume J (2018) Longitudinal findings of MRI and PET in West Syndrome with subtle focal cortical dysplasia. Am J Neuroradiol 39(10):1932–1937

Salamon N, Kung J, Shaw SJ, Koo J, Koh S, Wu JY (2008) FDG-PET/MRI co-registration improves detection of cortical dysplasia in epilepsy patients. Neurology 71:1594–1601

Sauer L, Pereira LD, Ciasca SM, Pestun M, Guerreiro MM (2006) Dichotic listening and spect in dyslexic children. Arq Neuropsiquiatr 64:108–111

Savic I, Ingvar M, Stone-Elander S (1993) Comparison of [11C]flumazenil and [18F]FDG as PET markers of epileptic foci. J Neurol Neurosurg Psychiatry 56:615–621

Savic I, Thorell JO, Roland P (1995) [11C]flumazenil positron emission tomography visualizes frontal epileptogenic regions. Epilepsia 36:1225–1232

Sayit E, Dirik E, Durak H, Uzuner N, Anal O, Cevik NT (1999) Landau-Kleffner syndrome: relation of clinical, EEG and Tc-99m-HMPAO brain SPECT findings and improvement in EEG after treatment. Ann Nucl Med 13:415–418

Schur S, Allen V, White A, Mirsky D, Stence N, O'Neill B, Handler M, Dudley R, Laoprasert P (2018) Significance of FDG-PET hypermetabolism in children with intractable focal epilepsy. Pediatr Neurosurg 53(3):153–162

Seo JH, Holland K, Rose D, Rozhkov L, Fujiwara H, Byars A, Arthur T, DeGrauw T, Leach JL, Gelfand MJ, Miles L, Mangano FT, Horn P, Lee KH (2011) Multimodality imaging in the surgical treatment of children with nonlesional epilepsy. Neurology 76:41–48

Shiraishi H, Takano K, Shiga T, Okajima M, Sudo A, Asahina N, Kohsaka S, Fukuhara M, Saitoh S (2007) Possible involvement of the tip of temporal lobe in Landau-Kleffner syndrome. Brain Dev 29:529–533

Siegel BV Jr, Asarnow R, Tanguay P, Call JD, Abel L, Ho A, Lott I, Buchsbaum MS (1992) Regional cerebral glucose metabolism and attention in adults with a history of childhood autism. J Neuropsychiatry Clin Neurosci 4:406–414

Sinclair DB, Snyder TJ (2005) Corticosteroids for the treatment of Landau-kleffner syndrome and continuous spike-wave discharge during sleep. Pediatr Neurol 32:300–306
Singer HS, Szymanski S, Giuliano J, Yokoi F, Dogan AS, Brasic JR, Zhou Y, Grace AA, Wong DF (2002) Elevated intrasynaptic dopamine release in Tourette's syndrome measured by PET. Am J Psychiatry 159:1329–1336
Spatola M, Dalmau J (2017) Seizures and risk of epilepsy in autoimmune and other inflammatory encephalitis. Curr Opin Neurol 30(3):345–353
Stern E, Silbersweig DA, Chee KY, Holmes A, Robertson MM, Trimble M, Frith CD, Frackowiak RS, Dolan RJ (2000) A functional neuroanatomy of tics in Tourette syndrome. Arch Gen Psychiatry 57:741–748
Sturm JW, Newton MR, Chinvarun Y, Berlangieri SU, Berkovic SF (2000) Ictal SPECT and interictal PET in the localization of occipital lobe epilepsy. Epilepsia 41:463–466
Suhonen-Polvi H, Kero P, Korvenranta H, Ruotsalainen U, Haaparanta M, Bergman J, Simell O, Wegelius U (1993) Repeated fluorodeoxyglucose positron emission tomography of the brain in infants with suspected hypoxic-ischaemic brain injury. Eur J Nucl Med 20:759–765
Swartz BE, Halgren E, Delgado-Escueta AV, Mandelkern M, Gee M, Quinones N, Blahd WH, Repchan J (1989) Neuroimaging in patients with seizures of probable frontal lobe origin. Epilepsia 30:547–558
Swartz BW, Khonsari A, Vrown C, Mandelkern M, Simpkins F, Krisdakumtorn T (1995) Improved sensitivity of 18FDG-positron emission tomography scans in frontal and "frontal plus" epilepsy. Epilepsia 36:388–395
Szelies B, Weber-Luxenburger G, Pawlik G, Kessler J, Holthoff V, Mielke R, Herholz K, Bauer B, Wienhard K, Heiss WD (1996) MRI-guided flumazenil- and FDG-PET in temporal lobe epilepsy. NeuroImage 3:109–118
Szelies B, Sobesky J, Pawlik G, Mielke R, Bauer B, Herholz K, Heiss WD (2002) Impaired benzodiazepine receptor binding in peri-lesional cortex of patients with symptomatic epilepsies studied by [(11)C]-flumazenil PET. Eur J Neurol 9:137–142
Sztriha L, al Suhaili AR, Prais V (1997) Cortical hypoperfusion in symptomatic West syndrome. A SPECT study. Eur J Radiol 25:20–25
Tae WS, Joo EY, Kim JH, Han SJ, Suh YL, Kim BT, Hong SC, Hong SB (2005) Cerebral perfusion changes in mesial temporal lobe epilepsy: SPM analysis of ictal and interictal SPECT. NeuroImage 24:101–110
Theodore WH, Rose D, Patronas N, Sato S, Holmes M, Bairamian D, Porter RJ, Di Chiro G, Larson S, Fishbein D (1987) Cerebral glucose metabolism in the Lennox-Gastaut syndrome. Ann Neurol 21:14–21
Theodore WH, Carson RE, Andreasen P, Zametkin A, Blasberg R, Leiderman DB, Rice K, Newman A, Channing M, Dunn B et al (1992) PET imaging of opiate receptor binding in human epilepsy using [18F]cyclofoxy. Epilepsy Res 13:129–139
Theodore WH, Sato S, Kufta CV, Gaillard WD, Kelley K (1997) FDG-positron emission tomography and invasive EEG: seizure focus detection and surgical outcome. Epilepsia 38:81–86
Thorngren-Jerneck K, Ohlsson T, Sandell A, Erlandsson K, Strand SE, Ryding E, Svenningsen NW (2001) Cerebral glucose metabolism measured by positron emission tomography in term newborn infants with hypoxic ischemic encephalopathy. Pediatr Res 49:495–501
Tien RD, Ashdown BC, Lewis DV Jr, Atkins MR, Burger PC (1992) Rasmussen's encephalitis: neuroimaging findings in four patients. AJR Am J Roentgenol 158:1329–1332
Tomás J, Pittau F, Hammers A, Bouvard S, Picard F, Vargas MI, Sales F, Seeck M, Garibotto V (2019) The predictive value of hypometabolism in focal epilepsy: a prospective study in surgical candidates. Eur J Nucl Med Mol Imaging 46(9):1806–1816
Uijl SG, Leijten FS, Arends JB, Parra J, van Huffelen AC, Moons KG (2007) The added value of [18F]-fluoro-D-deoxyglucose positron emission tomography in screening for temporal lobe epilepsy surgery. Epilepsia 48:2121–2129
Uthman BM, Reid SA, Wilder BJ, Andriola MR, Beydoun AA (1991) Outcome for West syndrome following surgical treatment. Epilepsia 32:668–671
Valenti MP, Froelich S, Armspach JP, Chenard MP, Dietemann JL, Kerhli P, Marescaux C, Hirsch E, Namer IJ (2002) Contribution of SISCOM imaging in the presurgical evaluation of temporal lobe epilepsy related to dysembryoplastic neuroepithelial tumors. Epilepsia 43:270–276

Van Bogaert P, Massager N, Tugendhaft P, Wikler D, Damhaut P, Levivier M, Brotchi J, Goldman S (2000) Statistical parametric mapping of regional glucose metabolism in mesial temporal lobe epilepsy. NeuroImage 12:129–138

Vera P, Kaminska A, Cieuta C, Hollo A, Stievenart JL, Gardin I, Ville D, Mangin JF, Plouin P, Dulac O, Chiron C (1999) Use of subtraction ictal SPECT co-registered to MRI for optimizing the localization of seizure foci in children. J Nucl Med 40:786–792

Volpe JJ, Herscovitch P, Perlman JM, Raichle ME (1983) Positron emission tomography in the newborn: extensive impairment of regional cerebral blood flow with intraventricular hemorrhage and hemorrhagic intracerebral involvement. Pediatrics 72:589–601

Volpe JJ, Herscovitch P, Perlman JM, Kreusser KL, Raichle ME (1985) Positron emission tomography in the asphyxiated term newborn: parasagittal impairment of cerebral blood flow. Ann Neurol 17:287–296

von Oertzen TJ, Mormann F, Urbach H, Reichmann K, Koenig R, Clusmann H, Biersack HJ, Elger CE (2011) Prospective use of subtraction ictal SPECT coregistered to MRI (SISCOM) in presurgical evaluation of epilepsy. Epilepsia 52:2239–2248

Wakamoto H, Chugani DC, Juhasz C, Muzik O, Kupsky WJ, Chugani HT (2008) Alpha-methyl-L-tryptophan positron emission tomography in epilepsy with cortical developmental malformations. Pediatr Neurol 39:181–188

Wang S, Tang Y, Aung T, Chen C, Katagiri M, Jones SE, Prayson RA, Krishnan B, Gonzalez-Martinez JA, Burgess RC, Najm IM, Alexopoulos AV, Wang S, Ding M, Wang ZI (2019) Multimodal noninvasive evaluation in MRI-negative operculoinsular epilepsy. J Neurosurg 12:1–11

Weiner HL, Carlson C, Ridgway EB, Zaroff CM, Miles D, LaJoie J, Devinsky O (2006) Epilepsy surgery in young children with tuberous sclerosis: results of a novel approach. Pediatrics 117:1494–1502

Werhahn KJ, Landvogt C, Klimpe S, Buchholz HG, Yakushev I, Siessmeier T, Muller-Forell W, Piel M, Rosch F, Glaser M, Schreckenberger M, Bartenstein P (2006) Decreased dopamine D2/D3-receptor binding in temporal lobe epilepsy: an [18F]fallypride PET study. Epilepsia 47:1392–1396

Willmann O, Wennberg R, May T, Woermann FG, Pohlmann-Eden B (2007) The contribution of 18F-FDG PET in preoperative epilepsy surgery evaluation for patients with temporal lobe epilepsy: a meta-analysis. Seizure 16:509–520

Wong DF, Brasic JR, Singer HS, Schretlen DJ, Kuwabara H, Zhou Y, Nandi A, Maris MA, Alexander M, Ye W, Rousset O, Kumar A, Szabo Z, Gjedde A, Grace AA (2008) Mechanisms of dopaminergic and serotonergic neurotransmission in Tourette syndrome: clues from an in vivo neurochemistry study with PET. Neuropsychopharmacology 33:1239–1251

Wu JY, Salamon N, Kirsch HE, Mantle MM, Nagarajan SS, Kurelowech L, Aung MH, Sankar R, Shields WD, Mathern GW (2010) Noninvasive testing, early surgery, and seizure freedom in tuberous sclerosis complex. Neurology 74:392–398

Wyllie E, Comair YG, Kotagal P, Bulacio J, Bingaman W, Ruggieri P (1998) Seizure outcome after epilepsy surgery in children and adolescents. Ann Neurol 44:740–748

Yacubian EM, Marie SK, Valerio RM, Jorge CL, Yamaga L, Buchpiguel CA (1997) Neuroimaging findings in Rasmussen's syndrome. J Neuroimaging 7:16–22

Yang WH, Jing J, Xiu LJ, Cheng MH, Wang X, Bao P, Wang QX (2011) Regional cerebral blood flow in children with autism spectrum disorders: a quantitative (9)(9)mTc-ECD brain SPECT study with statistical parametric mapping evaluation. Chin Med J 124:1362–1366

You SJ, Lee JK, Ko TS (2007) Epilepsy surgery in a patient with Lennox-Gastaut syndrome and cortical dysplasia. Brain Dev 29:167–170

Yum MS, Ko TS, Lee JK, Hong S, Kim DS, Kim J (2011) Surgical treatment for localization-related infantile spasms: excellent long-term outcomes. Clin Neurol Neurosurg 113:213–217

Zhai Q, Gui J, Zhang Y, Qiao H (2010) Children treated for epileptic encephalopathies show improved glucose metabolism. Pediatr Int 52:883–887

Zilbovicius M, Garreau B, Tzourio N, Mazoyer B, Bruck B, Martinot JL, Raynaud C, Samson Y, Syrota A, Lelord G (1992) Regional cerebral blood flow in childhood autism: a SPECT study. Am J Psychiatry 149:924–930

GPSR Compliance

The European Union's (EU) General Product Safety Regulation (GPSR) is a set of rules that requires consumer products to be safe and our obligations to ensure this.

If you have any concerns about our products, you can contact us on ProductSafety@springernature.com

In case Publisher is established outside the EU, the EU authorized representative is:

Springer Nature Customer Service Center GmbH
Europaplatz 3
69115 Heidelberg, Germany

Batch number: 10732535

Printed by Printforce, the Netherlands